To Dr. J. Binski
for his outstanding contribution
in the field of Limb Reconstruction
Surgery. C.N. Macizos XII. 07.
Larissa. Greece.

INFECTIONS of the HAND & UPPER LIMB

INFECTIONS of the HAND & UPPER LIMB

Editors
KONSTANTINOS N. MALIZOS
PANAYOTIS N. SOUCACOS

Foreword
MICHAEL J. PATZAKIS

Federation of the European
Societies for Surgery of the Hand

P.M.P. Paschalidis
Medical Publications

PMP (Paschalidis Medical Publications, Ltd.).
14th, Tetrapoleos str., Athens, 115 27, Greece
Tel.: 003-210-7789125, 003-210-7793012, Fax: 003-210-7759421,
e-mail:
orders: Paschalidis@Medical-Books.gr
© information: GP@Medical-Books.gr, CP@Medical-Books.gr

INFECTIONS OF THE HAND & UPPER LIMB

Contents

SECTION I

GENERAL PRINCIPLES IN MUSCULOSKELETAL INFECTIONS OF THE UPPER LIMB

Section II
Acute Soft Tissue Infections

Section III
Infections in Children and Chronic Osteomyelitis

Preface

We are quickly approaching the end of the Bone and Joint Decade, as declared by the World Health Organization. Musculoskeletal infections still comprise a major component of bone and joint disorders. Although enormous clinical and research efforts have focused on musculoskeletal diseases over the last 25 years, infections of the musculoskeletal system still remain a common cause of pain and disability having personal and socioeconomic consequences.

The hand and the upper extremity are easily and frequently injured during daily activities. Despite this, the upper limb appears to suffer from infections less than any other body part [1]. While trauma, mild or severe, facilitates introduction of pathogens to the hand, the compartmentalized anatomy of the hand appears to further promote the development and spread of infection. Most hand infections are the result of neglected minor wounds and if they are not appropriately diagnosed and treated, significant morbidity can result. In turn, these infections can have an enormous impact on patients' family lives and pose an increasing burden on Health Care systems. Infections of bones and joints are among the most devastating complications either post-traumatic, surgical, haematogenous or acute in nature. Despite the introduction of modern antibiotics, hand infections with a variety of organisms continue to be a source of morbidity and potential long-term disability [2, 3].

Over two decades of research in the field has clearly underscored that musculoskeletal infections are multifaceted diseases that require a multi-disciplinary approach for diagnosis and treatment. The purpose of this Instructional Course Lectures Book is to outline the current concepts regarding the pathophysiology of these diseases, and update on the diagnosis and mainly on the surgical treatment options. As such, pivotal to this effort is the tight collaboration among Hand Surgeons, Orthopaedic and Plastic Surgeons, Microbiologists, Infectious Disease Specialists, Molecular Biologists, Material Science Specialists, and others working within the field of Musculoskeletal Infections.

An International faculty from Europe and the United States, who span various disciplines, share their exper-

tise in this effort. This ICL Book has been divided into six sections. The first chapter reviews the historical milestones in the field of infection, while the second chapter delineates the socioeconomic burden imposed by infections of the upper extremity. An infection not only result in additional suffering of the patient, but also increases the expenses burdening the Health Care System, as well as frequently exhausts the efforts of the treating physician.

The section on the general principles relevant to musculoskeletal infections of the upper limb explores the characteristics of various infecting pathogens, the properties of the host and the source of the infection as well as the occurrence, type, severity and clinical prognosis of such infections. A special chapter explores the various species of microbes responsible for musculoskeletal infections and virulence factors of these pathogens, with particular focus on *Staphylococcus aureus,* the most commonly isolated bacterial species [4]. Hand infections can result in significant morbidity if they are not appropriately diagnosed and treated. Host factors, location, and circumstances of the infection are important guides to initial treatment strategies. Host factors including the normal immune response, as well as the defense against bacterial biofilms are discussed. The pathology of musculoskeletal infections and the various imaging modalities employed for the diagnosis are extensively described for children and adults. The chapters of this section, altogether, indicate that in order that physicians are able to choose the proper algorithm for treatment, underlying conditions that may affect care should be identified and appropriate cultures be obtained prior to antibiotic administration. Issues regarding antibiotic prophylaxis, local antibiotic delivery carriers, antimicrobial resistance and conditions mimicking infection are also included in this section [5-7].

The second section addresses various acute infections of the upper extremity. The most common infections are around and under nail (paronychia) and in the subcutaneous space of the distal phalanx (felon). Although they can be often treated by incision and spontaneous drainage, the authors detail various complications, as well as additional procedures which may be required in more complex cases [8]. Among the most severe acute infections are those of the tendon sheath, joint, web space and deep palmar space. Pyogenic flexor tenosynovitis and clenched-fist injuries are serious infections that often require surgical intervention [9, 10]. A clenched-fist injury usually is the result of an altercation and often involves injury to the extensor tendon, joint capsule, and bone. Wound exploration, copious irrigation, and appropriate antibiotics can prevent undesired outcomes. The authors indicate that when pus is present in such cases, there is no place for conservative treatment, only for operative treatment under clinical conditions [11]. Among the most devastating infections are septic arthritis, osteitis, gangrenous and necrotizing soft tissue and other life-threatening infections [12, 13]. Although rare, necrotizing and gangrenous soft tissue are a reality and they are associated with severe limb dysfunction, limb amputation or even death.

Despite their low incidence, surgeons should be aware of atypical infections of the hand, as well as fungal infections that are both being reported with increasing frequencies. Septic arthritis occurs more frequently in the large joints of the lower extremity, however it may be present in the upper extremity, being associated with high morbidity. Despite technical improvement in arthroplasty of the major joints of the upper extremity, complications are not uncommon and can be potentially catastrophic. Deep peri-prosthetic infection following total joint replacement of the shoulder or elbow is also a major complication resulting in significant morbidity [14]. Management options are discussed in order to improve both the functional outcome and satisfaction of the patient. One of the most serious complications in two-stage flexor tendon repair is infection in Stage I [15]. It is indicated that although each infectious process is unique, there are certain treatment principles that apply to all musculoskeletal infections [16]. These include prompt and accurate diagnosis, and timely medical and/or surgical intervention.

Basic surgical principles must be adhered to when managing infections of the upper extremity. The most important aspect in treating both acute and chronic infections is good debridement [17]. Knowledge of the anatomical features of the hand and upper extremity is essential for debridement of the infected areas and for proper surgical management. Taking that into consideration, the authors of the section on management of infections describe various surgical options for specific situations including, microvascular or pedicled flaps for the management of open contaminated wounds, vascularized fibular grafts for septic defects or osteomyelitis of the upper extremity, corticoperiosteal flaps for wrist arthrodesis in septic conditions, and distraction osteogenesis for managing septic non-union [18-23].

The work of clinicians and researchers in various fields over the last two decades has significantly augmented our knowledge regarding our understanding, diagnosis, and treatment of infections of the bones, joints, and soft tissues of the upper extremity. This ICL Book is designed to increase the reader's understanding of the etiology, diagnosis, basic treatment principles, as well as increase their awareness of the recent advancements, in order that they may achieve successful outcomes when faced with managing infections of the hand and upper extremity.

Konstantinos N. Malizos, MD
Professor and Chairman
Department of Orthopaedic Surgery and Musculoskeletal Trauma
School of Medicine
University of Thessalia

Panayotis N. Soucacos, MD
Professor and Chairman
Department of Orthopaedic Surgery
School of Medicine
University of Athens

REFERENCES

[1] Roth AI, Fry DE, Polk Jr, HC. Infections morbidity in extremity fractures. J Trauma 1986; 26: 757-761.

[2] Hausman MR, Lisser Sp. Hand infections. Orthop Clin North Am 1992; 23: 171-85.

[3] Moran GJ, Talan DA. Hand infections. Emerg Med Clin North Am 1993; 11: 601-19.

[4] Noble WC. Staphylococci in the skin. In: Noble WC (ed) The skin microflora and microbial skin disease. Cambridge University Press, Cambridge, UK. 1993; 135-152.

[5] Costerton JW. Biofilm theory can guide the treatment of device-related orthopaedic infections. Clin Orthop Relat Res 2005; 437: 7-11.

[6] Restrepo S, Gimenez CR, McCarthy K. Imaging of osteomyelitis and musculoskeletal soft tissue infections: current concepts. Rheum Dis Clin North Am 2003; 29: 89-109.

[7] Weed HG. Antimicrobial prophylaxis in the surgical patient. Med Clin N Am 2003; 87: 59-75.

[8] Jebson PJ. Infections of the fingertip. Paronychias and felons. Hand Clin 1998; 14: 547-55.

[9] Boles SD, Schmidt CC. Pyogenic flexor tenosynovitis. Hand Clin 1998; 14: 567-78.

[10] Griego RD, Rosaen T, Orengo IF, Wolf JE. Dog, cat and human bites: a review. J Am Acad Dermatol 1995; 33: 1019-29.

[11] Kelleher AT, Gordon SM. Management of bite wounds and infection in primary care. Cleve Clin J Med 1997; 64: 137-41.

[12] Kaandorp CJ, Krijnen P, Moens JH, Babbema JD, van Schaardenburg D. The outcome of bacterial arthritis: a prospective community-based study. Arthritis Rheum 1997; 40: 884-892.

[13] Theis JC, Rietveld J, Danesh-Clough T. Severe necrotizing soft tissue infections in orthopaedic surgery. J Orthop Surg 2002; 10: 108-113.

[14] Toms AD, Davidson D, Masri BA, Duncan DP. The management of peri-prosthetic infection in total joint arthroplasty. J Bone Joint Surg [Br]. 2006; 88: 149-55.

[15] Soucacos PN, Beris AE, Malizos KN, Xenakis T, Touliatos A, Soucacos PK. Two-stage treatment of flexor tendon ruptures. Silicon rod complications analyzed in 109 digits. Acta Orthop Scand Suppl 1997; 275: 48-51.

[16] Dellinger EP, Wertz MJ, Miller SD, Coyle MD. Hand infections. Bacteriology and treatment: a prospective study. Arch Surg 1988; 123: 745-50.

[17] Mastrokalos DS, Zahos KA, Korres D, Soucacos PN. Arthroscopic debridement and irrigation of periprosthetic total elbow infection. Arthroscopy 2006; 22: 1140-3

[18] Soucacos PN, Beris AE, Xenakis TA, Malizos KN, Touliatos AS. Forearm flap in orthopaedic and hand surgery. Microsurgery 1992; 13: 170-4.

[19] Mathes SJ, Feng LF, Hunt Tk. Coverage of The Infected Wound. Ann Surg 1983; 198: 420-9.

[20] Soucacos PN, Dailiana Z, Beris AE, Johnson EO. Vascularized bone grafts for the management of non-union. Injury 2006: Suppl 1: S41-50.

[21] Malizos KN, Zalavras DB, Soucacos PN, Beris AE. Urbaniak JR. Free vascularized fibular grafts for reconstruction of skeletal defects. J Am Acad Orthop Surg 2004; 12: 360-9.

[22] Walenkamp GH, Kleijn LL, Leeuw de, M. Osteomyelitis treated with gentamicin-PMMA beads: 100 patients followed for 1-12 years. Acta Orthop Scand 1998; 69: 518-522.

[23] Papagelopoulos PJ, Varogenis AF, Tsiodras S, Vlastou C, Giamarellou H, Soucacos PN. Calcium sulphate delivery system with tobramycin for the treatment of chronic calcaneal osteomyelitis. J Int Med Res 2006; 34: 704-12.

Foreword

Orthopaedic infections are both limb and life threatening and pose a major challenge to treating physicians. Over the past several decades, important advancements have been made in diagnostic modalities, surgical techniques, antibiotic therapy and delivery systems, microvascular bone and soft tissue transfers, bone transport procedures, and understanding the pathophysiological features of infections. Because of these significant worldwide advancements, limb salvage with excellent functional outcomes is now attainable.

The editors, Professor Konstantinos N. Malizos and Professor Panayotis N. Soucacos, introduce a superb book on infections of the hand and upper limb, and have asked outstanding authors to contribute their expertise into a state-of-the-art publication.

The section on General Principles is very comprehensive and encompasses historical, socioeconomic, anatomical, imaging, bacteriological and pathological aspects of musculoskeletal infections of the upper limb. The importance of biofilms and the understanding of its role in orthopaedic infections are presented.

The section on Acute Infections of the Upper Limb focuses on soft tissue, tendon, bone and joint infections and surgical principles of treatment.

The section on Chronic Infections of the Upper Limp emphasizes mycobacterial and fungal infections as well as tendon reconstruction following infection. In addition, the principles of treatment of the infected arthroplasty of the shoulder and elbow and arthroscopic debridement of elbow infections are presented.

In the section on Management and Adjunct Therapies, microvascular soft tissue and vascularized bone grafting, specialized soft tissue coverage, and distraction osteogenesis in the treatment of bone and soft tissue loss are emphasized. Resection arthroplasty in the upper extremity, the role of local antibiotic therapy and immunological therapy in infections, are included.

It is important to emphasize that all of the areas and principles presented by the authors in the management, treatment, and understanding of infection in the upper extremity are the same for treatment of orthopaedic infections affecting the lower extremity. This book gives the physician the necessary background to handle problematic complex infections of the upper extremity.

The contributors and editors should be congratulated for their contributions to this outstanding comprehensive book on infections of the hand and upper limb which gives the physician treating orthopaedic infections a strong foundation and understanding of the management of these serious entities.

Michael J. Patzakis, MD
Professor and Chairman
The Vincent and Julia Meyer Chair
Chief of Orthopaedic Surgery Service
USC University Hospital

Acknowledgments

We are grateful to those people who have done a superb job devoting enormous chunks of time and energy to contribute chapters to this book. Those surgeons believed that this project could come to fruition and gave us the chance to produce the book, putting aside their busy schedules to contribute their knowledge and experience in certain areas within the field of Infections of the Hand and Upper Extremity.

Vasiliki I. Boukouvala offered substantial help editing the manuscripts technically, collating and overseeing production to ensure a high level of quality of the book.

Special mention deserves Ass Prof Elizabeth O. Johnson who apart from contributing to this book as a writer, has overseen the project and assisted in the final editing of certain chapters.

We also wish to thank our colleagues from the Department of Orthopaedic Surgery, University of Thessalia, who have conducted the final review of the chapters, for their commitment, and time and effort they have spent to support us.

Acknowledgment must also be made of the participation of Christos Papanikolaou, painter, who generously shared his thoughts from an artistic point of view to finish this book and contributed his work "Hands" as the main theme of the book front cover.

To all those people we say a great THANKS !

List of Contributors

Roberto ADANI
Department of Orthopaedic Surgery, University of Modena and
Reggio Emilia, Policlinico, Modena, Italy

Sharon ADLER
Professor of English & Latin, Geneva, Switzerland

Kouroche AMINI
CHUV, Department of Plastic & Reconstructive Surgery,
Lausanne, Switzerland

Eleni APOSTOLAKI
Consultant Radiologist, University Hospital of Heraklion, Heraklion,
Greece

Konstantinos BARGIOTAS
Consultant, Department of Orthopaedic Surgery and Mus-
culoskeletal Trauma, University of Thessalia, School of
Medicine, Larissa, Greece

Bruno BATTISTON
Chief of Microsurgery Department, C.T.O. Hospital, Torino, Italy

Alexandros E. BERIS
Professor in Orthopaedics, Department of Orthopaedic Surgery,
University of Ioannina, Ioannina, Greece

Peter BRÜSER
Professor, Department of Hand- Plastic and Reconstructive
Surgery, Malteser Hospital, Bonn, Germany

Frank D. BURKE
Professor of Hand Surgery, The Pulvertaft Hand Centre,
Derbyshire Royal Infirmary, Derby, United Kingdom

Edward CALIF
Clinical and Research Fellow in Hand Surgery, Hand Surgery Unit,
Rambam Medical Center, Haifa, Israel

Dominique CASANOVA
Professor of Plastic Surgery, Department of Plastic and
Maxillo-facial surgery, Hôpital Nord, Chemin des Bourrely,
Marseille, France

Antonia CHARCHANTI
Lecturer, Department of Anatomy - Histology - Embryology,
University of Ioannina, School of Medicine, Ioannina,
Greece

Mauro CIOTTI
Department of Bone Infection, Codivilla-Putti Institute, Cortina
d'Ampezzo, Italy

Mauro CODELUPPI
Department of Medicine and Medical Specialities, Infectious
Disease Clinic, University of Modena and Reggio Emilia,
Modena, Italy

William J. COSTERTON
Professor, Director, Center for Biofilms, School of Dentistry,
University of Southern California, Los Angeles, CA, USA

Ferdinando DA RIN
Department of Bone Infection, Codivilla-Putti Institute, Cortina
d'Ampezzo, Italy

Zoe H. DAILIANA
Assistant Professor, Department of Orthopaedic Surgery and
Musculoskeletal Trauma, University of Thessalia, School of
Medicine, Larissa, Greece

Francisco DEL PIÑAL MATORRAS
Director, Instituto de Cirugia Plástica y de la Mano. Private practice.
Head, Unit of Hand-Wrist and Plastic Surgery, Hospital Mutua
Montañesa, Santander, Spain

Christian DUMONTIER
Associate Professor, Institut de la Main and SOS-Mains Orthopedic Department, Hôpital Saint Antoine, Paris, France

Daniel Vincent EGLOFF
Professor, CHUV, Department of Plastic & Reconstructive
Surgery, Clinique Longeraie, Lausanne, Switzerland

Pierre-Edouard FOURNIER
Infectiologist, Laboratoire de Bactérilogie Hôpital de la Timone,
Marseille, France

Maria Concetta GAGLIANO
Department of Emergency, Unit of Hand Surgery and
  Microsurgery, Policlinico, Modena, Italy

André GAY
Fellow, Department of Hand Surgery, Hôpital de la Conception,
  Marseille, France

Nikolaos E. GEROSTATHOPOULOS
Orthopaedic Surgeon, Head of Hand and Upper Extremity Surgery
  - Microsurgery Unit, KAT General Hospital, Athens, Greece

Helen GIAMARELLOU
Professor, 4th University Department of Internal Medicine,
  ATTIKON University Hospital, Athens, Greece

Efthymia GIANNITSIOTI
Consultant, 4th University Department of Internal Medicine,
  ATTIKON University Hospital, Athens, Greece

Alain GILBERT
Professor, Clinique Jouvenet, Institut de la Main, Paris, France

G. Maria HÄNSCH
Professor, Institut für Immunologie, Universität Heidelberg,
  Heidelberg, Germany

Michalis E. HANTES
Consultant, Department of Orthopaedic Surgery and Musculo-
  skeletal Trauma, University of Thessalia, School of Medicine,
  Larissa, Greece

Saiidy HASHAM
Clinical and Research Registrar in Hand Surgery, The Pulvertaft
  Hand Centre, Derbyshire Royal Infirmary, Derby, United Kingdom

Volkmar HEPPERT
Chief, Department of Septic Surgery, Berufsgenossenschaftliche
  Unfallklinik, Ludwigshafen, Germany

Peter HERRMANN
Department of Septic Surgery, Berufsgenossenschaftliche
  Unfallklinik, Ludwigshafen, Germany

Ioannis A. IGNATIADIS
Consultant, Hand and Upper Extremity Surgery - Microsurgery
  Unit, KAT General Hospital, Athens, Greece

Marco INNOCENTI
Chief of Microsurgery Department, C.T.O. Hospital, Firenze, Italy

John M. ITAMURA
Associate Professor, Department of Orthopaedic Surgery, Keck
  School of Medicine, University of Southern California,
  LAC+USC Medical Center, Los Angeles, CA, USA

Elizabeth O. JOHNSON
Associate Professor, Department of Anatomy - Histology -
  Embryology, University of Ioannina, School of Medicine,
  Ioannina, Greece

Theophilos KARACHALIOS
Associate Professor, Department of Orthopaedic Surgery and
  Musculoskeletal Trauma, University of Thessalia, School of
  Medicine, Larissa, Greece

Apostolos H. KARANTANAS
Associate Professor, Department of Radiology, University of
  Crete, Heraklion, Greece

Vasilios A. KONTOGEORGAKOS
Resident in Orthopaedics, Department of Orthopaedic Surgery,
  University of Ioannina, Ioannina, Greece

Anastasios V. KOROMPILIAS
Assistant Professor, Department of Orthopaedic Surgery,
  University of Ioannina, Ioannina, Greece

Alexandros S. KYRIAKOS
Resident in Orthopaedics - Fellow, Hand and Upper Extremity
  Surgery - Microsurgery Unit, KAT General Hospital, Athens,
  Greece

Antonio LANDI
Director, Unit of Hand Surgery and Microsurgery, Policlinico,
  Modena, Italy

Dominique LE VIET
Associate Professor, Institut de la Main, Paris, France

Roland LECLERCQ
Professor of Microbiology, Service de Microbiologie, Hôpital de la
  Conception, Universite de Caen, France

Régis LEGRÉ
Professor of Hand Surgery, Department of Hand Surgery, Hôpital
  de la Conception, Marseille, France

Andrea LETI ACCIARO
Hand Surgeon and Microsurgeon, Department of Emergency, Unit
  of Hand Surgery and Microsurgery, Policlinico, Modena, Italy

Lycurgus L. LIAROPOULOS
Professor of Health Economics, University of Athens, School of Nursing, Athens, Greece

Marios G. LYKISSAS
Resident in Orthopaedics, Department of Orthopaedic Surgery, University of Ioannina, Ioannina, Greece

Guy MAGALON
Professor of Plastic Surgery, Department of Plastic Surgery, Hôpital de la Conception, Marseille, France

Konstantinos N. MALIZOS (editor)
Professor and Chairman, Department of Orthopaedic Surgery and Musculoskeletal Trauma, University of Thessalia, School of Medicine, Larissa, Greece

Antonios MANIATIS
Professor, Department of Microbiology, University of Thessalia, School of Medicine, Larissa, Greece

Pierre MANSAT
Professor, Department of Orthopaedic Surgery and Traumatology, University Hospital -PURPAN, Toulouse, France

Dimitrios S. MASTROKALOS
Lecturer, Department of Orthopaedic Surgery, ATTIKON University Hospital, University of Athens, School of Medicine, Athens, Greece

Christophe MATHOULIN
Professor, Clinique Jouvenet, Institut de la Main, Paris, France

Gregory I. MITSIONIS
Assistant Professor of Orthopaedics, Department of Orthopaedic Surgery, University of Ioannina, Ioannina, Greece

Arrash MOGHADDAM
Department of Septic Surgery, Berufsgenossenschaftliche Unfallklinik, Ludwigshafen, Germany

Theophanis MORAITIS
Senior Consultant, Department of Orthopaedic Surgery and Musculoskeletal Trauma, University Hospital of Larissa, Larissa, Greece

Emanuele NASOLE
Hyperbaric Center - GyneProMedical, Bologna, Italy

Antonios PAPADOPOULOS
Lecturer in Pathology, 4th University Department of Internal Medicine, ATTIKON University Hospital, Athens, Greece

Dionysios PARIDIS
Resident in Orthopaedics, Department of Orthopaedic Surgery and Musculoskeletal Trauma, University of Thessalia, School of Medicine, Larissa, Greece

Efthimia PETINAKI
Assistant Professor of Microbiology, University of Thessalia, School of Medicine, Larissa, Greece

Lazaros A. POULTSIDES
Resident, Department of Orthopaedic Surgery and Musculoskeletal Trauma, University of Thessalia, School of Medicine, Larissa, Greece

Maria RAISSAKI
Lecturer in Radiology, Department of Radiology, University Hospital of Heraklion, University of Crete, School of Medicine, Heraklion, Greece

Antal RENNER
Professor, National Institute for Traumatology and Hand Surgery, Budapest, Hungary

Nikolaos RIGOPOULOS
Fellow, Department of Orthopaedic Surgery and Musculoskeletal Trauma, University of Thessalia, School of Medicine, Larissa, Greece

Nikolaos ROIDIS
Consultant, Department of Orthopaedic Surgery and Musculoskeletal Trauma, University of Thessalia, School of Medicine, Larissa, Greece

Khalid SALEM
Clinical & Research Registrar in Hand Surgery, The Pulvertaft Hand Centre, Derbyshire Royal Infirmary, Derby, United Kingdom

Stephen B. SCHNALL
Professor, Department of Orthopaedic Surgery, Keck School of Medicine, University of Southern California, Los Angeles, USA

Frances SHARPE
Orthopaedic Surgeon, Southern California Permanente Medical Group, Fontana, California, Los Angeles, USA

Panayotis N. SOUCACOS (editor)
Professor and Chairman, Department of Orthopaedic
  Surgery, University of Athens, School of Medicine,
  Athens, Greece

Sarantis G. SPYRIDONOS
Consultant, Hand and Upper Extremity Surgery - Microsurgery
  Unit, KAT General Hospital, Athens, Greece

Shalom STAHL
Clinical Associate Professor, Hand Surgery Unit, Rambam
  Medical Center, Haifa, Israel

Milan STEVANOVIC
Professor of Orthopedics and Surgery, University of Southern
  California, Keck School of Medicine, Los Angeles County
  Medical Center, USA

Zsolt SZABO
Associate Professor, Traumatology and Hand Surgery
  Department, B.A.Z. County University Teaching Hospital,
  Miskolc, Hungary

George S. THEMISTOCLEOUS
Department of Orthopaedic Surgery, Keck School of Medicine,
  University of Southern California, LAC+USC Medical Center,
  Los Angeles, CA, USA

Pierluigi TOS
Department of Orthopaedic Surgery, UOD Microsurgery -
  C.T.O. Hospital, Torino, Italy

Ioannis X. TSIONOS
Consultant, Hand and Upper Extremity Surgery -
  Microsurgery Unit, KAT General Hospital, Athens,
  Greece

Paraskevi A. TZORTZI
Resident in Orthopaedics - Fellow, Hand and Upper Extremity
  Surgery - Microsurgery Unit, KAT General Hospital, Athens,
  Greece

Sokratis E. VARITIMIDIS
Lecturer, Department of Orthopaedic Surgery and Musculoskeletal
  Trauma, University of Thessalia, School of Medicine, Larissa,
  Greece

Marios D. VEKRIS
Assistant Professor, Department of Orthopaedic Surgery,
  University of Ioannina, Ioannina, Greece

Bernd von MAYDELL
Department of Hand- Plastic and Reconstructive Surgery,
  Malteser Hospital, Bonn, Germany

Christof WAGNER
Professor, Department of Septic Surgery, Berufsgenossenschaftliche Unfallklinik, Ludwigshafen, Germany

Geert H.I.M. WALENKAMP
Professor of Orthopaedics, Chairman of Department of
  Orthopaedic Surgery, Academic Hospital Maastricht,
  Maastricht, the Netherlands

Vasileios C. ZACHOS
Department of Orthopaedic Surgery, Keck School of Medicine,
  University of Southern California, LAC+USC Medical Center,
  Los Angeles, CA, USA

Charalampos G. ZALAVRAS
Associate Professor, Department of Orthopaedic Surgery,
  University of Southern California Keck School of Medicine,
  LAC+USC Medical Center, Los Angeles, CA, U.S.A.

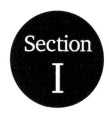

GENERAL PRINCIPLES IN MUSCULOSKELETAL INFECTIONS OF THE UPPER LIMB

General Principles in Musculoskeletal Infections of the Upper Limb

The History of Infections in Hand Surgery

Kouroche AMINI[a], Sharon ADLER[b], Daniel Vincent EGLOFF[c*]

[a]CHUV, Service de Chirurgie Plastique et Reconstruction, Lausanne , Switzerland

[b]Professor of English & Latin, Geneva, Switzerland

[c]CHUV, Service de Chirurgie Plastique et Reconstruction
& Clinique Chirurgicale et Permanence de Longeraie, Lausanne, Switzerland

"The basis of medicine is love, and not everyone can be a physician. Every surgeon should have three qualities, first as regards his own *person;* second, as regards the *patient,* and third, as regards his *art".*

Paracelsus (1493-1541)

Keywords: surgery; history; infection; hand.

1. INTRODUCTION

The history of surgery is that of an endless fight first for life and second for the integrity of the body. Throughout centuries this "art" has constantly struggled against conservatism, ignorance and religious superstition. Indeed, proficient surgery has always gone hand in hand with accurate knowledge of human anatomy. Therefore, one of the greatest challenges surgeons had to overcome was to get to know the human body well enough to treat it. Autopsies and dissections were taboo then, and still are today in some cultures. The human body was sacred in death. It could not be violated by dissection. Dissecting corpses became more common and tolerated after the Middle-Ages. Several anatomists/surgeons revolutionized surgery thanks to their discoveries during the Renaissance. Meanwhile, as old as the hills, it was wars that proved an excellent source of experience where the "medicine men" or "barbers" (later called surgeons) learnt their trade. War wounds were the best way to learn basic healing methods. It is unfortunate that wars provided such an impetus towards progress; yet it was a violent, but efficient teacher.

Among all surgical procedures, hand surgery stands apart from the others. It is a very thorough "art" that involves the repair of nerves, tendons and vessels, as well as osteosynthesis, and of course plastic surgery. In order to perform it properly, the surgeon needs to display wide-ranging experience and knowledge of all the surgical techniques cited above. This is just a glimpse of the know-how required to exercise this profession.

Ambroise Paré's definition of surgery parallels that of infections in hand surgery. He said that there are five objectives in surgery: "extracting morbid or foreign matter (pus, necrotic tissues, etc.), restoring damaged functions (tendinous gliding), separate what has been fixed together (adhesions), suturing what has been separated (skin),

*Corresponding Author
Service de Chirurgie Plastique et Reconstructive
1011 Lausanne (Switzerland)
Tel: +0041 21 314 22 11
Fax: +0041 21 314 25 30
e-mail: daniel.egloff@chuv.ch

and repairing the defects of nature (transplantation after amputation or prosthesis)".

2. HISTORY

The story of surgery begins with **Imhotep** (c. 2700 BC.) who was the first physician to be known by name in written history. He is credited of having founded **Egyptian medicine.** He probably wrote the first treaty on surgery. We unfortunately have only heard of it through other sources, because no original copies have ever been discovered. Some historians firmly believe that he was the author of the **Edwin Smith Papyrus** (c. 1700 BC), however there is no genuine proof of this. The original text of this treatise dates back to 3000-2500 BC. It differs from other medical papyri such as the **Ebers papyrus** because it primarily deals with surgery: forty-eight cases of surgery, mostly traumatic and orthopedic, are described. They detail anatomical observations, ailments and cures. They also indicate that Egyptian surgeons were already able to differentiate tubercular abscesses they did not incise, and septic ones for which they recommended incision. Edwin Smith Papyrus shows us that the state of scientific knowledge was remarkable for the time. Unlike other papyri, it contained no prayers, incantations, exorcisms or superstitious prescriptions which often appeared in other writings. This clearly indicates that its author was not a priest-physician, nor a member of a religious class.

Two notions of Egyptian medicine are particularly interesting. First of all, the importance of hygiene in their medical practice probably explains the success of their surgery. It is difficult to know if the Egyptians had understood the importance of hygiene in order to avoid infections or if they knew it instinctively. The second element is the Egyptians' highly specialized training. Medicine had reached such a degree of specialization that it led to absurd situations. An anecdote relates that one Pharaoh, Senusret, had a physician for his right eye and another for his left one. The Egyptians' knowledge of anatomy was mediocre and sometimes even dangerously wrong. For example, they believed that blood vessels made air, urine, semen and blood flow. In addition, they attributed the functions of conscience, thought and memory to the heart.

The great amount of information acquired during mummy preparation should have enlightened them on the subject. Yet, the embalming protocol was not as elaborate as could be thought. First, those who performed it were considered outcasts of society and were by no means physicians. Secondly, in order to extract the brain, they did not perform a craniotomy, but pulled it out through the nose with the help of an iron hook. As for the body, there was no real dissection: with only one incision on the side of the lower abdomen they removed the intestines and replaced them with some myrrh, cinnamon and other spices before sewing it back. Obviously, the process did not allow for any study.

The notion of **hygiene** or cleanliness can also be found in the Hindu texts of Sushruta, a surgeon who lived in ancient India (c. 6th century BC). It is still impossible today to date when the Sushruta Samhita, a textbook of surgery, was precisely written. The mere observation of the surgical instruments described in the Samhita, more than one hundred and twenty of them, leads us to believe that the therapeutic attitude in case of infection was extremely enlightened for that period. Sushrata is supposed to be the father of Plastic and Cosmetic Surgery. As proof of his inventivity and surgical understanding, let us remember that the Indian technique of forehead flap rhinoplasty is still used to this day as it was described in the Sushruta Samhita.

Around the same time in Greece, **Anaximenes of Miletus** (c. 585-525 BC), a Greek philosopher, taught that **air** was the principal element and the source of all that exists. Shortly after, **Hippocrates** (460-377 BC.) founded the Hypocratic School of Medicine and made a legitimate profession of practising medicine. Among his many contributions, some have influenced the development of medicine for close to a millennium. First and foremost, Hippocrates introduced the theory of "humorism" which assumed that any illness was the result of an imbalance of the four humours, blood, black bile, yellow bile and phlegm, in the body. Secondly, whereas contemporary physicians mainly focus on diagnosis and specialized treatment, Hippocrates was famous for his clinical doctrines of observation and preferred focusing on prognosis. Finally, he categorized diseases as acute, chronic, endemic and **epidemic.** He was the first to talk of **contamination and infection,** which he attributed to a foul air called "miasma". He hypothesized that there were particles likely to transmit an infection as he talked of "miasmata", meaning miasma in plural. This means it was not the air in itself which was harmful, but the extraneous elements altering it. This conception of foul air harmful to health became widespread. **Héliodorus,** a phoenician philosopher (4th century AD) says in the "Ethiopiques" that there are no means of protecting oneself: "...the air that is spread around us penetrates deep down in our body through the nose, the eyes, the mouth and other openings of the body, and brings with it external properties....".

This concept of contagious disease was reinforced by the observation of epidemics which the Greek historian **Thucydides** wrote about. He described the plague which decimated Athenians in 430 BC. Of course, he had not identified the phenomenon of contagion, but he had guessed the importance of its spreading, as had his compatriots. This is how he came to write that the disease caused its first ravages among doctors - the first in the line of fire. People instinctively tried to get away from the sick, in order to flee the foul air according to Hippocrates' tenet. A good example is when Galen fled

Rome as soon as the antonine plague began to rage (167 BC under Marcus-Aurelius).

In 30 AD, **Celsus** (53 BC-7AD) published "De re medica libri octo" of which the last two books deal with surgery. Among other topics, pus formation was mentioned and Celsus described methods of **tapping morbid pus** accumulation. We owe him the description of the inflammation: the famous "rubor, tumor, calor, dolor".

One of the most famous physicians of the Graeco-Roman period was **Galen of Pergamum** (129-200 AD) who revered Hippocrates and devoutly admired his work. He was keen on medicine just as much as on surgery and published a lot, more than four hundred works, among which a book on pathological swellings. For four years, Galen learnt practical surgery with the gladiators in Rome, a period which gave him wonderful opportunities for the practice of orthopedic and restorative surgery. However, his physiological views were chiefly based on animal experimentation, as he only dissected dogs and apes and very seldom human bodies. Moreover, he strongly believed that the movement of the blood originated from the liver. Although he was clearly a very efficient surgeon, Galen exerted a negative influence on the development of surgery because he believed that **suppuration was essential to the healing of a wound.** His posthumous influence dominated medicine for over fourteen centuries, even though some of his findings were based on erroneous ideas. His large body of writing became "canonized" to the extent that disagreeing with it was regarded as heresy.

Four centuries later, **Paul of Aegina** (607-690 AD) was the last of the classical Byzantine doctors. The sixth book of his "Abridgement of medicine in seven books" deals with surgery and was taken over by the Arabs, especially **Albucasis** (936-1013 AD). The latter suggested that in case of gangrene, amputation was the only means of saving the patient.

This belief of Galen, that suppuration was essential to the healing of a wound, remained a dogma for a thousand years, until **Ugo di Borgognoni** (c. 1160-1257) who founded the faculty of medicine of Bologna and his disciple, **Theodoric** (1205-1296), **refuted that wounds should go through a stage of infection before healing** "per intentio secundam". Unfortunately, only **Henri de Montville** (1260-1320) would adopt this heretical belief, so strong was the idea of "pus bonum and laudabile". However, he made France the leader in the field with his book "Chirurgie".

After Galen of Pergamum and Paul of Aegina, there would be practically no interesting discoveries in the medical world until **Benivieni** (1440-1502), almost a thousand years later. We owe him the knowledge of anatomical pathology thanks to his **autopsies.** By then, anatomical dissections had gradually become more commonly performed notably by Leonardo da Vinci, but especially by Vesalius who published the first book on anatomy.

Fifteenth century Renaissance artists became increasingly interested in the human form, so the study of human anatomy became a necessary part of the young artist's apprenticeship, especially in northern Italy. **Leonardo da Vinci** (1452-1519), however, was the first artist to consider **anatomy** for reasons beyond its practicality in depicting the human body. Leonardo himself made anatomical preparations from which he produced drawings, more than 750 of which are extant, representing the skeletal, muscular, nervous, and vascular systems. The illustrations were often supplemented with annotations of a **physiological** nature. Leonardo's scientific accuracy was greater than that of Vesalius, and his artistic beauty remains unchallenged. His correct assessment of the curvature of the spine went otherwise undiscovered for more than a hundred years. He depicted the true position of the fetus in utero and first noted certain anatomical structures. The sketches were seen by only a few contemporaries and were not published until the end of last century.

In the 16th century, knowledge became more widespread through the work of **Andreas Vesalius** (1514-1564), who was Flemish by birth. Vesalius made a monumental contribution to the field of anatomy, of which we are still the beneficiaries. He held a different point of view on the relation between diseases and the body structure. He refuted the theory of dyscrasia, and by doing so challenged the dogma of Galenism. One of the main reasons for his change of heart was the discovery of more than two hundred errors in the works of Galen. For instance he realized that Galen's work was based on the dissection of apes and not human bodies, therefore leading to many inaccuracies in the location of some organs. An anatomy teacher, Vesalius was one of the first to perform on his own public dissections in lecture halls of the University of Padua in Italy. Anatomy became based on the precise dissection of human cadavers rather than on animals, such as pigs, which the successors of Galen had had to be content with for more than thirteen centuries due to religious restrictions. Vesalius's research and study on human bodies allowed him to prepare a new book of the **complete human anatomy.** Thanks to his 663-page treaty "De humani corporis fabrica" published in 1543, he radically transformed anatomy from a primitive to a highly-developed science. The impact of this publication was outstanding, but also created quite a few enemies. Vesalius soon found himself in bitter controversy with his former teacher Jacques Sylvius. The latter was a die-hard Galenist imprisoned in scholastic tradition. His only retort upon learning of the differences between certain structures as seen by Vesalius and those as described by Galen was that mankind must have changed in the intervening twelve hundred years.

When talking about surgery, it is impossible to overlook **Ambroise Paré's** (1510-1590) deciding role in 16th century medical evolution. This French surgeon greatly influenced the acceptance and recognition of surgery, for long considered as a lowly form of "butchery" by all

Faculties of Medicine, as a respectable and noble profession. Paré's career began as an apprentice to a barber-surgeon until he met Laurent Collot and saw him perform a lithotomy on a patient. He then changed his career plan and decided he would focus on being a surgeon.

Paré was of a curious and observant nature and for him a prerequisite of surgery was a perfect knowledge of human anatomy. Consequently he became an anatomist just as much as a surgeon. Ambroise Paré's medical training was far from traditional. He undertook no formal studies, nor did he learn Latin or Greek. In 1533, at barely twenty, he completed his training in Paris under Jacques Goubli at the Hôtel Dieu. All Paré cared about was to relieve sick patients of their suffering. Most of them had been left to themselves, so Paré had ample opportunities to perfect his skills either with them or on dead bodies. Later, battlefields became his school. They were at the same time gruesome and a valuable source of experience. War injuries represented a new challenge for him. His aim was to prevent gunpowder from poisoning the wound. First he had learnt to cauterize wounds with boiling oil. However this procedure proved not only partially inefficient, but also excruciatingly painful for the injured soldiers. Paré then modified the treatment by applying a balm made of a mixture of egg yolk, honey and turpentine. To his surprise, this "homemade" ointment worked wonderfully. In between wars, Ambroise Paré had his civilian practice in Paris. He treated fractures, luxations, cataracts and became a pioneer in obstetrics. He also spent a lot of time writing books and treaties, and invented many prostheses and ortheses. Still, it was wartime with its dreadful atrocities, which enabled Paré to innovate and discover **vascular ligatures,** and these made him famous. He wrote at length about these techniques and it was recognized as one of the most revolutionary discoveries in surgery.

Throughout his life, Paré had always been more of a practitioner than a theoretician. It is mainly his knowledge in traumatology acquired on battlefields that allowed him to innovate and progress in his art of healing. Being the counselor and body surgeon of four successive kings brought Ambroise Paré both honor and respect, even from the College de Saint-Come, which is quite an achievement considering his lack of formal education. As for infections, Ambroise Paré advised incisions of abscesses, therefore drainage but amputation as well in cases of gangrenous evolution. One anecdote relates that King Charles IX once asked Ambroise Paré to please treat him better than his poor patients, Paré supposedly replied: "I treat all my patients like Kings".

A decisive step in the recognition of **the contagious character of infections** occurred only in the 19th century and was taken by **Ignaz Semmelweis** (1818-1865), a Hungarian physician. Semmelweis completed most of his medical education and training in Vienna in the mid 1840s. After graduating he became an assistant in the Obstetrical Clinic of the Vienna General Hospital, which was then a teaching hospital. While there, he noticed one of the two delivery rooms had a much higher incidence of puerperal fever and infections among its patients, thus often leading them to premature death. That specific room was the teaching service for medical students. Most of them had come there without washing their hands right after having performed autopsies or examining other patients, therefore increasing the maternal mortality rate to 18.27%. Let us not forget that back then, the act of examining a patient was done with bare hands, as the use of rubber gloves was not introduced before the end of the 19th century. The other delivery room was solely for the instruction of midwives who seldom came in contact with cadavers or other sick patients, hence the 2.03% mortality rate. Semmelweis also noticed that, if a woman arrived too late and had already given birth at home, or in a carriage, she seldom got childbed fever. It thus seemed that the infection was communicated during the actual birth in the clinic.

But the real clue appeared when a professor of criminal medicine, Kolletschka, cut his finger during an autopsy and got blood poisoning. Semmelweis later commented: "Day and night, the image of Kolletschka's illness pursued me. As we found identical changes in his body with those of the childbed women, it can be concluded that Kolletschka died of the same disease which caused the death of so many women. But we know what made Kolletschka ill: the wound he got from the autopsy knife, polluted with dead flesh. His death was not the result of the wound itself, but its pollution. Of course, Kolletschka was not the first to die in this way. I must therefore assume that if his disease and the women's are identical, it is quite likely that the cause of the women's death was the same as Kolletschka's. Consequently I must wonder: did dead flesh from autopsies enter the blood of all those whom I have seen die and cause their death? The answer is obviously "yes". So the explanation was discovered. What distinguished the two wards was that the medical students came straight from their autopsy exercises in the pathological institution, carrying infections from corpses on their hands.

In May 1847, Semmelweis made it compulsory to wash hands with chlorinated water before births. In two years, the mortality rate dropped to 1.27%, which was an astounding result. Unfortunately for Semmelweis, he proved unable to get the medical world's support, probably because his discoveries went against the conservatism of many eminent practitioners. Among some causes, the latter argued that washing their hands between treating patients would be too much trouble! In 1848 Semmelweis extended his washing protocol to all the instruments used during labour in the delivery rooms and reported having virtually eradicated puerperal fever. That same year a conservative movement came into power and Semmelweis was fired the following year. Semmelweis left for Pest in his native Hungary and took charge of the maternity ward of St Rochus Hospital from 1851 to 1857. There, his ideas were soon accepted and put into practice reducing the mortality rate from puerperal fever to 0.85%. In 1861 Semmelweis finally published his discovery in the book: "The Etiology, Concept and Prophylaxis of Childbed Fever." Again, Semmelweis had to face the incomprehension and the mockeries of the medical establishment rejecting his theory. His unbalanced, difficult temperament turned into mental illness, and he ended up in an asylum. Ironically, he died in the same manner as Kolletschka, from blood poisoning after a cut to his finger. Semmelweis' recognition was posthumous. Today he is considered as a pioneer in antiseptic policy and infections. Had his contemporaries taken him more seriously, many unnecessary deaths could have been prevented. He was one of the first physicians to use sodium hypochlorite as an antiseptic.

In 1881, **Robert Koch** proved the bacterial activity of hypochlorite. Dakin's solution, created by **Dakin** in 1915 as a disinfectant for war wounds, contained 0.45% to 0.50% of sodium hypochlorite.

Louis Pasteur (1822-1895) was one of the pioneers of microbiology. He undertook to demonstrate that fermentation was caused by the growth of **microorganisms** and that their growth in nutrient broths was not due to spontaneous generation, but came from outside, as spores on dust. He thus became of the few scientists to support the germ theory. At first, Pasteur focused his research on contaminated fermenting beverages such as milk and beer. He invented the process of heating liquids so that to kill most of their bacteria. He also distinguished between germs living with oxygen and those - anaerobiosis - capable of living and developing without oxygen or air. Later Pasteur concluded that micro-organisms also infected humans and animals, which further led Joseph Lister to develop antiseptic surgery. Pasteur's discovery of immunology and vaccination was serendipitous. At the time, in 1879, he was working on chicken cholera when a culture of the responsible bacteria had spoiled and failed to induce the disease to some chickens he was trying to infect. In fact, his assistant was instructed to inoculate the chickens while Pasteur was on holiday. Charles Chamberland, his assistant, failed to do so and went on vacation. When he came back, one month later, the assistant inoculated the chickens with the month-old cultures and instead of the infection being fatal to them, it just made them unwell. The chickens recovered completely and were now immune to the disease.

2.1. Immunization was discovered

In 1880, while Pasteur began researching rabies, he noticed that infected dried marrow could protect from the disease if inoculated to dogs. In 1885, Pasteur still hesitated to inoculate a human with the vaccine, even though his results were conclusive on animals. One day, along came a young boy infected with rabies, his death impending. After consulting several physicians about his dilemma, under their responsibility he inoculated the boy with the vaccine and saved his life.

2.2. Human vaccination was born

After the discovery of the germ by Pasteur but before Fleming's invention of antibiotics, the treatment for phlegmon was still the same as that of the Middle Ages: scarifications, draining, debridements and amputations (Chassaignac, Dupuytren (1777-1835), Hutchinson). The role of bacteria had not yet been formally recognized as such. **The Encyclopedic Dictionary of Medical Sciences of 1887** says the following about the etiology and of the pathogeny of phlegmons: the pathological anatomy shows us the presence of micro-organisms deep in the tissues infected by phlegmon; it must now be determined what role they play. Should they be considered as mere epiphenomenon or are they really the cause of the accidents? Nevertheless, the tendency was to recognize the pathogenic role of germs, as prevention by disinfection had been introduced for wounds, surgical interventions, blood-lettings, and like in Semmelweis's experience, a significant decrease in infections had been noticed.

Semmelweis's discoveries were not made in vain, in 1865 in Scotland; **Joseph Lister** (1827-1912) had come to the same conclusions. After reading one of Louis Pasteur's publications, he understood that "miasma" was not the reason why so many wounds got infected; putrefaction and fermentation occurred because of the presence of micro-organisms carried by the air. The only solution was to get rid of them in order to prevent them from accessing the wound. Lister decided to prove his theory right by experimenting on his own. His **antiseptic method** depended on one agent: carbolic acid. It is interesting to note that this agent had been in fact previously used but only to deodorize sewage. Lister began by sterilizing all surgical instruments as well as urging his colleagues to wash their hands with carbolic acid solutions before and after operating. He also disinfected operating rooms by spraying the solution and treated wounds or even abscesses particularly those of tubercular origin. Lister's second important contribution was to introduce sterile Catgut ligatures. The latter were absorbable sutures made by twisting together strands of purified collagen from bovine intestines. Thanks to this new material, deep suppuration would be prevented while ligatures would be cut short and safely left in the tissues. In 1867, Lister published a series of articles relating his various experiments and describing his antiseptic methods. Although, just like Semmelweis, he had to face tenacious questioning from his contemporaries, Lister's discoveries prevailed over the latter's ignorance. Today considered as "the father of modern antisepsis", Lister credited Semmelweis for his success: "Without Semmelweis, my achievements would be nothing".

Early in his career, at the beginning of the 20th century, **Allen B. Kanavel** (1874-1938), an American surgeon and researcher took a serious interest in hand infections. He revolutionized the basis for the type of care given to infections of the hand nowadays when he published "Infections of the hand: **the surgical treatment** of acute chronic suppurative processes in the fingers, hand and forearm" in 1912. The content was the result of twelve years of study on the spread of infection throughout the hand and on the proper means of draining pathways of the spread. In order to find which routes an infection could spread, Kanavel attempted experimental injections of red lead in the tendon sheaths. This study enabled him to first, establish the relations of the tendon sheaths and fascial spaces; secondly, to identify the possible locations where the infection might spread, and finally, the best sites of drainage of the infected areas. Today we still rely on Kanavel's anatomical description to drain infections of the hand. His general principles of treatment remain valid despite the access we now have to antibiotics: "When a patient presents himself with an infection of the hand, the surgeon's first obligation is to make a diagnosis as to the nature and location of the infection. A diffuse spreading infection in the subcutaneous tissues of hand or forearm, along the lymphatics or blood-vessels or in the deep fascial spaces, should first of all be controlled and localized by properly applied defensive measures. Many patients have lost their lives as a result of hasty and ill-advised incisions in the presence of a rapidly spreading streptococcic infection. On the other hand, a localized infection in the anterior closed space of the distal phalanx or in a tendon sheath must be incised promptly if bone involvement in the first case and tendon necrosis in the second are to be avoided. It is important therefore, to distinguish between a diffuse spreading infection in cellular tissue and a localized infection. In case of doubt, it is better to err on the side of conservatism and with the help of rest and warm moist dressings aid nature in effecting localization of the infectious process".

Fleming (1881-1955) was born the same year as Pasteur made the first group vaccination to a herd of sheep in 1881. He was a Scottish biologist and pharmacologist. After witnessing the death of many soldiers from septicaemia during World War I, Fleming looked for anti-bacterial agents. Unfortunately, the antiseptics killed the patient's immunological defences faster than they killed the bacteria, especially if they were used deep in the wounds. Indeed, the latter had the tendency to shelter anaerobic bacteria, and the antiseptics mainly removed beneficial agents that actually protected the patients. In 1928, Fleming was asked to write a chapter about staphylococci. He decided to repeat and confirm all the experiments described in medical literature. The concurrence of Fleming's summer holiday with the presence of Dr La Touche's mycology laboratory neighboring Fleming's will allow for one of the greatest discoveries of our century: penicillin. As Fleming was going on vacation, piled up in his laboratory he left Petri dishes containing cultures of *Staphylococcus aureus,* which became contaminated by spores of Penicillium notatum. He saw a zone around the fungus where the bacteria had not grown. Fleming isolated an extract from that zone and identified it as a new agent from the penicillium family that he named **Penicillin.** Thus, the era of antibiotherapy began in the most unexpected way. Fleming's publication in 1929 did not attract the attention of the medical and scientific world. It was only in 1940, at Oxford University, that Florey and Chain became interested in antibacterials and published their experimental works on penicillin. This publication was the starting point of modern antibiotherapy, and the first patients were treated with penicillin from 1941 onwards. Nevertheless, Fleming was well aware of the resistance of bacteria to Penicillin, whenever too little was used or for too short a period of time. He therefore cautioned not to use it carelessly unless the diagnosis was proven.

Broadly speaking, this is how the history of infections could be summarized: Hippocrates described the clinical observation of a patient leading to a diagnosis, Semmelweiss introduced the notion of contagion, Koch and Pasteur proved the existence of germs, Kanavel added the notions of anatomy to understand the physiopathology of hand infections and their treatment, and finally, Fleming discovered antibiotics. The following chapters are the state-of the-art treatments of hand infections. Their numbers illustrate the complexity of the specialty. Yet, the fundamental principle remains "**Ubi pus, ibi evacuat**".

The Socioeconomic Consequences of Upper Limb Infections

Lazaros A. POULTSIDES[a], Lycurgus L. LIAROPOULOS[b], Konstantinos N. MALIZOS[a*]

[a]*Department of Orthopaedic Surgery and Musculoskeletal Trauma, University of Thessalia, Larissa, Greece*
[b]*Centre for Health Services Management and Evaluation, Department of Nursing, University of Athens, Greece*

Musculoskeletal Infections are potentially devastating not only for the patient and health services, but society as well, as they may lead to functional impairment, long lasting disability, or even permanent handicap, inevitably incurring additional social and economic consequences. This increasing burden placed upon the patient, health services or society, may be both medical and socioeconomic. Infection commonly results in the need for re-operation, prolonged use of antibiotics, complications, extended rehabilitation and several outpatient follow-up visits wich incur additional costs. Total direct medical costs associated with revision of an infected joint arthroplasty are approximately three-fold higher compared to revision due to aseptic loosening and five-fold higher compared to primary joint arthroplasty. Infected total shoulder, elbow and wrist arthroplasties present the worst prognosis and poorer functional outcome, compared to infected arthroplasties of the lower limb. Accordingly, soft tissue infections and especially necrotizing ones have a profound economic impact on patients and health care systems. Identifying the basic components of the burden through "cost-of-illness" studies may assist in the decision-making process at policy and planning levels, facilitating in this way the process of setting appropriate priorities and adopting preventive strategies towards its reduction. Focusing on the three specific health care strategies, including the prevention, diagnosis and effective treatment of infection, physicians, members of society and health care policy makers need to critically evaluate musculoskeletal infections, not only from a medical standpoint, but also from the financial and the social-functional points of view.

Keywords: cost; infected joint arthroplasties; socioeconomic burden; cost-of-illness studies; economic evaluation; necrotizing fasciitis; hand infections.

1. MAGNITUDE AND PREDICTED TRENDS IN THE BURDEN OF DISEASE

Musculoskeletal disorders are the most common cause of severe chronic pain and physical disability, affecting millions of people. Their impact on the health-related quality of life of the individual, on society and on health care systems is enormous [1]. This impact will increase dramatically over the next years as the population ages and lifestyles change towards more mobility and recreational activities. The indirect costs related to morbidity and disability are higher in most European Union countries and in the United States, where total health expenditure rises faster than the gross domestic product [1]. However, disorders of the bone and joints have not been addressed yet as health care priorities. The established market economies allocate less than 5% of their national spending on research related to these conditions.

The burden of musculoskeletal infections parallels the increase in life expectancy, urbanization and motorization, incidence of trauma cases with their subsequent morbidity, expanding application of implants and new surgical innovations. The number of operated patients at risk of developing

*Corresponding Author
Professor and Chairman
Department of Orthopaedic Surgery and Musculoskeletal Trauma
University of Thessalia, School of Medicine
41110 Mezourlo, Larissa, Greece
Tel: +30 2410 682722
Fax: +30 2410 670107
e-mail: malizos@med.uth.gr

infection and other adverse outcomes is also increasing. At the same time, however, training for their management is lacking. The most common orthopaedic infections are those of the soft tissue, necrotizing fasciitis, gas gangrene, hematogenous osteomyelitis, septic arthritis, posttraumatic osteomyelitis and/or septic nonunion, as well as the infections that develop around arthroplasties and internal fixation devices. They can have a potentially devastating effect on the patient, as they may lead to functional impairment, long lasting disability or even permanent handicap [2]. Nowadays, overuse of antibiotics has led to increased bacteria resistance. Moreover, micro-organisms spread as patients are transferred among hospitals, making nosocomial infections a major threat. All these factors result in increased burden to the patient, health care services, and the society, as a whole.

2. Vulnerability and Mechanisms of Infection in the Upper Extremity

Although the hand, forearm and even the elbow are the most exposed anatomical regions of the upper extremity during daily activities, thus vulnerable to the inoculation of bacteria from the environment, they seem to suffer the ravages of infection less than other body parts [3]. Illicit drug use [4], delay in appropriate treatment [5], open fractures [6] and outbreaks of community-acquired infections [7], all contribute towards making infections of the hand and upper extremity a significant problem.

A solid understanding of the frequency of both aerobic and anaerobic infections (around 30%) [8], the increase in mixed infections (both gram-positive and gram-negative organisms) and the unique anatomical characteristics of the hand, is required for efficient management of upper limb infections and their relevant socioeconomic consequences. Wounds that can lead to particularly damaging patterns of infection are those that contaminate closed spaces of the hand, such as the digital pulp space, the nail bed area, the flexor tendon sheath, any of the deep spaces of the palm or thenar regions, and any of the joints of the fingers or the wrist. Infections involving these areas often need surgical debridement and a protracted course of IV antibiotics.

The acquisition of a nosocomial bacterial pathogen by a susceptible patient may occur via the hands of healthcare workers (HCWs), as handwashing policies are seldom adhered to [9, 10]. Furthermore, due to the fact that various bacterial species may persist more tenaciously on hands, handwashing alone may be ineffective for their removal. Bottone et al [11] reported that despite five 30-second handwashes, nosocomial bacterial pathogens persisted on the fingertips, and their complete removal was never achieved. This observation bears strongly on the transmissibility of nosocomial

pathogens in the hospital environment to the hands of HCWs, which may become contaminated after direct contact with an infected or colonized patient, after handling the specimens of infected or colonized patients, or from the environment [9]. The transmissibility of MRSA infections from an otherwise healthy individual with no apparent risk factors for MRSA acquisition, signals that MRSA epidemiology has changed and consists a present hazard imposing, without doubt, a great burden [12]. Although the concentration of bacteria acquired from a patient's setting may vary depending on the source of the contamination (i.e. wound, feces, or contaminated environment), the ability of the bacteria to persist means that within a short time they can be transmitted to another individual by contaminated hands, even if handwashing is performed, or that the same person can be infected, especially if the skin barrier is broken regionally due to trauma. This chain of transmission of nosocomial or community-acquired pathogens via the hands of HCWs or escorts of patients is a multifaceted problem and makes apparent the role of the hand and upper limb in the development of infection regionally or in remote sites of the human body.

3. Inevitable Burden of Upper Limb Orthopaedic Infections

3.1. Necrotizing soft tissue infections (mortality and treatment costs)

Necrotizing fasciitis is a life-threatening disease with reported mortality rates ranging from 6.1% to 43%. Early diagnosis and treatment is associated with lower mortality rates [13, 14]. The treatment of patients with necrotizing fasciitis incurs direct hospital in-patient costs, as well as post-discharge costs for survivors. The latter are related to expenses due to rehabilitation, and in some cases, long-term disability resulting from residual critical illness and tissue loss. Patients presenting clinical evidence of necrotizing fasciitis are managed by a multidisciplinary team consisting of surgeons, intensivists, and infectious disease and/or hyperbaric physicians. Treatment consists of early surgical debridement, broad spectrum intravenous antibiotics, hyperbaric oxygen treatment and intensive care as required.

Although necrotizing soft tissue infections of the abdomen and perineum have received much attention because of mortality rates of as high as 76% [15], the extremities are involved in more than half of necrotizing soft tissue infections [16, 17]. Descriptions of necrotizing soft tissue infections of the extremities have been limited to case reports, small series, and series of mixed anatomic sites. The mortality rates in these reports vary (range: 0-33%), with a combined rate of 19% (56 deaths in 293 patients) [16, 18-23]. Surprisingly, one large study found that necrotizing soft tissue infections in the extremities had a higher mortality risk than abdominal infections [16]. Despite previous reports, these infections remain difficult to diagnose. They may manifest few diagnostic or cutaneous signs early in the course of the infection, and frequently they can comprise a sub-acute variety which is hard to distinguish from usual soft tissue infections [23, 24]. As a result, clinicians who evaluate problems of the extremities may have difficulty in making a timely diagnosis. Orthopaedic surgeons should be familiar with necrotizing soft tissue infections. This is important as they are often the first to treat patients who are referred for treatment of cellulitis, fracture or soft tissue injury, and because time to surgery may affect the mortality rate [13, 14].

In a retrospective study, Ogilvie et al [25] analyzed 150 patients (average age: 41 years) with necrotizing soft tissue infections of the extremities treated at San Francisco General Hospital from 1993 to 1997. They reported an overall mortality rate of 9.3%, lower than the average rate for necrotizing soft tissue infections of the extremities indicated above (19%) [16, 18-23] and lower than the rate reported in a meta-analysis of mixed anatomic sites (26%) [26].

Widjaja et al [27] analyzed the cost of treating necrotizing fasciitis at an Australian tertiary referral hospital with extensive experience and well-developed financial expenditure systems and compared this with the current casemix-based government funding arrangements applied in Victoria, Australia. The extremities were involved in 42% of cases (77% lower limb and 23% upper limb). From the total number of patients, 87% were transferred from other hospitals; 27.5% of these were ventilated at the time of transfer, and 69% had undergone surgical debridement prior to transfer. Overall, 10 (11%) patients died; of these, 23% of patients who were ventilated at the time of the transfer. The mean hospital length of stay was 36 days (range: 1-132 days) for survivors. Five patients died within the first week of admission. Five died due to late complications after the acute processes had been controlled. The mean length of stay for non-survivors was 68 days. The average ICU length of stay was 11 days (range: 1-49 days) for the 63% of patients who required intensive care admission.

Using the Diagnosis-Related Group (DRG) coding as a basis to calculate the cost weights (in dollar value) of patient admissions for the 92 patients with case-mix funding translated into a funding dollar value of $3,208,664. The costs of care provided were nearly twice as this (i.e. $5,935,545). Only 10 patients attracted funding that exceeded the hospital costs, and the average shortage per case was $33,891. At a mean cost of $64,517 per patient, this is clearly an expensive condition, both in terms of dollars, as well as in terms of mortality and disability. One of the patients in this study incurred a total cost of $514,889 with 46 days in the ICU and 474 days in the hospital. Patients received an average of 10 hyperbaric oxygen treatment sessions which incurred an average cost of $7,597 per patient (range: $408 to $35,720). The total cost for the hyperbaric oxygen therapy (HBO) provided for the 92 patients was $698,902, comprising 12% of the total cost of care during hospitalization. The cost of treating necrotizing fasciitis (mean cost of AU $64,517 per patient) exceeded that published in the literature for a number of other medical conditions, particularly compared to carotid endarterectomy (US $9,577, AU$12,766, 1997) [28], coronary artery bypass surgery (US $15,987, AU $21,311, 1996) [29], one year of haemodialysis (US $28,666, AU $38,212, 1996) [30] and to surgical removal of small, operable cerebral arteriovenous malformations (CAN $33,022, AU $35,168, 1995) [31].

3.2. Soft tissue infections (morbidity and treatment costs)

Skin and soft tissue infections of the extremities are the cause of frequent visits to health care providers. Most of these infections are superficial and are readily treated with a regimen of local care and antibiotics. However, soft tissue infections may affect deeper structures including fascia and muscle. Infections tend to affect ischaemic, hypoxic or devitalized tissue and are encountered most commonly in immunocompromised or diabetic patients.

Charalambous et al [32] reported that from 142 consecutive admissions due to acute soft tissue infections of the extremities (3.5% of all acute orthopaedic trauma admissions) between 1996 and 2001, the majority were cellulitis (71/142) with a significant proportion being abscesses (43/142). Most soft tissue infections (43/142) developed secondary to penetrating trauma. These included human (15/142) and animal bites (14/142), and intravenous drug injection (25/142). Seventy-eight of 142 infections involved the hand, arm (2), elbow (5), forearm (10), foot (29), thigh (7), knee (4) and leg (7), revealing a predominance of upper extremity infections (70%). The 142 soft tissue episodes accounted for 748 hospital inpatient days. The average stay for each patient was 4 days (range: 1 - 44), which is similar to the post-operative stay following elective hip and knee joint replacement at the particular institution. Furthermore, these patients required 143 operations performed by orthopaedic specialists, again an important implication in planning financial support of medical resources. A total of 194 follow-up clinic appointments were devoted to this patient population. The cost of each episode of soft tissue infection was up to £1,011. Hospital services accounted for the majority (94%) of the expenses, as long as economic analysis referred to direct medical cost only, without taking into account the indirect or intangible costs and without discriminating between the costs referring to upper or lower limb soft tissue infections. Knowledge of these costs is important to the development of protocols that may reduce expenses.

3.3. Domestic animal bites to the hand (treatment costs depending on severity)

As the popularity of household pets continues to grow, the incidence of domestic animal bites has increased to epidemic proportions, posing major public health concerns to the United States [33]. It has been estimated that 2 million Americans are bitten by a domestic animal each year and that 50% of the Americans will be bitten in their lifetimes [34]. Animal bites currently constitute 1% of all emergency room visits in the US [35]. The estimated overall infection rate for dog bites, between 2% and 20%, is one of the lowest among mammals [36]. Bites to the hand and upper extremity comprise 18% to 68% of all dog bites and are associated with an increased risk for tenosynovitis, septic arthritis, and abscess formation [35]. Cat bites represent the second most common domestic mammalian bite in the United States and account for 5% to 15% of all domestic animal bites. The estimated annual incidence of domestic cat bites in the United States is 400,000 [37]. Of those with problematic bites who seek medical attention, about two-thirds have bites that affect the upper extremity [38]. The associated infection rate for domestic cat bites ranges from 30% to more than 50%, which is more than double the infection rate for dog bites [35, 36]. This can be explained from the fact that the sharp slender teeth of cats can penetrate joint capsule or bone easily, resulting in septic arthritis or osteomyelitis.

Benson et al [39] retrospectively reviewed the charts of 111 patients who had been treated for a domestic dog bite or cat bite from 1997 to 2003. The average time from injury to medical evaluation by a hand surgeon was 7.8 days. The bite locations for cat-related wounds were as follows: 20 finger wounds, 15 hand, 6 wrist, and 5 forearm wounds. The locations of the dog bites were as follows: 27 finger wounds, 42 hand, 2 wrist and 10 forearm wounds. Eighty-one patients were treated in the emergency room and 65 patients required hospital admission. The number of days of hospital admission for a cat bite ranged from 2 to 8 (average: 4.3 d) and for a dog bite ranged from 2 to 11 (average: 4.3 d). Bite injuries ranged from relatively minor wounds to major injuries that included open fractures, persistent deep infection including osteomyelitis, nerve laceration, tendon laceration or tissue loss. Approximately two thirds of the patients required hospital admission at least for intravenous antibiotics. Approximately one third of animal bite victims required at least one surgical procedure. Thirteen patients required long-term intravenous antibiotics and/or multiple surgeries.

The patients were grouped into 5 severity-of-injury categories based on the level of care necessary to treat their injuries (Table 1). It is particularly noteworthy that just 13 patients (categories 4 and 5 combined) accounted for 56% of the total cost of care for all 111 patients. Early treatment with antibiotics and wound care may help avoid the enormous expense associated with bone and joint infection, underlying the importance of delay in presentation. The total cost of care in this particular study [39] was estimated to be more than $1,8 million. Using this cost data to estimate both expenses and severity distribution, it can be projected conservatively that the cost of care for dog and cat bites just to the upper extremity in the United States is more than $850 million per year, reflecting the direct cost of medical care, without taking into account the economic and personal losses associated with time off work or permanent impairment of the hand function.

3.4. Septic arthritis and infected total shoulder and elbow arthroplasties

Bacterial septic arthritis is a serious health problem, as-

TABLE 1

Dog and cat bites to the hand: treatment and cost assessment. J Hand Surg [Am] 31(3):468-73.

Category	Clinical Scenario	Number of Patients	Estimated Cost of Care
1	ER visit with one IV antibiotic dose, 3 office visits, oral antibiotics	47	$1,880
2	ER visit, admitted to hospital for IV antibiotics for 72 hours, sent home on oral antibiotics, 4 subsequent office visits	30	$11,174
3	ER visit, admitted for soft-tissue debridement, 72 hours IV antibiotics, discharged on oral antibiotics, 4 office visits, 6 hand therapyvisits	21	$17,906
4	ER visit, admitted for bony debridement, PICC line placed for osteomyelitis, IV antibiotics for 6 weeks, 6 office visits, 10 hand therapy visits	7	$77,730
5	ER visit, admitted for bony debridement and nerve/tendon repair, PICC line, IV antibiotics for 6 weeks, 8 office visits, 16 hand therapy visits	6	$81,926

ER, emergency room
Source: Benson LS, Edwards SL, Schiff AP, Williams CS, Visotsky JL (2006)

sociated with considerable morbidity [40], usually involving the large joints of the lower extremity [41]. Septic arthritis of a large joint of the upper extremity is an uncommon clinical entity, with series of septic arthritis of the shoulder including only small numbers of patients treated over periods of several years. Specifically, the shoulder was involved in 4% to 12% of the patients with septic arthritis in these series, the elbow in 6% to 8% of the patients, and the wrist in 2% to 6% of the patients [41, 42]. Oxacillin-resistant Staphylococcus aureus (ORSA) is gradually emerging as a pathogen and community-acquired ORSA septic arthritis has been reported [43]. It should be remembered that septic arthritis may also result in death [44] and thus, extra care is necessary for the diagnosis of septic arthritis in a large joint of the upper extremity, irrespective of the patient's age and medical status.

Infection is a devastating complication of shoulder replacement surgery. The incidence rates range between 0% and 0.9% for primary arthroplasty and rises up to 15.4% for revision arthroplasty. The currently accepted treatment options have been adapted from experience gained from the treatment of infected hip and knee arthroplasty, and include antibiotic suppression, debridement with prosthesis retention, direct exchange arthroplasty, delayed reimplantation, resection arthroplasty, arthrodesis, and amputation [45, 46]. Infection control has been reported at approximately 90% for hip and knee arthroplasty [47, 48]. Codd et al [49] reported that three out of four patients who underwent delayed re-implantation were free of infection and had better function compared with patients treated with resection arthroplasty. The major disadvantage of this method is the time delay between stages, which is often associated with pain, reduced mobility and shoulder instability. Shoulder arthrodesis may be an option following resection arthroplasty if re-implantation cannot be performed due to insufficient bone stock. However, arthrodesis of the shoulder is rarely indicated or accepted by the patient [50]. Amputation for infected shoulder arthroplasty is extremely rare, but may be required to control life-threatening infection with severe loss of soft tissue and bone stock, or may result from vascular injury [50].

Despite multiple improvements in total elbow arthroplasty, infection has remained relatively common with reported rates of around 5% [51], remaining well above that of the arthroplasties of lower extremitiy, in part because of the high prevalence of severe rheumatoid arthritis or posttraumatic arthritis [52, 53]. In addition to being immunocompromised, patients with rheumatoid arthritis often exert a great deal of direct pressure on this subcutaneous joint. Following reported success of staged exchange arthroplasty for lower extremity indications, Yamaguchi and co-authors [54] report an 80% success rate for staged revision performed at Mayo Clinic, with the only failure occurring in patients infected with Staphylococcus epidermidis. Success rates of immediate exchange arthroplasty for infected total shoulder arthroplasty vary from 30% to 100% for eradication of sepsis [46, 55, 56], with improved results in cases with gram-positive non-glycocalyx-producing organisms. Resection arthroplasty has been the standard treatment for infected elbow arthroplasty and constitutes the largest treatment experience. Functional results are usually limited, but can be associated with a high satisfaction rate.

The number of primary total joint arthroplasties performed each year is increasing in the United States and in Europe, resulting unfortunately in a proportionate increase in the absolute number of infected total joint arthroplasties [57, 58]. Taking into account that the surgical algorithm for treating infected joint arthroplasties is almost the same for upper and lower extremity, along with the fact that there is lack of published data concerning cost of treatment of infected joint arthroplasties of upper extremity, we can obtain crucial information from cost evaluation studies referring to infected total knee and hip arthroplasties.

Whitehouse et al [59] studied surgical site infections after orthopaedic surgery and reported dramatically greater financial costs for the infected patients. They had twice as many hospitalizations and operative procedures as those of matched uninfected control patients, fourteen days longer hospital stay and four times higher median hospital costs. Infected patients also reported greater physical limitation and greater reduction in health-related quality of life. For an infected knee arthroplasty there was an average of 3.4 more operations and 2.4 more hospitalizations, with 3.7 times longer stay than that required for the primary arthroplasties and 2.7 longer stay than that necessary for an aseptic revision. The total operative time required for a two-stage revision of an infected knee is 3.4 times more than that required for a primary total knee replacement and 1.8 times more than that for an aseptic revision; infected patients received more units of blood [60, 61]. Bozic et al. [62] found that the total direct medical costs associated with revision of an infected total hip arthroplasty are 2.8 times higher than those associated with revision of aseptic total hip arthroplasty and 4.8 times higher than the direct medical costs associated with primary total hip arthroplasty and especially in terms of number and length hospitalizations, number of operations, outpatient visits, outpatient charges and complications.

Several other studies have further reiterated that the human labour and the system resources required for the treatment of an infected arthroplasty is three to four times more compared to that of a primary total joint replacement, and two to three times more than work and resources needed for an aseptic revision [60, 61, 63]. Revision procedures [60] require significantly more from the surgeon in terms of total work of treating and especially the time spent, mental effort, judgment, technical skill, physical effort, stress, preoperative planning and exposure to liability. On the other hand, this is not reflected in the differential in of reimbursements received by the surgeons. In addition, decreasing the length of stay and operative time requires more effort and probably a certain amount of increased risk on the part of the surgeon.

Although single-stage exchange revision has been proposed as a means to decrease costs and rehabilitation time and possibly to reduce the mechanical complications, this method is less likely to be more cost-effective than the two-stage exchange because of the higher risk of re-infection it carries [64]. Emotional burden should never be underestimated, because even in patients whose treatment is successful, 6-18 months are necessary in order that they regain function analogous to the pre-infection one [65]. Some patients may never return to pre-infection levels of function.

In the case of life threatening systemic sepsis and when local tissue conditions or the host's general health status becomes severely impaired, amputation is inevitable. Besides, the periprosthetic infections may rarely become lethal with an overall mortality rate ranging from 1 to 2.7% for patients around 65 years of age, but in patients older than 85 years it rises from 2 to 7%. In the first three months after resection arthroplasty, the probability of death increases twofold in cases of infected hip arthroplasties [66]. The lost opportunity for patients suffering from other health disorders due to bad resource utilization in the management of musculoskeletal infections is another important parameter, as treatment of infection necessitates disproportionate resource utilization.

4. Growing Burden on Hospitals and Health-care Systems

The direct association between hospital and surgical procedure volume and better clinical outcomes in terms of reducing re-admissions, re-operations, complications, and mortality rates referring to infected joint arthroplasties has been documented in several studies [67, 68]. The economic burden that results from disproportionate resource consumption and the lack of incremental reimbursement, further contributes to the financial problems of many tertiary-care referral centers [67]. The strong financial disincentives, resulting from current reimbursement patterns, have led certain high-volume joint replacement centers to restrict access to patients with an infected implant, with a detrimental impact on their care and clinical outcomes. Unfortunately, in most health care systems, the incentives are issued in order that "casemix losers" are avoided and "winners" are concentrated upon.

5. Malpractice

Malpractice insurance is most often obligatory and contributes to increasing treatment costs, as financial considerations are a significant motivation for malpractice suits in certain populations, or in areas with high concentrations of attorneys [69]. Malpractice claims may be related to either technical errors or problems with communication. The importance of strong physician-patient interaction and best possible communication with the patient and his relatives is the best protection against unwarranted litigation [70].

6. Is There a Solution to the Problem?

It is obvious that the treatment of infected implants, joint arthroplasties and skin and soft tissue infections of upper limb necessitate a team approach and especially the cooperation of surgeons specialized in musculoskeletal infections and reconstructive orthopaedic surgery, microbiologists, pathologists, radiologists and physiotherapists, in order to accomplish a functional outcome. In the process of cost identification, it is imperative that we should gain deeper insights of the considerable burden on the health care system, the surgeon or the physicians managing bone and joint infections, besides the patient's pain and suffering.

7. The Need for Estimating the Burden

In the last two decades, the number of reports examining the cost of musculoskeletal infections was small, considering the major financial cost, and the devastating human suffering. Very few studies adhered to the principles of sound economic analysis [71]. Most studies were actually retrospective cost-identification or cost-minimization analyses. As far as septic joint arthroplasties are concerned, none of the published studies calculates total costs and especially direct medical costs and non- medical or indirect costs to the patient and to society. There have been no papers in the literature evaluating cost, even direct, of septic total joints of upper extremity, except for direct medical costs in certain cases of soft tissue infections [27, 32, 39]. An important limitation of the study presented by Widjaia et al [27] was the use of existing financial systems to provide a best estimate of the costs of acute inpatient care, without identifying the costs of prior hospitalization or patient transfer by ambulance (direct non-medical costs) often including a medical escort, the building opportunity cost, postdischarge rehabilitation (some patients were transferred to other institutions for reconstructive surgery) [72, 73], or the intangible costs, or the indirect cost [72, 73] to the community in terms of lost productivity and reduction in the workforce (morbidity and mortality costs).

The opportunity cost of specialized training for each physician specialized in infectious diseases, although hard to quantify, must be identified and calculated as well. Also, limiting the analysis to data from a single institution and heterogeneous groups of patients and infections potentially limits the generalizability of the results.

Cost-of-illness (COI) studies provide a most comprehensive methodology to assess the scale and nature of musculoskeletal infections as a health problem, and raise the profile of the patient group suffering from them through identification of the three basic components of the burden: first, the direct medical and non-medical costs; second, the costs due to loss of productivity (morbidity and mortality costs); and third, psychosocial or intangible costs [72, 73], which represent deterioration in the quality of the patient's life, as well as the lives of their family members and friends. The suffering from disability, pain, reduced self-esteem, and feelings of non-well-being, is a factor extremely difficult to quantify.

8. REDUCING THE BURDEN AND FUTURE DIRECTIONS

The lowest reported rate of infection for total shoulder replacement is 0.4-0.9% [46] and for the total elbow is up to 5% [51]. Dedicated joint replacement surgical teams help in decreasing the infection rates, which have been higher in community-based hospitals [67]. The question is then whether it is only difficult or impossible to reduce infection rates. Following the process of clean room technology in the operative theatre environment, industry, technology and especially biomedical engineering, companies should proceed mainly to manufacturing of implants which are less vulnerable to bacterial attachment and apply procedures for more efficient prevention.

Control quality of practices and establishment of centers specialized in infectious diseases should be promoted by each health care system. All surgeons must be concerned with quality improvement as an integral part of patient care. As surgeons, we should never hesitate to diagnose an infectious complication in a surgical procedure, proceeding with the appropriate diagnostic approach and prompt management. From the patient's aspect, delays have particular implications to the cost of care. Early intervention is the best way to reduce the likelihood of infection spreading to deeper structures.

Focusing on the three specific health care strategies including prevention, diagnosis and effective treatment of infection, the wise use of antimicrobials and the prevention of transmission could make "the lowest rates" more easily established by all hospitals leading consequently to cost savings and less suffering. The establishment of dedicated teams to treat infections can allocate the resources to make the treatment not only clinically optimal, but also optimally efficient from a cost-of-care point of view.

Physicians should raise the awareness of the society members and health care policy makers to adopt a global viewpoint of the musculoskeletal infections to view not only the medical but also the socioeconomic consequences. Identifying the burden through further studying of orthopaedic infections and estimation of their epidemiologic indices is of crucial importance for evidence-based decision making towards prevention and effective management of the upper limb infections.

REFERENCES

[1] Liaropoulos L. Hellenic Representative. Organization of Economic Cooperation and Development (OECD). 2004. Ref Type: Personal Communication.

[2] Drummond MF, Richardson WS, O'Brien BJ, Levine M, Heyland D. Users' guides to the medical literature. XIII. How to use an article on economic analysis of clinical practice. A. Are the results of the study valid? Evidence-Based Medicine Working Group. JAMA 1997;277(19):1552-7.

[3] Roth AI, Fry DE, Polk HC, Jr. Infectious morbidity in extremity fractures. J Trauma 1986;26(8):757-61.

[4] Schnall SB, Holtom PD, Lilley JC. Abscesses secondary to parenteral abuse of drugs. A study of demographic and bacteriological characteristics. J Bone Joint Surg Am 1994;76(10):1526-30.

[5] Glass KD. Factors related to the resolution of treated hand infections. J Hand Surg [Am] 1982; 7(4):388-94.

[6] Patzakis MJ, Wilkins J. Factors influencing infection rate in open fracture wounds. Clin Orthop Relat Res 1989;(243):36-40.

[7] Crawford SE, Daum RS. Epidemic community-associated methicillin-resistant Staphylococcus aureus: modern times for an ancient pathogen. Pediatr Infect Dis J 2005;24(5):459-60.

[8] Spiegel JD, Szabo RM. A protocol for the treatment of severe infections of the hand. J Hand Surg [Am] 1988;13(2):254-9.

[9] Reybrouck G. Role of the hands in the spread of nosocomial infections. 1. J Hosp Infect 1983;4(2):103-10.

[10] Simmons B, Bryant J, Neiman K, Spencer L, Arheart K. The role of handwashing in prevention of endemic intensive care unit infections. Infect Control Hosp Epidemiol 1990;11(11):589-94.

[11] Bottone EJ, Cheng M, Hymes S. Ineffectiveness of handwashing with lotion soap to remove nosocomial bacterial pathogens persisting on fingertips: a major link in their intrahospital spread. Infect Control Hosp Epidemiol 2004;25(3):262-4.

[12] Chambers HF. The changing epidemiology of Staphylococcus aureus? Emerg Infect Dis 2001;7(2):178-82.

[13] McHenry CR, Piotrowski JJ, Petrinic D, Malangoni MA. Determinants of mortality for necrotizing soft-tissue infections. Ann Surg 1995;221(5):558-63.

[14] Voros D, Pissiotis C, Georgantas D, Katsaragakis S, Antoniou S, Papadimitriou J. Role of early and extensive surgery in the treatment of severe necrotizing soft tissue infection. Br J Surg 1993; 80(9):1190-1.

[15] Stone HH, Martin JD, Jr. Synergistic necrotizing cellulitis. Ann Surg 1972;175(5):702-11.

[16] Anaya DA, McMahon K, Nathens AB, Sullivan SR, Foy H, Bulger E. Predictors of mortality and limb loss in necrotizing soft tissue infections. Arch Surg 2005;140(2):151-7.

[17] Chen JL, Fullerton KE, Flynn NM. Necrotizing fasciitis associated with injection drug use. Clin Infect Dis 2001;33(1):6-15.

[18] Gonzalez MH, Kay T, Weinzweig N, Brown A, Pulvirenti J. Necrotizing fasciitis of the upper extremity. J Hand Surg [Am] 1996;21 (4):689-92.

[19] Sudarsky LA, Laschinger JC, Coppa GF, Spencer FC. Improved results from a standardized approach in treating patients with necrotizing fasciitis. Ann Surg 1987;206(5):661-5.

[20] Schecter W, Meyer A, Schecter G, Giuliano A, Newmeyer W, Kilgore E. Necrotizing fasciitis of the upper extremity. J Hand Surg [Am] 1982;7(1):15-20.

[21] Tang WM, Ho PL, Fung KK, Yuen KY, Leong JC. Necrotising fasciitis of a limb. J Bone Joint Surg Br 2001;83(5):709-14.

[22] Wang KC, Shih CH. Necrotizing fasciitis of the extremities. J Trauma 1992;32(2):179-82.

[23] Wong CH, Chang HC, Pasupathy S, Khin LW, Tan JL, Low CO. Necrotizing fasciitis: clinical presentation, microbiology, and determinants of mortality. J Bone Joint Surg [Am] 2003;85-A(8):1454-60.

[24] Wong CH, Wang YS. The diagnosis of necrotizing fasciitis. Curr Opin Infect Dis 2005;18(2):101-6.

[25] Ogilvie CM, Miclau T. Necrotizing soft tissue infections of the extremities and back. Clin Orthop Relat Res 2006;447:179-86.

[26] Callahan TE, Schecter WP, Horn JK. Necrotizing soft tissue infection masquerading as cutaneous abcess following illicit drug injection. Arch Surg 1998;133(8):812-7.

[27] Widjaja AB, Tran A, Cleland H, Leung M, Millar I. The hospital costs of treating necrotizing fasciitis. ANZ J Surg 2005;75(12):1059-64.

[28] Benade MM, Warlow CP. Costs and benefits of carotid endarterectomy and associated preoperative arterial imaging: a systematic review of health economic literature. Stroke 2002;33(2):629-38.

[29] Weintraub WS, Craver JM, Jones EL, Gott JP, Deaton C, Culler SD, Guyton RA. Improving cost and outcome of coronary surgery. Circulation 1998;98(19 Suppl):II23-II28.

[30] Whiting JF, Woodward RS, Zavala EY, Cohen DS, Martin JE, Singer GG, Lowell JA, First MR, Brennan DC, Schnitzler MA. Economic cost of expanded criteria donors in cadaveric renal transplantation: analysis of Medicare payments. Transplantation 2000;70(5):755-60.

[31] Porter PJ, Shin AY, Detsky AS, Lefaive L, Wallace MC. Surgery versus stereotactic radiosurgery for small, operable cerebral arteriovenous malformations: a clinical and cost comparison. Neurosurgery 1997;41(4):757-64.

[32] Charalambous CP, Zipitis CS, Kumar R, Lipsett PA, Hirst P, Paul A. Soft tissue infections of the extremities in an orthopaedic centre in the UK. J Infect 2003;46(2):106-10.

[33] Sacks JJ, Kresnow M, Houston B. Dog bites: how big a problem? Inj Prev 1996;2(1):52-4.

[34] Goldstein EJ. Management of human and animal bite wounds. J Am Acad Dermatol 1989;21(6):1275-9.

[35] Goldstein EJ. Bite wounds and infection. Clin Infect Dis 1992;14 (3):633-8.

[36] Griego RD, Rosen T, Orengo IF, Wolf JE. Dog, cat, and human bites: a review. J Am Acad Dermatol 1995;33(6):1019-29.

[37] Elenbaas RM, McNabney WK, Robinson WA. Evaluation of prophylactic oxacillin in cat bite wounds. Ann Emerg Med 1984;13 (3):155-7.

[38] Dire DJ. Emergency management of dog and cat bite wounds. Emerg Med Clin North Am 1992;10(4):719-36.

[39] Benson LS, Edwards SL, Schiff AP, Williams CS, Visotsky JL. Dog and cat bites to the hand: treatment and cost assessment. J Hand Surg [Am] 2006;31(3):468-73.

[40] Kaandorp CJ, Krijnen P, Moens HJ, Habbema JD, van SD. The outcome of bacterial arthritis: a prospective community-based study. Arthritis Rheum 1997;40(5):884-92.

[41] Kelly PJ, Martin WJ, Coventry MB. Bacterial (suppurative) arthritis in the adult. J Bone Joint Surg Am 1970;52(8):1595-602.

[42] Kaandorp CJ, Dinant HJ, van de Laar MA, Moens HJ, Prins AP, Dijkmans BA Incidence and sources of native and prosthetic joint infection: a community based prospective survey. Ann Rheum Dis 1997;56(8):470-5.

[43] Fridkin SK, Hageman JC, Morrison M, Sanza LT, Como-Sabetti K, Jernigan JA, Harriman K, Harrison LH, Lynfield R, Farley MM. Methicillin-resistant Staphylococcus aureus disease in three communities. N Engl J Med 2005;352(14):1436-44.

[44] Leslie BM, Harris JM, III, Driscoll D. Septic arthritis of the shoulder in adults. J Bone Joint Surg Am 1989;71(10):1516-22.

[45] Ramsey ML, Fenlin JM, Jr. Use of an antibiotic-impregnated bone cement block in the revision of an infected shoulder arthroplasty. J Shoulder Elbow Surg 1996;5(6):479-82.

[46] Sperling JW, Kozak TK, Hanssen AD, Cofield RH. Infection after shoulder arthroplasty. Clin Orthop Relat Res 2001;(382):206-16.

[47] Garvin KL, Hanssen AD. Infection after total hip arthroplasty. Past, present, and future. J Bone Joint Surg Am 1995; 77 (10): 1576-88.

[48] Hanssen AD, Rand JA, Osmon DR. Treatment of the infected total knee arthroplasty with insertion of another prosthesis. The effect of antibiotic-impregnated bone cement. Clin Orthop Relat Res 1994; (309):44-55.

[49] Codd TP, Yamaguchi K, Flatow EL. Infected shoulder arthroplasties: treatment with staged reimplantation versus resection arthroplasty. Orthop Trans 1996;20:59.

[50] Cofield RH, Edgerton BC. Total shoulder arthroplasty: complications and revision surgery. Instr Course Lect 1990; 39: 449-62.

[51] Little CP, Graham AJ, Carr AJ. Total elbow arthroplasty: a systematic review of the literature in the English language until the end of 2003. J Bone Joint Surg [Br] 2005;87(4):437-44.

[52] Poss R, Thornhill TS, Ewald FC, Thomas WH, Batte NJ, Sledge CB. Factors influencing the incidence and outcome of infection following total joint arthroplasty. Clin Orthop Relat Res 1984;(182):117-26.

[53] Wolfe SW, Figgie MP, Inglis AE, Bohn WW, Ranawat CS. Management of infection about total elbow prostheses. J Bone Joint Surg [Am] 1990;72(2):198-212.

[54] Yamaguchi K, Adams RA, Morrey BF. Infection after total elbow arthroplasty. J Bone Joint Surg [Am] 1998;80(4):481-91.

[55] Coste JS, Reig S, Trojani C, Berg M, Walch G, Boileau P. The management of infection in arthroplasty of the shoulder. J Bone Joint Surg [Br] 2004;86(1):65-9.

[56] Ince A, Seemann K, Frommelt L, Katzer A, Loehr JF. One-stage exchange shoulder arthroplasty for peri-prosthetic infection. J Bone Joint Surg [Br] 2005;87(6):814-8.

[57] Hsiao WC, Braun P, Dunn D, Becker ER. Resource-based relative values. An overview. 1988;JAMA 260(16):2347-53.

[58] Mendenhall S. 2002 Hip and knee implant review. Orthop Network News 2002;13(3):1-16.

[59] Whitehouse JD, Friedman ND, Kirkland KB, Richardson WJ, Sexton DJ. The impact of surgical-site infections following orthopedic surgery at a community hospital and a university hospital: adverse quality of life, excess length of stay, and extra cost. Infect Control Hosp Epidemiol 2002;23(4):183-9.

[60] Barrack RL, Hoffman GJ, Tejeiro WV, Carpenter LJ, Jr. Surgeon work input and risk in primary versus revision total joint arthroplasty. J Arthroplasty 1995;10(3):281-6.

[61] Barrack RL. Economics of revision total hip arthroplasty. Clin Orthop Relat Res 1995;(319):209-14.

[62] Bozic KJ, Ries MD. The impact of infection after total hip arthroplasty on hospital and surgeon resource utilization. J Bone Joint Surg [Am] 2005;87(8):1746-51.

[63] Barrack RL, Engh G, Rorabeck C, Sawhney J, Woolfrey M. Patient satisfaction and outcome after septic versus aseptic revision total knee arthroplasty. J Arthroplasty 2000;15(8):990-3.

[64] Jackson WO, Schmalzried TP. Limited role of direct exchange arthroplasty in the treatment of infected total hip replacements. Clin Orthop Relat Res 2000;(381):101-5.

[65] Economic analysis of health care technology. A report on principles. Task Force on Principles for Economic Analysis of Health Care Technology. Ann Intern Med 1995;123(1):61-70.

[66] Fisman DN, Reilly DT, Karchmer AW, Goldie SJ. Clinical effectiveness and cost-effectiveness of 2 management strategies for infected total hip arthroplasty in the elderly. Clin Infect Dis 2004;32(3):419-30.

[67] Katz JN, Barrett J, Mahomed NN, Baron JA, Wright RJ, Losina E. Association between hospital and surgeon procedure volume and the outcomes of total knee replacement. J Bone Joint Surg [Am] 2004;86-A(9):1909-16.

[68] Sharkey PF, Shastri S, Teloken MA, Parvizi J, Hozack WJ, Rothman RH. Relationship between surgical volume and early outcomes of total hip arthroplasty: do results continue to get better? J Arthroplasty 2004;19(6):694-9.

[69] Ries MD, Bertino JS, Jr., Nafziger AN. Distribution of orthopaedic surgeons, lawyers, and malpractice claims in New York. Clin Orthop Relat Res 1997;(337):256-60.

[70] Weycker DA, Jensen GA. Medical malpractice among physicians: who will be sued and who will pay? Health Care Manag Sci 2000;3(4):269-77.

[71] Saleh KJ, Gafni A, Macaulay WB, Miric A, Saleh L, Schatzker J. Understanding economic evaluations: a review of the knee arthroplasty literature. Am J Knee Surg 1999;12(3):155-60.

[72] How to read clinical journals: VII. To understand an economic evaluation (part B). Can Med Assoc J 1984;130(12):1542-9.

[73] How to read clinical journals: VII. To understand an economic evaluation (part A). Can Med Assoc J 1984;130(11):1428-34.

Bacterial Ecosystem
of the Upper Extremity

Efthimia PETINAKI[a], Konstantinos N. MALIZOS[b*]

[a]*Department of Microbiology, University of Thessalia, Larissa, Greece*
[b]*Department of Orthopaedic Surgery and Musculoskeletal Trauma*
University of Thessalia, Larissa, Greece

The role of the microbial flora of the body is important and well documented. The microorganisms that are part of the normal flora are involved in photosynthesis, production of vitamins and protection of the body from invasion of pathogenic bacteria. The destruction of bacterial flora has been associated with certain infections. For example, the absence of lactobacilli in the genitia results in the overgrowth of fungi. On the other hand, the presence of bacterial flora of the body does not remain stable, often changing due to various factors, such as climate, work environment, etc. We describe the normal flora of the upper extremity and its different compositions, which vary according to environmental factors. A comprehensive knowledge of the normal flora and, in particular, the flora of the upper extremity, significantly aids the clinician in selecting the appropriate management.

Keywords: microbial flora; upper extremity.

1. INTRODUCTION

In our daily lives we are surrounded by a wealth of microorganisms, the majority of which are inoffensive. Human existence would be impossible without these micro-organisms, since they play critical roles in processes so diverse as photosynthesis, nitrogen fixation, production of vitamins in the human intestine and decomposition of organic matter. Microorganisms are also the major driving force behind the evolution of life; they are the sole, true "recyclers" of our planet. They are involved in photosynthesis and respiration, and they mediate genome rearrangement in infected host cells.

*Corresponding Author
Department of Orthopaedic Surgery and
Musculoskeletal Trauma,
University of Thessalia
Larissa, Greece
Tel: +30 2410 682722
Fax: +30 2410 670107
e-mail: malizos@med.uth.gr

The indigenous flora or "normal flora" is found in any part of the body exposed to the outside environment, e.g. the mouth, nose and the oropharynx, the superficial part of the urethra and vagina and other moist areas of the skin [1, 2]. Although the human microbial population is especially dense in the large intestine, the skin is much less densely populated by the indigenous flora. Although the skin is impermeable by bacteria, a number of micro-organisms can penetrate it. Moreover, skin disruptions due to lacerations, insect bites or severe open deep tissue trauma may allow entry of pathogenic microbes into the body.

In addition to the three principal types of skin flora that have been described, i.e. the **resident,** the **transient** and the **temporary resident skin flora,** there is a fourth one, the **infectious flora,** which includes species, such as *Staphylococcus aureus* or beta-haemolytic streptococci that are frequently isolated from abscesses, whitlows, paronychia etc.

The **resident flora** consists of permanent inhabitans of the skin. They are found mainly on the surface of the skin and under the superficial cells of the stratum corneum. These bacteria are not regarded as pathogens on intact skin, but may cause infections in sterile body cavities, in the eyes, or on non-intact skin. Resident skin bacteria survive longer on intact skin than do gram-negative transient species. The protective function of the resident flora, the so-called "colonization resistance", has been demonstrated in various *in vitro* and *in vivo* studies. Its purpose is twofold: (i) microbial antagonism and (ii) the competition for nutrients in the ecosystem. Nevertheless, the interactions between bacteria and fungi on the skin are still inadequately understood. Many such interactions have been demonstrated experimentally. Skin flora provides a major mechanism for preventing the adherence of pathogens, but their contribution to the stability of the dermal ecosystem, remains unclear. The dominant species is *Staphylococcus epidermidis,* which is found on almost every hand. Nowadays, the incidence of oxacillin resistance among isolates of *S. epidermidis* is up to 64.3% and is higher for health care workers who have direct contact with patients than those who do not. Other regular residents are *Staphylococcus hominis* and other coagulase-negative staphylococci, followed by coryneform bacteria, such as propionibacteria, corynebacteria, dermabacteria, and micrococci. Among fungi, the most important genus of the resident skin flora is *Pityrosporum.* Viruses do not usually reside on the skin, but can proliferate within the living epidermis, where they may induce pathologic changes.

The transient skin flora consists of bacteria, fungi and viruses that may be found sometimes. They do not usually multiply on the skin, but they survive and occasionally multiply and cause disease. They may come from patients or inanimate surfaces. Between 4 and 16% of the hand surface is exposed by a single direct contact, and after 12 direct contacts, up to 40% of the hand surface may have been touched. The transmissibility of transient bacteria depends on the species, the number of bacteria on the hand, their survival on the skin, and the dermal water content.

In addition, there is the **temporary resident skin flora,** which persists and multiplies for a limited period on the skin. The definition is more or less identical to that of the transient skin flora because the duration of residence on human skin is unspecified and never permanent. In addition, the temporary resident skin flora often includes nosocomial bacteria and fungi.

2. COMPOSITION OF MICROBIAL FLORA OF THE HAND AND FACTORS INFLUENCING THE FREQUENCY OF SPECIES ISOLATION

Numerous studies have been reported on the composition of the bacterial flora of the hand [3, 4]. Most have resolved cutaneous bacterial populations into major groups or genera, e.g. *S. aureus,* coagulase-negative staphylococci, streptococci, nonlipophilic and lipophilic diphtheroids, propionibacteria, gram-negative bacilli, *Bacillus, Neisseria, Streptomyces,* and mycobacteria. Some have been more specific and have attempted to resolve species or even strains. As taxonomic and other systematic studies of microorganisms have progressed rapidly over the past few years, cutaneous bacteria have undergone changes in classification and new species have been recognized. A comprehensive study on the taxonomy of bacteria isolated from the hand has shown the diversity of these organisms. Indications are, however, that healthy individuals maintain a stable microbial flora which consists of predominantly gram-positive bacteria, even though there have been reports that in certain disease states there is an increase in the frequency of isolation of gram-negative bacteria. Many of the factors controlling the microbial flora of the hand are obscure owing to the complexity of the physiology of the skin, which is complicated by interaction with the environment with its variations in temperature and humidity. The relationship of the cutaneous microflora with the physiology of the skin on the one hand and with the environment on the other hand, has caused speculation as to the extent the environment can control the microbial flora of the skin. The effect of temperature and humidity on the microbial flora of the skin has been studied experimentally [5]; however, the influence of the environment on the microbial flora has not proven yet.

Factors that could influence the microbial composition of the hand flora are antibacterial soaps and deodorants; the majority of medical centers use those products and such use may be probably responsible for the existence of the lower bacterial populations that have been observed [6]. The increased use of antibacterial soaps and cosmetics cause concern that these compounds may upset the balance between gram-negative and gram-positive populations. Abnormal usage of antibacterials on the hand seems to result in a decline in the gram-positive population and an increase in colonization of the gram-negative [7]. Preliminary studies performed at the University Hospital of Larissa, showed that the medical personnel did not have a higher frequency of isolation of gram-negatives than healthy individuals, although in the axilla the relative proportions of gram-negative to gram-positive populations was higher. The medical personnel, however, had a higher frequency of gram-negative bacteria from the back, feet and axilla, and thus, the role of antibacterials is debatable [8]. According to our results, the axilla was the only site where gram-negative bacteria were isolated, and it is of interest that these organisms were isolated with equal frequency from individuals who did not use deodorant as compared to those who did. The main difference between deodorant users and non-users was a lower incidence of aerobic diphtheroids in the former group. Little is known of the incidence of fungi on the hand, but the incidence found in our study concerning the skin of the medical personnel would seem higher than the normal.

Even the healthy individuals, whose main activities involved exposure to soil (probably a source of these fungi), were found to have lower frequency of isolation than the medical personnel.

In conclusion, changes in the environment can cause fluctuation in the bacterial population of the hand, but the gram-positive character of the flora both in types and numbers of organisms is remarkably stable. Samples taken from the axillae usually contain fewer varieties of bacteria than those taken from the hand. Because of its position, the axillae is more naturally protected from environmental contamination and this may be a factor that helps to limit the number of the existing varieties.

3. DISTRIBUTION OF SPECIES OF MICROBIAL FLORA OF THE HAND AND THEIR EPIDEMIOLOGIC ROLE

The most predominant and persistent aerobic bacteria isolated from the hand belong to species such as *Staphylococcus, Micrococcus,* and *Bacillus,* followed by *Klebsiella, Enterobacter, E. coli,* and *Streptomyces.* Bacteria that are only occasionally isolated include *Neisseria, Flavobacterium, Mycobacterium, Nocardia, E. coli, Pseuromonas, Serratia, Moraxella* and some unclassified strains.

3.1. Gram-positive cocci

Staphylococci constitute a major component of the normal microflora of the hand; they usually constitute more than 50% of the bacteria isolated from the hand and the axilla and from 10 to 70% from the extremities. *S. epidermidis* followed by *S. aureus* and *S. hominis* are the most common gram-positive species that are isolated from the hands [9].

S. epidermidis usually comprises more than 75% of the staphylococci isolated from the hand and the axilla; this species together with *S. hominis* are the predominant species found in the axilla. Over the last two decades, there was an increase in the documentation of infections due to this microorganism. The infection rate was correlated with the increase in the use of prosthetic and indwelling devices and the growing number of orthopaedic patients using devices. It is well known that *S. epidermidis* is a major cause of implant infections. The first step in the establishment of this type of infection involves the adhesion of bacteria to biomaterials; this step is followed by the production of biofilm (slime) [10]. Clinical isolates that display a polysaccharide-adhesion are generally more adherent to catheters *in vitro,* and produce biofilm. Catheter-associated primary bloodstream infections are frequently caused by the species mentioned above [11]. In internsive care units, approximately one-third of all blood culture isolates from patients with nosocomial bloodstream infections are found to be coagulase-negative staphylococci.

Studies performed at the University Hospital of Larissa demonstrated genetic similarity between bacteria isolated from blood cultures of patients and those isolated from hand cultures of nurses; this finding indicates the potential role of microbial flora in a future infection. Furthermore, preliminary studies in our clinical setting demonstrated among coagulase-negative staphylococci isolated from hand cultures, a high prevalence of ica-operon genes involved in the biofilm biosynthesis [12, 13]. In turn, under specific conditions, these microorganisms, might be responsible for biofilm-related upper extremity infections.

S. aureus is a predominant species that is more frequently isolated from the nares of children than those of adults. This species is only occasionally isolated from the hands of healthy individuals. It is more frequently isolated from the hands of children. Isolation from the axilla is rare. However, colonization of on *S. aureus* heath care workers' hands has been described to range between 10.5% and 78.3%. Up to 24 million cells can be found per hand. The colonization rate of *S. aureus* was higher among doctors (36%) than among nurses (18%). The carrier rate may be up to 28% if the health care workers contact patients with an atopic dermatidis colonized by *S. aureus.* Methicillin-resistant *S. aureus* (MRSA) has been isolated in up to 16.9% of health care workers. These isolates are the most common gram-positive bacteria that cause nosocomial infections (NIs). The most common type of NIs is the surgical-site infection.

Nowadays, the emergence of *S. aureus* producing a variety of pathogenic-virulence factors poses a major problem worldwide. Among the virulence factors are the staphylococcal enterotoxins, the causative agents of food poisoning, the toxic shock syndrome toxin-1, which causes the staphylococcal toxin shock syndrome and the Panton-Valentin leukocidin genes, which are coded by the *PVL*-gene. The precise role of individual staphylococcal factors in invasive infections is difficult to assess, but the PVL production has been preferentially linked to furuncles, cutaneous abscesses and severe necrotic skin infections. In our country, 27% of *S. aureus* carries the *PVL-genes:* 45% of *MRSA* and 12% of *methicillin-sensitive S. aureus* [14]. The majority of *PVL*-positive MRSA isolates belong to a single clone, named clone C or MLST-80, that is also disseminated in Europe [15]. This clone has been found in our region to colonize the hands and the nares of healthy individuals, characterized by a great capacity to spread among persons in close contacts and cause disease, as has been observed mainly in otherwise healthy children or young adults. Recently, an outbreak of impetigo caused by this clone occurred in the Neonatal Unit of our hospital; hand cultures of two nurses revealed the presence of the same clone. To prevent infections by those strains, measures, such as repeated application of nasal mupirocin and simultaneous use of alcohol-based hand rubs are necessary.

3.2. Gram-negative bacteria

Gram-negative bacteria such as *Klebsiella* and *Enterobacter* are most commonly isolated from the hand and the axillae of adults (15-20%) and only occasionally from children. On the contrary, the colonization rate on the hand of the health care worker has been described as ranging from 21 to 86%. The number of gram-negative bacteria per hand may be as great as 13 million cells. Colonization of gram-negative bacteria is influenced by various factors. For example, it is higher before patient contact than after the work shift. In hands with artificial fingernails harbor gram-negative bacteria appear more often than in those without. Higher colonization rates of gram-negative bacteria also occur during periods of higher ambient temperature and high air humidity [16, 17]. Different species of gram-negative bacteria exhibit different colonization rates. For instance, the colonization rate of *Acintobacter baumanni* is 3% to 15%, 1.3% to 10% for *Pseudomonas areuginosa* etc. According to our studies, the occurrence of gram-negative bacteria followed a seasonal pattern; they were more frequently isolated during the warmer months of the year.

3.3. Corynebacterium

Corynebacterium usually constitutes 1-4% of the bacteria isolated from the hand. Adults have larger percentages of corynebacterium on their hands than most children [18].

3.4. Spore-forming bacteria

The main spore-forming bacterium isolated especially from the hands of health care workers is *Clostridium difficile*. The percentage of *C. difficile* on the hands correlates with the density of environmental contamination [19]. In one study, the hands of 59% of heath care workers who directly contacted *C. difficile* culture-positive patients were found to be colonized by this microorganism. In another study, cultures obtained from the hands of 14% of health care workers were found to be positive for *C. difficile*.

4. Conclusions

The outer part of the body is populated with microorganisms that reflect the contacts, habits, professions, as well as the environmental conditions in which a person lives [20]. A comprehensive knowledge of the normal flora, and in particular of the upper extremities, aids the clinicians significantly in the appropriate and accurate treatment, since microorganisms that are part of the flora of the upper extremities are frequently responsible for infections in those anatomic sites.

The most common microorganism associated with hands and upper extremity infections are staphylococci, which mirror the flora of these anatomic sites. These microorganisms, which are renowned for their multi-resistance to various antimicrobial agents, often carry virulence factors or genes responsible for biofilm production. Therefore, it is imperative for the orthopaedic clinician not only to be aware of, but also to have broad knowledge of the multi-resistance and genetic background of staphylococci in their geographic region. This will, in turn, assist in dealing with future infections and aid in avoiding unnecessary use of antibiotics.

References

[1] Allaker RP, Noble WC. Microbial interaction on skin. *In* WC Noble (ed), The skin microflora and microbial skin disease. Cambridge University Press, Cambridge, United Kingdom. 1993; p. 331-354.

[2] Mc Ewan P, Jenkins D. The basis of the skin surface ecosystem. *In* WC Noble (ed), The skin microflora and microbial skin disease. Cambridge University Press, Cambridge, United Kingdom 1993; p.1-32.

[3] Kownatzki E. Hand hygiene and skin health. J Hosp Infect 2003; 55:239-245.

[4] Larson EL, Gomez-Duarte C, Lee LV, Della-Latta P, Kain DJ, Keswick BH. Microbial flora of hands of homemakers. AM J Infect Control 2002;31:72-79.

[5] Aly R, Maibach HI. Factors controlling skin bacterial flora. In HI Maibach and R Aly (ed), Skin microbiology, relevance to clinical infection. Springer-Verlag, New York, NY 1981; p. 29-39.

[6] Albert RK, Condle F. Hand-washing patterns in medical intensive-care units. N Engl J Med 1981;304:1465-1466.

[7] Aiello AE, Cimiotti J, Della-Latta P, Larson E L. A comparison of the bacteria found on the hands of ''homemakers'' and neonatal intensive care unit nurses. J Hosp Infect 2003;54:310-315.

[8] Larson EL, Norton Hughes CA, Pyrak JD, Sparks SM, Cagatay EU, Bartkus JM. Changes in bacterial flora associated with skin damage on hands o health care personnel. Am J Infect Control 1998;26:51-521.

[9] Noble WC. Staphylococci in the skin. *In* WC Noble (ed), The skin microflora and microbial skin disease. Cambridge University Press, Cambridge, United Kingdom 1993; p. 135-152.

[10] Costerton JW. Introduction to biofilm. Int J Antimicrob Agents 1999;11 (3-4): 217-221.

[11] Cafiso V, Bertuccio T, Santagati M, Campanile F, Amicosante G, Perilli MG, Selan L, Artini M, Nicoletti G, Stefani S. Presence of the ica operon in clinical isolates of Staphylococcus epidermidis and its role in biofilm production. Clin Microbiol Infect 2004;10(12): 1081-8.

[12] Foka A, Chini V, Petinaki E, Kolonitsiou F, Anastassiou ED, Dimitracopoulos G, Spiliopoulou I. Clonality of slime-producing methicillin-resistant coagulase-negative staphylococci disseminated in the neonatal intensive care unit of a university hospital. Clin Microbiol Infect 2006;12(12):1230-3.

[13] Miyamoto H, Imamura K, Kojima A, Takenaka H, Hara N, Ikenouchi A, Tanabe T, Taniguchi H. Survey of nasal colonization by, and assessment of a novel multiplex PCR method for detection of biofilm-forming methicillin-resistant staphylococci in healthy medical students. J Hosp Infect 2003;53(3):215-23.

[14] Chini V, Petinaki E, Foka A, Paratiras S, Dimitracopoulos G, Spiliopoulou I. Spread of Staphylococcus aureus clinical isolates car-

rying Panton-Valentine leukocidin genes during a 3-year period in Greece. Clin Microbiol Infect 2006 Jan;12(1):29-34.

[15] Gerogianni I, Mpatavanis G, Gourgoulianis K, Maniatis A, Spiliopoulou I, Petinaki E. Combination of staphylococcal chromosome cassette SCCmec type V and Panton-Valentine leukocidin genes in a methicillin-resistant Staphylococcus aureus that caused necrotizing pneumonia in Greece. Diagn Microbiol Infect Dis 2006;56(2):213-6.

[16] Guenthner SH, Hendley JO, Wenzel R P. Gram-negative bacilli as nontransient flora on the hands of hospital personnel. J Clin Microbiol 1987;25: 488-490.

[17] Knittle MA, Eitzman DV, Baer H. Role of hand contamination of personnel in the epidemiology of gram-negative nosocomial infections. J Pediatr 1975;86: 433-437.

[18] Leyden JJ, McGinley K J. Coryneform bacteria, 1993; p. 102-117. The skin microflora and microbial ski disease. Cambridge University Press, Cambridge, United Kingdom.

[19] Mc Farland LV, Mulligan ME, Kwok RYY, Stamm WE. Nosocomial acquisition of *Clostridium difficile* infection. N Engl J Med 1989;320: 204-210.

[20] Brunetti L, Santoro E, De Caro F, Cavallo P, Boccia G, Capunzo M, Motta O. Surveillance of nosocomial infections: a preliminary study on hand hygiene compliance of healthcare workers. J Prev Med Hyg 2006;47(2):64-8.

Anatomy of the Normal Immune Response

Elizabeth O. JOHNSON[a*], Panayotis N. SOUCACOS[b]

[a]*Department of Anatomy-Histology-Embryology,*
University of Ioannina, School of Medicine, Ioannina, Greece
[b]*Department of Orthopaedic Surgery, University of Athens,*
School of Medicine, Athens, Greece

There are 2 levels of protection against infection. Innate or natural immunity is present from birth and is comprised of a variety of non-specific physical barriers, including the skin and mucous membranes, certain enzymes and phagocytic cells. If the defenses provided by the innate immune system fail to prevent infection, the adaptive or acquired immune response is triggered. Adaptive immunity, in contrast to innate immunity, is distinguished by a remarkable specificity for the foreign immunogen and memory. The hallmark of human immunity is the presence of a truly two-component immune system comprised of cellular immunity and humoral immunity (antibodies). The immune response is comprised of a complex cascade of events which is triggered by the introduction of an antigen or immunogen and usually ends with the elimination of the stimulus. The antigen is initially taken up and processed by antigen presenting cells. Antigen presenting cells express fragments of the antigen called immunogenic epitopes complexed with class II MHC (major histocompatibility complex) and present this complex to TH (T-helper) cells. The latter are able to recognize features of both the epitope and the class II molecule. In the end, the immune response generates a population of T lymphocytes and antibodies with specificity for recognizing an antigen in future encounters (memory). When the same antigen is subsequently encountered, several events may take place. These events are referred to as effector mechanisms, and include neutralization, cytotoxicity, cytostimulation and inflammation.

Keywords: lymphocyte; T-cell; B-cell; cell-mediated immunity; humoral immunity; infection; inflammation.

1. INTRODUCTION

The immune system provides a flexible and dynamic mechanism to specifically respond to a wide variety of foreign substances or antigens. The hallmark of human immunity is the presence of a truly two-component immune system comprised of cellular immunity and humoral immunity (antibodies). This bifunctional immune system is also characterized by a dual central lymphoid organ system. Cells are derived from the primary lymphoid organs, particularly the bone marrow and thymus, as well as the secondary lymphoid organs, which include the spleen, lymph nodes and mucosa-associated lymphoid tissue (MALT).

In an effort to protect the organism, the immune system is able to recognize and eliminate a large number of foreign molecules, microbes and aberrant autologous cells. In order to do this effectively, immune recognition must be selective and avoid attacking normal tissue and cell products. One of the primary functions of the immune response is to discriminate between self and non-self in order to be able to eliminate the latter. This is achieved by an elaborate network of cell subsets that interact in distinct microenvironments to re-

*Corresponding Author
Department of Anatomy-Histology-Embryology,
University of Ioannina, School of Medicine,
Ioannina Greece 45110
Fax: +30 26510 97861
e-mail: ejohnson@cc.uoi.gr or
          soukakos@panafonet.gr

gulate the immune response. Antigens are recognized by antigen specific lymphocytes, and this recognition, in turn, must lead to a variety of cellular responses. Specificity is derived from B cells that produce antibodies, and T cells which mediate the immune functions.

Immunogens are molecules that can induce an immune response in a particular host [1]. "Antigens", although often used interchangeably with "immunogens", refer to the ability of a molecule to react with antibodies. The more complex the foreign agent, the more distinct are the immunogens it contains. For example, bacteria are composed of many immunogens, each of which may elicit a unique immune response. Most immunogens are composed largely or exclusively of protein (lipoproteins, glycoproteins, nucleoproteins). The fate of an immunogen that penetrates the physical barriers of the innate immune system depends partially on its route of entry. For the most part, an immunogen may take 3 routes of entry into the human body. If it enters the bloodstream, it is carried to the spleen which in turn, becomes the principal site of the immune response. If the immunogen remains in the skin, a local inflammatory response ensues and it travels through afferent lymphatic channels to regional lymph nodes draining the affected area, which then serve as the major site of the immune response. Thirdly, the immunogen may enter the mucosal immune system that has lymphoid tissue for mounting an immune response. In this case, antibodies are produced and deposited locally.

2. THE CELLS OF THE IMMUNE SYSTEM

The immune system contains several cell types, including lymphocytes, mononuclear phagocytes (monocytes, macrophages) and granulocytes. Each cell type plays a distinct role in mediated immune function. They secrete various factors that play a role in regulating the immune system and inflammation.

An elaborate network of subsets of cells that interact in distinct microenvironments has evolved to regulate the immune response. The immune response depends primarily on 3 major cell types: the macrophages and the two predominant immunocytes, including the thymus-derived (T) lymphocytes and bone-marrow derived (B) lymphocytes. These cell types interact with one another, either directly or via interleukins. Specificity of the immune system is derived from the immunocytes; B cells which produce antibodies and T cells which mediate immune functions.

2.1. T Cells

Three distinct types of lymphocytes exist: T cells, B cells and natural killer (NK) cells. T cells are a special lineage of lymphocytes that arise from maturation of stem cells in the thymus. T cells are derived from hemapoietic cells and play a central role in regulating the immune re-

sponse. Various subpopulations of antigen-specific T-cells develop in the thymus, including helper, inducer, suppressor and cytotoxic cells [2, 3]. Even when matured T lymphocytes leave the thumus, they remain naive cells until they are exposed to an antigen. After maturation, each T-lymphocyte expresses a unique antigen-binding molecule on their cell surface. This is referred to as the T Cell Receptor (TCR). The TCR is comprised of 2 transmembrane molecules, and in contrast to antibodies on the cell surface of B lymphocytes which can only recognize antigen, most TCRs can recognize a complex ligand that includes an antigenic peptide bound to MHC [3].

T cells are the principal orchestrators and regulators of the immune response. They are able to recognize immunogens only together with the major histocompatibility complex (MHC) antigens on the surfaces of other cells, antigen presenting cells. The MHC is a cluster of genes located on chromosome 6, and in humans the MHC is referred to as HLA complex. These polymorphic membrane-bound glycoproteins play a fundamental role in intercellular recognition and the recognition between self and non-self. Presently, two classes of molecules are known to exist: Class I and Class II. Class I MHC molecules interact with CD8 cells and are expressed by nearly all nucleated cells. On the other hand, Class II MHC molecules interact with CD4 lymphocytes and are expressed only by antigen-presenting cells [4]. Overall, T cells initiate the immune response, mediate antigen-specific effector responses, and regulate the activity of other leukocytes by secreting soluble factors [5].

Mature T lymphocytes express either CD4 or CD8 molecules, and are identified as either CD4 T helper (TH) cells or CD8 cytotoxic T lymphocytes. TH cells produce cytokines that are necessary for initiating the humoral and cell-mediated immune response. Thus, activation of TH cells is tightly regulated. Naive CD4 cells become activated only when they encounter an antigen presented by HLA class II complex on the surface of an antigen-presenting cell (such as dendritic cells), along with the appropriate co-stimulatory molecules [6].

The cytotoxic T-cell is a direct attack cell that is capable of killing microorganisms (or even the body's own cells). The role of the CD8 T cell is to monitor all cells of the body, and be ready to destroy any that is a potential threat. These cells have receptor proteins on the cell surface that allows them to bind tightly to those organisms or cells that contain a specific antigen. They also kill virally infected cells, preventing them from releasing more of the viral pathogen.

Helper T-cells are the most numerous. They function to increase the activation of B cells, cytotoxic T cells and suppressor T cells. In the presence of IL-2 secreted by helper T cells, the activity of cytotoxic and suppressor T cells is increased. Helper T-cells also release macrophage migration inhibition factor that plays an important role in the macrophage response to invading organisms. This lymphokine inhibits the migration of macrophages that have been chemotactically attracted into the infected tissue area, thus resulting in a greater accumulation of macrophages. In addition, it activates the macrophages to phagocytose more effectively. Generally, it is believed that the naive T helper cell is activated as a result of a two-cell interaction between the TH cell and a dendritic cell. This process requires 3 signals [7]. The first or stimulation signal involves the recognition of antigenic peptides which are presented by the MHC class II molecule by the T cell receptor. The second or costimulation signal is the triggering of CD28 on the T cell by CD80 and CD86 molecules on the dendrititc cell. The third or polarization signal promotes T cell differentiation into various effector phenotypes, eg TH1 or TH2. There is recent support for the hypothesis that TH1 polarization requires interferon gamma (IFN-γ) from other innate immune cells, such as NK cells, mast cells, eosinophils, among others [7].

The differentiation of TH cells is tightly regulated by a small, potent sub-population of T cells. Suppressor T cells act to suppress the functions of both cytotoxic and helper T-cells. Their activity assists in avoiding excessive immune reactions that might be severely damaging to the body. Regulatory T cells and several types of induced suppressor T cells play key roles in the immune tolerance network, controlling both induction and effector phases of the immune response [8]. The recent identification of CD4(+) T cells that coexpress CD25 [(CD4(+)CD25(+) T cells; about 10% of CD4(+) cells] have been found to play a critical role in inhibiting TH 2 response [9].

2.2. B Cells

B cells express immunoglobulin on their cell surface membrane. B cells have a very efficient capture mechanism for specific antigens through their immunoglobulin (Ig) antigen receptors. This surface immunoglobulin is responsible not only for binding antigen, but also the subsequent cellular activation and the secretion of soluble immunoglobulins into the serum and tissues [10].

B cells also express MHC II molecules and, as such, are able to act as antigen presenting cells. Despite their ability to effectively bind antigens, B cells alone are relatively poor activators of the resting T cell. This is predominantly attributed to their inability to release activating factors, such as interleukins. Although they are not good activators, B cells require only one-thousandth as much immunogen for activating memory T cells [10, 11].

Recent evidence supports that at least three types of B lymphocytes are important for providing memory in a humoral immune response: memory cells that do not secrete immunoglobulin, long-lived plasma cells located in the bone marrow, and B-1 cells [11]. B-lymphocyte-induced maturation protein-1 (Blimp-1) appears to an important regulator of terminal B-cell differentiation and for memory cells to turn to plasma cells. In addition B-1

B lymphocytes and plasma cells appear to require Blimp-1 for immunoglobulin secretion [12].

3. THE IMMUNE RESPONSE

There are 2 levels of protection against infection. Innate or natural immunity is present from birth and is comprised of a variety of non-specific physical barriers, including the skin and mucous membranes, certain enzymes and phagocytic cells. Innate immunity lacks specificity and memory. Acquired or adaptive immunity is specific for the invading antigen, exhibits memory, and is based on the responses of T and B lymphocytes.

3.1. Innate Immunity

Body surfaces, particularly the skin, provide the first line of defense against microorganisms. If penetration does occur, other elements of the innate immune system may block the invading microorganism. Lysozyme is widely distributed in secretions and can damage the bacteria's cell wall. A variety of bacteria activate the alternative complement pathway which may result in lysis of the bacteria or facilitation of phagocytosis by macrophages. The innate response against viruses is implemented by natural killer (NK) cells and by interferons. NK cells are lymphocytes that are able to bind to and kill virus-infected and tumor cells and are activated by interferons. Both NK cells and interferons elevate the resistance of normal cells to viral infection and provide an early defense mechanism against several viruses.

3.2. Adaptive Immunity

If the defenses provided by the innate immune system fail to prevent infection, the adaptive or acquired immune response is triggered. Adaptive immunity, in contrast to innate immunity, is distinguished by a remarkable specificity for the foreign immunogen and memory. A foreign agent triggers a chain of events that leads to the activation of lymphocytes and the production of antibodies which are highly specific for the immunogen. Thus, two basic, but closely allied, types of acquired immunity exist: cell-mediated immunity and humoral immunity. Cell-mediated immunity is achieved through the formation of large numbers of activated lymphocytes that are specifically designed to destroy the foreign agent, while humoral immunity involves developing circulating antibodies which are globulin molecules that are capable of attacking the invading agent.

The principal players in the immune response are antigen-presenting cells (APC), and B and T lymphocytes. T cells produce soluble molecules with many effects and B cells eventually result in antibody formation. B and T cell populations differentiate at early stages into hundreds of thousands unique clones. Each clone has a different surface antigen receptor, and each for the most part, is committed to respond to a distinct antigen. As a result, most T and B cells exist before they are exposed to foreign factors. Thus, immunoregulation is directed at amplifying or suppressing specific cellular constituents.

The immune response is comprised of complex cascade of events. The cascade is triggered by the introduction of an antigen or immunogen and usually ends with the elimination of the stimulus.

The first steps in the immune response following entry of an immunogen involve capture and processing of the foreign body by antigen presenting cells (APC) [13]. A processed form of the immunogen is then presented in association with class II MHC (major histocompatibility complex) molecules to a subset of T cells, helper T (TH) cells. APCs include macrophages, dendritic cells in lymphoid tissue, Langerhans cells in the skin, Kupffer's cells in the liver and microglial cels in the central nervous system. B lymphocytes, the precursors of antibody-secreting cells, express class II MHC molecules and can also act as APC. Upon exposure, APCs phagocytose or pinocytose the immunogen. The immunogen is modified in endocytic vacuoles in the cytoplasm and then, where fragments (epitopes) become associated with class II molecules. Afterwards, the complex is transported to the cell surface for presentation. Although B cells can capture and present immunogens to T cells, they are not effect activators of the resting T cell. This is mostly because B cells are not able to produce activating factors, such as interleukins. Despite this, B cells require very little immunogen (about one-thousandth that of macrophages) for activating memory T cells. Thus, it is generally believed that macrophages probably play the predominant role as APCs in the primary immune response, whereas B cells play a major role in secondary (memory) response [1, 10].

TH cells are the principal orchestrators of the immune response. They are needed for the activation of the major effector cells in the response, particularly cytotoxic T (TC) cells and antibody-producing B cells. TH cells are activated quite early in the immune response cascade [4]. The process of activating TH cells requires 2 signals: 1) the class II MHC-antigen complex on the surface of the APC, and 2) interleukin-1 (IL-1) produced by the APC. These two signals, together, induce the expression of interleukin-2 (IL-2) receptors, as well as the production of various cell growth and differentiation factors (cytokines) that are essential for triggering B cells and activating macrophages. IL-2 functions predominantly to amplify the response initiated by the contact of the TH cells with APCs [14-17].

Activated TH cells are key to further steps along the immune pathway, where they regulate the activities of other lymphocytes through the secretion of soluble factors called lymphokines. IL-2 released by TH cells is the activating factor for TC cells. TC cells are able to recognize antigens in the context of Class I MHC molecules on target cells, and their primary function is the killing of cells that express foreign or non-self antigens [14].

TC cell is distinguished from the TH cell by the presence of CD8, rather than CD4. In addition, it recognizes foreign antigens in the context of class I rather than class II MHC molecules. TC cells also require two activating signals: 1) one is provided by the interaction of the T cell antigen receptors with a complex of a foreign epitope and class I MHC on the target cell; 2) IL-2 produced by the activated TH cell. In response to the presence of both signals, TC cells release cytotoxins that can kill the target cell.

TH cells also provide growth and differentiation factors for B cells, which in turn, differentiate into antibody-secreting plasma cells. Antibody production requires both the activation of B lymphocytes, as well as their differentiation into antibody-producing plasma cells. At least 2 lymphokines produced by TH cells are needed for growth and differentiation of B cells: 1) B cell growth factor (BCGF) which stimulates proliferation of B cells; 2) B cell differentiation factor (BCDF) which induces activated B cells to differentiate into antibody-producing plasma cells. A fraction of the activated B cells proliferate, but do not differentiate into plasma cells. These B cells form a pool of memory cells, which are able to respond to subsequent encounters with the same immunogen [15].

In summary, the immune response generates a population of T lymphocytes and antibodies with specificity for recognizing an antigen in future encounters. When the same antigen is subsequently encountered, several events may take place. These events are referred to as effector mechanisms, and include, neutralization, cytotoxicity, cytostimulation and inflammation. Neutralization refers to the ability of an antibody to block a toxic site on a chemical toxin or microorganism. This can take place either directly on the toxic site, or by steric hindrance. Cytotoxicity reflects lyses of the cell containing the antigenic epitope by the antibody using various mechanisms, including complement-induced lyses or antibody-dependent cellular cytotoxicity. An autoantibody may react with a host cell receptor to stimulate metabolic processes within the cell. This process is called cytostimulation. Inflammation takes place following the reaction of specific T lymphocytes or antibodies with the antigen and the subsequent recruitment of inflammatory cells and endogenous mediator chemicals [18].

4. INFECTION

Both immunologic and nonimmunologic defense mechanisms are responsible for maintaining the internal milieu free of microorgansisms and infection. Immunologic defenses against infection are those host defense mechanisms which have specificity toward the invading pathogen and which are augmented on second and subsequent exposures. Nonspecific, nonimmunologic defenses against infection include the body surface, inflammation and fever. Although the boundary between specific and nonspecific immune resistance to infection remains unclear, defenses against infection are characterized by considerable redundancy [19].

Specificity of immunologic defenses is determined by immunoglobulins and T lymphocytes, although nonspecific components, including complement and phagocytic cells can be recruited. Antibodies act to neutralize the biologic activity of the bacterial toxins, inhibit the activity of enzymes, block bacterial attachment to mucosal surfaces, and deter growth of certain prokaryotes. Although antibodies can also neutralize viruses, this is usually more effective in the presence of complement. Although the role of T lymphocytes is predominantly one of recruiting, facilitating and augmenting other effectors of the immune response, rather than directly attacking pathogens, T-lymphocytes do mediate attacks on virus-infected cells. The T-lymphocyte attack on virus-infected cells is mediated by CD8 cytotoxic T lymphocytes. Complement acts by inactivating microorganisms and by facilitating phagocytosis, both of which can be assisted by antibodies [20].

4.1. Bacterial Infection

Immunity to bacterial infection is mediated by both cellular and humoral mechanisms. Bacteria express many different surface antigens and secrete a variety of virulence factors or toxins that can trigger immune responses. Immunity to bacteria can be categorized into 3 principal types according to the characteristics of the bacterial infection: 1) toxigenic bacterial infections, 2) encapsulated bacteria, and 3) intracellular bacteria. Bacterial toxins, either exotoxins or endotoxins, play a significant role in the pathogenesis of certain diseases. Encapsulated bacteria, either gram-positive or gram-negative, evade phagocytosis by coating themselves with innocuous polysaccharide. Intracellular bacteria avoid immune responses by growing inside cells, particularly phagocytes. A similar mechanism of avoidance is also used by certain fungal and parasitic pathogens. Cellular immunity is mediated by macrophages that are activated by specific lymphocytes [21].

Because of the various virulence factors used by bacteria to enhance their survival, the immune response to bacterial infections, regardless of type, is extraordinarily complex, and includes antibody, complement, granulocytes, lymphocytes and macrophages. An initial nonspecific defense against bacterial infections is provided by granulocytes, which ingest and kill most potential pathogens. Specific immunity is needed for protection against encapsulated or intracellular bacteria. This requires the development of either antibodies that can enhance killing by its opsonic or complement-fixing activity or T-cell immunity that can activate the microbicidal activity of macrophages [22]. However, in many infections, a complex interaction of immune mechanisms is necessary to achieve immunity.

4.2. Viral Infections

Viruses are complex immunogens that can replicate within the host. During their replication, they are able to parasitize the cellular metabolic processes of the host and directly alter the host's cell structure and function. Viruses can activate both cellular and humoral immune response [23].

Because viruses are obligate, intracellular parasites, the clinical features of a viral infection are related to the particular cell type which is infected. Often, the host immune response to certain viral antigens induces other, additional injuries (immunopathic effects) [24].

4.3. Fungal Infections

Thousands of fungi are known in nature, although relatively few are pathogenic. Infectious diseases caused by fungi are called mycoses, and these can be grouped according to the predominant site of infection [25]. Superficial mycoses normally occur on the surface, external to normal immunologic processes. Cutaneous mycoses produce delayed hypersensitivity responses to the local presence of keratinolytic fungi; these organisms metabolize keratin. Subcutaneous and systemic mycoses successfully challenge the host's immunologic defense mechanisms. Subcutaneous infections are usually related to organisms of low virulence. Certain systemic mycoses are related to primary pathogens that are presumably able to infect anyone within the endemic area, while other mycoses are related to opportunistic pathogens [26]. Deep systemic infections are caused by organisms that have 2 stages to their life-cycle. They enter the body as spores, and then multiply in a different form. Although most primary invasive mycoses are acquired by inhalation of specialized forms, others have specialized forms that are more suitable for tissue invasion (dimorphic fungi) [27].

Immunity to mycoses is principally cellular, and involves neutrophils, macrophages, lymphocytes, among others. With rare exceptions, most mycoses are not susceptible to direct killing by an antibody and complement.

5. INFLAMMATION

One of the primary means by which the immune system functions in immunity is the inflammatory response. However, it is important to note that inflammation is a response that is not limited to just immunologic stimuli [28]. The mediators, chemical or cellular, of inflammation can be activated by various nonimmunologic events, including trauma, injury, heat, tissue-damaging chemicals, etc. The inflammatory response like the immune response can be generated by cells (neutrophils, esosinophils, basophils, macrophages, mast cells, platelets and endothelium), as well as by circulating proteins (factors from the complement, coagulation, fibrino-lysis or kinin pathways). Although immunologically induced inflammation begins with the specific recognition of the antigen, the subsequent events have no immuno-logic specificity. Three principal pathways of immuno-logically induced inflammation exist: 1) cell-mediated immunity, 2) immune complex-mediated inflammation, and 3) IgE-mediated inflammation [29, 30].

Cell-mediated immunity (often referred to as delayed hypersensitivity) involves T-cell mediated generation of cytokines. This cellular inflammatory response is a means by which the body defends against infection and repairs tissue damage. Inflammation is generated by the interaction of an antigen with the effector T-lymphocyte. The T-cell responds to exposure by generating lym-phokines that promote a mononuclear cellular inflam-mation. Specifically, the cells attracted by lymphokine-induced chemotaxis include monocytes, granulocytes, B and T lymphocytes and basophils. Vasodilation occurs, which enhances the availability of cells from the cir-culation, the coagulation-kinin system is activated so that fibrin is formed and deposited and the formation of granulomas is initiated [31, 32].

The microscopic appearance of cell-mediated im-munity is characteristic with mononuclear cellular in-filtration with monocytes and lymphocytes and granulo-cytes. The lymphocytes are often distributed perivas-cularly [33]. Fibrin is deposited, edema forms and tissue destruction takes place. The tissue can even be liquefied (caseation necrosis) in advanced lesions. The hallmark of cell-mediated immunity is the focal accumulation of monocytes, lymphocytes, neutrophils, plasma cells and epithelioid giant cells which form the granuloma [31, 33].

Immune complex-mediated inflammation involves the antigen-antibody complex-mediated generation of fac-tors derived from the complement system. In this case, the interaction of antigen with an antibody of certain im-munoglobulin isotypes activates the complement cas-cade. This ultimately generates a variety of chemotactic factors that induce neutrophilic inflammation and vas-culitis [18].

IgE-mediated inflammation involves IgE antibody-mediated release of active chemicals from mast cells. This response is initiated with the interaction of antigen with IgE antibodies occupying mast cell receptors. Ac-tivation of the mast cell releases mediators with effects on blood vessels, smooth muscles, and secretory glands, causing changes in vascular permeability and the functioning of visceral organs [29].

6. STRESS AND IMMUNE SYSTEM DYSFUNCTION

Physical, behavioral and inflammatory stress through the stimulation of the corticotropin releasing hormone (CRH) neuron, activate a final common neuroendocrine path-way: the hypothalamic-pituitary-adrenal (HPA) axis. The

final component of this axis is the release of glucocorti-coids from the adrenal cortex [34].

Corticosteroids represent one of the most potent endogenous anti-inflammatory agents known. They have the capacity to inhibit and suppress virtually all critical inflammatory and immune cell functions, even at physio-logical concentrations, and particularly during the early development of the immune/inflammatory response. At the molecular level, they inhibit the production of most inflammatory mediators including IL-1, TNF, phsopholi-pase A2 and prostaglandins. Hence, stress-induced en-hanced production and secretion of glucocorticoids ap-pears to counter-regulate and suppress excessive im-mune/inflammatory cell activation and mediator produc-tion that could otherwise result in self-induced tissue in-jury [35, 36]. This suggests a critical role for cortico-steroids in maintaining physiological homeostasis during the adaptive response to noxious stressors. On the other hand, it is noteworthy that IL-1 is also a potent stimulator of the hypothalamic-pituitary adrenal axis resulting in the release of corticosteroids. Cortico-steroids, in turn, feedback to inhibit macrophage release of IL-1. These interactions reflect the intricate communi-cation links between the immune and neuroendocrine system.

REFERENCES

[1] Goodman JW, Sercarz EE. The complexity of structures involved in T cell activation. Annu Rev Immunol 1983;1:465-98.
[2] Sanders ME, Makgoba MW, Shaw S. Human naive and memory T cells: reinterpretation of helper-inducer and suppressor-inducer subserts. Immunol Today 1988;9:195-9.
[3] Moss PA, Rosenberg WM, Bell JI. The human T cell receptor in health and disease. Annu Rev Immunol 1992;10:71-96.
[4] Andersen MH, Schrama D, Straten PT, Becker JC. Cytotoxic T cells. J Investigative Dermatol 2006;126:32-41.
[5] Miyajima A, Miyatake S, Schreurs J, De Vries J, Arai N, Yokota T, Arai K. Coordinate regulation of immune and inflammatory re-sponse by T cell-derived lymphokines. FASEB J 1988;2:2462-73.
[6] Stockwin LH, McGonagle D, Martin IG, Blair GE. Dendritic cells: immunological sentinels with a central role in health and disease. Immunol Cell Biol 2000;78:91-102.
[7] Corthay A. A three-cell model for activation of naive T helper cells. Scand J Immunol 2006;64:93-6.
[8] Becker C, Stoll S, Bopp T, Schmitt E, Jonuleit H. Regulatory T cells: present facts and future hopes. Med Microbiol Immunol (Berl) 2006;195:113-24.
[9] McHugh RS, Shevach EM. The role of suppressor T cells in regu-lation of immune responses. J Allergy Clin Immunol 2002;110:693-702.
[10] Kishimoto T, Hirano T. Molecular regulation of B lymphocyte re-sponse. Annu Rev Immunol 1988;6:485-512.
[11] Calame K. Transcription factors that regulate memory in humoral responses. Immunol Rev 2006;211:269-79.
[12] Duclos CA, Cattoretti G, Lin KI, Calame K. Commitment of B lym-

phocytes to a plasma cell fate is associated with Blimp-1 expression *in vivo*. J Immunol 2000;165:5462-5471.

[13] Jin Y, Fuller L, Ciancio G, Burke GW, Tzakis AG, Ricordi C, Miller J, Esquenzai V. Antigen presentation and immune regulatory capacity of immature and mature-endriched antigen presenting (dendritc) cells derived from human bone marrow. Hum Immunol 2004;65: 93-103.

[14] Marrack P, Kappler J. T cells can distinguish between allogeneic major histocompatibility complex products on different cell types. Nature 1988;332:840-3.

[15] Singer A, Hodes RJ. Mechanisms of T-cell B-cell interaction. Annu Rev Immunol 1983;1:211-41.

[16] Mizel SB, Kilian PL, Lewis JC, Paganelli KA, Chizzonite RA. The interleukin 1 receptor. Dynamics of interleukin 1 binding and internalization in T cells and fibroblasts. J Immunol 1987;138:2906-12.

[17] Smith KA. Interleukin-2: inception, impact and implications. Science 1988;240:169 - 76.

[18] Barnett EV. Circulating immune complexes: Their biologic and clinical significance. J Allergy Clin Immunol 1986;78:1089-96.

[19] Cohen S. Cell mediated immunity and the inflammatory system. Hum Pathol 1976;7:249-64.

[20] Mims CA. The pathogenesis of infectious diseases, 3rd ed. New York: Academic Press, 1986.

[21] Ahmed R, Canning WM, Kauffman RS, Sharpe AH, Hallum JV, Fields BN. Role of the host cell in persistent viral infection: coevolution of L cells and reovoirus during persistent infection. Cell 1981:25:325-32.

[22] McCuskey RS, McCuskey PA, Urbaschek B, Urbaschek R. Kupffer cell function in host defense. Rev Infect Dis 1987;9 (Suppl 5): S616-9.

[23] Fields BN. Studies of reovirus pathogenesis reveal potential sites for antiviral intervention. Adv Exp Med Biol 1992;312: 1-14.

[24] Notkins AL, Oldstone MB. Concepts in viral pathogenesis. New York: Springer Verlag, 1984.

[25] Cox RA. Immunology of the Fungal Diseases. New York: CRC Press, 1989.

[26] Reiss E. Molecular immunology of Mycotic and Actino-mycotic Infections. New York: Elsevier, 1986.

[27] Rippon JW. Medical Mycology. 3rd ed. Philadelphia: Saunders, 1988.

[28] Serafin WE, Austen KF. Current concepts. Mediation of immediate hypersensitivity reactions. N Engl J Med 1987;317:30-4.

[29] Ishizaka T, Ishizaka K. Activation of mast cells for mediator release through IgE receptors. Prog Allergy 1984;34:188-235.

[30] Bayon Y, Alonso A, Hernandex M, Nieto ML, Sanchex Crespo M. Mechanisms of cell signaling in immune-mediated inflammation. Cytokines Cell Mol Ther 1998;4:275-86.

[31] Galli SJ. Pathogenesis and management of anaphylaxis: current status and future challenges. J Allergy Clin Immunol 2005;115: 571-4.

[32] Unanue ER, Allen PM. The basis for the immunoregulatory role of macrophages and other accessory cells. Science 1987;236:551-7.

[33] Hanson PM, et al. Phagocytic cells: Degranulation and secretion. Chap 22. In: Gallin JI, Editor, Inflammation: Basic Principles and Clinical Correlates. Philadelphia: Raven Press, 1988, pp 363-390.

[34] Johnson EO, Kamilaris TC, Chrousos GP, Gold PW. Mechanisms of Stress: A Dynamic Overview of Hormonal and Behavioral Homeostasis. Neurosci Biobehav Rev 1992;16:115-130.

[35] Johnson EO, Moutsopoulos M. Neuroimmunological axis and rheumatic diseases. (Editorial) Eur J Clin Invest 1992;22 (S1):2-5.

[36] Johnson EO, Moutsopoulos HM. Neuroendocrine manifestations in Sjogren's syndrome. Relation to neurobiology of stress. Ann N Y Acad Sci 2000;917:797-808.

The Immune Defense Against Bacterial Biofilms: Dire Consequences for the Host

Christof WAGNER[a,b], Volkmar HEPPERT[a], G. Maria HÄNSCH[*b]

[a]Klinik für Unfall- und Wiederherstellungschirurgie, Berufsgenossenschaftliche Unfallklinik, Ludwigshafen, Germany

[b]Institut für Immunologie, Universität Heidelberg, Germany

Bacterial infections occurring after osteosynthesis or implantation of prostheses are serious complications in orthopaedic surgery. In the following chapter, the current knowledge and the most pertinent hypothesis regarding the etiology and the pathogenesis of implant-associated osteomyelits are delineated, with special reference to the role of the immune defense.

Keywords: bacterial biofilm; PMN; posttraumatic osteomyelitis; immune defense; osteolysis.

1. INTRODUCTION

Bacterial infections occurring after osteosynthesis or implantation of prostheses are serious complications in orthopaedic surgery. In the majority of cases, an antibiotic therapy is not successful. The infection persists and gives rise to a progressive, destructive inflammatory process with massive tissue injury, and eventually osteolysis, an entity known as implant-associated posttraumatic osteomyelitis (Fig. 1) [for review see 1-5]. In most cases, the removal of the implant with extensive debridement and intricate and costly reconstructive surgery is the only option. Hence, improvement of management and therapy is imperative, as is the development of means to prevent infection, first and foremost.

*Corresponding Author

Institut fur Immunologie der Universität Heidelberg

Im Neuenheimer Feld 305

69120 Heidelberg, Germany

Tel: +49 6221 564071

Fax: +49 6221 565536

e-mail: n50@ix.urz.uni-heidelberg.de

Since a thorough understanding of the underlying disease processes is the prerequisite for an adequate therapy and the design of a rational prophylaxis regimen, in the following chapter, the current knowledge and the most pertinent hypothesis regarding the etiology and the pathogenesis of the implant-associated osteomyelitis are delineated [6-8].

2. BACTERIAL BIOFILMS AS THE CAUSE OF PERSISTENT INFECTION

2.1. Bacterial biofilm formation

There is general agreement that the formation of bacterial biofilms on implant materials is the ultimate cause of persistent infection [3, 4, 7, 9, 10]. Biofilm formation is the result of an active, genetically driven process, which comprises the activation of defined sets of genes, e.g. of those coding for adhesion proteins, as well as the silencing of other genes that results in loss of certain features, e.g. of flagella, and hence of the mobility of the bacteria [11-14]. The most conspicuous feature of the biofilm, however, is the production of the extracellular polysaccharide substance (EPS) by the bacteria, which in some instances is visible even to the naked eye as "slime" or as the name-giving film (Fig.1).

In contrast to the mobile, single-living "planktonic" lifestyle, which until recently was thought to be prevalent, bacteria embedded in biofilms remain more or less stationary and are attached to surfaces. Occasionally, bacteria may be released from the biofilm, or pieces of the biofilm can tear off and form colonies at other locations.

In the ecosystem, living as a biofilm has its advantages for the bacteria: they are protected against flushing, predators, and unfavourable environmental conditions. Relevant to the human infection is the relative resistance to many antibiotics [15-17].

2.2. Formation of biofilms on artificial surfaces

As pointed out above, biofilm formation requires attachment of bacteria. Apparently artificial surfaces, including glass, metals, and all sorts of plastics, are especially suitable for adhesion. Most bacteria attach within hours, and at least *in vitro,* whereas visible biofilms are formed within days. From animal experiments it has been concluded that metal surfaces, as they are used for implants, are preferentially colonized by bacteria, and that less bacteria are needed to induce infection when im-

plants are present [18, 19]. Whether it is indeed the metal, which provides optimal conditions for the attachment, or is the artificial surfaces - in contrast to the lining endothelial or epithelial cells - that cannot interfere with bacteria adhesion, remains to be decided. Recently, it has been described that epithelial cells in culture inhibit biofilm formation of *Pseudomonas aeruginosa* by inactivating a relevant signalling molecule [20]. Though not a definite proof, it is an attractive hypothesis that living cells could interfere with biofilm formation [21].

Of importance is that the mucosa is not entirely protected against biofilm formation: the human gastrointestinal tract, for example, is colonized by bacterial biofilms in healthy individuals [22]. Moreover, nasal colonization by *S. aureus* is found in many healthy individuals [23-25]. Common to these infections is that they are confined to a location, and that they do not elicit an inflammatory immune response. Colonization by bacteria, such as S.aureus, however, enhances the risk of an infectious disease development, particularly when other factors contribute, compromising the host defense [26-30].

Numerous chronic infectious diseases can be attributed to biofilm formation, e.g. otitis media, airway infections, chronic sinusitis or periodontal disease [31-36]. For example, in patients with cystic fibrosis, the formation

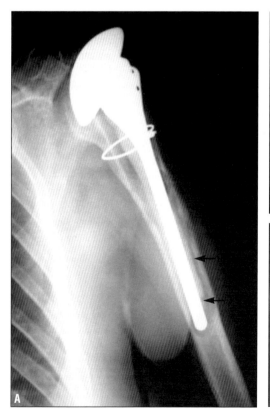
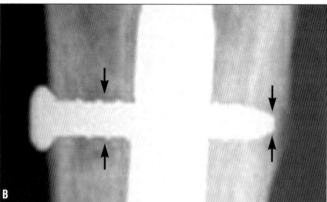
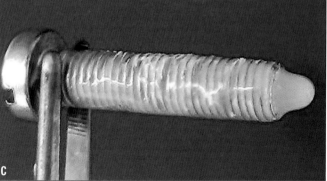

FIGURE 1. Examples of osteolysis and biofilm formation: osteolysis around a prosthesis **(A)** or a screw **(B)** is shown (zones of lysis are marked by the arrows). **(C)** A biofilm becomes visible after obtaining a few-day culture of an explanted screw.

of bacteria biofilms of *P. aeruginosa* in the lung greatly contributes to an increase in the mortality rate [37-40].

2.3. Biofilm formation on orthopaedic implants

The overall rate of infection of primary prostheses or implants ranges between 1 and 2%. The incidence increases with re-implants (e.g. 3.2% in hip replacement, 5.6% in knee replacement, and particularly, after trauma with open fractures and extensive soft tissue injury [1, 2, 41-43].

It is worth noting that the time span between primary surgery and the clinically apparent infection varies among patients. In some patients, the infection occurs within weeks after surgery, while in others, after years (Fig. 2). Obviously, there are different routes of infection: while an early infection points to contamination during surgery (by either exogenous bacteria or by endogenous, e.g. skin colonizing bacteria), late-occurring infections could be due to bacteria contracted by the host on a later date. Even if these bacteria use a different site of entry, it is feasible for them to finally attach to privileged sites such as an implant. Moreover, also "harmless" bacteria colonizing the skin or the epithelium (e.g. in the nose) could become invasive for reasons that are unknown so far [24, 28, 44].

In our experience, the frequency of infections around implants varies with regard to the location, with a preference for the lower extremities. As for the upper extremities, the rate of infection is reported to be higher for the elbow joint (7.7%) than for the wrist (2.39%) or the shoulder (1.06%) (endoprostheses) [45].

In the majority of patients with implant-associated osteomyelitis, bacteria can be isolated from the infected site or the implant. According to the literature, staphylococci species are prevalent [46], which proved true also for our patients: in 55% staphylococci were found, with S.aureus being the most prevalent. Streptococci (6.5%) and enterococci (11.5%) were also found, the latter always together with other bacteria, particularly with staphylococci. A mixture of 2 to 4 bacteria species was identified in 16.4% of the patients. Also in accordance with the literature, in 27% of patients, no bacteria from swabs taken from the infected site could be cultivated. Whether the patients examined were indeed "aseptic" cannot be deduced from these data, because bacteria grown in biofilms may escape detection through use of the routine laboratory test, due to their altered growth characteristics [47, 48].

3. THE PATHOGENESIS OF IMPLANT-ASSOCIATED POSTTRAUMATIC OSTEOMYELITIS

While biofilms are generally considered as the ultimate cause of osteomyelitis, the molecular process leading to tissue damage and osteolysis has not been clarified yet. In principle, two possibilities have to be considered: either products released from the bacterial biofilm are cytotoxic or cause noxious conditions for the surrounding tissue, or otherwise, the bacterial biofilm induces an inflammatory response with the infiltration of leukocytes, which in turn attack not only the biofilm but also the adjacent tissue.

The examination of the infected sites, e.g. during surgery for removal of the implant, clearly supports the latter possibility: pus is always found locally, and in extreme cases, there is also purulent discharge. Since pus is nothing but dead leukocytes, tissue debris and serum, there is no doubt that leukocytes infiltrate the infected site. Moreover, in a recent series of experiments we characterized the infiltrated cells as *polymorphonuclear neutrophils* (PMN) comprising 65-85% of the cellular infiltrate, T-lymphocytes (5 to 15%), natural killing (NK) - cells (5-15%), B-cells (<1%), and monocytes (<1%) [49, 50].

3.1. Host defense mechanisms versus inflammation: the dual role of PMN

PMN are considered as the "first-line defense" against bacterial infection; for this task, the cells are equipped with receptors recognizing bacteria-typical structures, such as lipopolysaccharides, lipoteichoic acids, peptidoglycans, the so-called "pattern-recognition" receptors, and in addition, receptors of the bound antibodies (Fcγ-receptors CD16, CD32, CD64) or complement C3 (com-

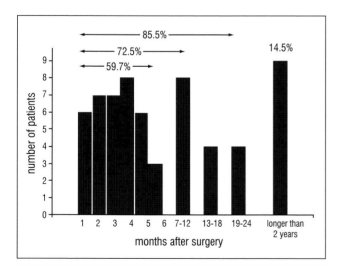

FIGURE 2. Time interval between the first application of the implant and the removal of the implant due to infection: for 62 patients, the time interval is shown in months or years, respectively. As calculated from the data, 59.7% of the patients with implant-associated osteomyelitis required removal of the implant after the first 6 months; 72.5% within the first year, and 85.5% within the first 2 years. In 14.5% of the patients the time interval ranged from 25 months to 13 years.

plement receptors CR 1-4). Moreover, PMN are able to migrate in a directed manner (chemotaxis) towards bacteria or a source of chemotactic cytokines [51-53].

Phagocytosis of bacteria and intracellular killing by oxygen radicals is supposedly the major bactericidal mechanism of PMN. Extensive *in vitro* studies, predominantly on planktonic bacteria, but also data from patients with severe congenital PMN defects (particularly those resulting in failure to generate oxygen radicals, or defect in the expression of adhesion proteins) lead to delineation of the following reaction sequence (Fig. 3): in case of an infection, chemokines (e.g. platelet activating factor PAF or complement C5a) are generated at the infected site and diffuse into the tissue. The nearby endothelial cells become "sticky" by up-regulating special-

ized adhesion proteins, which sequentially capture the leukocytes, predominantly PMN, from the peripheral blood. The PMN "roll" on the endothelial cells becomes further activated to allow them to attach firmly. They squeeze between the endothelial cells and migrate actively towards the source of infection. Then, phagocytosis of the bacteria occurs, followed by intracellular killing. Oxygen radicals production by PMN is thought to be the predominant, though not the only mechanism [52, 54-56]. Successful phagocytosis initiates the programmed cell death of PMN, which in turn are phagocytosed by macrophages. Thereby, spilling of the cytotoxic content is prevented [57-59]. Thus, bactericides and the accompanying inflammation is a well-contained, self-limiting process, which eventually results in

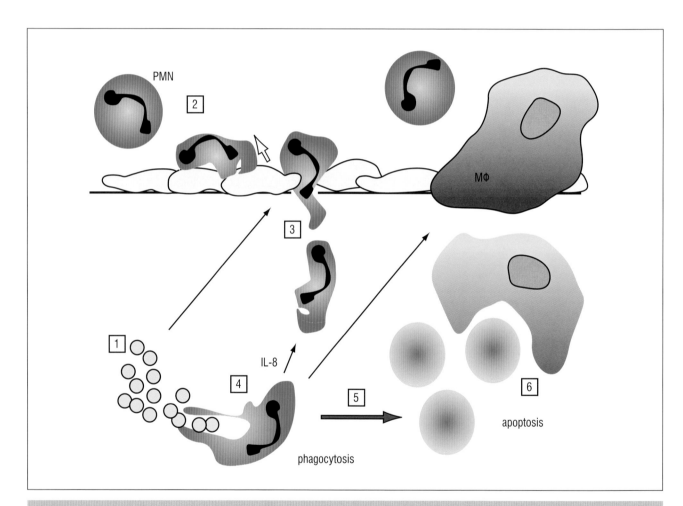

FIGURE 3. The role of PMN in bacterial defense: to efficiently combat bacteria, PMN have to migrate from the blood vessel into the infected tissue at an approriate site. This is accomplished through a complex and well-regulated sequence of events, which are depicted here schematically. **(1)** From the infected site, mediators are emitted, which act on the close-by endothelium. **(2)** The endothelial cells up-regulate adhesion proteins that capture the PMN, which then bind to the endothelial cells, and finally **(3)** transmigrate in-between the epithelial cells towards the site of infection. **(4)** Having reached the site, the PMN take up the bacteria. Simultaneously, the PMN release cytokines, such as interleukin (IL)-8, which attracts more PMN, or the monocytes attractant MCP-1. The phagocytosis results in killing the bacteria, and also **(5)** induces the programmed cell death ("apoptosis") of the PMN. **(6)** Apoptotic PMN are cleared by the invaded monocytes (different from macrophages), which limits the inflammatory process in a time- and site-dependent manner.

clearing of the infected site, which is a prerequisite for healing and regeneration [56, 57, 60].

An old observation is that PMN during phagocytosis also release their cytotoxic and bactericidal entities to the surroundings. Moreover, enzymes, such as elastase, are released, maybe to blaze a trail through the connective tissue. Given the large variety of substrates for elastase, extensive tissue damage could ensue when a large number of PMN are activated [61]. In addition to the accidental driveling, PMN are also known to release the content of lysosomal vesicles in an attempt to phagocytose very large particles. This phenomenon, termed "frustrated phagocytosis", is thought to account for tissue damage, e.g. in autoimmunity with organ-specific autoantibodies [62-64]. Thus, PMN on the one hand are crucial for the host defense against bacteria; on the other hand, due to the fact that PMN release their cytotoxic and proteolytic entities in an undirected manner, they can also deteriorate the tissue in the immediate vicinity.

It is also important to realize that the infiltrating leukocytes and the surrounding tissue produce and release a fair amount of cytokines, which, depending on the activation status of the cells, can support the inflammatory response e.g. by eliciting a further cell influx. Creating a "proinflammatory" environment might also promote tissue destruction and bone resorption, while simultaneously, regeneration and healing is prevented. A chronic-destructive inflammatory process ensues [56, 63, 64].

3.2. The host defense against bacteria in biofilms

A popular belief is that bacteria in biofilms are rather resistant to host defense mechanisms. Taking into account the mere dimensions of a biofilm, phagocytosis, which is central to the bacterial defense, appears unlikely to take place. Since there is "frustrated phagocytosis" release of the PMN content into the surrounding area might not be efficient regarding the killing of bacteria, but could contribute to the tissue damage.

Our own data appear to support that assumption: in a study of 70 patients, we found evidence for activation of immunocompetent cells and their infiltration into the site of infection. Considerable up-regulation of the activation-associated receptors CD14, CD11b, CD18, CD64 on PMN was detected, as well as priming for an enhanced oxygen radical synthesis. Thus, the infiltrated PMN were well equipped for their bactericidal activity (as an example, data for CD14 are shown in Fig. 4). Nevertheless, in the majority of patients, living bacteria could be recovered from the same site, indicating that PMN had not been able to control the infection [49, 50, 65].

It is worth mentioning our observation that the ability of the infiltrated PMN to migrate in a directed manner was greatly reduced. This observation is in line with *in vitro* data, showing that exposure of PMN to proinflammatory cytokines or excessive amounts of chemokines reduced their chemotactic activity, while phagocytosis is preserved [50] (Fig. 4).

3.3. Interaction of PMN with bacterial biofilms

Whether or not PMN recognize bacterial biofilms cannot be delineated from the *in vivo* observations, but require *in vitro* studies with cultivated biofilms and cells of healthy donors. From two published studies [66, 67] it was deduced that leukocytes adhere to biofilms but they are unable to take up the bacteria.

In contrast to these experiments, we could show phagocytosis of S.aureus in biofilms; the major difference between the published data and ours was that human serum was used as a source of antibodies and a complement (Fig. 5). These findings are in line with the well-known fact that phagocytosis, as studied with planktonic bacteria or other particulate materials, is most efficient after "opsonisation" with serum, since triggering the Fcγ receptors and the complement receptors provides the optimal signal for the PMN for phagocytosis and killing [68].

Since the killing of bacteria in biofilms is obviously possible, the question remains, why biofilms persist in patients. One explanation, which is not only true for biofilms, is the classic saying "too little - too late". In the case of patients with implants, it is quite feasible that due to the local conditions (reduced blood circulation, scarred tissue) infiltration of PMN is initially rather slow, so biofilms can form undisturbed, particularly, since the implants are considered to be a privileged site for bacteria adhesion and biofilm formation. Moreover, since PMN lose their migratory capacity when arriving at the infected site (Fig. 4), they cannot infiltrate into the biofilm. Consequently, phagocytosis and killing occur only on the surface, while the bulk of the biofilm would persist.

The persistence of the biofilm has serious consequences: first, as a permanent source of bacteria, it would continuously attract PMN, and eventually, other leukocytes as well; secondly, the PMN are not cleared, because the decisive signal for the programmed cell death, i.e. the phagocytosis, is lacking. The PMN persist and eventually release their cytotoxic content in an uncontrolled fashion. Tissue damage ensues, which per se is a considerable trigger for an inflammatory response.

3.4. The mechanism of osteolysis

Osteolysis is the hallmark of osteomyelitis. The link between bacterial infection and osteolysis, however, has not been established yet. While direct effects of bacteria cannot be ruled out, bone loss as a consequence of the persistent inflammation is presumed, at least in diseases like rheumatoid arthritis [69-72]. The most likely mechanism is enhanced synthesis and/or activation of the bone-resorbing osteoclasts. Osteoclasts are generated from monocytes; pro-inflammatory cytokines, such as tumor necrosis factor (TNF) α or interleukin 8 promote the differentiation of osteoclasts, as does the interaction with activated T-lymphocytes [73-77]. Since (i) these cytokines are generated at the site of infection, (ii) the

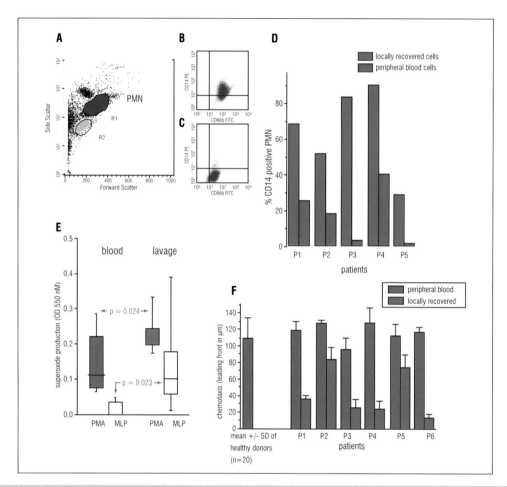

FIGURE 4. Analysis of the infiltrated leukocytes in patients with implant-associated osteomyelitis. **A.** By extensive lavage of the infected site, leuko-cytes could be recovered. By forward-side scatter analysis, two major cell populations were identified, i.e. PMN (blue, in this particular patient 76% of the leukocytes) and T-lymphocytes (green, 12%). **B.** The PMN (CD66b positive cells) of the lavage are expressed as CD14, but not the cells of the peripheral blood **(C)** which were taken immediately prior to surgery. In **D**, data of five other patients are summarised: in all CD14 was seen on the locally recovered cells (blue), but none or much less on the PMN of the peripheral blood (red). **E.** The synthesis superoxide was measured in PMN of the peripheral blood (red) or of the lavage (blue), respectively. When a strong stimulus was used, such as phorbol ester (PMA), the pro-duction of superoxides was enhanced by cells of the lavage. Similarly, the PMN of the lavage also responded to a weak stimulus, the bacterial pep-tide fMLP, indicating a preconditioning or "priming" of the cells (here data of 6 patients are summarised and depicted as box-and whiskers blot). **F.** Chemotaxis towards complement C5a was measured of PMN of the peripheral blood (red) and compared to that of PMN recovered from the lavage. In six individual patients (P1-P6) a reduction of chemotaxis was seen.

osteolysis is regularly localized in the immediate vicinity of the implants (compare to Fig. 1), and (iii) osteoclasts could be identified at the infected site, it can be assumed that in implant-associated osteomyelitis, mono-cytes are differentiated locally to osteoclasts with bone resorbing activity [5].

4. CONCLUSION

From the published data and our own experience we support the following hypothesis: the formation of bacte-rial biofilms elicits a local inflammatory response, hall-marked by the infiltration of leukocytes, predominantly

PMN and T-cells. We do not know whether the defense against a bacterial biofilm could be successful, because only infections having escaped the immune defense will become clinically apparent, as in the case of osteomyeli-tis, with a progressive, destructive inflammatory process. Based on accumulating knowledge regarding the role of leukocytes, particularly of PMN, in inflammation, it is most probable that these cells are responsible for the destructive process. If indeed the PMN cannot phago-cytose the biofilm efficiently, e.g. because they cannot migrate into the film under *in vivo* conditions, the signal for programmed cell death ("apoptosis") will not be tran-smitted.

Eventually, PMN will undergo necrotic cell death, resulting in release of their cytotoxic and proteolytic enti-

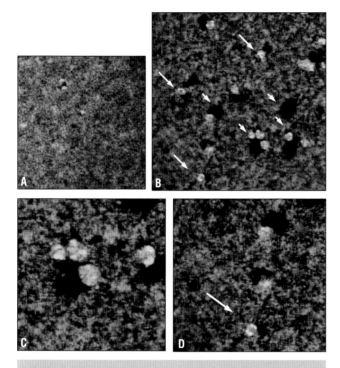

FIGURE 5. Phagocytosis of bacterial biofilms by PMN: **A.** *S. aureus* was grown as a homogenous biofilm and stained (green fluorescence) **(B).** PMN, labelled red (arrows) were added and after 60 minutes, the biofilm was examined by confocal Laserscan Microscopy. Bacteria-free zones became apparent around the PMN (arrow heads). **C** and **D** show blow-ups. The yellow colouring indicates uptake of bacteria into the PMN as result of an overlay of red and green.

with a synthesis of cytokines, e.g. of interleukin 8, which in turn, may attract more leukocytes, but also can cause the differentiation of monocytes to osteoclasts. Thus, the microenvironment created by the infiltrating leukocytes would, on the one hand, perpetuate the inflammatory process, and on the other hand, promote osteolysis resulting in the progression of tissue destruction (this hypothesis is summarized in Fig. 6).

Acknowledgements

This study was supported by a grant (WA1623/1-4) of the Deutsche Forschungsgemeinschaft (DFG).

REFERENCES

[1] Lew DP, Waldvogel FA. Osteomyelitis. N Engl J Med 1997;363: 999-1007.
[2] Tsukayama DT. Pathophysiology of posttraumatic osteomyelitis. Clin Orthop 1999;360:22-9.
[3] Costerton JW, Stewart PS, Greenberg EP. Bacterial biofilms: a common cause of persistent infections. Science 1999;284:1318-26.
[4] Donlan RM. Biofilms and device-associated infections. Emerg Infect Dis 2001;7:277-81.
[5] Wagner C, Obst U, Hansch GM. The implant-associated posttraumatic osteomyelitis: collateral damage by the local host defence? Int J Artif Organs 2005;28:1172-80.
[6] Costerton W, Veeh R, Shirtliff M, Pasmore M, Post C, Ehrlich G. The application of biofilm science to the study and control of chronic bacterial infections. J Clin Invest 2003;112:1466-77.
[7] Costerton W, Montanaro L, Arciola CR. Biofilm in implant infections: its production and regulation. Int J Artif Organs 2005;28: 1062-8.

ties into the environment, which will cause tissue damage. The escape from apoptosis is also associated

FIGURE 6. The pathogensis of the implant-associated osteomyelitis. Our hypothesis is that the bacterial biofilm attracts the PMN, which attach but cannot migrate into the biofilm, because they have lost their migratory capacity. Since they are highly activated, they release their cytotoxic content (e.g. superoxides, ROS, as well as proteolytic enzymes), which in turn cause tissue destruction; simultaneously, the PMN release cytokines, which attract more PMN, and also monocytes. The latter can differentiate from osteoclasts with bone resorbing activity.

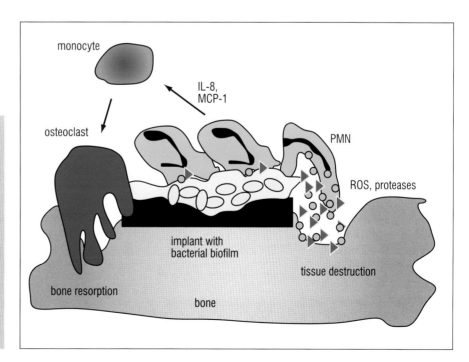

[8] Fitzpatrick F, Humphreys H, O'Gara JP. The genetics of staphylococcal biofilm formation-will a greater understanding of pathogenesis lead to better management of device-related infection? Clin Microbiol Infect 2005;11:967-73.

[9] von Eiff C, Jansen B, Kohnen W, Becker K. Infections associated with medical devices: pathogenesis, management and prophylaxis. Drugs 2005;65:179-214.

[10] Vinh DC, Embil JM. Device-related infections: a review. J Long Term Eff Med Implants 2005;15:467-88.

[11] Watnik P, Kolter R. Biofilm, City of microbes. J Bact 2000;182: 2675-9.

[12] Davey ME, O'Toole GA. Microbial biofilms: from ecology to molecular genetics. Microbiol Mol Biol Rev 2000;64:847-67.

[13] Dunne WM. Bacterial adhesion: seen any good biofilms lately? Clin Microb Rev 2002;15:155-66.

[14] Arciola CR, Campoccia D, Gamberini S, Donati ME, Baldassami L, Montanaro L. Occurrence of ica genes for slime synthesis in a collection of Staphylococcus epidermis strains from orthopedic prosthesis infections. Acta Orthop Scand 2003;74:617-21.

[15] Gilbert P, Das J, Foley I. Biofilms susceptibility to antimicrobials. Adv Dent Res 1997;11:160-7.

[16] Lewis K. Riddle of biofilm resistance. Antimicrobial Agents and Chemotherapy 2001;45:999-1007.

[17] Fux CA, Costerton JW, Steward PS, Stoodley P. Survival strategies of infectious biofilms. Trends in Microbiology 2005;13:34-40.

[18] Chang CC, Merrit K. Infection at the site of implanted materials with and without pre- adhered bacteria. J Orthop Res 1994;12: 526-31.

[19] Ward KH, Olson ME, Lam K, Costerton JW. Mechanism of persistent infection associated with peritoneal implants. J Med Microbiol 1992;36:406-13.

[20] Chun CK, Ozer E, Welsh MJ, Zabner J, Greenberg EP. Inactivation of a Pseudomonas aeruginosa quorum-sensing signal by human airway epithelia. Proc Natl Acad (USA) 2004;101:3587-90.

[21] Hastings JW. Bacterial quorum-sensing signals are inactivated by mammalian cells. PNAS 2004;101:3993-4.

[22] Probert HM, Gibson GR. Bacterial biofilms in the human gastrointestinal tract. Curr Issues Intest Microbiol 2002;3:23-7.

[23] Nulens E, Gould I, MacKenzie F et al. Staphylococcus aureus carriage among participants at the 13th European Congress of Clinical Microbiology and Inectious Diseases. Eur J Clin Microbiol Infect Dis 2005;24:145-8.

[24] Creech CB 2nd, Kernodle DS, Alsentzer A, Wilson C, Edwards KM. Increasing rates of nasal carriage of methicillin-resistant Staphylococcus aureus in healthy children. Pediatr Infect Dis J 2005;24: 617-21.

[25] Miyamoto H, Imamura K, Kojima A, et al. Survey of nasal colonization by, and assesment of a novel multiplex PCR method for detection of biofilm-forming methicillin-resistant staphylococci in healthy medical students. J Hosp Infect 2003;53:215-23.

[26] Dougherty SH, Simmons RL. Endogenous factors contributing to prosthetic device infections. Infect Dis Clin North Am 1989;3:199-209.

[27] Wertheim HF, van Leeuwen WB, Snijders S, et al. Associations between Staphylococcus aureus Genotype, Infection, and In-Hospital mortality: A nested case-control study. J Infect Dis 2005a;192: 1196-200.

[28] Wertheim Hf, Melles DC, Vos MC, van Leeuwen W, van Belkum A, Verbrugh HA, Nouwen JL. The role of nasal carriage in Staphylococcus aureus infections. Lancet Infect Dis 2005b;5:751-62.

[29] Keene A, Vavagiakis P, Lee MH, Finnerty K, Nicolls D, Cespedes C, Quagliarello B, Chiasson MA, Chong D, Lowy FD. Staphylococcus aureus colonization and the risk of infection in critically ill patients. Infect Control Hosp Epidemiol 2005;26:622-8.

[30] Bess J. Infection control. First your nose. Hosp Health Netw 2005; 79:18-20.

[31] Post JC. Direct evidence of bacterial biofilms in otitis media. Laryngoscope 2001;111:2083-94.

[32] Cryer J, Schipor I, Perloff JR, Palmer JN. Evidence of bacterial biofilms in human chronic sinusitis. ORL J Otorhinolaryngol Rel Spec 2004;66:155-8.

[33] Sanclement JA, Webster P, Thomas J, Ramadan HH. Bacterial biofilms in surgical specimens of patients with chronic rhinosinusitis. Laryngoscope 2005;115:578-82.

[34] Kobayashi H. Airway biofilms: implications for pathogenesis and therapy of respiratory tract infections. Treat Respir Med 2005;4: 241-53.

[35] Leung KP, Crowe TD, Abercombie JJ, et al. Control of oral biofilm formation by an antimicrobial decapeptide. J Dent Res 2005;84: 1172-7.

[36] Pihlstrom BL, Michalowicz BS, Johnson NW. Periodontal diseases. Lancet 2005;366:1809-20.

[37] Pedersen SS, Kharazmi A, Espersen F, Hoiby N. Pseudomonas aeruginosa alginate in cystic fibrosis and the inflammatory response. Infect Immun 1990;58:3363-8.

[38] Pier GB. Peptides, Pseudomonas aeruginosa, polysaccharides and lipopolysaccharides-players in the predicament of cystic fibrosis patients. Trends Microbiol 2000;8:247-50.

[39] Rogan MP, Taggart CC, Greene CM, Murphy PG, O'Neill SJ, McElvaney NG. Loss of microbicidal activity and increased formation of biofilm due to decreased lactoferrin activity in patients with cystic fibrosis. J Infect Dis 2004;190:1245-53.

[40] Garcia-Medina R, Dunne WM, Singh PK, Brody SL. Pseudomonas aeruginosa acquires biofilm-like properties within airway epithelial cells. Infect Immun 2005;73:8298-305.

[41] Ehrlich GD, Hu FZ, Lin Q, Costerton JW, Post JC. Intelligent implants to battle biofilms. ASM News 2004;70:127-33.

[42] Gustillo RB, Anderson JT. Prevention of infection in the treatment of 1025 open fractures of long bones: retrospective and prospective analysis. J Bone Joint Surgery (Am) 1976;58:453-458.

[43] Schmidt AH, Swiontkowski MF. Pathophysiology of infections after internal fixations of fractures. J Am Acad Orthop Surg 2000;8:285-291.

[44] Frebourg NB, Cauliez B, Lemeland JF. Evidence for nasal carriage of methicillin-resistant staphylococci colonizing intravascular devices. J Clin Microbiol 1999;37:1182-5.

[45] Rand JA, Morrey BF, Bryan RS. Management of the infected total joint arthroplasty. J Bone Joint Surg [Am] 1983;64:491-504.

[46] Arciola CR, An YH, Campoccia D, Donati ME, Montanaro L. Etiology of implant orthopedic infections. A survey on 1027 clinical isolates. Int J Artif Organs 2005;28:1091-100.

[47] Nelson CL, Mc Laren AC, MCLaren SG, Johnson JW, Smeltzer MS. Is aseptic loosening truly aseptic? Clin Orthopaedics and related research. 2005;437:25-30.

[48] Neut D, van Horn JR, van Kooten TG, van der Mei HC, Busscher HJ. Detection of biomaterial-associated infections in orthopaedic joint implants. Clin Orthop 2003;413:261-8.

[49] Wagner C, Kondella K, Bernschneider T, Heppert V, Wentzensen A, Hansch GM. Post-Traumatic osteitis: analysis of inflammatory cells recruited into the site of infection. Shock 2003;20:503-10.

[50] Wagner C, Kaksa A, Muller W, Denefleh B, Heppert V, Wentzensen A, Hansch GM. Polymorphonuclear neutrophils in posttraumatic os-

teomyelitis: cells recovered from the inflamed site lack chemotactic activity but generate superoxides. Shock 2004;22:108-15.

[51] Wagner C, Hansch GM. Born to kill- bound to die: the role of leukocytes in host defence. Quaderne di infezioni osteoarticolari 2005;4:3-9.

[52] Kubes P, Ward PA. The leukocyte recruitment and the acute inflammatory response. Brain Pathol 2000;10:127-35.

[53] Melnikoff MJ, Horan PK, Morahan PS. Kinetics of changes in peritoneal-cell populations following acute inflammation. Cell Immunol 1989;118:178-91.

[54] Rubin RH, Ferraro MJ. Understanding and diagnosing infectious complications in the immunocompromised host. Current issues and trends. Hematol Oncol Clin North Am 1993;7:795-812.

[55] Takagi J, Springer TA. Integrin activation and structural rearrangement. Immunol Rev 2002;186:141-63.

[56] Kaplanski G, Marin V, Montero-Julian F, Mantovani A, Farnarier C. IL-6: a regulator of the transition from neutrophil to monocyte recruitment during inflammation. Trends Immunol 2003;24:47-52.

[57] Savill J. Apoptosis in resolution of inflammation. J Leuko Biol 1997;61:375-80.

[58] Sendo F, Tsuchida H, Takeda Y, et al. Regulation of neutrophil apoptosis - its biological significance in inflammation and the immune response. Hum Cell 1999;9:215-22.

[59] Kobayashi SD, Voyich JM, Buhl CL, Stahl RM, DeLeo FR. Global changes in gene expression by human polymorphonuclear leukocytes during receptor-mediated phagocytosis: cell fate is regulated at the level of gene expression. Proc Natl Acad Sci USA 2002;99: 6901-6.

[60] Savill J, Wyllie AH, Henson JE, Walport MJ, Henson PM, Haslett C. Macrophage phagocytosis of aging neutrophils in inflammation. Programmed cell death in the neutrophil leads to its recognition by macrophages. J Clin Invest 1989;83:865-75.

[61] Tremblay GM, Janelle MF, Bourbonnais Y. Anti-inflammatory activity of neutrophil elastase inhibitors. Curr Opin Investig Drugs 2003; 4:556-65.

[62] Gardiner EE, Mok SS, Sriratana A, et al. Polymorphonuclear neutrophils release 35S-labelled proteoglycans into cartilage during frustrated phagocytosis. Eur J Biochem 1994;22:871-9.

[63] Dallegri F, Ottonello L. Tissue injury in neutrophilic inflammation. Inflamm Res 1997;46:382-91.

[64] Ward PA, Lentsch AB. The acute inflammatory response and its regulation. Arch Surg 1999;134:666-9.

[65] Zimmermann F, Lautenschlager K, Heppert V, Wentzensen A, Hansch GM, Wagner C. Expression of elastase on polymorphonuclear neutrophils in vitro and in vivo: Identification of CD11b as ligand for the surface-bound elastase. Shock 2005; 23:216-23.

[66] Leid JG, Shirtliff ME, Costerton JW, Stoodley AP. 2002. Human leukocytes adhere to, penetrate, and respond to Staphylococcus aureus biofilms. Infect Immun 70:6339-6345.

[67] Jesaitis AJ, Franklin MJ, Berglund D, et al. Compromised host defense on Pseudomonas aeruginosa biofilms: characterization of neutrophil and biofilm interactions. J Immunol 2003;171:4329-39.

[68] Nimmerjahn F, Ravetch JV. Fc-gamma receptors: old friends and new family members. Immunity 2006;24:19-28.

[69] Nair SP, Meghji S, Wilson M, Krisanavane R, White P, Henderson B. Bacterially induced bone destruction: mechanisms and misconceptions. Infect Immun 1996;64:2371-80.

[70] Hendersen B, Nair SP. Hard labour: bacterial infection of the skeleton. Trends in Microbiology 2003;11:570-7.

[71] Goldring SR. Inflammatory mediators as essential elements in bone remodeling. Calcif Tissue Int 2003;73:97-100.

[72] Walsh NC, Gravellese EM. 2004. Bone loss in inflammatory arthritis: mechanisms and treatment strategies. Current Opinion in Rheumatology 2004;16:419-27.

[73] Horowitz MC, Lorenzo JA. The origins of osteoclasts. Curr Opin Rheumatol 2004;16:456-64.

[74] Bendre MS, Montague DC, Peery T, Akel NS, Gaddy D, Suva LJ. Interleukin-8 stimulation of osteoclastogenesis and bone resorption is a mechanism for the increased osteolysis of metastatic bone disease. Bone 2003;33:28-37.

[75] Boyle WJ, Simonet WS, Lacey DL. Osteoclast differentiation and activation. Nature 2003;423:337-42.

[76] Kudo O, Fujikawa Y, Itonaga I, Sabokbar A, Torisu T, Athanasou NA. Proinflammatory cytokine (TNFalpha/IL-1 alpha) induction of human osteoclast formation. J Pathol 2002;198:220-7.

[77] Theill LE, Boyle WJ, Penninger JM. RANK-L and RANK: T cells, bone loss, and mammalian evolution. Annu Rev Immunol 2002; 20:795-823.

Biofilms and Orthopaedic Infections

Charalampos G. ZALAVRAS[a], William J. COSTERTON[b*]

[a]Department of Orthopaedic Surgery, University of Southern California, Keck School of Medicine, LAC + USC Medical Center, Los Angeles, CA, USA
[b]Center for Biofilms, University of Southern California, School of Dentistry, Los Angeles, CA, USA

A biofilm is a highly structured community of bacterial cells that adopt a distinct phenotype, communicate with cell-cell signals, and are enclosed in a self-produced polymeric matrix consisting primarily of polysaccharides. Biofilm formation is a key pathogenetic feature of chronic orthopaedic infections. In biofilm-associated infections the diagnostic usefulness of traditional microbiological culture techniques is questionable and negative results do not indicate the absence of pathogens growing in biofilms. Novel diagnostic methods for detection of biofilm infections include microscopic methods, molecular methods, and immunological assays. Antibiotic therapy alone is ineffective and radical debridement with removal of implants and dead bone remains the cornerstone of management. Prevention of biofilm formation may be achieved by elimination of organic debris from orthopaedic implants, killing of planktonic cells prior to biofilm development, and inhibition of bacterial quorum-sensing communication.

Keywords: biofilm; chronic infection; osteomyelitis.

1. INTRODUCTION

Study of natural ecosystems has demonstrated that individual floating (planktonic) bacteria are rare; instead, bacteria grow predominantly in biofilm formations [1]. A biofilm is a highly structured community of bacterial cells that adopt a distinct phenotype [2], communicate with cell-to-cell signals [3], and are enclosed in a self-produced polymeric matrix (slime) consisting primarily of polysaccharides [4, 5]. Formation of this community undergoes various stages that include initial attachment of bacteria to an inert or living surface, microcolony formation, maturation of attached bacteria into differentiated biofilm, and subsequent detachment of planktonic cells [1, 4, 6, 7].

This chapter will present the role of biofilm formation in chronic orthopaedic infections and will discuss current concepts in the diagnosis, management, and prevention of biofilm-associated infections.

2. BIOFILMS IN CHRONIC INFECTIONS

Biofilm formation has been shown to be a key pathogenetic feature of chronic bacterial infections, which now comprise 65% of bacterial and fungal infections in the industrial world [5]. The biofilm constitutes a protected form of bacterial growth that allows survival in a hostile environment; compared to planktonic cells, sessile biofilm cells are less susceptible to antibiotics and host immune responses. Protective mechanisms include incomplete biofilm

*Corresponding Author
University of Southern California, School of Dentistry
925 West 34th St.
Los Angeles, CA 90089, USA
Tel: +1 213 740 2538
Fax: +1 213 740 5715
e-mail: costerto@usc.edu

penetration by antibiotics and antibodies, altered chemical microenvironment, slow-growing or starved state of biofilm cells, and development of resistant phenotypes as an adaptive response to stress [5, 8, 9].

Therefore, biofilm formation offers an explanation to the distinct features and persistent nature of chronic bacterial infections: presentation is usually less pronounced (or even subclinical), diagnosis with traditional microbiological methods is unreliable, and antibiotic therapy is ineffective [5].

3. BIOFILMS IN CHRONIC ORTHOPAEDIC INFECTIONS

Gristina and Costerton demonstrated the association of musculoskeletal prosthetic infections with biofilm formation using scanning and transmission electron microscopy. [10] Subsequent direct examination of tissue and biomaterials retrieved from patients with chronic musculoskeletal infections yielded similar findings [11, 12]. Biofilm formations adherent to foreign bodies were present in 76% (19/25) of foreign body infections in general and in 59% (10/17) of orthopaedic implant-related infections [12].

Mayberry-Carson et al. experimentally induced *Staphylococcus aureus* osteomyelitis in rabbit tibiae in the presence of a foreign body, and demonstrated by direct microscopic techniques the extensive formation of glycocalyx adhering to the bone and implant [13]. Additional investigations described biofilm formation as a key feature of experimental foreign-body-associated osteomyelitis [14, 15].

Therefore, in chronic osteomyelitis and implant-associated infections bacteria grow in biofilms attached on the surface of dead bone or foreign material. This protective mode of growth shields bacteria from antibiotics and host defense mechanisms, leading to persistence of infection [5, 8, 9]. The widespread occurrence and the challenging management of chronic orthopaedic infections urge both basic scientists and clinicians to employ concepts and methods of modern biofilm microbiology to the diagnosis, management, and prevention of these biofilm-associated diseases.

4. DIAGNOSIS OF ORTHOPAEDIC BIOFILM INFECTIONS

Chronic biofilm infections present a diagnostic challenge, because they elicit a less pronounced inflammatory response compared to infections due to planktonic bacterial cells; biofilm infections may even follow a subclinical course without eliciting symptoms for months or years [16, 17].

Even when symptoms do occur, traditional microbiological diagnostic techniques may not be accurate because these techniques depend on isolation and culture of planktonic bacteria [16, 17]. In contrast, biofilm cells

grow poorly, if at all, on agar plates. Therefore, in biofilm infections the diagnostic usefulness of culture techniques is questionable. It has been shown that cells of *Staphylococcus aureus* growing in biofilms in the human vagina cannot be detected by swab recovery and plating on appropriate agar media [18].

Dobbins et al. investigated the presence of occult infection in orthopaedic devices removed for reasons other than infection [19]. Cultures of metallic scrapings after sonication were positive for coagulase-negative *Staphylococcus* in 58% (15/26) of cases, whereas swab cultures were positive in only 12% (3/26).

Tunney et al. reported that, after sonication, quantifiable numbers of bacteria were cultured from 22% (26/120) of total hip implants examined during revision surgery [20]. The same bacterial species were cultured by routine microbiological techniques from corresponding tissue samples in only 4% of cases (5/120). In 18 of the 26 culture-positive cases, there were adequate tissue samples for pathologic examination, which showed the presence of inflammatory cells. In 12 of these 18 patients the preoperative diagnosis was aseptic loosening; the remaining 6 patients had a history of infection but preoperative aspiration cultures were negative in 4.

Similarly, bacterial biofilms were detected on 8 of 10 acetabular cups removed for aseptic loosening while bacterial cultures from either hip aspirates or from removed devices were negative [16]. These findings cast doubt on the preoperative diagnosis of "aseptic" loosening and on the value of traditional microbiological methods in the setting of chronic orthopaedic implant-related infections. We must remember that negative results do not indicate the absence of pathogens growing in biofilms. Neut et al. pointed out that "the search for infecting organisms in excised tissue, as currently done, can be compared with the search for a needle in a haystack, although it is known where the needle can be found: on the biomaterial surface of the prostheses" [21]. Novel diagnostic methods for detection of biofilm infections are now available to assist us in the "search for the needle", and they include microscopic methods, molecular methods, immunological assays, and combinations thereof [16, 22].

4.1. Molecular and microscopic methods

The synthesis of molecular and microscopic methods will produce an increment in understanding that will transform Microbiology. Specially designed probes conjugated to fluorescent stains allow direct visualization of biofilm bacteria. Nucleic-acid-targeted probes stain all microorganisms present in a biofilm, irrespective of their viability. Combined with confocal scanning laser microscopy (CSLM) this technique visualizes the sample in three dimensions and provides information on aspects of biofilm structure, such as thickness and presence of water channels.

Fluorescent in situ hybridization (FISH) uses rRNA-targeted probes and with CSLM allows for detection of organisms within a biofilm. Non-specific FISH probes can locate all bacterial cells, in broad categories, in their correct spatial relationships to physical surfaces and co-colonizing or host eukaryotic cells. We can then use species-specific 16 S rRNA FISH probes and fluorescent antibodies to subdivide the broad bacterial categories, and to identify and locate cells of known bacterial species in their correct spatial relationships to each o-ther. In these molecular based techniques for direct microscopy we can see and count individual bacterial cells, in relation to cells of other species and to host cells, and we can detect both bacterial and host re-actions to these juxtapositions.

Fluorescent probes can also evaluate the viability of microorganisms within a biofilm. The Live/Dead Bac-Light viability assay (Molecular Probes Inc., Eugene, OR) differentially stains microbial cells based on the integrity of the cell membrane, thereby staining living bacteria green and dead ones red; this will let us determine the extent to which anti-bacterial agents have killed bacterial cells in biofilms.

Multiple displacement amplification (MDA), using a unique Phi 29 phage enzyme, now allows us to amplify the DNA from very small numbers (1-10) of prokaryotic or eukaryotic cells, and to obtain sufficient DNA for full genomic characterization of these cells [23]. Further-more, mRNA can also be obtained from larger numbers (1,200-1,500) of prokaryotic or eukaryotic cells, and this pivotal nucleic acid can be used for quantitative analy-ses of the expression of known genes by clonal aggre-gates of these cells.

The development of these new molecular techniques can now be linked to the equally explosive parallel de-velopment of new microscopic methods, by the simple expedient of existing "capture" technologies that allow us to excise and recover cells for molecular analysis. Specifically, the new Zeiss 2-photon confocal micro-scope with PALM micro-dissection capability (Carl Zeiss MicroImaging, Inc., Thornwood, NY) will allow us to visualize bacteria in natural and pathogenic ecosystems, and then to recover clonal aggregates of either bacteria or eukaryotic cells for genomic or expressomic analysis, leading to an even deeper understanding of the struc-ture and function of natural and pathogenic communi-ties.

Differential Gradient Gel Electrophoresis (DGGE) yields very practical semi-quantitative data on the pre-dominant species present in an ecosystem, and the re-finement of this technique, (Denaturing High Perfor-mance Liquid Chromatography [DHPLC]), in which de-natured DNA is separated on an HPLC column, has im-proved resolution and enabled us to recover the DNA for analysis using specific primers. Two new technology streams now converge in that we can extract DNA from whole ecosystems and identify the predominant species present, and we can visualize bacterial cells in situ in ac-tual ecosystems and amplify their DNA following precise micro-dissection of clonal aggregates. Both of these methods yield DNA from cells that have not been iso-lated, and may never have been cultured, but we can identify their entire genomes, determine their 16 S rRNA sequences, and construct FISH probes to identify the in-dividual cells in the mixed species ecosystem. These technical developments will remove cultures from the equation, in that predominant organisms and organisms of special interest can be identified without ever having been isolated or cultured and their 16 S rRNA "sig-natures" can be added to the database that will serve all fields within Microbiology.

4.2. Immunologic methods

Biofilm bacteria produce surface proteins that are dis-tinct from those on the surfaces of planktonic cells of the same species [2]. Therefore, the hypothesis was gene-rated that the humoral immune system will react to the presence of immunogenic epitopes on the surfaces of biofilm bacteria by producing antibodies specific for these bacteria. Selan et al. [24] demonstrated that these distinct immunologic interactions between biofilm bacte-ria and the host could form the basis for a novel dia-gnostic technique. The authors identified a surface epitope, the Staphylococcal Slime Polysaccharide Anti-gen (SSPA), which is produced by biofilm cells of *Sta-phylococcus aureus* and *Staphylococcus epidermidis,* but not by their planktonic counterparts. Subsequently, they developed an enzyme-linked immunosorbent assay (ELISA) test with very high sensitivity and specificity for detection of antibodies to this epitope in patients who had received vascular grafts [24]. This immunodiagnos-tic technique, if shown to be sensitive and specific for or-thopaedic biofilm infections, has the potential to greatly enhance our ability to diagnose and treat these infec-tions, before they even become clinically apparent. As a next step, anti-biofilm antibiodies may be tagged with "opacity markers" for various types of scans and deter-mine the location of infection.

5. TREATMENT OF ORTHOPAEDIC BIOFILM INFECTIONS

Antibiotic therapy is effective against planktonic bacteria that are released from biofilms but not against bacteria within a biofilm; thus, resolution of acute symptoms - caused by planktonic bacteria - may take place, but the sessile biofilm bacteria will remain unaffected, leading to exacerbations of the infection at a future time. Similarly, host defense mechanisms attack the biofilm, triggering inflammation, but remain ineffective in this siege warfare against an apparently impenetrable fortress.

Various therapeutic approaches have been ex-plored but without conclusive results. High-dose com-bined administration of tobramycin and piperacillin eradicated *in vitro* young biofilm cells of Pseudomonas aeruginosa but not old biofilm cells [25, 26]. Clari-thromycin has shown promising results [27]. Very high doses of antibiotics may improve action against biofilm bacteria; local delivery will avoid systemic toxicity, however issues that need to be addressed include the mode of delivery and the potential for osteoblastic adverse effects.

Proteolytic enzymes, direct current, and ultrasound application have shown a beneficial effect when administered concurrently with antibiotics. Serratiopeptidase enhanced the activity of ofloxacin against sessile bacteria and inhibited biofilm formation [28]. Application of direct current electrical field increased the bactericidal action of tobramycin against Pseudomonas aeruginosa growing in biofilms [29, 30]. Ultrasound application enhanced the action of vancomycin and gentamicin against biofilms of *Staphylococcus epidermidis* and *E. coli,* respectively [31, 32]. However, *Pseudomonas aeruginosa* biofilms treated with gentamicin did not demonstrate a significant ultrasound-enhanced reduction in the number of viable bacteria [31].

During this elusive search for the Achilles heel of formed biofilms, the time-tested principle of aggressive surgical debridement remains the cornerstone of management of chronic biofilm-associated infections of the musculoskeletal system [33-35]. All dead bone should be debrided and all foreign material should be removed, thereby removing the attached biofilm and initiating a new "race for the surface" [36].

6. PREVENTION OF ORTHOPAEDIC BIOFILM INFECTIONS

Prevention of orthopaedic biofilm infections is an exciting new concept that can be pursued via elimination of organic debris from orthopaedic implants, killing of planktonic cells prior to biofilm development, and inhibition of bacterial cell communication that precedes biofilm formation.

6.1. Surface cleaning of orthopaedic implants

Research in the water industry has shown that contamination of surfaces by organic materials (especially residual biofilm matrices) accelerates the process of planktonic cells attraction and biofilm formation by at least tenfold [1]. The presence of any residual biofilm matrix on a biomaterial surface favors colonization and infection; therefore, plastic or metal biomaterials must be perfectly clean prior to implantation. Orthopaedic prostheses are manufactured by machining techniques that favor biofilm development and simple sterilization (e.g. ethylene oxide) kills the bacteria in these biofilms, but fails to remove the residue of their matrices. Removal of these deposits before the devices are implanted offers a possibility to intervene preventatively. The combined administration of enzymes and chemical agents (alkaline detergent and sodium hypochlorite solution) has been shown to eradicate biofilm both *in vitro* and in a clinically used dialysis machine [37].

6.2. Killing of planktonic cells prior to biofilm development

Another strategy for the prevention of colonization and consequent biofilm formation on biomaterials is the use of materials and coatings that release conventional antibiotics into the surrounding tissues and fluids, in order to kill planktonic cells before they can initiate biofilm formation on the biomaterial. Elution of antibiotics from currently available local antibiotic delivery systems (e.g. PMMA cement) follows a biphasic pattern with an initial rapid phase and a secondary slow phase [38]. This may prevent colonization of implants during the early postoperative period; however, subinhibitory antibiotic concentrations may favor the development of resistant strains of bacteria.

These concerns may be alleviated by a novel drug delivery vehicle, which consists of a polymer hydrogel matrix coated with ordered methylene chains that form an ultrasound-responsive coating [39]. This system was able to retain ciprofloxacin inside the polymer in the absence of ultrasound but showed significant drug release when low-intensity ultrasound was applied. *In vitro* experiments demonstrated that accumulation of Pseudomonas aeruginosa biofilms was significantly reduced on ciprofloxacin-loaded hydrogels with ultrasound-induced drug delivery compared to biofilms grown in control experiments [39]. Future development of medical devices sensitive to external ultrasonic impulses and capable of preventing biofilm growth via "on-demand" release of antibiotics may be a useful addition to the orthopaedic surgeon's armamentarium.

6.3. Quorum sensing inhibition

Bacterial cell-cell signaling (quorum sensing) is a key event preceding formation of a biofilm. Bacteria produce and release chemical signaling molecules, the concentration of which increases as a function of cell density [3]. The signals that exercise this control are simple acyl-homoserine lactones (AHLs), in the case of gram-negative bacteria [40], and simple cyclic octapeptides in gram-positive bacteria [41]. When the concentration of these signaling molecules - and therefore the bacterial population - exceeds a threshold, distinct patterns of gene expression are promoted and biofilm formation is initiated.

The discovery that the development of microbial biofilms is controlled by the quorum sensing process offers a new approach to the prevention of chronic biofilm infections. It has been shown that natural and synthetic molecules that mimic these signals, react with the cognitive signal receptor proteins, and attenuate biofilm formation [42-45].

Seaweeds are devoid of advanced immune systems but are resistant to colonization by both prokaryotes and eukaryotes due to the production of furanones, which, amongst other functions, inhibit AHL-mediated quorum sensing [43]. Synthetic furanones were able to reduce the virulence of *Pseudomonas aeruginosa* and increased biofilm susceptibility to both tobramycin and immune mechanisms [42].

Similary, virulence factor synthesis and biofilm formation by *Staphylococcus aureus* is controlled by a regulatory RNA molecule (RNAIII), which is inhibited by the naturally occurring and synthetically available RNAIII-inhibiting peptide (RIP) [41]. Balaban et al. demonstrated that the RIP prevents biofilm formation by *Staphylococus aureus* and *Staphylococcus epidermidis* [44, 46]. This inhibition of biofilm formation was shown in elegant animal models of device-related infection and the inhibitor was shown to be especially effective in infection control if it was combined with an antibiotic (mupurocin) [44]. The recently reported synergistic action of RIP with antibiotics may improve not only prevention but also treatment of staphylococcal infections [47].

7. CONCLUSION

In conclusion, the new developments in diagnosis, treatment, and prevention of biofilm-associated bacterial growth offer the tools for a revolutionized approach towards these challenging infections. Close collaboration between microbiologists and surgeons is essential to optimize efficiency of these tools and maximize benefit to the patients with chronic orthopaedic infections.

REFERENCES

[1] Costerton JW, Lewandowski Z, Caldwell DE, Korber DR, Lappin-Scott HM. Microbial biofilms. Annu Rev Microbiol 1995;49:711-745.

[2] Sauer K, Camper AK, Ehrlich GD, Costerton JW, Davies DG. Pseudomonas aeruginosa displays multiple phenotypes during development as a biofilm. J Bacteriol 2002;184(4):1140-1154.

[3] Davies DG, Parsek MR, Pearson JP, et al. The involvement of cell-to-cell signals in the development of a bacterial biofilm. Science 1998;280(5361):295-298.

[4] Stoodley P, Sauer K, Davies DG, Costerton JW. Biofilms as complex differentiated communities. Annu Rev Microbiol 2002;56:187-209.

[5] Costerton JW, Stewart PS, Greenberg EP. Bacterial biofilms: a common cause of persistent infections. Science 1999;284 (5418):1318-1322.

[6] Stoodley P, Wilson S, Hall-Stoodley L, et al. Growth and detachment of cell clusters from mature mixed-species biofilms. Appl Environ Microbiol 2001;67(12):5608-5613.

[7] Costerton JW. Introduction to biofilm. Int J Antimicrob Agents 1999;11(3-4):217-221; discussion 237-219.

[8] Fux CA, Costerton JW, Stewart PS, Stoodley P. Survival strategies of infectious biofilms. Trends Microbiol 2005;13(1):34-40.

[9] Stewart PS, Costerton JW. Antibiotic resistance of bacteria in biofilms. Lancet 2001;358(9276):135-138.

[10] Gristina AG, Costerton JW. Bacterial adherence and the glycocalyx and their role in musculoskeletal infection. Orthop Clin North Am 1984;15(3):517-535.

[11] Marrie TJ, Costerton JW. Mode of growth of bacterial pathogens in chronic polymicrobial human osteomyelitis. J Clin Microbiol 1985;22(6):924-933.

[12] Gristina AG, Costerton JW. Bacterial adherence to biomaterials and tissue. The significance of its role in clinical sepsis. J Bone Joint Surg [Am] 1985;67(2):264-273.

[13] Mayberry-Carson KJ, Tober-Meyer B, Smith JK, Lambe DW, Jr., Costerton JW. Bacterial adherence and glycocalyx formation in osteomyelitis experimentally induced with Staphylococcus aureus. Infect Immun 1984;43(3):825-833.

[14] Lambe DW, Jr., Ferguson KP, Mayberry-Carson KJ, Tober-Meyer B, Costerton JW. Foreign-body-associated experimental osteomyelitis induced with Bacteroides fragilis and Staphylococcus epidermidis in rabbits. Clin Orthop Relat Res 1991;(266):285-294.

[15] Buxton TB, Horner J, Hinton A, Rissing JP. *In vivo* glycocalyx expression by Staphylococcus aureus phage type 52/52A/80 in S. aureus osteomyelitis. J Infect Dis 1987;156(6):942-946.

[16] Costerton JW. Biofilm theory can guide the treatment of device-related orthopaedic infections. Clin Orthop Relat Res 2005; (437):7-11.

[17] Fux CA, Stoodley P, Hall-Stoodley L, Costerton JW. Bacterial biofilms: a diagnostic and therapeutic challenge. Expert Rev Anti Infect Ther 2003;1(4):667-683.

[18] Veeh RH, Shirtliff ME, Petik JR, et al. Detection of Staphylococcus aureus biofilm on tampons and menses components. J Infect Dis 2003;188(4):519-530.

[19] Dobbins JJ, Seligson D, Raff MJ. Bacterial colonization of orthopedic fixation devices in the absence of clinical infection. J Infect Dis 1988;158(1):203-205.

[20] Tunney MM, Patrick S, Gorman SP, et al. Improved detection of infection in hip replacements. A currently underestimated problem. J Bone Joint Surg [Br] 1998;80(4):568-572.

[21] Neut D, van Horn JR, van Kooten TG, van der Mei HC, Busscher HJ. Detection of biomaterial-associated infections in orthopaedic joint implants. Clin Orthop Relat Res 2003;(413):261-268.

[22] Donlan RM. New approaches for the characterization of prosthetic joint biofilms. Clin Orthop Relat Res 2005;(437):12-19.

[23] Raghunathan A, Ferguson HR, Jr., Bornarth CJ, et al. Genomic DNA amplification from a single bacterium. Appl Environ Microbiol 2005;71(6):3342-3347.

[24] Selan L, Passariello C. Microbiological diagnosis of aortofemoral graft infections. Eur J Vasc Endovasc Surg 1997;14 Suppl A:10-12.

[25] Anwar H, Costerton JW. Enhanced activity of combination of tobramycin and piperacillin for eradication of sessile biofilm cells of Pseudomonas aeruginosa. Antimicrob Agents Chemother 1990;34(9):1666-1671.

[26] Anwar H, Strap JL, Chen K, Costerton JW. Dynamic interactions of biofilms of mucoid Pseudomonas aeruginosa with tobramycin and piperacillin. Antimicrob Agents Chemother 1992;36(6):1208-1214.

[27] Sano M, Hirose T, Nishimura M, et al. Inhibitory action of clarithromycin on glycocalyx produced by MRSA. J Infect Chemother 1999;5(1):10-15.

[28] Selan L, Berlutti F, Passariello C, Comodi-Ballanti MR, Thaller MC. Proteolytic enzymes: a new treatment strategy for prosthetic infections? Antimicrob Agents Chemother 1993;37(12):2618-2621.

[29] McLeod BR, Fortun S, Costerton JW, Stewart PS. Enhanced bac-

terial biofilm control using electromagnetic fields in combination with antibiotics. Methods Enzymol 1999;310:656-670.

[30] Blenkinsopp SA, Khoury AE, Costerton JW. Electrical enhancement of biocide efficacy against Pseudomonas aeruginosa biofilms. Appl Environ Microbiol 1992;58(11):3770-3773.

[31] Carmen JC, Roeder BL, Nelson JL, et al. Treatment of biofilm infections on implants with low-frequency ultrasound and antibiotics. Am J Infect Control 2005;33(2):78-82.

[32] Carmen JC, Roeder BL, Nelson JL, et al. Ultrasonically enhanced vancomycin activity against Staphylococcus epidermidis biofilms in vivo. J Biomater Appl 2004;18(4):237-245.

[33] Patzakis MJ, Zalavras CG. Chronic posttraumatic osteomyelitis and infected nonunion of the tibia: current management concepts. J Am Acad Orthop Surg 2005;13(6):417-427.

[34] Costerton W, Veeh R, Shirtliff M, et al. The application of biofilm science to the study and control of chronic bacterial infections. J Clin Invest 2003;112(10):1466-1477.

[35] Zalavras CG, Patzakis MJ, Thordarson DB, et al. Infected fractures of the distal tibial metaphysis and plafond: achievement of limb salvage with free muscle flaps, bone grafting, and ankle fusion. Clin Orthop Relat Res 2004;(427):57-62.

[36] Gristina AG, Naylor P, Myrvik Q. Infections from biomaterials and implants: a race for the surface. Med Prog Technol 1988;14(3-4):205-224.

[37] Marion K, Pasmore M, Freney J, et al. A new procedure allowing the complete removal and prevention of hemodialysis biofilms. Blood Purif 2005;23(5):339-348.

[38] Zalavras CG, Patzakis MJ, Holtom P. Local antibiotic therapy in the treatment of open fractures and osteomyelitis. Clin Orthop Relat Res 2004;(427):86-93.

[39] Norris P, Noble M, Francolini I, et al. Ultrasonically controlled release of ciprofloxacin from self-assembled coatings on poly (2-hydroxyethyl methacrylate) hydrogels for Pseudomonas aeruginosa biofilm prevention. Antimicrob Agents Chemother 2005; 49(10):4272-4279.

[40] Fuqua WC, Winans SC, Greenberg EP. Quorum sensing in bacteria: the LuxR-LuxI family of cell density-responsive transcriptional regulators. J Bacteriol 1994;176(2):269-275.

[41] Balaban N, Goldkorn T, Nhan RT, et al. Autoinducer of virulence as a target for vaccine and therapy against Staphylococcus aureus. Science 1998;280(5362):438-440.

[42] Hentzer M, Wu H, Andersen JB, et al. Attenuation of Pseudomonas aeruginosa virulence by quorum sensing inhibitors. Embo J 2003;22(15):3803-3815.

[43] de Nys R, Givskov M, Kumar N, Kjelleberg S, Steinberg PD. Furanones. Prog Mol Subcell Biol 2006;42:55-86.

[44] Balaban N, Giacometti A, Cirioni O, et al. Use of the quorum-sensing inhibitor RNAIII-inhibiting peptide to prevent biofilm formation in vivo by drug-resistant Staphylococcus epidermidis. J Infect Dis 2003;187(4):625-630.

[45] Balaban N, Stoodley P, Fux CA, et al. Prevention of staphylococcal biofilm-associated infections by the quorum sensing inhibitor RIP. Clin Orthop Relat Res 2005;(437):48-54.

[46] Balaban N, Gov Y, Bitler A, Boelaert JR. Prevention of Staphylococcus aureus biofilm on dialysis catheters and adherence to human cells. Kidney Int 2003;63(1):340-345.

[47] Giacometti A, Cirioni O, Ghiselli R, et al. RNAIII-inhibiting peptide improves efficacy of clinically used antibiotics in a murine model of staphylococcal sepsis. Peptides 2005;26(2):169-175.

chapter
7

Prophylaxis from Musculoskeletal Infection in Upper Limb Surgery

Antonios PAPADOPOULOS, Helen GIAMARELLOU*

4th University Department of Internal Medicine, "ATTIKON" University Hospital, Athens, Greece

Postoperative surgical site infection remains a major problem in orthopaedic and especially in upper limb surgery. The identification of patient and operation characteristics and risk factors, which can influence the risk of infection, are crucial in order to implement efficient prevention measures. Antibiotic prophylaxis is one of the most effective measures in both elective and emergency hand surgery. It is recommended mostly in elective procedures involving implants and procedures of long duration (>2 hours), while in dirty complex open hand wounds, animal or human bites and open fractures it might be considered as therapy. First or second generation cephalosporins (or alternatively hemisynthetic penicillins, clindamycin and in special circumstances, glycopeptides) are used, but in cases of Gram negative or anaerobic bacteria contamination, an aminoglucoside or high dose penicillin must be added. Antibiotics must be administered 1-2 hours preoperatively, and if possible, during induction of anesthesia and generally for no more than 24 hours. In any case, antimicrobial prophylaxis cannot be a substitute to a good clinical technique.

Keywords: antibiotic prophylaxis; surgical prophylaxis; upper limb surgery; hand surgery.

1. INTRODUCTION

Despite the advances in modern surgery, postoperative surgical site infection (SSI) remains a major cause of operative morbidity and mortality and this fact is applied to every surgical sub-specialty, including orthopaedic surgery [1]. Prevention of SSI must take into account many variables, including host response, wound environment and bacterial burden introduced into the surgical wound [2]. Various prophylactic and critical measures must be taken, such as the assessment of the patient's risk factors, the application of proper preoperative planning, a meticulous surgical technique, as well as careful postoperative care [3]. The administration

of systemic antibiotics immediately before surgery (antibiotic prophylaxis, AP) is the most effective prophylactic measure and it is now well established that it significantly reduces the incidence of postoperative SSI in all surgical categories [2]. AP has become the standard of care in surgical procedures involving foreign materials, grafts or prosthetic devices or implants, but its use in clean non-implant wounds is still controversial [4]. These principles are also applied in orthopaedic and especially in upper limb surgery, but many issues concerning prevention of infection remain unresolved. Moreover, it must always be remembered that AP is not a substitute for good surgery.

2. PERIOPERATIVE INFECTION AND ANTIBIOTIC PROPHYLAXIS IN ORTHOPAEDIC SURGERY

2.1. Pathogenesis of infection and responsible microorganisms

Microorganisms can be introduced into the wound from the skin flora, from the operating room en-

*Corresponding Author
4th University Department of Internal Medicine
"Attikon" University Hospital
1 Rimini St, Haidari, Athens 12462
Tel: +30210 5831990
e-mail: hgiama@forthnet.ath.gr

vironment, from postoperative contamination, and haematogenously, from a remote anatomic site [5]. In orthopaedic surgery *S.aureus* and coagulase-negative staphylococci (CNS), particularly *S.epidermidis,* are responsible for up to 70-90% of postoperative infections [4]. In clean procedures *S.aureus* is the predominant pathogen. In infected joint arthroplasty *S.epidermidis* (and other CNS) and *S.aureus* are the most common pathogens, with reported frequency of 20-40% and 20-35%, respectively [6-8]. Less common pathogens include aerobic and anaerobic streptococci, diphtheroids, *Corynebacterium* spp, *Bacillus* spp, *C.perfrigens,* enterobacteriaceae and *Bacteroides* spp. Mixed infections can occur, especially in open, contaminated wounds [4, 6]. The same microorganisms are isolated in patients with closed fractures, use of nails, bone plates and other internal fixation devices, functional repair without implant, and in trauma [9]. In upper limb surgery the isolated (or possibly acting) microorganisms are the same as in other types of orthopaedic surgery [10].

2.2. Goals and principles of antibiotic prophylaxis

The goals of AP are: (i) to reduce the incidence of postoperative SSIs and the subsequent morbitity and mortality, (ii) to minimize the effect of antibiotics in the patient's normal microbial flora and prevent the appearance of adverse events and bacterial resistance in particular, and (iii) to reduce the duration and cost of health care [8, 11].

AP refers to a very brief course of an antimicrobial agent initiated just before the beginning of an operation, and better, upon induction of anesthesia [9]. It is limited to operations with a high infection rate or serious consequences of infection, such as the implantation of prosthetic material [1]. It is not an attempt to sterilize tissues but rather to reduce the microbial flora of intraoperative contamination to a level that it can be effectively managed by the host defenses [9]. It is directed against the most likely infecting organism and does not need to eradicate every potential pathogen [1, 9, 12]. AP inhibits growth of contaminant bacteria and their adherence to prosthetic implants [11].

Here are some general principles that govern the administration of AP in orthopaedic surgery:
(a) Ideally, the antimicrobial agent should be administered as near to the incision time as possible, to achieve lower SSI rates [13]. The optimal timing of antibiotic administration is 30-60 minutes prior to incision and within 2 hours if vancomycin is indicated [2, 3, 9, 11, 13-15]. There is enough evidence that the administration of the drug at the time of anesthesia induction is safe and effective [8, 13, 16]. The risk of SSI increases 2- to 6-fold when AP is given too early or too late (>2 hours prior to or >2 hours after the initial incision respectively) [14, 17]. Whenever a proximal tourniquet is required, the entire antimicrobial dose should be administered before the tourniquet is inflated [2, 11, 13, 18].

(b) Current consensus among various guidelines is on discontinuation of AP within 24 hours after the end of the operation [3, 8, 13, 15]. A single prophylactic dose is normally sufficient and postoperative doses are usually unnecessary and should not be given [11-13]. Most studies showed no benefit of additional doses, when single doses were compared with multiple ones [13]. If the antimicrobial agent has a short half-life (eg. 2 hours for cefazolin) and the duration of the operation is more than 3-4 hours or above 1-2 times the half-life of the drug, or if there is major blood loss during the operation (eg. >1500 ml), then additional doses of the drug may be justified during the procedure [1, 9, 11, 13, 15]. Medical literature also does not support the continuation of antimicrobial agents until all drains or catheters are removed, and provides no evidence of benefit when they are continued for more than 24 hours [2, 15].
(c) Antimicrobial agents should be administered intravenously and in the same dose as that for the therapy of infection [11]. The dose should be based on the patient's weight or body mass index - larger doses are needed for morbidly obese patients [2, 9, 13, 15].

2.3. Choice of appropriate antimicrobial agent

Many different antibiotics are appropriate for AP and the selection of a drug should take into account not only comparative efficacy but also local epidemiological and resistance patterns [8, 11, 12]. Numerous older, relatively narrow-spectrum agents (eg. first or second generation cephalosporins, hemi-synthetic penicillins) are suitable for use, while newer, broad-spectrum drugs should be avoided (eg. third generation cephalosporins) or restricted and used under certain circumstances (eg. glycopeptides) [1, 12, 13].

The first and second generation cephalosporins (eg. cefazolin, cefuroxime) exhibit a time-dependent bactericidal action and demonstrate a reasonably broad spectrum of activity, good pharmacokinetics, low rate of allergic responses, limited adverse events (mostly diarrhea and occasionally *C.difficile*-associated colitis) and acceptable cost [4, 9]. Cefazolin (1-2 g) is a good choice for clean operations and provides adequate blood and tissue concentration above the MIC of common SSI microorganisms. Some second generation cephalosporins, eg. cefuroxime (1.5 g) or cefamandole (2 g) have been shown more effective *in vitro* than cefazolin against some strains of methicillin-sensitive S. aureus (MSSA) and should be considered at least as appropriate as cefazolin for AP in clean surgery [2, 8, 13, 18]. This recommendation is endorsed by various societies [13]. In cases of allergy, clindamycin or a glycopeptide (eg. vancomycin) can be used [9]. The third and fourth generation cephalosporins are contraindicated for AP because: (i) they are less active than cefazolin against staphylococci, (ii) their spectrum of activity includes microorganisms rarely encountered in elective orthopaedic surgery, (iii) their use promote the emergence of resistant microorganisms, especially enterococci, and (iv) they are more expensive than other alternatives [1, 8, 12]. For practically the same reasons, fluoroquinolones should not be used in AP.

The routine use of glycopeptides (vancomycin or teicoplanin) in AP is not recommended for any kind of operation [2, 9, 11]. No prospective comparative data exist on the clinical efficacy of cephalosporins or hemisynthetic penicillin compounds versus a glycopeptide for prevention of infections associated with prosthetic implants [2, 19]. Clinical trials have failed to show an advandage of glycopeptide over β-lactam antibiotics despite the high prevalence of methicillin-resistant S.epidermidis (MRSE) in those infections [11]. Due to absence of evidence of clinical benefit from glycopeptides, and for fear of the increase in the prevalence of vancomycin-resistant enterococci (VRE) and S.aureus (VRSA) their overuse may cause, coupled with the fact that glycopeptides are inferior antistaphylococcal agents for methicillin-sensitive strains (compared to cephalosporins and penicillinase-resistant penicillins), various guidelines are against the use of those agents in AP [2, 8, 11, 12].

However, surgeons increasingly use vancomycin due to:
(i) the rising prevalence of methicillin-resistant S. aureus (MRSA) combined with the fact that most CNS are methicillin-resistant,
(ii) the high incidence of methicillin-resistant staphylococci that have been reported in total joint arthroplasty (TJA), eg. in Italy in SSIs following clean prosthetic procedures, over 50% of S. aureus and over 60% of CNS strains were methicillin-resistant, and
(iii) some guidelines (eg. of the Hospital Control Practices Advisory Committee, HICPAC, USA) which suggest that the high frequency of MRSA infection at an institution should promptly require vancomycin use for AP [2, 13, 14, 19].

There is no consensus on what constitutes a high prevalence of methicillin-resistance [2, 13]. Wiesel and Esterhai, as well as others, recommend use of vancomycin at an institution with MRSA prevalence >10-20% [2, 20]. Other investigators propose that the use of glycopeptides should be restricted to major prosthetic orthopaedic procedures, in departments where the prevalence of MRSA and MRSE is as high as 20-30% [18]. It is likely that with the increasing prevalence of both health-care associated and community-acquired MRSA in some institutions, some high risk patients would benefit from use of glycopeptides for AP.

It is evident that the decision to use glycopeptides should take into consideration: a) the SSI rates of particular orthopaedic operations and the local prevalence of MRSA isolates, b) the infection prevention practices and an effective SSI surveillance system that would isolate and determine pathogens and antimicrobial agent susceptibilities, and c) consultation between orthopaedic surgeons and infectious disease experts [5].

It is suggested [8, 9, 15, 21] that glycopeptides can be used only in:
(1) institutions with a significant prevalence (eg. >10-20%) of MRSA and MRSE among orthopaedic patients;
(2) facilities with recent MRSA or incisional MRCNS outbreaks;
(3) history of MRSA infection;
(4) known MRSA colonization; and
(5) history of life-threatening allergy to β-lactam antibiotics.

3. HOSPITAL INFECTIONS IN HAND SURGERY

3.1. Nature and magnitude of the problem

Surgical infections after hand surgery are probably less common than other types of orthopaedic surgery [6]. Duncan et al showed an infection rate of 13%, 15%, 21% and 38% in response to a standardized bacterial inoculum in human arms, back, thighs and legs respectively [6].

The hand is less vulnerable to infection than most sites of the body, in part due to its rich blood supply [5]. Neutrophil chemotaxis to standardized wounds of the upper extremity is 3 times stronger than the lower extremity chemotaxis [6]. But once a wound infection becomes established, it can easily spread to underlying structures such as bone, tendon sheaths, blood vessels and deep spaces [6]. Rapidly spreading soft tissue infections can occur, such as necrotizing fasciitis or other catastrophic infection, eg. due to C. perfrigens [6]. Toxic shock syndrome, caused by (a) toxin(s) produced by certain strains of S. aureus, has been rarely reported [6]. Postoperative pneumonia or urinary tract infections have well been recognized [5].

The infection rate in hand surgery reported in the literature varies considerably (0.1-15%). In a survey conducted by the French Society for surgery of the hand, the infection rate for hand surgery was estimated to be around 0.1% (21/22,000 patients), but this rate could be an underestimation for several reasons [10].

Few studies deal enough with orthopaedic operations of the hand and are eligible for statistical analysis [5]. Even fewer look specifically at infection rate for elective clean hand surgery procedures. The incidence of infection without AP appears to be low [3]. For carpal tunnel release, infection rates range from 0.25% to 6%, and are higher in men, in longer procedures, in steroid administration at surgery, and with tenontosynovectomy or use of drains [5, 6, 22]. In a retrospective review of 3,620 carpal tunnel releases (>80% did not receive AP) the infection rate was 0.47% [3]. No infection was observed in 31 patients undergoing delayed flexor tendon repair [3]. In operations against Dupuytren's contracture the reported infection rate was 2% [22]. A low rate of infection has also been reported in arthroplasties of the small joints of the hand with silastic prostheses [5]. In a large series of metacarpophalangeal (MCP) and proximal in-terphalangeal (PIP) arthroplasties the reported rates are 0.6 - 2.6% and 0.36%, respectively [3, 22, 23]. The low rate of infection is due to the small surface area of the implant and the decreased adhesion of bacteria to silastic, when compared to metal [6]. Larger joints carry a higher risk of infection, eg. in total joint arthroplasty of the elbow and the shoulder, the incidence of infection is 7-9% and 4-7%, respectively [3, 24].

In a study of 2,458 patients, who were followed up for at least 30 days after hand surgery, the infection rate was 1.3% in 2,311 clean wounds (without a drain, as classi-fied by the authors) and 4.8% in 147 clean-contaminated wounds with a drain [5]. In a retrospective study of pin fixation of hand and wrist fractures and dislocations, the pin-tract infection rate was 7%, mainly after prolonged pin placement, and no difference was found between biodegradable and metallic pins [5, 6].

Percutaneous Kirschner wires are well known to de-velop pin track infections [22]. In a large review of the literature, external fixators were associated with an infec-tion rate of 8.3% [6].

Higher wound infection rates are expected in emer-gency surgery, with anticipated contaminated wounds. Infection rates ranging from 1.1 to 11% have been re-ported after treated hand lacerations [22].

Much of the variation in reported infection rates is due to variation in the definition used by several authors, or due to problems associated with wound surveillance [5, 6]. It is often difficult to distinguish between superfi-cial and deep infection in the hand, where there is no deep fascial layer that is routinely closed [22]. In addi-tion, the majority of SSIs after hand surgery become ap-parent after hospital discharge, and consequently, the actual infection rate can be underestimated [5].

3.2. Antimicrobial prophylaxis in hand surgery

There is a limited number of studies that consider care-fully AP in patients undergoing hand surgery. Specifical-ly, there is a paucity of prospective randomized, placebo-controlled clinical studies, which require a standard defi-nition of infection, take into consideration co-morbidities and risk factors, report drug adverse events and use strong and valid statistics [3]. Therefore, the role of AP in both elective and emergency hand surgery in several in-stances remains equivocal [3]. Many suggestions repre-sent extrapolations from studies published in the or-thopaedic and plastic surgery literature and referred to other parts of the body, and especially, to the lower limbs. For example, various studies and reviews demon-strate a reduction of the incidence of SSIs to 0.5-1% for total hip arthroplasty, 1-4% for total knee arthroplasty and 4-7% for shoulder prostheses, while firm and specific data for elbow or wrist arthroplasty are lacking [3, 24, 25]. The incidence of SSIs is also generally reduced by 50-80% in patients with closed fractures treated with in-ternal fixation by nails, plates, screws or wires [3, 11].

It is rather difficult to prove the efficacy of AP in elec-tive hand surgery, since a very large number of patients should participate in clinical trials to demonstrate any significant difference in outcome [3]. In a randomized placebo-controlled trial of 715 patients (including 35 patients with hand surgery, not separately analyzed), who received preoperatively cefamandole intravenously or placebo, the postoperative infection rate was 1.6% versus 4.2% in the placebo group and the difference was noted mainly in patients with operations lasting more than 2 hours [3, 26]. In another early historical ran-domized placebo-controlled trial of 1591 patients who received cephaloridine preoperatively and during the operation, postoperative infection rate was 2.8% versus 5% of the placebo group. However, in a subgroup of patients who underwent a hand, wrist, forearm or elbow procedure the findings were not statistically significant compared to the placebo group [3]. In a more recent study, Platt and Page prospectively analyzed 112 patien-ts with elective hand surgery over a 4-month interval [22]. Multiple AP regimens were used by many sur-geons. The same postoperative infection rates were found in 48 patients who received prophylaxis, and in 64 patients who did not receive any antibiotic. These results do not support the use of AP in elective hand surgery, but the study had some drawbacks, such as the small population size and the lack of randomization [3].

The role of AP in patients undergoing implantation of a prosthetic device in the hand is not clear. There is lack of studies evaluating the efficacy of AP in total elbow or wrist arthroplasty [3]. Nevertheless, in a French survey, 81% of orthopaedic surgeons administered AP in opera-tions involving implantation of a prosthetic device [10]. This tendency seems to be justified by extrapolation of positive results of AP in total joint arthroplasty elsewhere in the body, and especially, in the hip or the knee.

The use of AP in traumatic hand surgery seems to be dependent on the type of the injury. The use of AP in simple lacerations was studied in several prospective randomized placebo-controlled trials, which demon-strated no benefit derived from its use [3]. In a prospec-tive controlled trial of 250 patients with sharp soft tissue lacerations, who received amoxicillin / clavulanic acid, the infection rate was 5% in the antibiotic group and 3.2% in the group which did not receive any antibiotic. Careful surgical debridement was performed in every patient [27]. In another recent prospective randomized, double-blind placebo-controlled clinical study, a total of 180 patients with clean incised hand injuries, which in-cluded trauma to skin, tendon and nerve, were recruited into three trial groups to receive oral placebo or in-travenous flucloxacillin upon induction of anesthesia with or without an oral flucloxacillin course [28]. The in-fection rates were 15%, 4% and 13% respectively, but there was no statistically significant difference was de-monstrated among the groups.

The use of antibiotics in the management of open long bone fractures in the extremities is well accepted

chapter 7

and documented in several prospective randomized, double-blinded and not blinded clinical studies [5, 29]. Data from 913 participants in seven studies have shown that the use of antibiotics had a protective effect against early infection compared with no antibiotics or placebo (RR 0.41, 95% CI 0.27 - 0.63) [30]. The issue of AP especially in complex hand trauma, involving bone, joint, tendon and neurovascular structures is still controversial, since information on this topic is less abundant [3]. Patzakis et al conducted a prospective randomized trial in 310 patients (89 with open forearm and hand fractures). The infection rate was 13.9% in the placebo group and 2.3% in patients receiving a 10-day course of intravenous cephalothin [3, 31]. In this study 12 of 115 tibia fractures became infected compared to 10 out of 218 open fractures elsewhere in the body. In another open prospective randomized study in patients with open fractures of the distal phalanx, seen within 6 hours after injury, 3 out of 10 patients who did not receive antibiotics developed an infection, compared to 2 out of 75 patients who received prophylaxis (p=0.02) [3]. The best regimen was 1g of intravenous cephradine preoperatively and 1g orally, postoperatively. Madsen et al. conducted a prospective randomized, double-blind placebo-controlled clinical study of 599 patients with a traumatic wound located distally to the wrist or ankle joint (570 patients had a hand injury). They were allocated to receive a single intravenous dose of penicillin or penicillin tablets for 6 days or placebo, and the infection rates were 4.9%, 6% and 10% respectively. The difference in infection rate was significant only among patients who received intravenous penicillin and placebo [32].

On the other hand, Peacock conducted a prospective randomized study in 87 patients with a wide variety of hand injuries that were distal to the distal radio-ulnar joint, treated predominantly on an outpatient basis [3]. Patients were randomized to receive placebo or intravenous cefamandole during the operation and for 3 days postoperatively. Only 1 patient developed infection in the placebo group and none in the drug group. In another open prospective study of 91 open finger fractures distal to the metacarpophalangeal joint (68 of which involved the distal phalanx) patients received a 3-day course of dicloxacillin, erythromycin or first generation cephalosporin, and 4 patients in each group developed infection [33].

It is obvious that controversy persists regarding the efficacy of AP in complex hand trauma, and therefore, the lower incidence of infection in complex hand trauma requires a well designed study with a large number of patients to definitely answer this question. In any case we must note again that, as all studies emphasize, thorough debridement of an open wound is the cornerstone of open fracture treatment, and antibiotics are not a substitute for the meticulous surgical technique [3].

In mutilating hand injuries, including high velocity gun shots and blast and fragment injuries, the administration of antibiotics are technically not prophylactic, since bacterial contamination in the mutilating hand wound occurs early and before the drug delivery [32, 34]. When the injury occurs at home or industry, the infecting microorganisms are mainly Gram-positive cocci (eg. staphylococci) at a 70% rate. In a farm implement injury the responsible pathogens are 60% Gram-negative bacteria and 40% Gram-positive cocci or anaerobic Clostridium spp [32, 34]. Tetanus prophylaxis is mandatory in this setting and in patients with unknown history of tetanus immunization (or <3 doses of tetanus and diphtheria toxoids adsorbed vaccine - Td) involves the immediate and simultaneous administration of Td antitetanus human immune globulin (TIG). If 3 or more doses have been definitely administered, a Td dose is indicated if more than 5 years have elapsed since the last booster dose [35].

Defining the incidence of infection after the latter injuries is difficult, and prospective randomized, placebo-controlled clinical studies are lacking for a variety of reasons, including small number of patients and many different kinds of injury. The role of AP in these injuries is also not clear [32].

The administration of antibiotics in animal or human bite wounds can also be considered therapy rather than prophylaxis, because the majority of patients present several hours or days after wound contamination by animal or human saliva [12]. A distinction must be made between contaminated bite wounds and established infections. In cat bites the usual pathogens are Pasteurella multocida and S.aureus, while in dogs, additional pathogens may be Bacteroides spp, Capnocytophaga spp etc. [12]. A meta-analysis of 8 randomized controlled trials demonstrated a reduced risk of infection in patients with dog bite wounds treated with oral penicillin or penicillinase-resistant penicillin compared with control subjects (RR 0.56, 95% CI 0.38 - 0.82). A sub-analysis of hand wounds also demonstrated the protective effect of antibiotics [3]. The same protective role of antibiotics was also shown in a small prospective study of 11 patients with cat wounds [3].

In human bites the responsible pathogens are mainly viridans streptococci, S.epidermidis, Corynebacterium spp, S.aureus, Bacteroides spp, peptostreptococci and Eikenella corrodens. Bites on the hand have a higher rate of infection [35, 36]. A specific type with a high rate of infection is the clenched or closed-fist injury ("fight bite"), which usually involves a small and not alarming initial laceration directly over the index or long finger of the metacarpophalangeal joint. But the victim's teeth penetrate the extensor mechanism and the joint capsule resulting in wound contamination. An established infection appears within 1-2 days [3]. Many retrospective and without control group studies as well as a prospective randomized, placebo-controlled clinical study of 48 patients who received a 5-day course of penicillin plus cefazolin or cefaclor or placebo, suggest a short course of "prophylactic" antibiotics for patients with human bite wounds [3]. Tetanus prophylaxis is also necessary. One may also consider anti-rabies prophylaxis (immune globulin plus vaccine) in dog bite wounds. Aggressive irrigation and wound debridement is also necessary, while primary closure of the wound should be avoided [3, 36].

4. RECOMMENDATIONS FOR ANTIBIOTIC PROPHYLAXIS IN HAND SURGERY

As has already been noted, the role of AP in both elective and emergency hand surgery is still not clearly defined [3, 28]. Definite guidelines are not practically available but taking into account the available data, expert opinions and a few consensus statements, some suggestions can be made, concerning the use of AP in upper limb surgery in the following situations:
1) *Elective procedures involving implants (metal and silastic)* [3, 6, 22, 35]. This is based on limited data and extrapolation studies conducted in other body sites. Some authors believe that this suggestion is valid only for total wrist prosthesis implantation and that there are not available data to support the use of AP for other implants [33].
2) *Dirty complex open hand wounds* with severe soft tissue injury and gross contamination (this can also be considered as therapy) [3, 6, 22].
3) *Human or animal bites* (this can also be considered as therapy) [3, 6].
4) *High-velocity (>2000 feet per second) gun shot injuries or intraarticular gun shot injuries* [37]. In injuries caused by low-velocity gun shots the literature shows no clear advantage in administering AP, unless the wound is grossly contaminated.
5) *Open fractures* [22, 29, 30, 38]. AP is applied preoperatively and as soon as possible after injury (best if administered within 3 hours) to all types of open fracture wounds (Gustilo types I, II and III). In types I and II antibiotics are discontinued 24 hours after closure and in type III they are administered for no more than 72 hours (this can also be considered as therapy). Some authors believe that in open fractures with a risk of 1% (eg. type I open fracture) AP is not indicated (unless the operation lasts >2 hours) [33].
6) *Procedures of long duration* (>2 hours) [3, 10, 22].
7) Some authors also recommend AP in procedures involving bone or soft tissue reconstruction with large flaps [3, 6], in elective hand surgery with preexisting major disease (eg. diabetes mellitus, rheumatoid arthritis, patients on steroids or other immunosuppression) [22] and in elective procedures with Kirschner wires [22].

Controversy persists over the use of AP in closed fractures treated with osteosynthesis [10, 35]. There are data supporting its use and it seems that many surgeons would administer AP in this setting [39]. Others believe that its use is not justified [33].

AP does not appear warranted in: a) clean elective operations lasting fewer than 2 hours, because the low infection rate make small differences difficult to determine, and b) in routine hand lacerations or simple soft tissue injuries [10, 22, 35, 40].

5. PROPHYLACTIC ANTIBIOTIC CHOICE IN HAND SURGERY

As a rule, the surgeon should follow the aforementioned principles, which are applied in general orthopaedic surgery, i.e. the antibiotic should be administered intravenously preoperatively (within 1-2 hours before incision), and if possible, upon induction of anesthesia for a brief period of time, mostly during the operation period [3, 10].

In hand surgery the possible infective microorganisms are the same as in any other type of orthopaedic surgery. In **total joint arthroplasty** in the hand, in elective clean surgery of long duration and in placement of an internal fixation, the most common pathogens are *S.aureus* and *S.epidermidis* [3]. In those operations a first or a second generation cephalosporin (cefazolin, cefuroxime, cefamandole) are recommended as the first choice, and a semisynthetic penicillinase-resistant penicillin (eg. flucloxacillin) as an alternative agent [3, 6, 10, 22]. In cases of β-lactam, allergy clindamycin or a glycopeptide (eg. vancomycin or teicoplanin) can be used. A glycopeptide may be indicated in special situations, as mentioned above [6, 10]. In cases of open reductions of **closed fractures** with internal fixation, some authors suggest the use of ceftriaxone (2 g iv / im once) based in one prospective, randomized, placebo-controlled study (the Dutch Trauma Trial) [35, 41]. According to the authors, ceftriaxone was chosen because of its broad spectrum of activity and pharmacokinetic profile, including high serum levels and long elimination half-life ensuring bactericidal concentrations for 24 hours. However, it should be pointed out that ceftriaxone does not cover MRSA, which nowadays are endemic in most tertiary hospitals.

Data has documented the benefit of timely (if possible within in <3 hours after trauma) AP in long bone (including hand and digits) **open fractures** [29]. Agents against *S.aureus* (eg. first generation cephalosporins or a glycopeptide in specific situations) seem to be appropriate for Gustilo I and II open fractures. In Gustilo III wounds, after the initial debridement and since various Gram-negative microorganisms are often cultured from the wounds, a broader anti-Gram-negative coverage should be attempted through the addition of an aminoglycoside [29]. However, it should be noted that aminoglycosides are poorly concentrated in the bone tissue. A second generation cephalosporin with a broader coverage (eg. cefuroxime) might be a reasonable alternative. In cases of suspected fecal/clostridial contamination, such as farm-related injuries, a high dose of penicillin should be added [25, 29].

Some trials have suggested that the combination of cefamandole plus gentamicin is superior to monotherapy with clindamycin, cloxacillin or ciprofloxacin [25]. In another prospective randomized study, ciprofloxacin was found equivalent to the combination of cefamandole and gentamicin in type I and II, but not in type III open fractures [38]. Fluoroquinolones can be used (in combination with a first or second generation cephalosporin) instead of an aminoglycoside, because they are bactericidal, broad spectrum antibiotics with good oral bioavailability, bone penetration and tolerability. However, these agents inhibit osteoblast activity and experimental bone healing and promote the emergence of resistance, and therefore, their use must be very limited [38].

In **complex or mutilating hand trauma** occurring at home or in an industrial environment, the combination of a first or a second generation cephalosporin or semisynthetic penicillin plus an aminoglycoside is recommended. In cases of injuries occurring in an agricultured or garden setting, the addition of penicillin is appropriate [3, 32]. The duration of prophylaxis / treatment is arbitrary but it should not extend beyond 5 days [3]. In high velocity and intra-articular gunshot injuries, as well as in blast and fragments injuries, the same regimens can be applied for no more than 48-72 hours [37]. In all cases tetanus prophylaxis is necessary.

In **bite wounds** cleaning, irrigation and debridement are the most important prophylactic measures. Primary closure, especially in case of human bite wound, should be avoided [3]. It also seems reasonable to recommend a 3-5 day course of prophylaxis / treatment. In all bite wounds amoxicillin/clavulanic acid 875/125 mg bid or 500/125 mg tid po is recommended. Alternative regimens include cefuroxime axetil 500 mg po bid or doxycycline 100 mg po bid for human or cat bites and clindamycin 600 mg po tid plus a fluoroquinolone for dog bites [3, 35, 36]. Anti-rabies prophylaxis may be considered in certain dog wounds.

6. OTHER METHODS OF PREVENTING INFECTION

Besides AP, many other measures have been tried and tested in an attempt to further reduce the incidence of SSI. These measures have not been tested specifically in hand surgery, and conclusions can be drawn only by extrapolation and may in part be arbitrary. Briefly, these measures are [2, 3, 6, 9, 13]:

1) Identification of patient characteristics and risk factors that could be positively influenced by various interventions, eg. effective preoperative control of diabetes or rheumatoid arthritis, etc.

2) Identification and optimization of operation characteristics, eg. preoperative antiseptic showering and hair removal by clipping, proper skin preparation and surgeon hand antisepsis and strict adherence to aseptic and meticulous surgical techniques. Although local antibiotic irrigation is a common clinical practice among surgeons, this technique cannot be recommended [19, 32].

3) Implementation of a suitable SSI surveillance system. Each hospital infection control committee in co-operation with orthopaedic surgeons should establish such a program [9].

The role of antibiotic-impregnate bone cement (AIBC) in AP, and especially in hand surgery, remains unclear. In spite of potential benefits, controversies remain regarding its use and no established guidelines exist for use for AP [2, 13]. Perhaps AIBC has a more definite prophylactic role in high risk patients, as the immunocompromised, the elderly and those requiring revision surgeries, but this has to be proven in large prospective clinical trials [2].

7. CONCLUSIONS

The increasing number of orthopaedic upper limb operations render the application of proper prophylaxis mandatory for the prevention of postoperative musculoskeletal infection in this kind of surgery. The general principles of antibiotic prophylaxis in orthopaedics are also applied in hand surgery but established guidelines are not widely available. Large prospective well-controlled studies are needed to reinforce and complement existing data on prophylaxis. In any case, good surgical techniques is paramount to avoid postsurgical infections in the hand.

REFERENCES

[1] Weed HG. Antimicrobial prophylaxis in the surgical patient. Med Clin N Am 2003;87:59-75.

[2] Marculescu CE, Osmon DR. Antibiotic prophylaxis in orthopaedic prosthetic surgery. Infect Dis Clin N Am 2005;19:931-46.

[3] Hoffman DR, Adams BD. The role of antibiotics in the management of elective and post-traumatic hand surgery. Hand Clin 1988;14:657-66.

[4] Mini E, Nabili S, Periti P. Does surgical prophylaxis with teicoplanin constitute a therapeutic advance? J Chemother 2000;12 (Suppl 5):40-55.

[5] Calkins ER. Nosocomial infections in hand surgery. Hand Infect 1998;14:531-45.

[6] Shapiro DB. Postoperative infection in hand surgery. Hand Clin 1998;14:669-81.

[7] Sia IG, Berbari E, Karchmer AW. Prosthetic joint infections. Infect Dis Clin N Am 2005;19:885-914.

[8] Morita K, Smith K. Antimicrobial prophylaxis in orthopaedic surgery. Orthopaedics 2005;28:749-51.

[9] Mangram AJ, Horan TC, Pearson ML, Silver LC, Jarvis WR. Guidelines for prevention of surgical site infection 1999. Centers for Disease Control and Prevention (CDC) Hospital Infection Control Practices Advisory Committee. Infect Control Hosp Epidemiol 1999;20:250-78.

[10] Dumontier C, Lemerle JP. L' antibioprophylaxie en chirurgie de la main: 'a la recherche d'un consensus. Chirurgie de la main 2004; 23:167-77.

[11] Scottish Intercollegiate Guidelines Network. Antibiotic prophylaxis in Surgery. A National Clinical Guideline, July 2000 (http://www.sign.ac.uk / pdf).

[12] Anonymous. Antibiotic prophylaxis in surgery. The Medical Letter on Drugs and Therapeutics 2001;43:W1116-1117B.

[13] Bratzler DW, Houck PM for the Surgical Infection Prevention Guidelines Writers Workgroup. Antibiotic prophylaxis for surgery: An advisory statement from the National Surgical Infection Prevention Project. Clin Infect Dis 2004;38:1706-15.

[14] Burke JP. Maximizing appropriate antibiotic prophylaxis for surgical patients: an update from LDS Hospital, Salt Lake City. Clin Infect Dis 2001;33 (Suppl 2):S78-83.

[15] Advisory Statement. Recommendations for the use of intravenous antibiotic prophylaxis in primary total joint arthroplasty. American Association of Orthopaedic Surgeons. June 2004 (http://www.aaos.org/wordhtml/papers/advistmt/1027.htm.

[16] Waddell TK, Rotstein OP. Antibiotic prophylaxis in surgery. Can Med Assoc J 1994;151:925-31.

[17] Classen DC, Evans RS, Pestonik SL et al. The timing of prophylactic administration of antibiotics and the risk of surgical-wound infection. N Engl J Med 1992;326:281-6.

[18] DeLalla F. Surgical prophylaxis in practice. J Hosp Infect 2002;50 (Suppl A):S9-12.

[19] Darouiche RO. Antimicrobial approaches for preventing infections associated with surgical implants. Clin Infect Dis 2003;36;1284-89.

[20] Wiesel BB, Esterhai J. Prophylaxis in musculoskeletal infection. In: Calhoun J, Mader JT, editors. Musculoskeletal infections. New York: Marcel Dekker 2003, p. 115-29.

[21] Advisory Statement. The use of prophylactic antibiotics in orthopaedic medicine and the emergence of vancomycin-resistant bacteria. American Association of Orthopaedic Surgeons. February 2002 (http://www. aaos.org/wordhtml/papers/advistmt/1016.htm.

[22] Platt AJ, Page RE. Post-operative infection following hand surgery. Guidelines for antibiotic use. J Hand Surg [Br] 1995;20B(5):685-90.

[23] Blair WF, Shurr DG, Buckwalter JA. Metacarpophalangeal joint implant arthroplasty with a silastic spacer. J Bone Joint Surg 1984; 66A(3):365-70.

[24] Munoz P, Bouza E. Acute and chronic adult osteomyelitis and prosthesis-related infections. Bailliere's Clinical Rheumatology 1999;13:129-47.

[25] Jaeger M, Maier D, Kern W, Sudkamp NP. Antibiotics in trauma and orthopaedic surgery - a primer of evidence-based recommendations. Injury 2006;37:S74-80.

[26] Henley BM, Jones RE, Wyatt RW, Hofman A, Cohen RL. Prophylaxis with cefamandole nafate in elective orthopedic surgery. Clin Orthop 1986;209:249-56.

[27] Cassell OC, Ion L. Are antibiotics necessary in the surgical management of the upper limb lacerations? Br J Plast surg 1997;50: 523-9.

[28] Whittaker JP, Nancarrow JP, Sterne GD. The role of antibiotic prophylaxis in clean incised hand injuries: a prospective randomized placebo controlled double blind trial. J Hand Surg [Br] 2005; 30B(2):162-7.

[29] EAST Practice management guidelines workgroup. Practice management guidelines for prophylactic antibiotic use in open fractures, 2000. http://www.east.org/tpg/openfrac.pdf.

[30] Gosselin RA, Roberts I, Gillespie WJ. Antibiotics for preventive infection in open limb fractures. Cochrane Database Syst Rev 2004; 1:CD 003764.

[31] Patzakis MJ, Harvey P, Ivler D. The role of antibiotics in the management of open fractures. J Bone Joint Surg [Am] 1974;56:532-41.

[32] Hoffman DR, Adams BD. Antimicrobial management of multilating hand injuries. Hand Clin 2003;19:33-9.

[33] Suprock MD, Hood JM, Lubahn JP. Role of antibiotics in open fractures in the finger. J Hand Surg [Am] 1990;10:796-805.

[34] Covey DC. Blast and fragment injuries of the musculoskeletal system. J Bone Joint Surg [Am] 2002;84:1221-34.

[35] The Sanford Guide to Antimicrobial Therapy 2006, Antimicrobial Therapy Inc, Sperryville, 2006.

[36] Daniels JM, Zook EG, Lynch JM. Hand and Wrist Injuries: Part II. Emergent evaluation. Am Fam Phys 2004;69:1949-56.

[37] Simpson BM, Wilson R, Grand R. Antibiotic therapy in gunshot wound injuries. Clin Orthop Rel Res 2003;408:82-5.

[38] Zalavras C, Patzakis M, Holtom PD, Sherman R. Management of open fractures. Infect Dis Clin. N Am 2005;915-29.

[39] Gillespie WS, Walenkamp G. Antibiotic prophylaxis for surgery for proximal femoral and other closed long bone fractures. Cochrane Review In: The Cochrane Library, Issue 4, 2004.

[40] Hunfeld KP, Wichelhaus TA, Schafer V, Rittmeister. Evidence-based antibiotic prophylaxis in aseptic orthopedic surgery. Orthopade 2003;32:1070-7.

[41] Boxma H, Broekhuizen T, Patka P, Oosting H. Randomised controlled trial of single-dose antibiotic prophylaxis in surgical treatment of closed fractures: the Dutch Trauma Trial. Lancet 1996; 347:1133-7.

Antimicrobial Resistance
of Gram–positive Cocci:
New Therapeutic Alternatives

Roland LECLERCQ

Service de Microbiologie, CHU Côte de Nacre, Universite de Caen Basse Normandie, France

Staphylococci are major causes of bone and joint infection. Oxacillin or related beta–lactams, fluoroquinolones, rifampicin (used in combination) and clindamycin are commonly used antimicrobials for first–line therapy of *Staphylococcus aureus* infections. Staphylococci are becoming increasingly resistant to antimicrobials and methicillin–resistant *S. aureus* is currently spreading in the community. This has led to the proposal of alternative therapies, based mostly on the use of vancomycin or teicoplanin. New antimicrobials, which are active against multiply resistant gram–positive organisms, such as quinupristin–dalfopristin (an injectable streptogramin), linezolid (an injectable or oral oxazolidinone), tigecycline (glycylcycline) and daptomycin (cyclic lipopeptide), have recently been introduced in therapy. Some of these new drugs have favourable properties for the treatment of bone infections, although they have not been approved for this use. As such, only small series of bone infections treated with these new drugs are available for analysis. Moreover, linezolid has adverse effects when treatment is prolonged, hence limiting the use of this antibiotic.

Keywords: Staphylococcus aureus; linezolid; vancomycin; resistance; nosocomial infections. ■

1. INTRODUCTION

Bone and soft tissue infections of the upper extremities are frequently due to microorganisms that are part of the flora of these sites (see chapter 2 by Petinaki and Malizos). This is the reason why staphylococci that are predominantly commensal bacteria of the skin are also the major cause of infection. In particular, *Staphylococcus aureus* is the most common organism causing osteomyelitis and septic arthritis [1, 2]. Coagulase-negative sta-

phylococci (CoNS) followed by *S. aureus* are implicated in prosthetic joint infections which is an uncommon complication following mostly hip and knee replacement, although a large variety of microorganisms may be isolated. Beta-haemolytic streptococci are also responsible for septic arthritis and bone infection as a consequence of direct trauma or haematogenous spread. Group A septic arthritis may be observed at all ages, whereas group B osteomyelitis may be found in neonates. Enterococci and viridans streptococci may also be a cause of prosthetic joint infections. Septic arthritis of the upper extremity following animal bites is often polymicrobial, and may involve anaerobes [3]. Gram-negative organisms are responsible for a small proportion of bone and joint infections, particularly in patients that are predisposed to specific Gram-negative infections (patients with diabetes and intravenous drug abuse).

High failure rates may follow antibiotic treatment of bone infection. Inadequate initial debridement, the presence of prosthetic material, duration

*Corresponding Author
CHU de Caen, Service de Microbiologie
Avenue Côte de Nacre, 14033 Caen Cedex, France
Tel: +33 02 31 06 45 72
Fax : +33 02 31 06 45 73
e-mail: leclercq-r@chu-caen.fr

of infection and previous treatment failure are major risk factors for poor outcomes. The initial choice of antibiotics depends on the suspected or documented causal pathogen and its sensitivity pattern. Among these organisms, staphylococci are remarkable not only for their frequency, but also for their propensity to develop multiple antibiotic resistance. In contrast, β-haemolytic streptococci and anaerobes currently remain susceptible to most antibiotics commonly used for the treatment of bone and joint infections. In this chapter, we will discuss the possible alternative antimicrobial treatments for infections which are due to multiple resistant Gram-positive cocci.

2. Antibiotics Used in the Treatment of Bone Infections

Oxacillin, cloxacillin or related beta-lactams are commonly used for first-line therapy of *S. aureus* infection. The fluoroquinolones, e.g. ciprofloxacin, ofloxacin and pefloxacin, have been studied extensively for bone and joint infections. These antimicrobials have several favourable properties, combining an effect on adherent bacteria, penetration into macrophages and neutrophils [4], high bone:serum concentrations after oral administration [5] and a low side-effect profile. The effect of rifampicin in combination with various antibiotics has been very encouraging in clinical practice and this antibiotic is often part of treatment protocols for bone infections. This is due to favourable pharmacokinetic characteristics in terms of penetration in bone, tissues and phagocytic cells. However, the use of rifampicin is limited by the rapid development of resistance and this antibiotic must therefore be combined with a second agent. Against methicillin-susceptible staphylococci, rifampicin has been combined with penicillins and cephalosporins, and with quinolones [6, 7]. Clindamycin, with high bone:serum ratios is an interesting alternative therapy when the patient is discharged from hospital while continuing with oral therapy [8]. In children, it has been shown to be comparable to standard parenteral therapy [8]. Although pseudomembranous colitis may occur in elderly patients, such patients are also at risk of developing *Clostridium difficile* diarrhoea while receiving other parenteral antibiotics, in particular cephalosporins.

3. Antibiotics for Infections Due to Multiply Resistant Gram-Positive Organisms

The increasing prevalence of multiple antibiotic resistance in staphylococci is a limitation to the use of the classical antimicrobials. Although methicillin-resistant *S. aureus* (MRSA) are traditionally associated with hospital-acquired

infections and are mostly isolated from post-operative knee or hip infections, emergence of community-acquired MRSA (CA-MRSA) may change the patterns of acute hematogenous osteomyelitis and septic arthritis [9]. Cases of CA-MRSA have been documented in healthy community-dwelling persons without established risk factors for MRSA acquisition [10]. They have been reported worldwide, including Europe, and predominantly infect young and healthy patients. The bacterial isolates produce Panton-Valentine leucocidin (PVL) and harbour a type IV staphylococcal chromosomal cassette *mec* (SCC*mec*) element that contains the *mec*A gene that is responsible for the resistance. Their incidence varies greatly depending on the country. In some areas of the United States, MRSA isolates account for the majority of *S. aureus* infections acquired in the community [11]. Skin and soft-tissue infections are the predominant types of CA-MRSA infections, but it is the invasive and life-threatening infections that produce major concerns. In a recent 3-year survey of CA-MRSA infections, osteomyelitis and septic arthritis were among the most common invasive infections caused by CA-MRSA isolates [12] (Table 1). Usually, acute osteomyelitis affects mostly the long bones. Strains producing Panton-Valentine leucocidin are more often associated with complications of osteomyelitis than those of isolates without the toxin for example, deep venous thrombophlebitis, which has been rarely reported to affect children with *S. aureus* osteomyelitis, or the development of chronic osteomyelitis [13].

The glycopeptides, vancomycin and teicoplanin have become the major therapeutic alternative for MRSA infection, although there remains some discussion as to

TABLE 1

Sites and types of infection with community-acquired *Staphylococcus aureus* in children [adapted from 12].

Site or type of infection	No. of Cases	
	MRSA	MSSA
Abscess		
Epidural	3	1
Lung	2	0
Paraspinal	1	1
Renal	1	0
Sacral	1	0
Osteomyelitis	54	28
Septic arthritis	9	10
Bacteraemia	7	7
Empyema	9	2
Lymphadenitis	7	16
Myositis	8	7
Pneumonia	14	2
Others	1	3
Total	*117*	*76*

what would be the best choice. Some consider that vancomycin is a superior treatment option for staphylococci with more rapid bacterial killing due to lower protein binding than teicoplanin [14]. However, teicoplanin has been particularly useful, as it allows patients to be discharged from the hospital while continuing with parenteral therapy. It can be given by bolus injection once daily, or even less frequently and is associated with lower nephrotoxicity at high serum concentrations compared to vancomycin [15]. Adverse side effects have also been observed with teicoplanin. High-dose (>60 mg/L) and prolonged therapy with teicoplanin has been associated with thrombocytopenia and neutropenia [16]. A small percentage of coagulase-negative staphylococci are intermediate or resistant to teicoplanin, but remain susceptible to vancomycin. Diminished susceptibility or resistance of *S. aureus* to teicoplanin and/or vancomycin is rare, but must be examined [17]. A summary of non-comparative studies (n = 23) has demonstrated an efficacy between 50% and 100% for bone infections (median success rate: 83%) [18] including, however, initial studies using lower doses with decreased efficacy [19]. Higher doses that give high serum concentrations appear necessary to treat deep-seated staphylococcal bone infections and 12 mg/kg is recommended for septic arthritis [19].

Since rifampicin and clindamycin may remain active against multiply resistant staphylococci, they are still useful. However, susceptibility of the isolate should be examined. Oral minocycline (with and without rifampicin) has been shown to be useful in the treatment of MRSA infection, including osteomyelitis [20]. High-dose oral co-trimoxazole has also been used to treat MRSA prosthetic infections as an alternative to glycopeptides. After prolonged high-dose therapy, the overall cure rate at 6 years was 66.7%, but side effects led to discontinuation of this therapy in eight patients [21].

4. NEW ANTIMICROBIALS

Difficulties in the management of infections due to MRSA have challenged clinicians and microbiologists to find new antibiotics or combinations that are not only effective against deep infection, but also tolerable over prolonged treatment courses [19]. Treatment of bone infections is not an approved indication for new antibiotics administration and only small series of treated infections are available for analysis.

Quinupristin/dalfopristin (Synercid ®) is a streptogramin consisting of a combination of quinupristin (streptogramin factor B) and dalfopristin (streptogramin factor A) [22]. This bactericidal streptogramin combination inhibits protein synthesis by binding to the 50S ribosome subunit. It has activity against *Enterococcus faecium,* including vancomycin-resistant strains and *S. aureus* (including MRSA). It is not active against *E. faecalis.* However, quinupristin/dalfopristin requires admini-

stration via a central line with dextrose infusion three times daily, which is a significant limitation for its use. The most important side effect is myalgia, which may necessitate cessation of the treatment. In a study of 40 patients treated for MRSA bone and joint infections (mean duration: 42 days), clinical and bacteriological success was observed in 77.5% and 69%, respectively, of those who were evaluated [23]. Caution must be taken if a *Staphylococcus* sp. is resistant to clindamycin as, this antibiotic may be only inhibitory, but not bactericidal due to cross-resistance of the MLS$_B$ type. [24].

A recent addition to the antibiotics directed against the resistant Gram-positive organisms is **linezolid.** It is the first available member of a new class of antibiotics, the oxazolidinones. Linezolid is a bacteriostatic antibiotic which is administered intravenously and that is also available in an oral formulation with almost 100% bioavailability. Linezolid inhibits bacterial protein synthesis by binding a specific site on the 50S ribosomal subunit and has no cross-resistance to other antibiotics commonly used for treatment of bone infections. It is approved for the treatment of soft tissue infection and pneumonia. The activity spectrum of linezolid covers Gram-positive bacteria, including staphyloccoci, enterococci and streptococci, but this drug is inactive against Gram-negative bacteria [25].

S. aureus, a major cause of bone infections, is nearly always susceptible to linezolid. The MIC$_{50/90s}$ of linezolid against methicillin-resistant and susceptible *S. aureus* were reported to be 1-2/2-4 mg/l, in various studies collecting strains from various parts of the world [26, 27, 28]. Linezolid has similar activity against coagulase negative staphylococci. In all preclinical and early studies, all strains tested were found to be susceptible to linezolid at a breakpoint of 4 mg/l, whether the staphylococci were susceptible or resistant to methicillin. It was also shown that vancomycin intermediate or resistant strains were susceptible to linezolid (MIC=1 mg/l) [29].

Enterococci that are rarely involved in bone infections have developed resistance to most antibiotics, including high-level resistance to aminoglycosides, and especially in the species *E. faecium,* to penicillins and glycopeptides. *In vitro* studies have shown that linezolid is active against enterococci. The MIC$_{50/90}$ of linezolid is similar to that against staphylococci [26, 27]. Again, resistance to glycopeptides and penicillins does not affect susceptibility to linezolid.

Although only few cases of bone infections treated with linezolid have been published, this antibiotic displays several favourable properties, including penetration of the bone and excellent bioavailability of the oral form. Linezolid concentrations measured in bone samples from 10 individual patients ranged from 3.3 to 17.4 mg/kg (mean: 8.5 mg/kg) [30]. Penetration of linezolid into bone and joint tissues was also studied in 13 patients suffering from implant-associated infections with MRSA [31]. Mean concentrations of linezolid in infected tissues were greater than 10 mg/liter after administration of the preoperative dose, except in bone specimens, where they reached 3.9 ± 2.0 mg/liter.

Unfortunately, linezolid may interact with other drugs, e.g. monoamine oxidase inhibitors, and most importantly, may cause reversible anaemia or thrombocytopenia with continued use, as well as neuropathy. Currently, the treatment should not exceed 28 days. Due to the requirement of prolonged therapy in bone infections, there are a few reports of longer use with or without adverse effects. In all cases, if used for prolonged treatment, careful observation of adverse effects is required.

Successful treatment for MRSA has been reported in three cases of post-traumatic hand *Staphylococcus aureus* osteomyelitis [32], and several cases of osteomyelitis and prosthetic joint infections [33 - 36]. However, in an animal study comparing 25 mg/kg of linezolid given twice or three times daily intraperitoneally with 50 mg/kg of cefazolin given intramuscularly three times daily for *S. aureus* osteomyelitis, the results of linezolid treatment were not significantly different from those of untreated controls, while cefazolin treatment was significantly more effective than no treatment or linezolid treatment [37]. As linezolid offers the only option for oral treatment for some of the most resistant Gram-positive organisms, additional studies are needed.

Other recently developed antibiotics, in particular **daptomycin** and **tigecycline,** might be of interest, provided that more clinical studies are conducted. Daptomycin is a cyclic lipopeptide with activity against MRSA that has been approved for the treatment of complicated skin and skin structure infections. It may be useful in systemic or local treatment of chronic osteomyelitis. In a recent rat model of experimental osteomyelitis, daptomycin was administered at a dose of 50 mg/kg subcutaneously twice daily, as well as at 60 mg/kg subcutaneously twice daily. These were compared to vancomycin given intraperitoneally at 50 mg/kg twice daily. All systemic anti-infectives studied were more active than no treatment at all, while systemic daptomycin was as active as vancomycin [38].

Tigecycline is a glycylcycline. This bacteriostatic antibiotic is active against multiply resistant staphylococci. The efficacy of tigecycline and vancomycin with or without rifampicin were recently studied in a rabbit model of MRSA osteomyelitis. Rabbits that received tigecycline and oral rifampicin therapy (n=14) showed a 100% infection clearance. Rabbits treated with tigecycline (n=10) and rabbits treated with vancomycin and oral rifampicin (n=10) both showed 90% clearance. Rabbits treated with vancomycin (n=11) showed 81.8% clearance, while untreated controls (n=15) demonstrated only 26% clearance.

5. CONCLUSION

The emergence of resistance to antimicrobials, particularly in staphylococci, complicates the treatment of bone infections. Alternative protocols of treatment are available, although they have several limitations. In particular, few of the alternative antibiotics are orally available. New drugs aimed at treating infections that are due to Gram-positive organisms have been recently introduced for therapy. All these antimicrobials are bacteriostatic and although some seem to be promising, more clinical data are required.

REFERENCES

[1] Waldvogel FA, Vasey H. Osteomyelitis: the past decade. N Engl J Med 1980;303:360-370.
[2] Houshian S, Seyedipour S, Wedderkopp N. Epidemiology of bacterial hand infections. Int J Infect Dis 2006;10:315-319.
[3] Goldstein EJC. Bite wounds and infection. Clin Infect Dis 1991; 14:633-640.
[4] Hooper DC, Wolfson JS. Fluoroquinolone antimicrobial agents. N Engl J Med 1991;324:384-394.
[5] Desplaces N, Acar JF. New quinolones in the treatment of joint and bone infections. Reviews in Infectious Diseases 1988;10 (Suppl. 1): S179-183.
[6] Zimmerli W, Widmer AF, Blatter M, Frei R, Ochsner PE. Role of rifampin for treatment of orthopedic implant-related staphylococcal infections: a randomized controlled trial. Foreign-Body Infection (FBI) Study Group. JAMA 1998;279:1537-1541.
[7] Widmer AF, Gaechter A, Ochsner PE, Zimmerli W. Antimicrobial treatment of orthopedic implant-related infections with rifampin combinations. Clin Infect Dis 1992;14:1251-1253.
[8] Kaplan SL, Mason EO, Feign RD. Clindamycin versus nafcillin or methicillin in the treatment of Staphylococcus aureus osteomyelitis in children. Southern Medical Journal 1982;75:138-142.
[9] Crum NF. The emergence of severe, community-acquired methicillin-resistant Staphylococcus aureus infections. Scand J Infect Dis 2005;37:651-656.
[10] Vandenesch F, Naimi T, Enright MC, Lina G, Nimmo GR, Heffernan H, Liassine N, Bes M, Greenland T, Reverdy ME, and Etienne J. Community-acquired methicillin-resistant Staphylococcus aureus carrying Panton-Valentine leukocidin genes: worldwide emergence. Emerg Infect Dis 2003;9:978-984.
[11] Sattler CA, Mason EO Jr., Kaplan SL. Prospective comparison of risk factors and demographic and clinical characteristics of community-acquired, methicillin-resistant versus methicillin-susceptible Staphylococcus aureus infection in children. Pediatr Infect Dis J 2002;21:910-917.
[12] Kaplan SL, Hulten KG, Gonzalez BE, Hammerman WA, Lambert HL, Versalovic J, Mason EO Jr. Three-year surveillance of community-acquired Staphylococcus aureus infections in children. Clin Infect Dis 2005;40:1785-1791.
[13] Martinez-Aguilar, G, Avalos-Mishaan A, Hulten K, Hammerman W, Mason EO, Kaplan SL. Community-acquired, methicillin-resistant and methicillin-susceptible Staphylococcus aureus musculoskeletal infections in children. Pediatr Infect Dis J 2004;23: 701-706.
[14] Bailey EM, Ryback MJ, Kaatz GW. Comparative effect of protein binding on the killing activities of teicoplanin and vancomycin. Antimicrobial Agents and Chemotherapy 1991;35:1089-1092.
[15] Wood M. The comparative efficacy and safety of teicoplanin and vancomycin. Journal of Antimicrobial Chemotherapy 1996;37: 209-222.

[16] Del Favero A, Menichetti F, Guerciolini R, Bucaneve G, Baldelli F, Aversa F, Terenzi A, Davis S, Pauluzzi S. Prospective randomized clinical trial of teicoplanin for empiric combined antibiotic therapy in febrile, granulocytopenic acute leukemia patients. Antimicrob Agents Chemother 1987;31:1126-1129.

[17] Wootton M, Macgowan AP, Walsh TR, and Howe RA. A multicenter study evaluating the current strategies for isolating Staphylococcus aureus strains with reduced susceptibility to glycopeptides. J Clin Microbiol 2007;45:329-332.

[18] Gruneberg RN. Anti-Gram-positive agents: what we have and what we would like. Drugs 1997;54 (Suppl. 6):29-38.

[19] Darley ES, MacGowan AP. Antibiotic treatment of gram-positive bone and joint infections. J Antimicrob Chemother 2004;53:928-935.

[20] Yuk, JH, Dignani MC, Harris RL, Bradshaw MW, Williams Jr TW. Minocycline as an alternative antistaphylococcal agent. Reviews in Infectious Diseases 1991;13:1023-1024.

[21] Stein, A, Bataille JF, Drancourt M, Curvale G, Argenson JN, Groulier P, Raoult D. Ambulatory treatment of multidrug-resistant Staphylococcus aureus-infected orthopaedic implants with high dose oral co-trimoxazole (trimethoprim-sulfamethoxazole). Antimicrobial Agents and Chemotherapy 1998;42:3086-3091.

[22] Leclercq R, Courvalin P. Streptogramins: an answer to antibiotic resistance in gram-positive bacteria. Lancet 1998;352:591-592.

[23] Drew RH, Perfect JR, Srinath L, Kurkimilis E, Dowzicki M, Talbot GH. Treatment of methicillin-resistant Staphylococcus aureus infections with quinupristin-dalfopristin in patients intolerant or failing prior therapy. Journal of Antimicrobial Chemotherapy 2000; 46:775-784.

[24] Clarebout G, Nativelle E, Bozdogan B, Villers C, Leclercq R. Bactericidal activity of quinupristin-dalfopristin against strains of Staphylococcus aureus with the MLS(B) phenotype of resistance according to the erm gene type. Int J Antimicrob Agents 2004;24: 444-449.

[25] Diekema J, Jones RN. Oxazolidinone antibiotics. Lancet 2001; 358:1975-1982.

[26] Gemmell CG. Susceptibility of a variety of clinical isolates to linezolid: a European inter-country comparison. J Antimicrob Chemother 2001;48:47-52.

[27] Bolmstrom A, Ballow CH, Qwarnstrom A, Biedenbach DJ, Jones RN. Multicentre assessment of linezolid antimicrobial activity and spectrum in Europe: report from the Zyvox antimicrobial potency study (ZAPS-Europe). Clin Microbiol Infect 2002;8: 791-800.

[28] Hoban DJ, Biedenbach DJ, Mutnick AH, Jones RN. Pathogen of occurrence and susceptibility patterns associated with pneumonia in hospitalized patients in North America: results of the SENTRY Antimicrobial Surveillance Study (2000). Diagn Microbiol Infect Dis 2003;45:279-285.

[29] Bozdogan B, Esel D, Whitener C, Browne FA, Appelbaum PC. Antibacterial susceptibility of a vancomycin-resistant Staphylococcus aureus strain isolated at the Hershey Medical Center. J Antimicrob Chemother 2003;52:864-868.

[30] Rana B, Butcher I, Grigoris P, Murnaghan C, Seaton RA, Tobin CM. Linezolid penetration into osteo-articular tissues. Journal of Antimicrobial Chemotherapy 2002;50:747-750.

[31] Kutscha-Lissberg F, Hebler U, Muhr G, Koller M. Linezolid penetration into bone and joint tissues infected with methicillin-resistant staphylococci. Antimicrob Agents Chemother 2003;47:3964-3966.

[32] Pasticci MB, Altissimi M, Azzara A, Di Candilo F, Lapalorcia LM, Giustelli G, Pea F, Baldelli F Treatment of post-traumatic hand Staphylococcus aureus osteomyelitis with oral linezolid. J Chemother 2006;18:425-429.

[33] Melzer M, Goldsmith D, Gransden W. Successful treatment of vertebral osteomyelitis with linezolid in a patient receiving hemodialysis and with persistent methicillin-resistant Staphylococcus aureus and vancomycin-resistant Enterococcus bacteraemia. Clinical Infectious Diseases 2000;31:208-209.

[34] Till M, Wixson, RL, Pertel PE. Linezolid treatment for osteomyelitis due to vancomycin-resistant Enterococcus faecium. Clinical Infectious Diseases 2002;15:1412-1414.

[35] Rao N, Ziran BH, Hall RA, Santa ER. Successful treatment of chronic bone and joint infections with oral linezolid. Clin Orthop Relat Res 2004;427:67-71.

[36] Razonable RR, Osmon DR, Steckelberg JM. Linezolid therapy for orthopedic infections. Mayo Clin Proc 2004 Sep;79 (9):1137-1144.

[37] Patel R, Piper KE, Rouse MS, Steckelberg JM. Linezolid therapy of Staphylococcus aureus experimental osteomyelitis. Antimicrobial Agents and Chemotherapy 2000;44:3438-3440.

[38] Rouse MS, Piper KE, Jacobson M, Jacofsky DJ, Steckelberg JM, Patel R. Daptomycin treatment of Staphylococcus aureus experimental chronic osteomyelitis. J Antimicrob Chemother 2006;57: 301-305.

Local Antibiotic–loaded Carriers in Upper Extremity Surgery

Geert H.I.M. WALENKAMP*

*Department of Orthopaedic Surgery, Academic Hospital Maastricht,
Maastricht, the Netherlands*

Antibiotic–loaded bone cement was developed in the 1970s as a prophylactic and therapeutic tool that would act against orthopaedic infections. The admixture of antibiotics with polymethyl methacrylate seems to be effective in local release of antibiotics, but for the treatment of osteomyelitic cavities beads seem to be necessary. As far as the pharmacokinetic properties are concerned, in the present essay it is explained how a larger carrier surface, as in beads, is responsible for increased local antibiotic concentrations. Moreover, the practical aspects in the use of beads are described and the results of the treatments presented.

Keywords: local antibiotic carriers; osteomyelitis; pharmacokinetics; gentamicin beads.

1. INTRODUCTION

Local antiseptics have been used since the end of the 19th century after the discovery of bacteria. Lister used antiseptics not only to prevent post-operative infections, but also therapeutically in the treatment of open fractures: he applied tampons with carbolic acid and plaster. Later on, he and others treated infections with carbolic acid or cod liver oil in plaster [1,2]. Thus, long before the discovery of antibiotics, application of antibacterial agents to a carrier was already being practised for the treatment and prevention of orthopaedic infections. In irrigation systems, antiseptics were applied locally at the beginning of the 20th century [3,4], whereas antibiotics were applied as soon as they became available, i.e. after the Second World War [5]. Coleman was at that time the first to admix antibiotics into bone grafts [6]. Therefore, as soon as antiseptics and antibiotics became available, local application with a carrier was practised for therapeutic purposes.

Such antibiotic-carrier combinations were also used for the prevention of wound infection. Buchholz used antibiotic-containing solutions for frequent lavage during the operation, and he sutured cloths soaked in antibiotics and applied them to the fascia. In his search for more effective reduction of postoperative deep infections of hip prostheses (3%), he found that bone cement could be used as a means to achieve sustained release of various substances such as the residual monomer and CuS (copper sulphate). Therefore, in a pilot study, he admixed four heat stable antibiotic powders with bone cement and found that except for tetracycline, antibiotics indeed were released by a diffusion process for at least 2 weeks in a bactericidal concentration [7]. The Kulzer and Merck companies (Germany) developed commercially available gentamicin bone cement (Refobacine Palacos®) in the time period from 1970 to 1978. Since then, many combinations of antibiotics and bone cements have been studied. In general, it was found that when gentamicin was chosen, the combination with Palacos® resulted in the best release [8].

*Corresponding Author
Department of Orthopedic Surgery
Academic Hospital Maastricht, Maastricht
Postbox 5800, 6202 AZ Maastricht, the Netherlands
Tel: +31 43 387 5038.
e-mail: gwa@sort.azm.nl

2. ANTIBIOTIC-LOADED CARRIERS: PHARMACOKINETIC PROPERTIES

Bone cement is based on methyl methacrylate and made by mixing the liquid monomer with the polymer powder (PMMA). During the curing process, a network of newly formed PMMA chains are formed. Various substances such as antibiotics can be mixed and will be incorporated in-between those PMMA chains. They can be released by diffusion when the PMMA absorbs water, which is a process determined by the hydrophobicity of the cement. The antibiotic release is influenced by the porosity and roughness of the cement. The release of antibiotics is limited to a depth of 100 μm [9]. The initial high release is a surface phenomenon which lasts for some hours. Then a sustained release starts, a bulk phenomenon, that depends on the penetration of fluid through connected pores into the cement [10].

Once the antibiotic-loaded cement was on the market, it was also used to treat osteomyelitis. Filling bone cavities after debridement of the infection, however, did not appear to be effective in clinical practice [11-13], which was confirmed later on in animal experiments [14]. Therefore, Klaus Klemm started in 1972 to knead small beads of bone cement mixed with antibiotics to treat osteomyelitis. Since 1976, they had been manufactured at the Kulzer company (Wehrheim, Germany) and distributed by Merck (Darmstadt, Germany) (Fig. 1).

Many antibiotics and many bone cements have been tested, and still new combinations are produced. In vitro and in vivo studies of the combinations are not standardized, so it is difficult to decide which products would be the best choice.

In in vitro studies, the release of the antibiotic diffused out of the carrier can be quantified. The tests, however, are not standardized. Two methods are used more frequently.

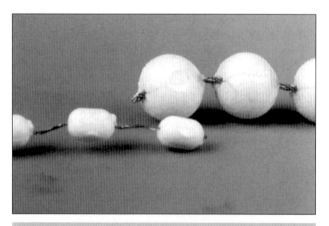

FIGURE 1. Large and mini PMMA beads with gentamicin. The large beads have a diameter of 7 mm and contain 7.5 mg of gentamicin. The minibeads are 3×5 mm and contain 2.8 mg of gentamicin. They are suitable for hand surgery.

Elution of an antibiotic out of the carrier can be measured by changing the bath fluid every hour or day, and this results in a curve with rapid decrease of the eluted antibiotic per time unit. The largest quantity is released within the first hours. The curve will be a type of decreasing logarithmic curve. The second method leaves the bath fluid around the test vehicle undisturbed, except for some relatively very small samples of the fluid that are taken and replaced. The concentration around the carrier will increase gradually, and the resulting curve will be a comparable increasing logarithmic curve.

The in vivo reality will be in-between the two methods of in vitro tests. In the in vivo state there will be more or less replacement of the surrounding fluid (depending on the vascularization, and/or the haematoma), not so much as compared with the first in vitro test method, and more or less as at the second in vitro test method. Because the elution is a diffusion process, the maximum release occurs at the very beginning (first hours and days) when the gradient that appears between the carrier and its surrounding is the highest. The elution will diminish in time when this gradient decreases, and the "motor" of the diffusion loses power.

This diffusion process is the mechanism of spreading antibiotics into the tissues around the implantation area. The antibiotic concentration in these tissues will decrease within the postoperative weeks, as well as with an increasing distance between the implantation area and the carriers increases. In general, gentamicin beads will not be able to create high antibiotic concentrations more than 2 weeks after the time of implantation and at a distance of more than a few centimetres from the beads, depending on the kind of tissue. Such pharmacokinetics in vivo can only be measured in animal experiments and in treated patients. Tissue concentration has been studied in a dog osteomyelitis case by Wahlig et al. [15]. They have proven that the concentration in the haematoma and the tissues decreases in the weeks following implantation. They also demonstrated that the more solid the structure of the tissue, the lower the concentration. The kinds of tissue examined were fibrous tissue, cancellous and cortical bone (Table 1).

It appeared that it was not necessary that the bone be alive: Elson proved that dead bone, too, is well-penetrated and diffused by antibiotic released by bone cement [16]. We could confirm the above mentioned relation of concentration with time and distance from the carrier by conducting animal experiments involving sheep [17] and rabbits.

When collagen is used in combination with gentamicin, attention must be paid to the different properties of the different products. First, gentamicin collagen was compared with gentamicin PMMA beads. In that in vitro study the gentamicin was immediately released, i.e. within a few hours [18], resulting in very high local concentration in the exudate, which lasted for a very short period only. To produce delayed release, another pro-

TABLE 1

Tissue concentrations of gentamicin following implantation of gentamicin PMMA beads in a diaphyseal bone of a dog osteomyelitis model (according to Wahlig et al. [15])

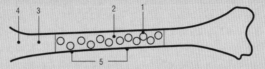

Canine Nr	Number of beads	Postop days	Genta conc in hematoma	Genta conc in connective tissue	Genta conc in spongiosa at level 1	Genta conc in spongiosa at level 2	Genta conc in spongiosa at level 3	Genta conc in cortex
1	17	3	148.0		17.8		3.6	6.8
2	15	3	112.0		15.2		3.6	13.0
3	13	7	200.0		24.0	14.5	4	20.1
4	16	7	212.0		16.4		6.6	14.1
5	18	14	124.0		8.2	5.9	0.6	1.8
6	17	14	101.0		5.2	2.1	0.8	3.8
7	14	28	9.1	9.1	2.9		0.4	1.6
8	14	28		7.5	4.9		0.2	0.4
9	19	42		16.1	8.4	0.34	0.2	0
10	19	42		7.7	4.9	0.9	0.5	0
11	7	63		4.4	0.4	0.2	0.2	0
12	14	63		4.4	0.9	0	0	0
13	28	116		5.6	5.1	1	0.7	0
14	37	116		5.4	2.6	0.2	0.2	0
15	30	116		2.2	1.1	0.8	0	0

Experiment performed in 15 dogs. Concentrations measured at different postoperative periods (3-116 days), in haematoma, connective tissue, spongiosa at 3 levels (see schedule) and in cortical bone.

duct was developed (which would give protracted release). This was achieved by replacing the gentamicin sulfate partly with the inactive gentamicin crobophat. This is transformed to the active sulfate form in a period of some weeks, resulting in a longer period of high release and local concentration.

3. HOW TO USE LOCAL ANTIBIOTIC CARRIERS IN PATIENTS

In general, antibiotic-loaded carriers can be used for the prevention, as well as for the therapeutic treatment of infection. For prevention, high local antibiotic concentration will be effective, even if it lasts for a short period of time only. One or two days, even a few hours may be enough for effective use of antibiotics for prophylaxis, since in such a case, they are used systemically. When the antibiotics are used for therapeutic purposes, the carrier may be more effective when the antibiotic concentration remains high for a longer period, preferably

for 2-4 weeks. The diffusion of the antibiotic into the infected tissues needs time, and the process of killing the bacteria, too.

There is some evidence which suggests that long-term treatment, even over several months, with systemic use of antibiotics, is more effective than repetitive short-term treatments when we have to treat cases with osteomyelitis. So the indication for use of *preventive* local antibiotics may be resorbable carriers with a short half-life, such as some gentamicin collagen products or hand-mixed combinations inserted into autologous bone grafts. For *therapeutic* application, products that are able to maintain high antibiotic concentration for weeks are preferable.

When gentamicin PMMA beads are used in patients, the highest gentamicin concentration can be achieved in a cavity, provided that this cavity is filled with as many beads as possible throughout the whole available space, since the release depends on the surface in relation to the surrounding volume of the haematoma. When the haematoma is properly handled, the local gentamicin concentration will increase immediately after implantation, and achieve a maximum level circa on the third day [19,20]. This maximum contribution can be 50-100 times higher than the MIC value of the causative bacteria. When the distance between the beads and the infected area increases, the antibiotic concentration decreases considerably, thus the effectiveness of the antibiotics: at a distance of 2-3 cm their effectiveness will be largely reduced. Therefore, the beads must be placed densely throughout the whole infected or contaminated space (Fig. 2).

A haematoma is needed to make the elution of the antibiotic possible and antibiotics are released because the place in the PMMA carrier of the antibiotics is replaced by watery solutions. Therefore, PMMA beads will be less effective when they act in subcutaneous, lipophilic tissue. The haematoma should be in an optimal situation not larger than the volume of the beads which cover it. In that case the concentration will be the highest.

Therefore, wound drains must be used with special attention. For example, in the case of infected total hip removal, the best effect will be achieved by use of two drains: one deep, inserted into the centre of the cavity, and the other into the tightly closed fascia. The deep drain must be changed to work as an overflow drainage, once the drain is filled with blood by inserting a needle into the bottle to remove the vacuum. This process is followed to prevent too much antibiotic loss during the first days. When there is not much production left, the vacuum is restored for a short period, to minimize the haematoma, and then removed. In the meantime, the subcutaneous drain should permanently function as vacuum drainage that would remove the haematoma from the subcutaneous layers. In this way, a disturbing

large subcutaneous haematoma will be avoided, and should stop long lasting wound drainage. This drain is removed one day after the first deep drain removal.

In case of collagen carriers, the vacuum drains will suction the collagen too, so they must be used as overflow from the beginning.

PMMA beads are able to occupy space in cavities of osteomyelitis and removed prostheses, and can easily be removed after 2-4 weeks through a part of the original incision, depending on the local anatomy. However, when they are inserted into soft tissue and/or into a stretched form, they will be encapsulated. In that case, the beads must be removed earlier. Permanent implantation of the beads is possible, but the danger of persistence of germs on the beads is always present, so removal of the beads is advisable.

If no reconstruction of the infected area is necessary, beads can also be placed in it, with the end of the chain protruding from the skin. The chain of beads can be removed by simply pulling the end of the chain. In my experience, the best approved option is: to start pulling 1 week after implantation, about 3-5 beads at a time, every other day. The chain should be implanted in a meandering manner, not stretched, and protrude the skin through a separate incision, which should be sufficientlyy wide enough. Special attention must always be paid in checking that the last bead is present at the end of the chain has not slid off.

Patients should not be sent home with beads in a joint cavity, because the chains will break. In such cases of reimplantation with a long-term interval, a spacer could be used. In osteomyelitic cavities, chains with beads can be removed after a longer period if they are not intra-medullary: then they are fixed after 4-6 weeks.

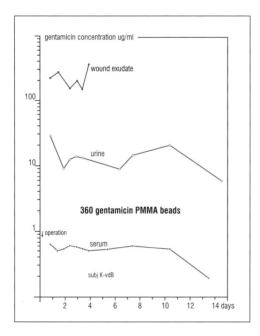

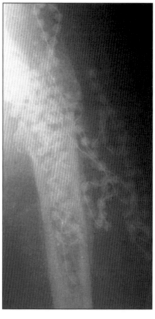

FIGURE 2. Concentrations of gentamicin in exudate, urine and serum in a 64-year-old patient. The Y-axis is logarithmic. After total extraction of an infected prosthesis, 360 gentamicin beads are implanted throughout the entire contaminated area. The local exudate concentration of gentamicin can increase up to several hundreds of µg/ml in this kind of treatment [19].

The solid, not resorbable PMMA beads are easy to use in cases where at a second intervention reconstruction is planned, as bone grafting, osteosynthesis or prosthesis reimplantation. The philosophy is to heal the infection first, and then to reconstruct. It depends on the experience of the clinician in dealing with the calculated risk of healing versus non-healing, and whether the problems that may arise when a relapse occurs after reconstruction are acceptable. It may be wise to let some time pass observing the healing of infection before moving on to the next treatment stage.

So far there is not much experience in the use of resorbable bone substitutes in combination with antibiotics. At this moment, there are only few products on the market. One of the best options at present is admixing yourself antibiotics in the bone graft, autologous or homologous. In *in vitro* and in *in vivo* experiments, as well as in clinical use, bone grafts could give protracted release of admixed antibiotics over several weeks [21,22]. This is a promising application, and, thus important in prosthesis revision and osteomyelitic reconstructions.

When bone substitutes such as Hydroxylapatite, $CaSO_4$, and Tricalciumphosphate are used, wound infections may result in extensive infections of these biomaterials, necessitating the complete removal of all implanted bone substitutes. Coating the substitutes or admixing them with antibiotics by the producer or by the surgeon himself seem to be the most advisable procedure. The advantage is that the choice of the antibiotic is free. However, the disadvantage is that there is never enough evidence that good release will be the result of such home-made antibiotic-loaded biomaterial.

4. Results

The results of the prophylactic use of antibiotics are best documented in primary total hip prostheses. In experimental studies, admixed antibiotics into bone cement have proven to provide protection not only against infection in case of contaminated wounds, but also against haematogenous infection which may appear within a period of 6 weeks after implantation of a prosthesis. This may be an important period in which deep infections may occur due to concomitant pneumonia, decubitus ulcers or urine infection in patients with compromised immune status.

The good therapeutic results of the use of antibiotic-loaded cement in the case of one-stage revisions are due to its letnal effect on the bacteria that are present in the entire wound bed, as inoculants after explantation of a prosthesis loosened by infection, recognized or not. This application may be regarded as a line in-between prophylactic and therapeutic use.

In prophylactic, as well as in therapeutic use, one may expect better results after local antibiotic application rather than after systemic antibiotic use, because the higher local antibiotic concentrations should kill more bacteria in tissues, also when the perfusion of the tissue is less. The proof in randomized clinical trials (RCT), however, appeared difficult. The many clinical variables involved in osteomyelitis make clinical studies difficult to design and to evaluate.

A RCT to achieve FDA approval in the US failed to demonstrate significantly better results in the application of gentamicin PMMA beads in osteomyelitis cases versus parenteral antibiotic treatment. Participating surgeons worried about whether the results would be optimal for the patients in the gentamicin-beads group, who had been administered parenteral antibiotics in addition to the PMMA beads. However, the treatment with gentamicin-beads alone was significantly cheaper [23].

In a series of RCT conducted in 77 open fractures no significant difference was found between local and parenteral antibiotic treatment (by self-made beads) when compared, due to the small-scale of the study [24].

Numerous open cohort studies have been published with the clinical results of the treatment of osteomyelitis, prosthesis infection and other orthopaedic infections. Results in general have been expressed as "healing percentages" at some period after the treatment. An infection will then be considered as healed when all clinical symptoms have disappeared, including and laboratory values have normalized. It may be difficult to judge in case of persistent pain whether that is related to low-grade persistent infection. The same applies in the case of a high ESR value in rheumatoid patients or patients with other infections.

Two proverbs express the prevalent pessimistic view on the healing of osteomyelitis: "Once osteomyelitis, always osteomyelitis" and "Osteomyelitis is a time-bomb that always ticks". However, the literature and my own experience indicate that this pessimism is not justified any more. The results presented in the literature of aggressive operative and medical treatment in cases of early postoperative infection of prosthesis indicate that a healing percentage of 80-90% can be achieved. Most relapses will be recognizable a few months after discontinuation of systemic antibiotic therapy. In osteomyelitis cases, the results of treatment have improved over years: they have increased from 30-50% to 80-90% in the last century (Fig. 3).

Healing, however, should not be expressed as a mere percentage (%), but rather, a detailed survival analysis should be conducted, as in the case of oncological treatment. We studied the healing rate in 100 consecutive patients with osteomyelitis (acute and chronic) and found 19 relapses. When those were treated through another treatment course (operations, eventually followed by postoperative systemic antibiotic treatment) followed over a specific time period, the overall healing success rate after 1-12 years was 92% [25].

The survival analysis showed that the relapses al-

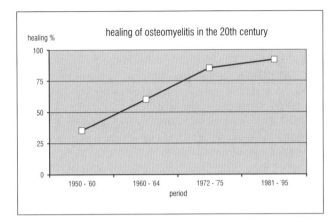

FIGURE 3. Increase of the healing percentage of osteomyelitis in the 20th century. Graph constructed by the author based on interpretation of the literature.

most always occurred in the first postoperative months or year. Based on these data patients are no longer followed at the out patient clinic after the period of 2 years follow up has passed.

5. Conclusions

In the beginning of the use of local antibiotic treatment for soft tissue infections and osteomyelitis, surgeons seriously doubted whether they should go on to a primary closure of the wound. Ever since, it has been advocated that infected wounds should be treated open after debridement. Closure after thorough debridement and implantation of a local antibiotic delivery system was a surgical revolution. However, surgeons still appear to have problems with this innovative approach, as illustrated by the upcoming vacuum-assisted wound treatment. The primary wound closure, necessary to keep the antibiotic inside the wound, however, has graetly improved the comfort of the patient and decreased significantly the workload for the nurses, the time spent in hospital, antibiotic use and the cost of treatment [26].

Antibiotic-loaded carriers are able to create local effective high antibiotic concentrations. This route of administration is more effective: due to the higher antibiotic concentrations in the haematoma and tissues, more resistant bacteria can be killed and better penetration of scarred tissues is possible. Since in the circulation the antibiotics are hardly detectable, systemic side effects are not present when the carriers are used in a proper way. Additional systemic antibiotic treatment is often not necessary anymore.

A prerequisite for the use of local antibiotic carriers is the surgeon's understanding of the pharmacokinetic mechanism. Antibiotic carriers should not be implanted as a kind of magic tool. Only when used in a proper

way are they effective and of great benefit to the patient.

References

[1] Dreesmann H. Über Knochenplombirung, Zentr bl 1896;20:55-56.
[2] Löhr W. Die Behandlung der akuten und der chronische Osteomyelitis der Röhrenknochen mit dem Lebertrangips, Arch Klin Chir 1934;180:206-222.
[3] Carrel A et al. Traitement abortif de l'infection des plaies, Bull Acad Med Paris 1915;74:361.
[4] Dakin H. On the use of certain antiseptic substances in the treatment of infected wounds, Br Med J 1915;2:318.
[5] Willenegger H. Therapeutische Möglichkeiten und Grenzen der antibakteriellen Spüldrainage bei chirurgischen Infektionen, Langenbecks Arch Chir 1963;304:670-672.
[6] Coleman HM, et al. Cancellous bone grafts for infected bone defects, Surg Gynec Obstet 1946;83:392-398.
[7] Buchholz HW, Gartmann HD. Infektionsprophylaxe und operative Behandlung der schleichende tiefen Infektion bei der Totalen Endoprothese, Chirurg 1972;43:446-453.
[8] Wahlig H et al. Über die Freisetzung von Gentamycin aus Polmethylmethacrylat. II. Experimentelle Untersuchungen *in vivo*, Langenbecks Arch Chir 1972;331 (3):193-212.
[9] Schurman DJ et al. Antibiotic-acrylic bone cement composites, J Bone Jt Surg 1978;60-A:978-984.
[10] Belt van der H et al. Surface roughness, porosity and wettability of gentamicin-loaded bone cements and their antibiotic release, Biomaterials 2000;21:1981-1987.
[11] Jenny G et al. Utilisation de billes de ciment acrylique à la gentamycine, Rev Chir Orthop Repar Appar Mol 1977;63:491-500.
[12] Voorhoeve A, Stöhr Chr. Ergebnisse bei der Behandlung der chronischer-eitrigen Ostemyelitis mit einem Palacos-gentamycin Gemisch, Munsch med Wschr 1973;115:924-930.
[13] Klemm K. Die Behandlung chronischer Knocheninfektionen mit Gentamycin-PMMA-Keten und -Kugeln, in: Contzen H (Ed.), Gentamycin-PMMA-Kette. Gentamycin-PMMA-Kugeln. Symposium Munchen 12 November 1976, VLE Verlag, 1977;20-25.
[14] Fitzgerald RH. Experimental osteomyelitis: description of a canine model and the role of depot administration of antibiotics in the prevention of sepsis, J Bone Jt Surg 1983;65-A (3):371-380.
[15] Wahlig H et al. The release of gentamicin from polymethylmethacrylate beads. An experimental and pharmacokinetic study, J Bone Jt Surg 1978;60-B (2):270-275.
[16] Elson RA et al. Antibiotic loaded acrylic cement, J Bone Joint Surg 1977;59-B (2):200-205.
[17] Kaarsemaker S, Walenkamp GH, Bogaard van der AE, New model for chronic osteomyelitis with *Staphylococcus aureus* in sheep, Clin Orthop 1997;vol 1997:246-252.
[18] Sandberg Soerensen T, Ibsen Soerensen A, Merser S. Rapid release of gentamicin from collagen sponge: *in vitro* comparison with plastic beads, Acta Orthop Scand 1990;61 (4):353-356.
[19] Walenkamp GHIM. Gentamicin PMMA beads. A clinical, pharmacokinetic and toxicological study: Thesis Katholieke Universiteit Nijmegen, 1983.
[20] Walenkamp GHIM. Chronic osteomyelitis. How I do it, Acta Orthop Scand 1997;68 (5):497-506.
[21] Witsoe E et al. Cancellous bone as an antibiotic carrier, Acta Orthop Scand 2000;71 (1):80-84.

[22] Witsoe E et al., Adsorption and release of antibiotics from morselized cancellous bone. *In vitro* studies of 8 antibiotics, Acta Orthop Scand 1999;70 (3):298-304.

[23] Blaha JD et al. Comparison of the clinical efficacy and tolerance of gentamicin PMMA beads on surgical wire versus combined and systemic therapy for osteomyelitis, Clin Orthop Relat Res 1993;295:8-12.

[24] Moehring HD et al. Comparison of antibiotic beads and intra-venous antibiotics in open fractures, Clin Orthop Relat Res 2000;372:254-261.

[25] Walenkamp GH, Kleijn LL, Leeuw de M. Osteomyelitis treated with gentamicin-PMMA beads: 100 patients followed for 1-12 years, Acta Orthop Scand 1998;69 (5):518-522.

[26] Hoök M, Lindberg L. Treatment of chronic osteomyelitis with gen-tamicin-PMMA beads. A prospective study in Nepal, Trop Doct October 1987;157-163.

Imaging of Musculoskeletal Infections of the Upper Limb in Children

Maria RAISSAKI*, Eleni APOSTOLAKI

Department of Radiology, University of Crete, Heraklion, Greece

The mechanism and site of upper limb musculoskeletal infection, pathogens, clinical and laboratory findings at presentation and the response from the growing skeleton may be different in neonates and children compared to adults. Complications, such as skeletal deformities and recurrent or difficult to treat, chronic lesions, may be avoided if infection is diagnosed early and treated adequately. Imaging findings in pediatric musculoskeletal infection correlate with the pathogenesis and pathophysiology of disease. Imaging can often help us to confirm the clinical diagnosis of musculoskeletal infection, to evaluate the site and extent of disease and to determine the most appropriate mode of therapy. Knowledge of the potential and limitations of each imaging modality should guide the radiologist to avoid tests that require ionizing radiation, and consider issues regarding special technique. Ultrasonography plays an increasingly important role in all kinds of acute musculoskeletal infections of the upper extremities in children.

Keywords: osteomyelitis; septic arthritis; soft tissue infection; upper limb; imaging; child.

1. INTRODUCTION

Osteoarticular infection in children consists of bone, intra-articular and soft tissue infection. Upper-limb osteomyelitis and septic arthritis are less common than lower-limb osteoarticular infections [1,2] and comprise approximately 15-25% of cases of pediatric osteoarticular infections involving the limbs [3, 4]. In tropical countries upper limb joints of younger children may be more commonly affected, while in older children lower limb joint septic arthritis is more common [5].

The mechanism and site of infection, pathogens, clinical and laboratory findings at presentation, and the response from the growing skeleton may be different in neonates and children compared to adults. Complications, such as skeletal deformities and recurrent or difficult to treat chronic lesions, may be avoided if the infection is adequately diagnosed and treated within one week from the onset of symptoms [6].

In most cases, clinical presentation will be fairly typical. However, clinical assessment may be difficult, especially when these children present with systemic upset, nonspecific pseudoparalysis or persistent pain, or in cases where the course of the disease has been altered by antibiotic administration. Imaging is often able to confirm or contribute to early diagnosis. It should be undertaken early to evaluate the site and extent of disease, to determine the most appropriate mode of therapy and to monitor the response to treatment.

Imaging is only justified after thorough clinical examination, including laboratory studies [7]. Various imaging techniques can be effectively used, but no single modality is superior in every clinical situation. Understanding the strengths and limitations of different techniques, as well as the natural history of infection, allows appropriate timing of the correctly chosen technique [8].

*Corresponding Author
Department of Radiology,
University Hospital of Heraklion,
University of Crete, Heraklion, Greece
Tel: +30 2810 392542
Fax: +30 2810 542095
e-mail: mariarai@her.forthnet.gr

2. CLASSIFICATION OF PEDIATRIC MUSCULOSKELETAL INFECTION

Musculoskeletal infections in children comprise osteomyelitis, septic arthritis and soft tissue infection. According to the clinical setting, infection may be characterized as acute (lasting less than 2 weeks), sub-acute (2-6 weeks) and chronic (more than 6 weeks). The source of the infection may be (i) hematogenous, (ii) inoculation from a penetrating wound or (iii) direct spread from adjacent structures. The majority of osteoarticular infections in otherwise healthy children are of hematogenous origin [9]. Sporadic cases of post-traumatic osteomyelitis associated with foreign bodies, clavicular osteomyelitis following central catheter placement and radial osteomyelitis following venous cannulation have also been described [10, 11]. Depending on the causative organism, musculoskeletal infections are divided into congenital and acquired. Congenital infection may be due to syphilis or viral agents including rubella, CMV and varicella. Acquired infection may be due to bacteria, mycobacteria (TB), fungi and may also be idiopathic, a condition known as Chronic Recurrent Multifocal Osteomyelitis.

3. ORGANISMS

Acute osteoarticular infection is usually a bacterial infection. Mycobacterial infections of the upper extremities are extremely rare, usually causing chronic or multifocal osteomyelitis [12]. Fungal infections are also rare. *Staphylococcus aureus* is the predominant cause of acute hematogenous osteomyelitis and septic arthritis (40%-90% of cases), especially in children older than 2 years [13]. *Group A-hemolytic Streptococcus* (GABHS) is the next in frequency, followed by *Streptococcus pneumonia*. Both organisms tend to affect preschool and early school-aged children [13]. *Haemophilus influenzae* type b is less and less frequently associated with acute hematogenous osteomyelitis. *Kingella kingae* is increasingly being associated with acute osteomyelitis and septic arthritis in younger children, up to 3 years old [14]. *Salmonella* is the main pathogen of osteomyelitis in children with sickle cell disease [15] and may cause septic arthritis following gastroenteritis and bacteremia in otherwise healthy infants. *Y. Enterocolitica* has been found in patients with thalassemia and osteomyelitis or septicemia [1]. The most common pathogens in soft tissue infections are *Staphylococcus aureus, Clostridium novyi* and *Clostridium perfigens*. Pseudomonas species and Gram-negative bacteria may arise from penetrating injuries [16, 17]. Anaerobic bacteria are responsible for infections following human or animal bites [18].

4. SPECIAL TECHNIQUE ISSUES IN CHILDREN

Successful scanning in children depends on meticulous technique. For optimal results, images should be carried out by personnel accustomed to dealing with children and viewed by pediatric radiologists, considering all scans from various imaging techniques and pertinent clinical parameters.

In scintigraphy, high resolution images are required; coarse matrix digital images are unsatisfactory. Limbs must be imaged separately so that count rates are adequate for the diagnosis [19]. Ideally a three-phase bone scan increases the sensitivity of the test. In small infants a two-phase scan omitting the arterial phase is usually performed.

For radiographs and CT, justification of tests on diagnosis and follow-up, as well as the ALARA principle (As Low As Reasonably Achievable) should be meticulously applied. Recommended exposures for extremities (elbow down - knees down) include 120 kV, 21mAs for children under 15 kg, 35 mAs for children 15-34 kg and 55 mAs for children 35-54 kg. Reconstruction in three planes is mandatory. Automated exposure control techniques have been applied in pediatric musculoskeletal imaging [20].

Ultrasonography (US) is preferred for its availability, lack of ionizing radiation and low cost. Following clinical examination, comparative views between the limbs and careful evaluation of the entire circumference of the bone using linear, high frequency probes should be employed [21]. In painful situations and non-cooperative children, the water bath technique could prove helpful for adequate US imaging [22].

MRI scans should be performed under sedation in non-cooperative children, employing small field-of-view, thin section, high resolution scans with reduced echo-train lengths on Turbo Spin-echo sequences, reduced RF angle in refocusing pulses (<180º) in Spin echo sequences, use of GRE sequences and fast turbo spin echo rather than spin echo sequences for cartilage imaging, and finally, minimization of imaging time [23]. The entire involved limb should be scanned within extremity or phased-array coils rather than body coils. Small flexible or surface coils may be used for imaging the pediatric hand or wrist [24]. Older children are positioned prone and the limb above the head, while younger children are positioned supine and the limb at the side of the body. Post-contrast scans may determine necrotic areas requiring decompression.

5. SOFT TISSUE INFECTION

Soft tissue infections of the upper limb in children rarely require imaging. They most commonly result from penetrating injuries and hematogenous spread but are also seen as a complication of systemic disorders, mainly diabetes. The radiologist's interest focuses on exclusion of foreign bodies complicating cellulitis, differentiation of cellulitis from septic arthritis and/or osteomyelitis, exclusion of abscess formation and pyomyositis, and on follow-up. Imaging may also guide drainage and aspiration for cultures.

5.1. Cellulitis

Cellulitis is a clinical diagnosis and refers to acute inflammation/infection without suppuration of the skin and subcutaneous tissue. It presents with localized pain, erythema, swelling and heat, having a predilection for the extremities in children [25, 26]. Cellulitis may progress to necrosis, cavitation and micro- or macro- abscess formation; occasionally with hemorrhage. The value of imaging is helping to rule out an abscess or cellulitis complicated with fasciitis and to differentiate cellulitis from septic arthritis and/or osteomyelitis. US is the imaging modality of choice [25], showing thickening of the skin and subcutaneous tissues, loss of architecture of the subcutaneous fat with increased echogenicity (Fig. 1) progressing to hypoechoic strands between hyperechoic fat lobules, the so-called "cobblestone appearance" (Fig. 2). Poor ultrasound penetration of tissues and blurring of tissue planes may also occur. Increased vascularity at color or power Doppler may suggest an infectious cause [25, 27]. Cultures are more likely to grow bacteria if fluid is aspirated from anechoic strands, provided that a minimal fluid will not be masked by excessive transducer compression. CT and MRI are more sensitive in identifying and mapping edematous regions and for abscess exclusion. CT, usually performed for other reasons, may reveal cellulitis as increased subcutaneous fat density at narrow window settings and rarely subtle gas formation. MRI may show scattered ill-

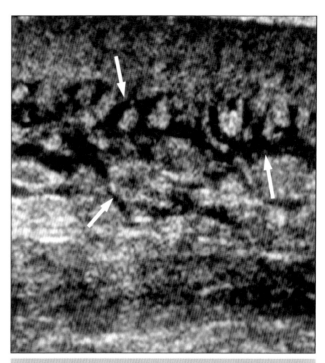

FIGURE 2. Cobblestone appearance: anechoic strands (arrows) among fat lobules.

defined hypointense areas on T1-weighted sequences (Fig. 3a), a striated pattern of hyperintensity on T2-weighted images, more conspicuous on STIR or T2w fat saturated sequences (Fig. 3b). These areas enhance diffusely (Fig. 3c).

5.2. Soft tissue abscess

Bacterial infections may develop into an abscess depending on the patient's immunologic status. On plain radiographs a soft tissue mass with distortion of fascial planes can be seen, occasionally containing air. US, imaging modality of choice for superficial abscesses, shows cystic structures containing multiple echoes (Fig. 4). The margins may be relatively sharp, blend with surrounding cellulitis or may be outlined by an echogenic rim. The liquefied contents may be anechoic, hypoechoic, hyperechoic or isoechoic to surrounding tissues. Posterior acoustic enhancement is helpful but often absent. Gentle compression with the probe may reveal motion of the liquefied material, the so called "swirling sign" or "ultrasonographic fluctuation" [25, 28]. Color Doppler may show fluid collections that lack flow, surrounded by hyperemia [28]. CT, indicated when US cannot identify suspected abscesses, may show a rim-enhancing fluid collection with a wall of varying thickness. On MRI, abscesses are hypointense on T1w and hyperintense on T2w sequences. A low signal intensity rim is seen on T2w sequences (Fig. 3b). Post contrast images show rim enhancement (Fig. 3c).

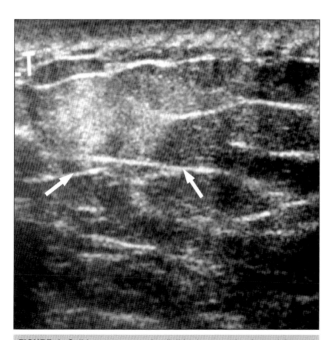

FIGURE 1. Solid appearance of cellulitis: increased echogenicity and distorted fat lobules (arrows).

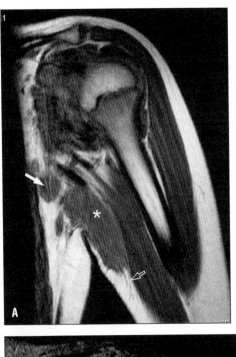

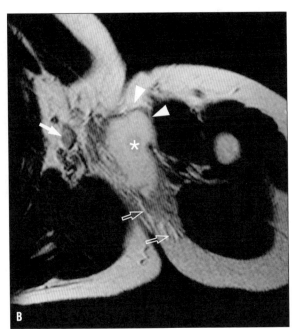

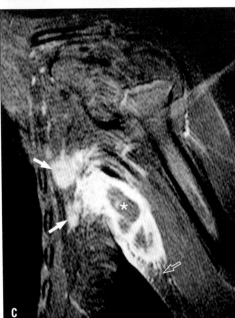

FIGURE 3. A. Coronal T1w and **B.** axial T2w sequences in a 6-year-old female with cat-scratch disease. Enlarged axillary nodes (white arrows). A hypointense on T1w and hyperintense on T2w sequences ovoid area (*), represents an abscess, surrounded by a low intensity rim (arrowheads). Subcutaneous fat stranding (open arrows) represents cellulitis. **C.** T1w fat saturated post-contrast coronal image. Nodes (arrows) enhance homogeneously. There is peripheral abscess enhancement, central necrosis (*) and adjacent cellulitis (open arrow).

5.3. Fasciitis/Necrotizing fasciitis (NF)

Fasciitis, an inflammatory process of the superficial fascia spares the skin and muscles initially. Fasciitis may evolve to necrotizing fasciitis that is a rare, life-threatening condition [29] with gangrenous infection of the subcutaneous fat and fascia. A severe toxic state and pain disproportionate to skin appearances suggest NF. In 20-40% of NF cases, myositis coexists. Predisposing factors reported in up to 50% of pediatric NF include malnutrition, immunosuppression and acute leukemia [16, 30]. Surgical resection of necrotic tissue is life-saving and should not be delayed by imaging. On US, NF is characterized by subcutaneous

edema and thickened, distorted fascial planes, occasionally containing turbid fluid and eventually gas. CT or MRI may inconstantly demonstrate gas in the anatomic region of fasciae and/or fluid collections locally [26]. Mild forms cause thickening of fasciae with mild or no enhancement and cellulitis-like changes of the subcutaneous fat. Adjacent muscles usually demonstrate ill-defined edema.

5.4. Myositis/Pyomyositis (PM)

Pyomyositis, possibly the sequela of myositis, is an intramuscular suppuration caused by bacterial infection which rarely affects muscles of the upper extremity. One

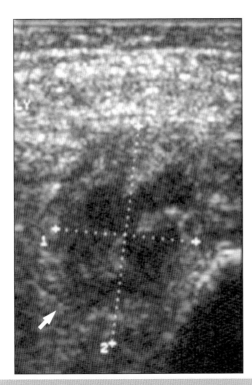

FIGURE 4. Cursors denote an inhomogeneous abscess, containing multiple echoes. Margins are relatively sharp superficially, ill-defined posteriorly and blend with surrounding cellulitis (arrow).

third of PM cases are children, both in tropical and non-tropical regions [31]. Contributing factors include trauma, diabetes mellitus, steroid therapy, sickle cell anemia, acute lymphocytic leukemia, connective tissue disorders and immunosuppression [16]. The disease is characterized by localized muscle edema followed by abscess formation. On US, early findings comprise poorly defined, hypoechoic or hyperechoic areas with preservation of stranding in one or more muscles with or without fascial thickening. Axial imaging demonstrates non-specific muscle enlargement and edema: hypodense non-enhancing muscles on CT, hyperintense on T2w sequences, non-enhancing muscles on MRI. Biopsy is usually required. Subsequently, liquefaction occurs and an intramuscular abscess-looking structure is identified by all modalities. The inconstant presence of air is best appreciated with CT.

5.5. Tenosynovitis

Acute suppurative tenosynovitis most commonly involves the tendon sheaths of the digital flexor muscles and usually follows penetrating injuries, human or animal bites. The examiner should exclude an associated foreign body, ideally with US, especially if it is non-radiopaque. All foreign bodies are initially hyperechoic. Wooden foreign bodies may become less echoic over time [32]. An acoustic shadow, alone or in con-

junction with reverberation artifacts increases conspicuity. A hypoechoic halo corresponds to surrounding fluid, pus or granulation tissue (Fig. 5). On US, acute tenosynovitis appears as fluid within the tendon sheath, thickening of synovial membrane (Fig. 6a, 6b, 7a) and increased Power Doppler signal within the area of local swelling, indicating that the hypoechoic rim around the tendon is partly vascularized synovium (Fig. 7b). MRI depicts fluid signal intensity around affected tendons [27, 32].

5.6. Bursitis

Bursitis may be caused by repetitive trauma, infection and inflammatory arthropathy. Infectious bursitis is rare in childhood [33] and almost exclusively involves the pre-patellar and olecranon bursa. Septic and nonseptic bursitis cause fluid collections in specific locations. Septic bursitis can be excluded in the absence of swelling of bursa and surrounding soft tissues. During US-guided aspiration, the needle tip can be guided away from synovial hypertrophy and at fluid collections within the bursa. Moreover, when infectious bursitis is mistaken for infectious arthritis, US will identify the bursa as the infected structure and will prevent contamination of a normal joint [25].

6. SEPTIC ARTHRITIS

Septic arthritis (SA) of childhood is not common, but remains an important and serious disease because of

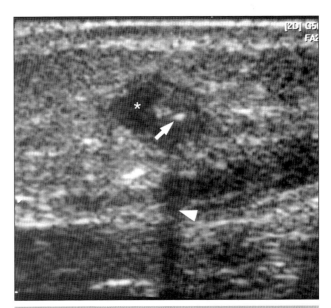

FIGURE 5. Echogenic wood splinter (arrow) casting an acoustic shadow (arrowhead), surrounded by a hypoechoic rim (*), probably granulation tissue.

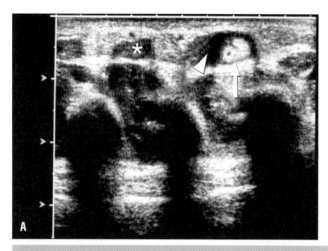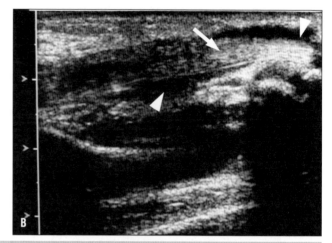

FIGURE 6. A: Axial and **B:** longitudinal view of the flexor tendon of the 4th finger revealing tenosynovitis in a 14-year-old guitar player. The tendon is echogenic and thickened (arrows) compared to adjacent tendons (*). The thickened sheath is hypoechoic (arrowheads).

potential permanent disability, especially when occurring in neonates and infants [34]. The shoulder, elbow, and wrist joints are involved in about 25% of SA cases; small joints are uncommonly infected. Septic arthritis is monoarticular in 90% of cases [14]. Multifocal osteoarticular involvement is encountered in gonnococcal infections and neonatal osteomyelitis [9].

6.1. Pathogenesis

The majority of SA cases in otherwise healthy children results from hematogenous inoculation to the hypervascular synovium. Preceding trauma locally or distally is less common in SA compared to osteomyelitis. Interventional and surgical procedures have also been incriminated. Synovial membrane receptors for certain bacteria may also play a role in pathogenesis [9]. Proteolytic enzymes and cytokines have the potential to destroy the articular cartilage. Degradation of cartilage begins within 8 hours after the onset of infection, with the breakdown of glycosaminoglycans and collagen [35].

6.2. Clinical findings

In SA, neonates may present with redness, swelling, peudoparalysis or pain on movement of the affected extremity. Older children usually have fever and localized signs. Nonspecific disseminated infectious syndrome is seen with multifocal osteoarticular disease, usually due to *S. aureus* [9]. ESR and C-reactive protein are usually elevated. If SA is suspected, urgent aspiration and culture are mandatory. Bacteria are isolated from one or more cultures of blood, joint fluid, pus or bone in 70% of patients [4]. Arthrotomy is used when aspiration has failed. Surgical or arthroscopic joint washout and antibiotics have been employed for shoulder SA [36]. Complications include avascular necrosis, ambulatory disability, limb-length discrepancy, abnormal skeletal growth, sepsis and meningitis [34].

6.3. Imaging findings

Radiographs may be normal or may reveal soft tissue

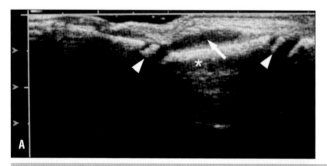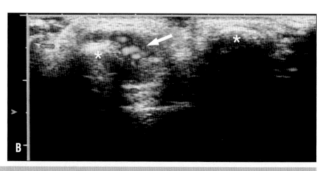

FIGURE 7. A: longitudinal and **B:** axial power Doppler view of the palmar surface of the 4th finger. The thickened tendon sheath is hypoechoic (arrow) abutting the adjacent phalangeal diaphysis (*). Arrowheads: epiphyses. B: Color (arrow) indicates inflammatory tissue.

swelling due to capsule swelling, fat pad elevation at the lateral elbow radiographs, fat pat obliteration due to soft tissue edema joint space widening and periarticular osteoporosis [37]. Joint space narrowing occurs after several days due to cartilage destruction, rarely with subluxation and dislocation. Subchondral bone erosion and destruction appear within 14 to 19 days.

US may detect small amounts of intra-articular fluid up to 1 ml and guide aspiration [25]. Absence of effusion virtually excludes septic arthritis. The size and echogenicity of fluid can not distinguish infectious from noninfectious causes. Increased power Doppler flow suggests infection while normal blood flow does not exclude infection [25].

Technetium 99m methylene diphosphonate (Tc^{99m} MDP) bone scan is useful in doubtful diagnoses, can accurately identify SA in 90% of patients and may differentiate bone from joint involvement. Isolated septic arthritis may appear as non-specific diffuse increased uptake around the joint. A totally photopenic epiphysis may indicate early avascular necrosis due to increased intracapsular pressure [38].

CT and MRI may detect joint effusions. CT is generally avoided. MRI is reserved for complex cases with multiple compartment involvement and may reveal joint effusion, thickening and enhancement of synovium. Subchondral areas of edema, seen as abnormal signal intensity with homogeneous enhancement, occasionally seen in SA, do not necessarily correspond to osteomyelitis and are helpful for differenting SA from idiopathic synovitis [16]. The sensitivity and specificity of MRI employing fat saturated T1w post contrast sequences may be 100% and 77%, respectively [39].

7. OSTEOMYELITIS

7.1. Clinical findings

Signs and symptoms of upper limb pediatric osteomyelitis may be nonspecific and include localized swelling, redness, focal tenderness, motion-induced pain, decreased range of motion, fever and failure/refusal to use the affected arm [3, 16]. Erb's palsy shortly following delivery may rarely be secondary to neonatal osteomyelitis, due to soft tissue edema compressing the brachial plexus [40], or due to ischemic neuropathy from inflammation of the vasa nervorum [41]. Infection may be silent in neonates. Laboratory studies may assist the diagnosis. ESR is increased in 70-100% of cases [3], C-reactive protein in 82-98% of children hospitalized for infection and white cell count in 52-92% of cases. Blood cultures are positive in about half of patients [3]. Chronic osteomyelitis may be clinically present with discharging sinuses and low-grade fever [16].

7.2. Site of involvement depending on patient's age

Hematogenous osteomyelitis is closely related to the osseous blood supply [21]. It may occur following trauma in about one third of patients [9] and also following transient bacteremia. The vascular supply of tubular bones is age-dependent: vessels penetrate the growth plate during infancy, while during childhood they do not extend across the growth plate. Transphyseal vessels disappear by the 12th-18th month of age [7]. Metaphyseal vessels form slow-flowing sinusoidal lakes and predispose to local hematogenous colonization. The shoulder and elbow joints may be secondarily affected because the joint capsule inserts below the epiphyseal growth plate. Therefore, in neonates, hematogenous osteomyelitis, often accompanied by septic arthritis, may be seen at the metaphysis, epiphysis, or both. In children, the metaphysis is the commonest, typical site of hematogenous osseous infection. Metaphyseal-equivalent sites include the periphery of the scapula, the proximal and distal humerus by its secondary ossification centers and the wrist bones. Epiphyseal osteomyelitis in children is rare [7] and is more likely the result of retrograde infection from adjacent septic arthritis.

7.3. Pathogenesis

Following inoculation of the organism, inflammatory exudates result in increased intraosseous pressure, blood flow stasis, thrombosis with potential bone necrosis and resorption, uplifting of the periosteum and penetration of the periosteal membrane [42]. Subperiosteal spread and abscess formation is easier in children due to loose periosteal attachment. Complications include SA with subsequent subluxation and avascular necrosis, growth plate arrest/deformity, chronic infection, slipped epiphyses and pathological fractures. Subacute osteomyelitis is characterized by a localized pyogenic process surrounded by granulation tissue and sclerosis, the Brodie's abscess. Chronic osteomyelitis is characterized by a sequestrum, a piece of necrotic bone embedded in inflammation. An involucrum consists of periosteal new bone around dead bone. An opening connecting the necrotic medullary cavity to the surrounding soft tissues is called "cloaca" [43] and may continue to the skin with a sinus tract.

7.4. Imaging findings

7.4.1. Plain Radiography

The main utility of radiographs is to provide a global view of the affected skeletal area and to exclude other entities [21]. X-rays may be normal within the first 10 days of symptom appearance. Osteomyelitis may manifest with osteopenia with or without soft tissue swelling, fat plane loss and/or displacement, followed by development of an ill-defined area of trabecular and subsequently cortical bone destruction (Fig. 8). Periosteal reaction may never appear or may be noted within the

10th-14th day of infection (Fig 9), depending on the efficacy of treatment. A permeative or sclerotic (Fig. 10) pattern is a characteristic feature of subacute or chronic osteomyelitis. A Brodie's abscess is seen as an elongated radiolucent lesion in the long bones, measuring 1-4 cm in length with surrounding sclerosis, occasionally extending from the metaphysis to the epiphysis (Fig. 11). Brodie's abscesses, when cortical, may simulate osteoid osteomas. Pus penetrates the cortex via a cloaca, may elevate the periosteum or extend beneath it, causing vascular deprivation and dense periosteal reaction, known as involucrum (Fig. 12). A sequestrum is seen as devitalized radiodense bone within osteopenic areas. Complications such as growth plate distortion may be radiographically detected.

7.4.2. Scintigraphy

A three-phase Tc99m MDP bone scan may detect infection within 14-72 hours, days to weeks earlier than radiographs in up to 60% of cases [2]. Scintigraphy will effectively demonstrate lesions about the scapula that are difficult to recognize radiographically. Bone scintigraphy is more than 90% sensitive [44], relatively non-specific and

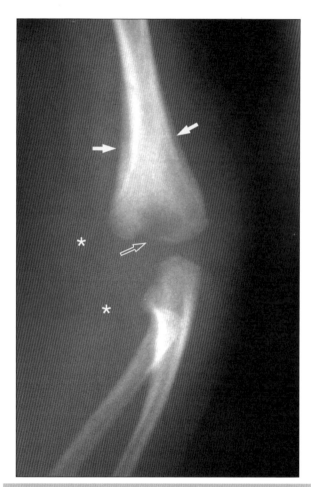

FIGURE 9. Elbow radiograph of a 1-month-old male with upper limb pseudoparalysis shows trabecular rarefaction, cortical disruption at the olecranon fossa (open arrow), periosteal reaction (white arrows) and soft tissue swelling (*).

unable to differentiate osteomyelitis from malignancy or trauma. A known limitation is that false negative Tc99m MDP scans can occur [45]. This has been attributed to the destructive pattern of neonatal osteomyelitis, with lack of bony repair. Osteomyelitis may be multifocal in 22-47% of neonatal cases, thus whole body scintigraphy is imperative [46].

In acute osteomyelitis all three phases of Tc99m MDP scans show increased uptake with the abnormal "hot" area being well-defined and matched, while in septic arthritis and cellulitis, bone scans show increased uptake in the first two phases only [16]. In metaphyseal infection, loss of the sharp demarcation of the normal growth plate is accompanied by a flare of increased activity in the shaft. A 4th-phase scan, 24 hours after injection, may reveal further increased activity in equivocal 3-phase scans.

Gallium 67 citrate scans may more accurately detect osteoarticular infections. However, it carries a high radiation dose and is reserved for difficult cases when the bone scan is negative [2] and for the differential diagno-

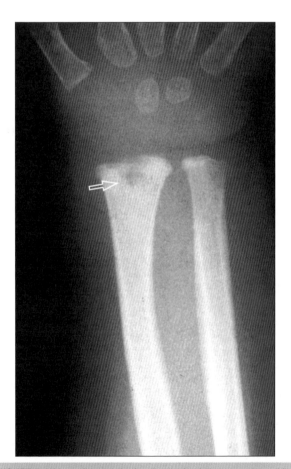

FIGURE 8. Wrist radiograph for localized pain shows metaphyseal ill-defined lucency (open arrow).

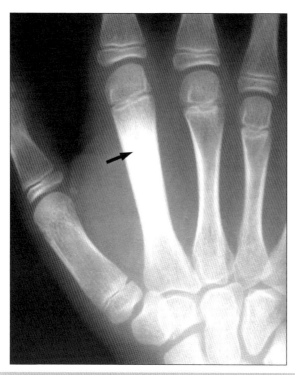

FIGURE 10. Hand radiograph in an 11-year-old male with pain for 2 years, shows sclerosis and mild diaphyseal expansion of the second metacarpal. A lucent moth-eaten area (arrow) proved to be a medullary abscess containing a sequestrum.

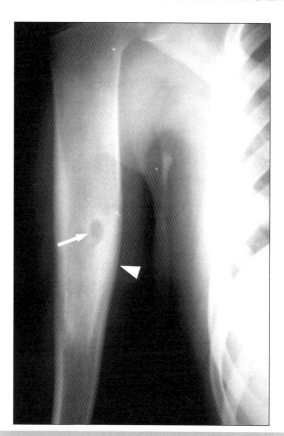

FIGURE 11. X-ray of an 11-year-old female with low grade fever for 1 month shows diffuse sclerosis and cortical thickening (arrowhead), containing a lucent, well-defined, oblong lesion (arrow).

sis of bone infarct and chronic osteomyelitis in patients with sickle-cell disease [47].

7.4.3. Ultrasonography
Deep soft tissue swelling may be the earliest US sign of acute osteomyelitis and may persist through the course of infection. Periosteal reaction may be seen in long bones as echogenic periosteum elevated by 2-3 mm, occasionally accompanied by a thin layer of subperiosteal anechoic fluid. Subperiosteal abscesses are seen as periosteal elevation >3mm and a spindle-shaped fluid collection along the cortex of bone with decreased or increased echogenicity (Fig. 13) [25, 48]. On color Doppler, peripheral hyperemia may not be demonstrated around abscesses until the 4th day of symptom appearance [49, 50, 51]. Cortical erosions may be detected within the 2nd-4th week as progressively increased transmission of sound through the bone due to calcium absorption and echoes within the medullary cavity [50]. US may show soft tissue multifocal osteomyelitis, intra-articular fluid collections, may guide drainage or fluid aspiration [21, 50] and may observe treated collections [48, 52]. US findings usually resolve within 4 weeks.

7.4.4. Computed Tomography
CT should not be performed routinely in acute osteomyelitis due to radiation burden and should be reserved

for the evaluation of the subacute and chronic stages of infection, for cortical lesions (Fig. 14a) and for radiographically hidden sites including the sterno-clavicular junction and shoulder bones. Increased bone marrow density may be due to purulent material replacing normal fatty marrow (Fig. 14b). CT accurately accesses features of sequestrae (Fig. 15), involucrum, cloaca and abscesses.

7.4.5. MRI
MRI offers excellent contrast resolution and depicts changes in the bone marrow, joints and soft tissue. Its sensitivity in diagnosing early osteomyelitis is equal to or greater than scintigraphy [3] and could be considered a substitute for scintigraphy in cooperative children. However, in a series of children with acute osteomyelitis, who underwent both scintigraphy and MRI, in no instance was the diagnosis of osteomyelitis indicated only by MRI [53]. In practice, MRI is reserved for difficult clinical diagnoses, in cases with poor response to treatment and for preoperative planning.

Imaging findings of acute osteomyelitis include areas in the bone marrow exhibiting hypointensity on T1w sequences and hyperintensity on T2w and inver-

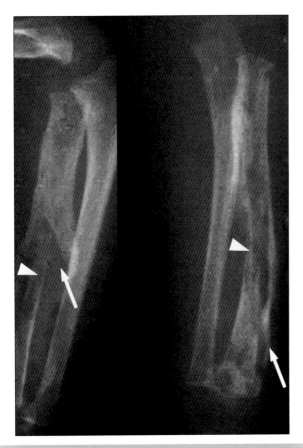

FIGURE 12. Chronic osteomyelitis and involucrum. A dense bony layer is seen (arrow) around the disorganized native bone (arrowhead), consistent with living bone below the elevated periosteum surrounding the dead native bone.

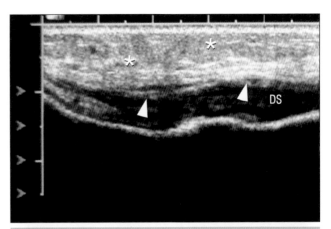

FIGURE 13. US of a drained subperiosteal abscess showing deep soft tissue swelling (DS) at the left forearm, elevated echogenic periosteum (arrowheads) and increased echogenic subcutaneous fat, consistent with cellulitis (*).

sion recovery sequences (Fig. 16) [7, 24]. These changes represent edema, inflammation and/or purulent material. Inflammatory tissue enhances, whereas purulent material does not [16]. As opposed to malignancies, in acute osteomyelitis, the zone of transition at T1w sequences is wide due to interspersed fatty islands. Subperiosteal fluid collections and intraosseous, subperiosteal, or soft tissue abscesses may exhibit hypointensity on T1w and hyperintensity on T2w sequences, surrounded by zones of low signal intensity on T2w sequences. Fluid collections and abscesses may appear as non-enhancing or rim-enhancing areas,

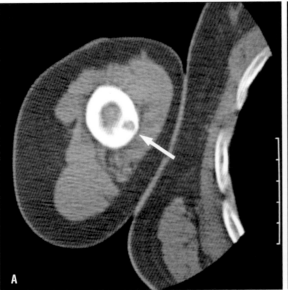

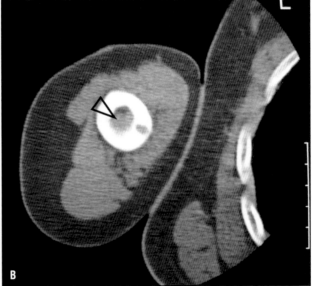

FIGURE 14. A: CT of same patient as in Fig. 11, demonstrates the cortical location of a Brodie's abscess (arrow). B: Increased medullary density due to inflammatory tissue (arrowhead).

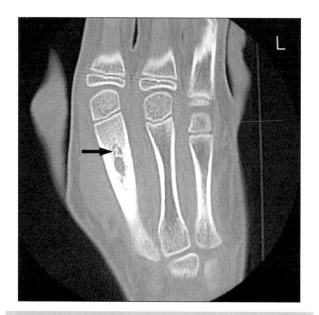

FIGURE 15. CT shows bony sclerosis around an area of medullary destruction that contains a piece of sclerotic bone (arrow), which is indicative of a sequestrum.

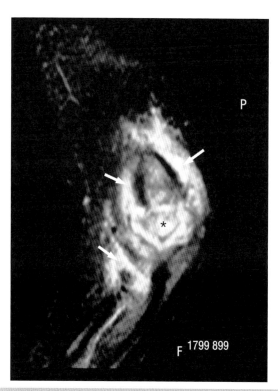

FIGURE 16. STIR sequence of same patient in Fig. 9. Hyperintensity of soft tissues (arrows) and humeral epiphysis (*) is attributed to soft tissue edema and epiphyseal osteomyelitis, respectively.

respectively. The penumbra sign describes the characteristic MRI appearance of a Brodie's abscess [54] as a central area of hypointensity on T1w sequences, surrounded by an isointense-to-muscle rim of granulation tissue, surrounded by hypointense fibrous tissue. The rim of granulation tissue is the single enhancing part. Sequestra appear as hypointense in all sequences, non-enhancing bony structures within enhancing inflammatory tissue.

8. DIFFERENTIAL DIAGNOSIS

In most cases, infection is clinically suspected prior to imaging and there are no differential diagnostic problems except for permeative lesions, suggestive of aggressive processes and sclerotic lesions suggestive of chronic osteomyelitis. Many of these occasions may require biopsy. Differential diagnosis of osteomyelitis comprises septic arthritis, cellulitis, bacteremia, acute rheumatic fever, aseptic bone necrosis or infarcts in children with sickle cell disease, indolent fractures and malignancy [18, 38]. Malignant conditions that may mimic osteomyelitis, clinically and radiologically, include LCH, Ewing's Sarcoma, leukemia, osteosarcoma and metastatic neuroblastoma.

Differential diagnosis for suppurative arthritis depends on the child's age and the number of joints involved. In monoarticular involvement, cellulitis, pyomyositis, other infectious arthritides (viral, mycoplasma, mycobacerial, fungal, Lyme disease), sickle-cell disease, hemophilia, trauma, collagen vascular

diseases, and Henoch Schönlein purpura should be clinically considered. In polyarticular involvement, rheumatic fever, serum sickness, Henoch-Schönlein purpura and collagen vascular disease must be considered [9]. Differentiation from malignancy should be based on the entire clinical situation. Imaging criteria favoring osteomyelitis could include metaphyseal location of the focus, with the exception of chronic osteomyelitis, while malignancies tend to be diametaphyseal with the exception of leukemia. On CT and MRI, osteomyelitis may cause a rather inhomogeneous process with cavities and active change peripherally, while in tumors the tissue is relatively more homogeneous [16].

9. PATHWAYS FOR IMAGING INVESTIGATION IN CHILDREN

Comprehensive protocols have been recommended [55] (Fig. 17). When osteomyelitis is suspected, all patients may undergo an AP and lateral radiograph of the affected region and if positive, prompt treatment is initiated. If radiographs are negative, and the area in question is the long bones, a positive US prompts initiation of treatment, while a negative US indicates further investigation with scintigraphy and/or MRI. MRI should

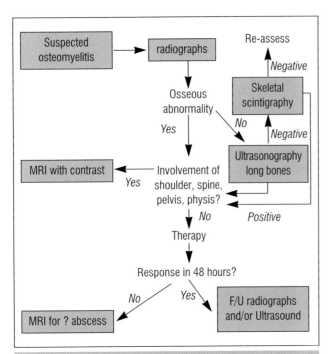

FIGURE 17. Imaging pathway in pediatric osteomyelitis.

be performed following a positive scintigram if response to treatment is slow [53]. In neonates with negative scintigraphy, MRI may be performed. CT is reserved for preoperative planning in chronic osteomyelitis and for differentiating cortical lesions.

When septic arthritis is suspected, plain radiographs are performed to exclude osteomyelitis or other diagnoses. US may identify or exclude joint effusion. In cases of positive radiographic (osteolysis) or negative US findings, the patient should be reassessed and evaluated for osteomyelitis with scintigraphy. In cases of joint effusion, aspiration and cultures of fluid should be performed. Treatment should be instituted without further imaging or, alternatively, the patient could simultaneously undergo MRI in order to identify lesions in the vicinity of the joint [55].

When dealing with soft tissue infections, US is considered the best initial imaging modality [25]. US may be negative in early infections, exclude an abscess, guide aspiration and therapeutic drainage and may reveal signs of osteoarticular infection. Plain radiographs are not usually performed. CT is reserved for cases of unavailability of contrast-enhanced MRI. MRI is considered the gold standard for the evaluation and preoperative planning of rapidly progressing and/or complex soft tissue infections.

10. CONCLUSIONS

Imaging findings in pediatric musculoskeletal infections correlate with the pathogenesis and pathophysiology of disease. The diagnosis should be based on the combi-

nation of clinical, imaging and laboratory findings. Osteomyelitis is a great mimic of benign and malignant conditions. Knowledge of the potential and limitations of each modality, should guide the radiologist to avoid tests that require ionizing radiation and consider issues of special technique when imaging pediatric musculoskeletal infection. Ultrasonography plays an increasingly important role in all kinds of acute musculoskeletal infections of the upper extremities in children.

REFERENCES

[1] Goergens ED, McEvoy A, Watson M, Batterr IR. Acute osteomyelitis and septic arthritis in children. J Pediatr Child Health 2005; 41:59-62.
[2] Kao HC, Huang YC, Chiu CH, et al. Acute hematogenous osteomyelitis and septic arthritis in children. J Microbiol Immunol Infect 2003;36:260-5.
[3] Bonhoeffer J, Haeberle B, Schaad UB, Heininger U. Diagnosis of acute haematogenous osteomyelitis and septic arthritis: 20 years experience in the University Children's Hospital Basel. Swiss Med Wkly 2001;131:575-81.
[4] Caksen H, Ozturk MK, Uzum K, Yuksel S, Ustunbas HB, Per H. Septic arthritis in childhood. Pediatr Int 2000;42(5):534-40.
[5] Lavy CB, Thyoka M, Pitani AD. Clinical features and microbiology in 204 cases of septic arthritis in Malawian children. J Bone Joint Surg [Br] 2005;87(11):1545-8.
[6] Petersen S, Knudsen FU, Andersen EA, Egeblad M. Acute haematogenous osteomyelitis and septic arthritis in childhood. A 10-year review and follow-up. Acta Orthop Scand 1980;51(3):451-7.
[7] Blickman J G, van Die CE, de Rooy JWJ. Current imaging concepts in pediatric osteomyelitis. Eur Radiol 2004;14:L55-L64.
[8] Abernethy LJ, Carty H. Modern approach to the diagnosis of osteomyelitis in children. Br J Hosp Med 1997;58:464-8.
[9] Nelson JD. Osteomyelitis and suppurative arthritis. In: Bergman R, Kliegman R, Benson H (eds), Nelson textbook of pediatrics-16th edition, Saunders WB, 2000.
[10] Peters V, Rubin L, Gloster ES, Aprin H. Foreign-body osteitis of the metacarpal bone. Clin Orthop Relat Res 1992;278:69-72.
[11] Straussberg R, Harel L, Bar-Sever Z, Amir J. Radial osteomyelitis as a complication of venous cannulation. Arch Dis Child 2001;85(5):408-10.
[12] Wang CT, Sun JS, Hou SM. Mycobacterial infection of the upper extremities. J Formos Med Assoc 2000;99(9):710-5.
[13] Ibia EO, Imoisili M, Pikis A. Group A β-Hemolytic Streptococcal Osteomyelitis in Children. Pediatrics 2003;112:22-6.
[14] Yagupsky P, Bar-Ziv Y, Howard CB, Dagan R. Epidemiology, etiology, and clinical features of septic arthritis in children younger than 24 months. Arch Pediatr Adolesc Med 1995;149(5):537-40.
[15] Norris CF, Smith-Whitley K, McGowan KL. Positive blood cultures in sickle cell disease: time to positivity and clinical outcome. J Pediatr Hematol Oncol 2003;25(5):390-5.
[16] Harvey EL, Teo J. Musculoskeletal infections in children. In: Carty H, Brunelle F, Stringer DA, Kao SCS, (eds), Imaging Children, 2nd Edition, Elsevier 2005.
[17] Marin C, Sanchez-Alegre ML, Gallego C, et al. Magnetic resonance imaging of osteoarticular infections in children. Curr Probl Diagn Radiol 2004;33(2):43-59.

[18] Vazquez M. Osteomyelitis in children. Current Opinion in Pediatrics 2002,14:112-115.

[19] Carty H. Radionuclide bone scanning. Arch Dis Child 1993; 69:160-5.

[20] Salamipour H, Jimenez RM, Brec SL, Chapman VM, Kalra MK, Jaramillo D. Multidetector row CT in pediatric musculoskeletal imaging. Pediatr Radiol 2005;35:555-64.

[21] Schmit P, Glorion C. Osteomyelitis in infants and children. Eur Radiol 2004;14 Suppl 4:L44-54.

[22] Blaivas M, Lyon M, Brannam L, Duggal S, Sierzenski P. Water bath evaluation technique for emergency ultrasound of painful superficial structures. Am J Emerg Med 2004;22(7):589-93.

[23] Gordon AC, Friedman L, White PG. Pictorial review: Magnetic Resonance Imaging of the Paediatric Elbow. Clinical Radiology 1997; 52:582-8.

[24] Azouz ME, Babyn PS, Mascia AT, Tuuha SE, Decarie J. MRI of the abnormal paediatric hand and wrist with plain film correlation. J Comp Assist Tomogr 1998;22(2):252-61.

[25] Robben SGF. Ultrasonography of musculoskeletal infections in children. Eur Radiol 2004;14:L65-L77.

[26] Chao H, Lin S, Huang Y, Lin T. Sonographic evaluation of cellulitis in children. J Ultrasound Med 2000;19:743-9.

[27] Cardinal E, Bureau N, Aubin B, Chem R. Role of ultrasound in musculoskeletal infection. Radiol Clin North Am 2001;39:191-201.

[28] Loyer EM, DuBrow RA, David CL, Coan JD, Eftekhari F. Imaging of superficial soft-tissue infections: sonographic findings in cases of cellulitis and abscess. AJR 1996;166:149-52.

[29] Brook I. Aerobic and anaerobic microbiology of necrotizing fasciitis in children. Pediatr Dermatol 1996;13:281-4.

[30] Fustes-Morales A, Gutierrez-Castrellon P, Duran-Mckinster C, Orozco-Covarrubias L, Tamayo-Sanchez L, Ruiz-Maldonado R. Necrotizing fasciitis: report of 39 pediatric cases. Arch Dermatol 2002;138(7):893-9.

[31] Chiedozi LC. Pyomyositis: review of 205 cases in 112 patients. Am J Surg 1979;137:255-9.

[32] Breidahl WH, Newman JS, Taljanovic MS, Alder RS. Power Doppler sonography in the assessment of musculoskeletal fluid collections. AJR 1996;166(6):143-6.

[33] Harwell JL, Fisher D. Pediatric septic bursitis: case report of retrocalcaneal infection and review of the literature. Clin Infect Dis 2001;32:E102-4.

[34] Wang CL, Wang SM, Yang YJ, Tsai CH, Liu CC. Septic arthritis in children: relationship of causative pathogens, complications and outcome. J Microbiol Immuol Infect 2003;36:41-6.

[35] Shaw BA, Casser JR. Acute septic arthritis in infancy and childhood. Clin Orthop 1990;212-25.

[36] Forward DP, Hunter JB. Arthroscopic washout of the shoulder for septic arthritis in infants. A new technique. J Bone Joint Surg 2002;84-B:1173-1175.

[37] Lim-Dunham JE, Ben-Ami TE, Yousefzadeh DK. Septic arthritis of the elbow in children: the role of sonography. Pediatr Radiol 1995; 25:556-9.

[38] Wright RER, Majury CW. The child with a limp. In: Carty H (Ed), Emergency Pediatric Radiology, Springer 2002.

[39] Lee SK, Suh KJ, Kim YW, et al. Septic arthritis versus transient synovitis at MR imaging: preliminary assessment with signal intensity alterations in bone marrow. Radiology 1999; 211(2):459-65.

[40] Estienne M, Scaioli V, Zibordi F, Angelini L. Enigmatic osteomyelitis and bilateral upper limb palsy in a neonate. Pediatr Neurol 2005;32(1):56-9.

[41] Lejman T, Strong M, Michno P. Septic arthritis of the shoulder during the first eighteen months of life. J Pediatr Orthop 1994; 15:172-5.

[42] Capitanio MA, Kirkpatrick JA. Early roentgen observations in acute osteomyelitis. AJR 1970;108:488-96.

[43] Santiago Restrepo C, Gimenez GR, McCarthy K. Imaging of osteomyelitis and musculoskeletal soft tissue infections: current consepts. Rheum Dis Clin North Am 2003;29:89-109.

[44] Bressler EL, Conway JJ, Weiss SC. Neonatal Osteomyelitis examined by Bone scintigraphy. Radiology 1984;152:685-8.

[45] Sullivan DC, Rosenfield NS, Ogden J, Gottschalk A. Problems in the scintigraphic detection of osteomyelitis in children. Radiology 1980;135:731-6.

[46] Asmar BI. Osteomyelitis in the neonate. Infect Dis Clin North Am 1992;6:117-32.

[47] Amundsen TR, Siegel MJ, Siegel BA. Osteomyelitis and infarction in sickle cell hemoglobinopathies: Differentiation by combined technetium and gallium scintigraphy. Radiology 1984;153:807-12.

[48] Mnif J, Khannous M, Ayadi K, et al. Ultrasonography of acute osteomyelitis of the long bones in children. Diagnostic and prognostic value. J Radiol 1997;78(4):275-81.

[49] Cheon JE, Chung HW, Hong SH, et al. Sonography of acute osteomyelitis in rabbits with pathologic correlation. Acad Radiol 2001;8:243-9.

[50] Kaiser S, Rosenborg M. Early detection of subperiosteal abscesses by ultrasonography. Pediatr Radiol 1994;24:336-9.

[51] Chao HC, Lin SJ, Huang YC, Lin TY. Color Doppler ultrasonographic evaluation of osteomyelitis in children. J Ultrasound Med 1999; 18:729-36.

[52] Mah ET, LeQuesne GW, Gent RJ, Paterson DC. Ultrasonic features of acute osteomyelitis in children. J Bone Joint Surg [Br] 1994; 76(6):969-74.

[53] Connolly LP, Connolly SA, Drubach LA, Jaramillo D, Treves ST. Acute hematogenous osteomyelitis of children: assessment of skeletal scintigraphy-based diagnosis in the era of MRI. J Nucl Med 2002;43(10):1310-6.

[54] Grey AC, Davies AM, Mangham DC, Grimer RJ, Ritchie DA. The "penumbra sign" on T1-weighted MR imaging in subacute osteomyelitis: frequency, cause and significance. Clin Radiol 1998; 53(8):587-92.

[55] Jaramillo D, Treves ST, Kasser JR, Harper M, Sundel R, Laor T. Osteomyelitis and septic arthritis: appropriate use of imaging to guide treatment. AJR 1995;165:399-403.

Imaging of Musculoskeletal Infections of the Upper Limb in Adults

chapter
11

Apostolos H. KARANTANAS

Department of Radiology, University of Crete, Heraklion, Greece

Musculoskeletal infections of the upper limb are rare. In the clinical indication of acute osteomyelitis, plain radiography is the method of choice for initial evaluation, followed by MRI if the results are negative. Scintigraphy should be performed if there is no definite clinical localization of the lesion. Contrast-enhanced MRI is important in differentiating active from inactive chronic osteomyelitis. CT is indicated in patients with contraindications for MRI or claustrophobia. Early infectious arthritis has no specific findings with any imaging modality. Soft tissue infection should be initially investigated with ultrasonography followed by MRI in equivocal cases.

Keywords: infections; musculoskeletal; upper limb; imaging; MRI.

1. INTRODUCTION

Musculoskeletal infection is a common clinical disorder provoking tissue alterations which can be visualized in detail with various imaging techniques. Infections of the upper limb though, are rare. Direct local invasion by trauma or previous operation is more common as opposed to hematogenous spread. The vast variety of imaging findings depends on both the immune competence of the host and the virulence of the microorganism. Infections of the musculoskeletal system are divided into the following, depending upon the tissue or structure involved: osteomyelitis (bone), infectious arthritis (joint) and cellulitis-myositis-abscess (soft tissue). Plain radiographs show low sensitivity and specificity in the early depiction of the whole spectrum of musculoskeletal infection [1]. The present chapter will focus on the imaging findings of upper limb musculoskeletal infections with emphasis on the optimal application of each imaging modality.

2. IMAGING METHODS

2.1. Magnetic resonance imaging (MRI)

The focus of infection, either in bone or soft tissues, will appear early in the disease process with a low signal intensity on T1-w and high signal intensity on fat-suppressed T2-w and STIR images [2, 3]. MRI, due to its superb tissue contrast and multiplanar capability, is the method of choice in investigating bone marrow infection with associated sinus tracts and soft tissue abscesses [4]. Fat-suppressed contrast-enhanced MRI shows increased sensitivity (88%) and specificity (93%) in diagnosing osteomyelitis compared to bone scintigraphy and plain

*Corresponding Author
Department of Radiology
University Hospital of Heraklion
University of Crete
Stavrakia 71110
Heraklion, Greece
e-mail: apolsen@yahoo.com
       karantanas@med.uoc.gr

MRI [5]. MRI is contraindicated for patients with claustrophobia or heart pacemakers whereas metallic implants in the region of interest may produce focal artefacts which decrease the image quality [6].

2.2. Computed tomography (CT)

The major advantage of CT is its ability to demonstrate sequestration, calcification, cortical disruption and gas within the marrow or soft tissues. The advent of multidetector CT further increased the role of CT in imaging infections of the musculoskeletal system by means of better spatial resolution and multiplanar capability. In addition, aspiration or biopsy could be performed by CT guidance [7]. Major limitation of CT is the presence of artefacts due to presence of metal in or near the area of bone infection which result in substantial loss of image quality.

2.3. Ultrasonography (US)

The major advantages of US are the wide availability, low cost and lack of radiation. Its role is limited to imaging only the structures that are quite superficial, such as the soft tissues and joints [8]. Therefore, US is ideal for the upper limb where no deep structures exist. A significant contribution of US in approaching the correct diagnosis is its ability to discriminate various soft tissue causes of pain or swelling, such as cellulitis, thrombophlebitis, bursitis, hematoma, tenosynovitis or abscess, either subcutaneous or adjacent to infected bones, in clinically suspected osteomyelitis [9].

2.4. Radionuclide imaging

Bone scintigraphy using ^{99m}Tc-MDP and ^{99m}Tc-HMDP is very sensitive in detecting osteomyelitis [10]. All three phases show increased uptake. However, specificity is low as the increased uptake may also be seen in osseous fractures, healed osteomyelitis and diabetic neuroarthropathy. In addition, cases with aggressive infectious process with pus formation may show decreased uptake due to impaired vascularity. The exact anatomic location of the lesion occasionally can not be defined, due to limited resolution. Nevertheless, a negative bone scan excludes osteomyelitis in more than 90% of cases. Diagnostic accuracy is lower in elderly patients [7]. However, the three-phase bone scan is independent of orthopaedic implants and can differentiate between soft tissue and bone infection. FDG PET scan improved resolution, and studies have shown an accuracy of 94% in diagnosis of musculoskeletal infections [11]. Others showed sensitivity of 100% and specificity of 92% in diagnosing chronic osteomyelitis [12].

3. OSTEOMYELITIS

The infectious organism can reach the bone via a) hematogenous spread from a remote site of infection, b) contiguous spread from the soft tissues, and c) direct inoculation because of a previous trauma. The shaft of a long bone is a common site of infection in adults, where infection is usually dispersed by contiguous spread or direct implantation. Acute hematogenous osteomyelitis is rarely found in the upper limb in adults. Osteomyelitis is divided into pyogenic and non-pyogenic types.

3.1. Acute and chronic pyogenic osteomyelitis

Within 1-2 days after the onset of infection, soft tissue edema and loss of fat planes are the earliest signs to detect by the use of plain radiographs [13]. MRI and scintigraphy are able to demonstrate early changes. In the upper limb, contamination of a wound is the usual mechanism of infection and MRI shows early soft tissue changes followed by cortical abnormalities and marrow edema. A destructive lytic lesion is obvious on plain radiographs within 7 to 10 days and an aggressive process manifested with further destruction of the cortical and medullary bone, endosteal sclerosis and periosteal reaction is obvious within 2 to 6 weeks. Necrotic bone, also known as sequestra, is usually apparent within 6-8 weeks [14]. At this stage, a draining sinus tract can occur and the disorder is called "chronic osteomyelitis".

At a very early stage when radiographs are negative, MRI shows the infective lesion as low-signal intensity on T1-w and high on T2-w and STIR images because of hyperemia, edema and inflammation (Fig. 1). MRI can also evaluate the cortical bone and the intramedullary sequestration. However, CT is by far superior to MRI in assessing subtle changes such as sequestra, calcification, gas, and cortical destruction. CT is not able, though, to discriminate suppuration from granulation tissue, edema or fibrosis [15]. The activity of chronic osteomyelitis with MRI is established by edematous changes in the bone marrow and surrounding soft tissues. Contrast-enhanced MRI is more accurate in differentiating active from inactive chronic osteomyelitis (Fig. 2).

Postoperative infection may occur in any surgical or interventional procedure. In general, the diagnosis is delayed as the clinical symptoms are masked by the tissue trauma. Therefore, persistent symptoms lead clinicians to refer patients for imaging. Periosteal formation and sequestration are not common in those cases as the surgical decompression of the bone does not allow the intramedullary pressure to increase. Bone lysis, intracortical fistula formation and soft tissue changes may coexist. The correct diagnosis often requires a combination of plain radiographs, scintigraphy, arthrography, CT and MRI. A potential pitfall with MRI occurs within one year postoperatively, since the resulting fibrovascular tissue may show similar signal changes and contrast enhancement to inflammatory bone marrow edema [16]. Combined bone scintigraphy and immunoscintigraphy may improve the accuracy of diagnosis within this period. In addition, scintigraphy may help in equivocal cases

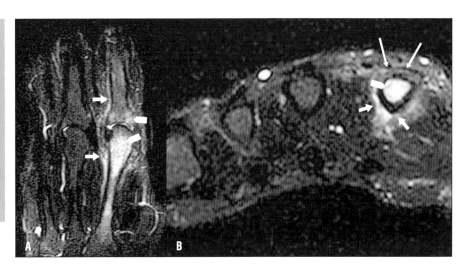

FIGURE 1. Acute osteomyelitis and septic arthritis in a 55-year-old female with a recent superficial injury during gardening. Both the STIR **(A)** and the T2-w fat-suppressed TSE **(B)** sequences show increased signal in the soft tissues (small arrows), the cortical bone (thin arrows), and the bone marrow of the 2nd metacarpal bone and the proximal phalanx (arrowheads). There is also moderate effusion in the 2nd metacarpophalangeal joint in keeping with septic arthritis.

where susceptibility artefacts are found in MRI from tiny metallic residues.

MRI is more sensitive in the case of low-grade infections and may prevent false positive interpretations of immunoscintigraphy due to ectopic hematopoietic bone marrow. Postoperatively, it is important to interpret films in comparison with previous ones, as changes such as new linear periosteal reaction, osteolysis, and cortical irregularity are suspicious of active infection. Sensitivity and specificity of the above findings are only 14% and 70%, respectively. Sequestration is the only reliable finding distinguishing active bone infection in a postoperative situation [17]. Delayed union of a fracture is an additional indication of underlying infection [18]. After application of an external fixation device, infection is typically demonstrated on plain radiographs as a circular lytic zone around the percutaneously applied pin (Fig. 3). Infectious osteolysis surrounding the metal area is usually irregular in shape and has blurred borders, while there is no normal fine sclerotic rim, normally confining a drill hole. On the contrary, metal loosen-

ing results in a well-defined halo surrounded by a sclerotic rim [19].

A specific pattern of osteomyelitis occurs in patients with bone infarcts. Marrow infarction and osteomyelitis may coexist in certain patient population, such as those with sickle-cell anaemia, systemic lupus erythematosus, and human immunodeficiency disease, as well as patients who have undergone renal transplantation [20]. MRI has proven to discriminate those two entities [21]. It has been hypothesized that the infarcts may act as "giant sequestra" providing the medullary culture medium for bacterial growth [22]. Necrotic bone is better appreciated by use of CT (Fig. 4). Cortical penetration usually leads to a soft tissue abscess because the periosteum is firmly adhered to the bone and subperiosteal extension is rare [23].

3.2. Subacute osteomyelitis - Brodie's abscess

Either due to low virulence or to good immune response, acute osteomyelitis may be contained. The

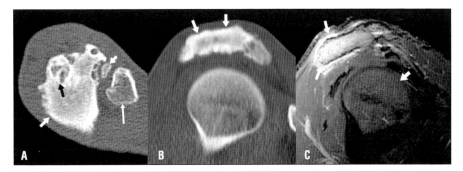

FIGURE 2. Chronic Garre sclerosing osteomyelitis in a 30-year-old female, who has a history of injections, starting 7 years before due to persistent rotator cuff symptoms. A biopsy revealed Staphylococcus Warneri. The MDCT in **(A)** the axial and **(B)** the oblique sagittal planes show generalized marrow sclerosis of the acromion (arrows) associated with lucencies (black arrow). For comparison, the normal appearance of the trabecular bone marrow is shown in the clavicle (long arrow). Os acromiale (short arrow) represents an anatomic variation. **(C)** Fat suppressed contrast-enhanced T1-w MR image in oblique sagittal plane, shows increased bone marrow signal in the acromion together with surrounding soft tissue enhancement (arrows). The normal marrow of the humeral head exhibits low signal intensity (thick arrow).

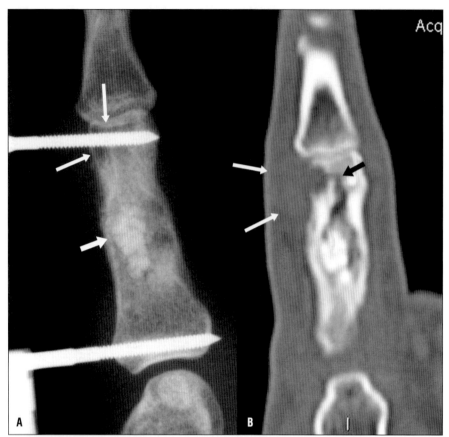

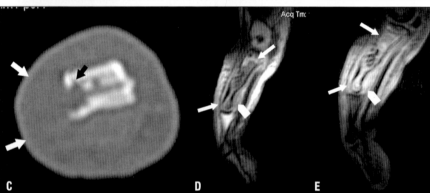

FIGURE 3. Chronic active postoperative osteomyelitis in a 31-year-old female physician, operated with bone grafting and external fixation for a pathologic fracture secondary to a medullary enchondroma. (A) Plain radiograph shows a lytic zone around the percutaneously applied pin (arrows). Bone graft is seen in the medullary cavity (thick arrow). (B) Coronal CT reformatted image after removal of the fixation device shows a soft tissue swelling (arrows) and a draining sinus (black arrow). (C) Axial CT image shows the soft tissue swelling (arrows) and the bone lysis at the site of the previous pin (black arrow). (D) Sagittal MRI with T1-w and (E) fat-suppressed contrast-enhanced T1-w images show the abnormal signal and enhancement of the diaphyseal bone marrow (arrows) as well as the associated soft tissue infectious changes (arrowheads).

Brodie's abscess is often localized in the tibial or femoral metaphysic and rarely in the upper limb, surrounded by reactive sclerosis on plain radiographs. In general, there are no sequestra, but a radiolucent tract extending from the medullary cavity to the cortex or through the cortex to the soft tissues, may be seen. Rarely, the Brodie's abscess can be located in the cortex with a typical lysis, which is seen well with CT (Fig. 5). MRI is able to evaluate cortical bone, that normally shows low signal intensity in all sequences, and intracortical lesions which almost always show areas of increased signal intensity on fat-suppressed T2-w and STIR images. Periostitis and soft tissue involvement is better depicted in MRI, particularly when applying fat-suppressed techniques.

3.3. Non-pyogenic bone infections

Non-pyogenic infections are usually the result of Tb mycobacterium, and infrequently, fungi and spirochete *Treponema pallidum* (syphilis). Tuberculous bone infection usually results from hematogenous spread from a primary focus point, such as the lung. The joints in adults are more commonly affected, with or without associated osteomyelitis (Fig. 6, 7). Progressive medullary destruction and abscess formation associated with osteopenia are the common radiological signs. Fungal infections are of a low grade, associated with abscesses and draining sinuses, their location being usually at a point of bony prominence. The most common radiological finding

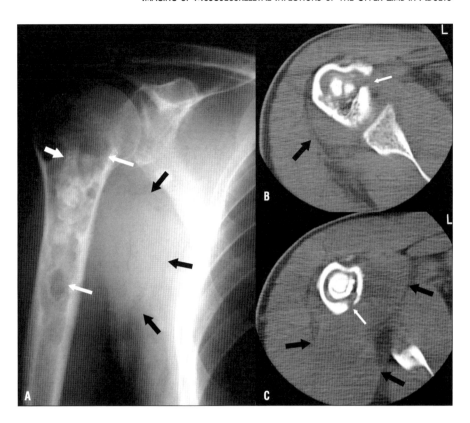

FIGURE 4. Chronic active osteomyelitis with soft tissue abscess formation in a 61-year-old male patient with a history of renal transplantation. **(A)** The AP plain radiograph of the right shoulder shows an old metaphyseal medullary infarct (thick white arrow), mixed osteolytic (white arrows) and osteoscrerotic lesions of the proximal humeral diaphysis, and a soft tissue axillary mass (black arrows). **(B, C)** Axial CT images at two levels shows intramedullary osteosclerosis representing the old infarct and necrotic bone, cortical disruption (white arrows) and the soft tissue abscess (black arrows).

seen is a lytic and well-marginated lesion in long or flat bones. Rarely, a permeative pattern of bone destruction may be present.

4. INFECTIOUS ARTHRITIS

An infectious organism can involve the joint by the same mechanisms as in osteomyelitis. In most cases, the scintigram is positive and the radiological findings include joint effusion and joint space narrowing. Pyogenic or septic arthritis usually involves a single joint. Periarticular osteopenia and joint effusion are the early radiological signs, whereas joint space narrowing with destruction of the subarticular plates are later signs. MRI shows synovial thickening with enhancement, perisynovial edema and joint effusion [24]. Prompt

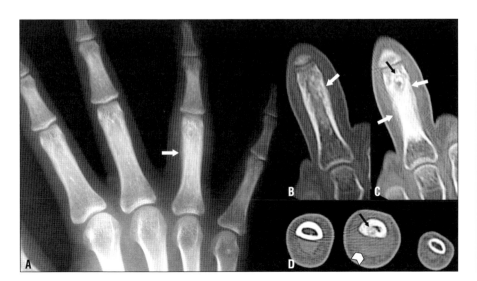

FIGURE 5. Subacute osteomyelitis involving the 4th proximal phalanx of the hand in a 19-year-old female with unknown previous trauma. Both the plain radiograph **(A)** and the coronal high resolution CT **(B, C)** show soft tissue swelling, thick periosteal reaction and marrow sclerosis (arrows). A small sequestrum is seen distally (black arrow). **(D)** The axial CT image shows a lytic lesion in the cortex corresponding to intracortical abscess (black arrow) and soft tissue swelling surrounding the flexor tendons (arrowhead).

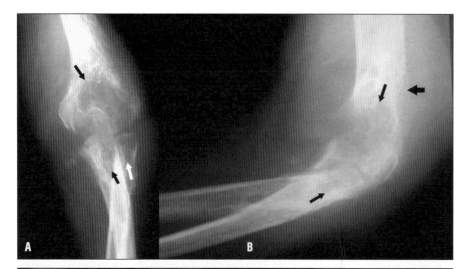

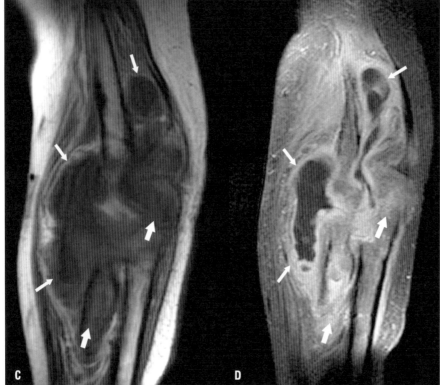

FIGURE 6. Tuberculous arthritis and osteomyelitis in a 39-year-old female with known active lung tuberculosis. Plain **(A)** anteroposterior and **(B)** lateral radiographs show soft tissue swelling, loss of the normal joint space, osteolytic appearance of the distal humerus and proximal ulna and radius (arrows) and cortical disruption of the distal humeral metaphysis (thick arrow). **(C)** The sagittal MR T1-w and **(D)** the contrast-enhanced fat-suppressed T1-w images show the extensive joint effusion with thick synovial enhancement corresponding to Tb arthritis (arrows) and abnormal signal intensity and intense enhancement of the bone marrow (thick arrows) corresponding to osteomyelitis.

puncture of the joint effusion should be performed for an early diagnosis. US guidance might be of help in this respect. Bone marrow signal changes adjacent to a known form of septic arthritis may be erroneously diagnosed as osteomyelitis in up to 60% of cases [2].

Non-pyogenic arthritides are rare and usually less aggressive. The most common is Tuberculous arthritis (Fig. 6, 7), which presents radiologically with the *Phemister's triad:* (i) periarticular osteopenia, (ii) peripherally located bony erosion, and (iii) gradual diminution of the joint space. Both MDCT and MRI can be quite helpful in identifying subtle and early erosions.

5. SOFT TISSUE INFECTION

Soft tissue inflammation and infection usually result from the skin and disperse by direct spread of the infectious agent. Diabetic patients are prone to such disorders due to a combination of causes including skin ulceration and local ischemia. MRI, with its inherent superior soft tissue contrast, is able to discriminate diffuse cellulitis and myositis from focal abscess formation.

Cellulitis is seen with US as diffuse thickening and increased echogenicity of the skin and subcutaneous tis-

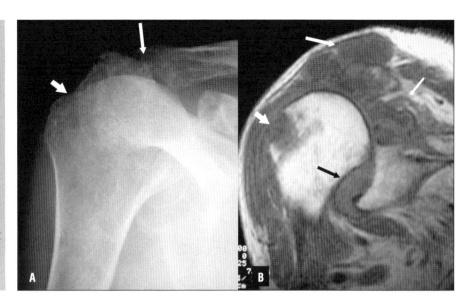

FIGURE 7. Tuberculous arthritis and osteomyelitis in a 64-year-old male with not-yet-diagnosed lung tuberculosis. **(A)** Plain anteroposterior radiograph shows soft-tissue swelling, cranial displacement of the humerus, a destructive process in the acromioclavicular joint in keeping with infectious arthritis (arrow) and a focal osteolysis of the greater tubercle suggesting osteomyelitis (short arrow). **(B)** The oblique coronal T1-w MR image shows the extensive joint effusion (black arrow), synovial effusion over the acromioclavicular joint (white arrow), and the focal osteomyelitis in the proximal humerus (short arrow). There is also retraction and atrophy of the supraspinatus tendon due to complete rupture (thin white arrow).

sues, occasionally having a cobblestone appearance with anechoic strands randomly traversing the subcutaneous tissues [25].

Septic bursitis most frequently involves the olecranon bursa in the upper limb (Fig. 8). US demonstrates a fluid collection in the expected location of the bursa. The walls of the bursa may or may not be thickened, and there may be debris or septa within. Color Doppler US may show hyperemia in the walls but does not allow accurate differentiation between an infected bursa and posttraumatic bursitis or inflammatory bursitis. Aspiration may be required in this respect and can be performed under US guidance.

Acute suppurative tenosynovitis most frequently involves the tendon sheaths of the digital flexor muscles [26]. It is usually the result of a penetrating injury (e.g. human / animal bite or puncture wound) and may be complicated by the presence of foreign bodies. Early diagnosis and treatment are crucial to prevent compli-

cations such as tendon necrosis and tear as well as contamination of adjacent joints and surrounding soft tissues. US can be diagnostic, but MRI shows to better advantage the proteinaceous content of the fluid and the abnormal enhancement [27] (Fig. 9).

Abscesses may appear as an anechoic, diffusely hypoechoic with increased through transmission hyperechoic or isoechoic lesions relative to surrounding tissues, with or without septa formation [25]. In addition, the lesions may be well-defined or blend in with the surrounding tissues, occasionally associated with an echogenic rim. Internal echoes may represent debris or gas. Color Doppler imaging is able to demonstrate peripheral hyperemia and absence of central flow as well as the possible presence of a foreign body. MRI is able to demonstrate the abnormal enhancement of the lesion and the relation to surrounding structures (Fig. 10).

Pyomyositis represents a primary muscle abscess, often with non-specific clinical presentation, seen in im-

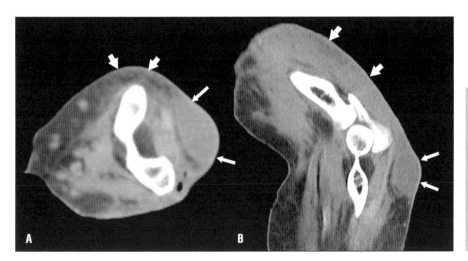

FIGURE 8. Soft-tissue infection in a 50-year-old male patient with a history of chronic renal failure and diabetes. The **(A)** axial and **(B)** sagittal reformatted CT images show the olecranon bursitis (arrows) and the increased density in the subcutaneous fat corresponding to cellulitis (short arrows). Focal air in (A) is due to previous aspiration which revealed staphylococcus aureus.

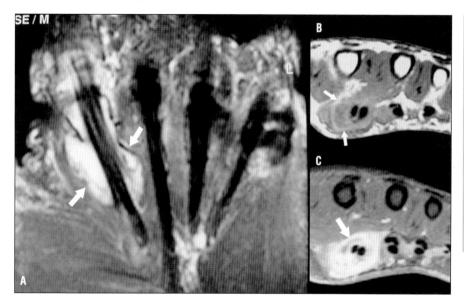

FIGURE 9. Septic tenosynovitis in a 68-year-old female patient with a history of a minor cat bite. **(A)** The coronal STIR MR image shows extensive effusion surrounding the flexor tendons of the 2nd finger (arrows). **(B)** The axial T1-w Spin Echo MR image demonstrates thick wall and moderate signal intensity of the effusion (arrows), slightly higher than the surrounding muscles, suggesting proteinaceous content. **(C)** The contrast enhanced fat-suppressed T1-w MR Spin Echo image shows intense enhancement of the effusion (arrow) in keeping with infection.

munocompromised patients and intravenous drug abusers. US contributes significantly to the correct diagnosis by demonstrating an ill-defined hypoechoic area within one or more muscles corresponding to the initial phlegmon. Later in the course, an intramuscular fluid collection corresponding to a mature abscess is detected.

6. PATHWAYS FOR IMAGING INVESTIGATION OF THE IMPLANT-RELATED INFECTIONS

The management of infected shoulder prostheses has not been standardised because most patients complain of stiffness or pain, without any clinical signs of infection.

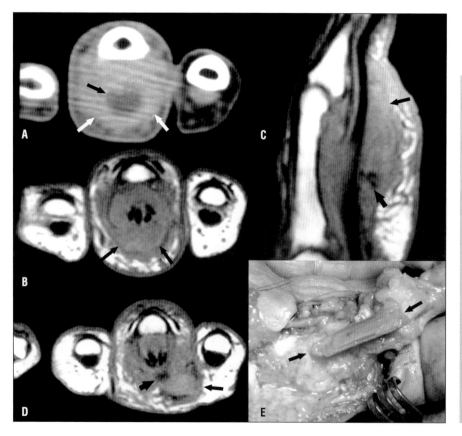

FIGURE 10. Chronic granulomatous infection in a patient with no definite history of previous injury and painless swelling of the 3rd finger. **(A)** The axial CT image shows a soft tissue swelling in the palmar site (white arrows), edema of the subcutaneous fatty tissue and a central hypodense focal area (black arrow) compatible with either abscess formation or a foreign body. **(B)** The axial T1-w MR imaging confirms the soft tissue swelling (arrows) surrounding the flexor tendons. **(C)** The sagittal T1-w MR image, shows to better advantage the lesion surrounding the tendons (arrow) and a focal low signal intensity area suggesting a foreign body (thick arrow). **(D)** The contrast-enhanced axial T1-w MR image shows moderate enhancement of the lesion (arrow) and the non-enhancing foreign body (thick arrow). **(E)** Intraoperative picture confirms the presence of a wooden foreign body which caused the infection.

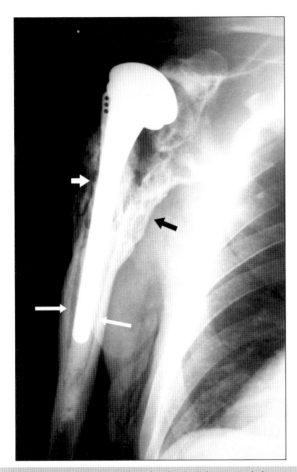

FIGURE 11. Infectious loosening of an implant due to staphylococcus epidermidis in a 59-year-old man operated 3 months after a fracture of the humerus. There was successful response to conservative treatment with antibiotics. The anteroposterior plain radiograph shows cortical disruption (short white arrow), a complete lucent line >2 mm around the implant (thin white arrows), and a thick periosteal reaction (black arrow).

nostic accuracy [19, 31]. FDG PET is not able to distinguish an infected from an aseptically loosened prosthesis since in both conditions it is characterized by increased periprosthetic uptake due to presence of inflammation [32]. In equivocal cases, MRI might be helpful, provided that operation was performed at least 1 year before.

7. CONCLUSIONS

Although rare, musculoskeletal infections of the upper limb in adults are a challenge for both the clinician and the radiologist. In the clinical indication of acute osteomyelitis, plain radiography is the method of choice for initial evaluation, followed by MRI in the case the results are negative. Scintigraphy should be performed if there is no definite clinical localization of the lesion. Computed tomography no longer plays a role in the early detection of acute osteomyelitis. In chronic osteomyelitis, MRI is the most accurate means of depicting the activity of the disease and the extension in the marrow and soft tissues, which is important for treatment planning. Postoperatively, plain radiographs should be used in the initial examination. Leukocyte scintigraphy is superior to MRI in establishing reactivation of osteomyelitis, particularly during the first 12 months after surgery. CT is indicated only for depicting sequestration. Soft tissue infection should be initially investigated with ultrasonography followed by MRI in equivocal cases. Ultrasonography is also important in enabling real-time guidance for aspiration of effusions in the soft tissues. Even with advanced imaging methods, findings may remain inconclusive, particularly in complicated cases such as those of postoperative patients. Understanding the clinical question is mandatory for the proper use of the available imaging methods and augments diagnostic confidence and efficiency.

In addition, infected prostheses are rare with an incidence of less than 2% for primary and 4% for revision replacements [28]. Plain radiographs should be the initial imaging examination. The main radiological findings consist of loosening, defined as a complete lucent line >1 mm around the implant, and periosteal reaction [10]. Nevertheless, loosening alone may not be associated with infection. Conventional radiography does not usually allow this differentiation unless a cortical disruption exists (Fig. 11). CT and MRI are of somewhat limited value because of metallic implants resulting in degradation of the images.

A normal bone scan is able to rule out septic or aseptic loosening with very high probability [29]. Increased metabolism of the periprosthetic bone during the healing process may persist for months or years postoperatively resulting in poor specificity of bone scintigraphy in differentiation between septic and aseptic loosening [30]. A combination of the three-phase bone scintigraphy with leukocyte scintigraphy increases diag-

REFERENCES

[1] Butt WP. The radiology of infection. Clin Orthop 1973;96:20-30.
[2] Erdman WA, Tamburro F, Jayson HT, Weatherall PT, Ferry KB, Peshock RM. Osteomyelitis: characteristics and pitfalls of diagnosis with MR imaging. Radiology 1991;180:533-9.
[3] Tehranzadeh J, Wang F, Mesgarzadeh M. Magnetic resonance imaging of osteomyelitis. Crit Rev Diagn Imaging 1992;33:495-534.
[4] Unger E, Moldofsky P, Gatenby R, Hartz W, Broder G. Diagnosis of osteomyelitis by MR imaging. AJR Am J Roentgenol 1988;150:605-10.
[5] Morrison WB, Schweitzer ME, Bock GW, et al. Diagnosis of osteomyelitis: utility of fat-suppressed contrast-enhanced MR imaging. Radiology 1993;189:251-7.
[6] Modic MT, Pflanze W, Feiglin DH, Belhobek G. Magnetic resonance imaging of musculoskeletal infections. Radiol Clin North Am 1986;24:247-58.

[7] Sammak B, El Bagi A, Al Shahed M, et al. Osteomyelitis: a review of currently used imaging techniques. Eur Radiol 1999;9:894-900.

[8] Bureau NJ, Chhem RK, Cardinal E. Musculoskeletal infections: US manifestations. Radiographics 1999;19:1585-92.

[9] Abiri MM, Kirpekar M, Ablow RC. Osteomyelitis: detection with US. Radiology 1989;172:509-11.

[10] Sciuk J. Scintigraphic Techniques for the Diagnosis of Infectious Disease of the Musculoskeletal System. Sem Musculoskelet Radiol 2004;8:205-13.

[11] De Winter F, Vogelaers D, Gemmel F, Dierckx RA. Promising role of 18-F-fluoro-D-deoxyglucose positron emission tomography in clinical infectious diseases. Eur J Clin Microbiol Infect Dis 2002;21:247-57.

[12] Guhlmann A, Brecht-Krauss D, Suger G, et al. Chronic osteomyelitis detection with FDG PET and correlation with histopathologic findings. Radiology 1998;206:749-54.

[13] Bohndorf K. Infection of the appendicular skeleton. Eur Radiol 2004;14:53-63.

[14] Restrepo S, Gimenez CR, McCarthy K. Imaging of osteomyelitis and musculoskeletal soft tissue infections: current concepts. Rheum Dis Clin North Am 2003;29:89-109.

[15] Gold RH, Tong DFJ, Crim JR, Seeger LL. Imaging the diabetic foot. Skeletal Radiol 1995;24:563-71.

[16] Kaim A, Ledermann HP, Bongartz G, Messmer P, Muller-Brand J, Steinbrich W. Chronic post-traumatic osteomyelitis of the lower extremity: comparison of magnetic resonance imaging and combined bone scintigraphy/immunoscintigraphy with radiolabelled monoclonal antigramulocyte antibodies. Skeletal Radiol 2000;29:378-86.

[17] Tumeh SS, Aliabadi P, Weissman BN, Mc Neil BJ. Disease activity in osteomyelitis: role of radiology. Radiology 1987;165:781-84.

[18] Kaim AH, Gross T, von Schulthess GK. Imaging of chronic posttraumatic osteomyelitis. Eur Radiol 2002;12:1193-202.

[19] Buhne KH, Bohndorf K. Imaging of Posttraumatic Osteomyelitis. Semin Musculoskel Radiol 2004;8:199-204.

[20] Epps CH, Bryant DD, Coles MJM, Castro O. Osteomyelitis in patients who have sickle cell disease. J Bone Joint Surg Am 1991;73-A:1281-94.

[21] Umans H, Haramati N, Flusser G. The diagnostic role of gadolinium enhanced MRI in distinguishing between acute medullary bone infarct and osteomyelitis. Magn Reson Imaging 2000;18:255-62.

[22] Blacksin MF, Finzel KC, Benevenia J. Osteomyelitis originating in and around bone infarcts: giant sequestrum phenomena. AJR Am J Roentgenol 2001;176:387-91.

[23] Shirtliff ME, Mader JT. Imaging in osteomyelitis and septic arthritis. Curr Treat Options Infect Dis 2003;5:323-35.

[24] Karchevsky M, Schweitzer ME, Morrison WB, Parellada MA. MRI findings of septic arthritis and associated osteomyelitis in adults. AJR Am J Roentgenol 2004;182:119-22.

[25] Loyer EM, DuBrow RA, David CL, Coan JD, Eftekhari F. Imaging of superficial soft-tissue infections: sonographic findings in cases of cellulitis and abscess. AJR Am J Roentgenol 1996;166:149-52.

[26] Canoso JJ, Barza M. Soft tissue infections. Rheum Dis Clin North Am 1993;19:293-309

[27] Brooke RJ Jr, Laing FC, Schechter WP, Markison RE, Barton RM. Acute suppurative tenosynovitis of the hand: diagnosis with US. Radiology 1987;162:741-2

[28] Coste JS, Reig S, Trojani C, Berg M, Walch G, Boileau P. The management of infection in arthroplasty of the shoulder. J Bone Joint Surg [Br] 2004;86-B:65-9.

[29] Al Sheikh W, Sfakianakis GN, Mnaymneh W, et al. Subacute and chronic bone infections: diagnosis using In-111, Ga-67 and Tc-99m MDP bone scintigraphy and radiography. Radiology 1985;155:501-6.

[30] Williamson BRJ, McLaughlin RE, Wang GJ, Miller CW, Teates D, Bray ST. Radionuclide bone imaging as a means of differentiating loosening and infection in patients with a painful hip prosthesis. Radiology 1979;133:723-5

[31] Sciuk J, Puska/s C, Greitemann B, Schober O. White blood cell scintigraphy with monoclonal antibodies in the study of the infected prosthesis. Eur J Nucl Med 1992;19:497-502.

[32] Stumpe KD, Notzli HP, Zanetti M, et al. FDG PET for differentiation of infection and aseptic loosening in total hip replacements: comparison with conventional radiography and three-phase bone scintigraphy. Radiology 2004;231:333-341.

Primary Histological Features in Acute and Chronic Infections

Antonia CHARCHANTI[a]*, Panayotis N. SOUCACOS[b], Elizabeth O. JOHNSON[a]

[a]*Department of Anatomy-Histology-Embryology, University of Ioannina, School of Medicine, Ioannina, Greece*
[b]*Department of Orthopaedic Surgery, University of Athens, School of Medicine, Athens, Greece*

The upper extremity consists of various potential spaces that can become infected by a wide variety of organisms, which in turn, induce specific and non-specific defense responses. For descriptive purposes, infections can be divided according to the tissue compartment they have infected into three major categories: infections of the soft tissue, infections of the joints and infections of the bone. Despite the growing wealth of information regarding the immune response cascade involved in infections, relatively little information is available on the morphological and histologic changes that accompany infections of the musculoskeletal system. The primary purpose of the inflammatory response is to eliminate the pathogenic insult and remove injured tissue components. This process accomplishes either regeneration of the normal tissue architecture and return of physiological function or the formation of scar tissue to replace what cannot be repaired. The hallmarks of acute inflammation include accumulation of fluid and plasma components in the affected tissue, intravascular stimulation of platelets, and the presence of polymorphonuclear leukocytes. In contrast, the characteristic cell components of chronic inflammation are lymphocytes, plasma cells, and macrophages.

Keywords: lymphocyte; T-cell; b-cell; cell-mediated immunity; humoral immunity; infection; inflammation. ■

1. INTRODUCTION

The organism recruits both immunologic and non-immunologic defense mechanisms to help maintain the internal milieu free of infection. Immunologic defenses are characterized by specificity that is determined by immunoglobulins and T-lymphocytes [1]. Non-immunologic defenses that are non-specific in nature, include inflammation and fever [2]. The upper extremity consists of various potential spaces that can become infected by a wide variety of organisms, which in turn, induce specific and non-specific defense responses. For descriptive purposes, infections can be divided, according to the tissue compartment they have infected, into three major categories: infections of the soft tissue, infections of the joints and infections of the bone. Despite the growing wealth of information regarding the immune response cascade involved in infections, relatively little information is available on the morphological and histologic changes that accompany infections of the musculoskeletal system.

*Corresponding Author
Department of Anatomy-Histology-Embryology,
University of Ioannina, School of Medicine,
Ioannina, Greece 45110
Fax: +30-26510-97861
e-mail: acharcha@cc.uoi.gr

2. INFECTIONS OF SOFT TISSUES

Soft tissue infections may be either acute or chronic. These may involve the subcutaneous tissues, referred to as cellulites, and/or deeper structures, including muscle tendons and ligaments. It is noteworthy that infections of the bones or joints may spread to involve the soft tissues. On the other hand, it is less common that a soft tissue infection extends to involve bones and joints [3-6].

The involvement of the soft tissues in an infectious process usually results from the direct extension from cutaneous, visceral, or osseous foci or as a complication of trauma or surgery. Soft tissue infections rarely have a hematogenous source. The severity of the inflammatory reaction and the type of tissue response observed depend on various parameters, including the type, dose and virulence of the infecting organism, the resistance of the host tissue, the presence or absence of necrotic tissue, hematoma or foreign body, and the anatomic features of the infected area.

Pyogenic and necrotizing infections produce acute inflammatory tissue reactions which are indistinguishable microscopically. Granulomatous inflammation of soft tissue include tuberculosis, atypical mycobacteriosis, actinomycosis, blastomycosis, coccidiomycosis, sporotrichosis and dirofilariasis [7]. Chronic pyogenic infection, granulomatus inflammation, or encysted hematoma of soft tissue can often mimic clinically a soft tissue tumor.

The various clinical entities of infections processes, such as hemolytic streptococcal gangrene, necrotizing fasciitis, and Meleney's "synergistic gangrene", can be differentiated by clinical appearance and bacteriologic study. This requires a proper search for microorganisms with special stains and cultures.

2.1. Cellulitis

Cellulitis is an inflammatory infection of the subcutaneous tissues, usually due to *staph* or *strep* (and Haemophilus in children). It is a spreading infection of the skin and subcutaneous tissues, usually deeper than erysipelas, which is characterized by marked swelling, pain and erythema. In addition to the local erythema, tenderness, and occasional lymphangitis/lymphadenopathy, the clinical picture may progress quite rapidly. Most mild cases of cellulitis can be treated with an oral penicillinase-resistant penicillin or cephalosporin, while patients with high fever, systemic toxicity, poor host resistance, or underlying skin diseases should be admitted for IV antibiotic therapy.

Although swelling, pain and heat are the hallmarks of cellulites, care must be taken to differentiate these features from those of vascular insufficiency, as indicated by poor pulses and deep venous thrombosis [3]. The later are sometimes very difficult to discriminate.

Cellulitis may progress to necrosis with cavitation. Haemorrhage may also occur in the course of some of the more fulminant disease processes. As the organisms become established, collections of pus may develop in microabscesses; these may coalesce to create a macroscopic abscess. In due course, an untreated abscess may point to the surface and discharge either onto the skin or into a viscus. As a result of this process, potential cavities, such as bursae or tendon sheaths, may become infected. However, collections of fluid in these locations are more commonly the result of repetitive injury or inflammatory joint disease. Chronic soft tissue involvement may lead to indurated and woody change, especially in the case of the more indolent fungal infections. Calcification may occur in soft tissues secondary to local necrosis or in the wall of treated abscesses.

2.2. Necrotizing fasciitis

Necrotizing fasciitis is a life-threatening condition that often commences with trauma. The trauma may even be minor in nature, including a cut or insect bite. Although group-A *Streptococcus* is the most common bacterial isolate, a polymicrobial infection with a variety of gram-positive, gram-negative, aerobic, and anaerobic bacteria is more common. In necrotizing fasciitis, large areas of soft tissue and muscle are destroyed and devitalized. Gas formation in soft tissues may be present, but its absence does not exclude infection. Aggressive surgical debridement and broad-spectrum antibiotics are essential to manage this potentially devastating disease [4, 5, 6].

There is very rapid progression of the infection with necrosis of skin and subepidermal fascia, which may also extend to involve the deeper muscle layers. Death may occur within hours without immediate treatment. Necrotizing fasciitis is an aggressive, life-threatening fascial infection that is often associated with underlying vascular disease (especially diabetes).

---

3. Infections of Joints

Septic arthritis is usually a monarticular infection that tends to occur in infants and adults. Children are rarely affected. It usually involves the hip in infants and young children, and the knee in older children and adults [8]. Factors predisposing to bacterial arthritis are contiguous osteomyelitis, particularly after closure of the growth plate; contiguous soft tissue infection; penetrating injury into the joint; hematogenous spread from a remote infection, intra-articular injections and arthroscopic and prosthetic joint surgery.

The essential histological manifestations in the affected joints include, changes in the synovium, cartilage, and in the subchondral bone, similar to those observed in osteoarthritis. The longer the delay in diagnosis, the more irreversible is the damage to the articular cartilage. Synovitis precedes actual septic arthritis and destructive changes. As a result, the cartilaginous and bony changes following effusions take weeks to develop [9].

Inflammatory and immune processes have several damaging effects on the synovial membrane. The phagocytes of inflammation, including neutrophils and macrophages, ingest the immune complexes. This process results in the release of powerful enzymes that degrade synovial tissue and articular cartilage. Inflammation results in hemorrhage, coagulation, and fibrin deposits on the synovial membrane, in the intracellular matrix, and in the synovial fluid. Over denuded areas of the synovial membrane, fibrin develops into granulation tissue called *pannus*. Pannus is the earliest tissue produced in the healing process. The role of pannus inflammation of the joints is not clear. It has been hypothesized that as the disease progresses, the pannus extends from the synovial membrane into adjacent articular cartilage and destroys the cartilage. On the other hand, it has also been proposed that pannus forms on articular cartilage after the cartilage has been destroyed by inflammation. In any case, pannus formation does not lead to synovial or articular regeneration, but rather to formation of scar tissue that immobilizes the joint.

3.1. Synovium

The normal histologic appearance of the synovium includes a discrete layer of cells in the intimal lining. Beneath this lining lies a rich vascular layer of loose connective tissue. Hyperplasia and/or hypertrophy of the cells in the synovial lining may occur focally or diffusely. Acute inflammatory lesions characteristically show infiltration of polymorhonuclear leukocytes. Late stages of chronic inflammatory lesions, on the other hand, show infiltration of mononuclear cells, including lymphocytes and plasma cells [10, 11].

3.2. Articular cartilage

Normally, articular cartilage is an organized structure with an even spatial distribution of chondrocytes. Articular cartilage is characterized by its avascularity. It is sparsely cellular at the surface of the joint, and cellularity increases significantly towards the subchondral bone.

In infections of the joint, articular cartilage damage can be observed resulting initially from effusion-driven increased intraarticular pressure and later from leukocytosis-driven enzymatic degradation. Histologic evidence of cartilage damage, such as cartilage softening, chondrolysis, and fissure, is notable at 1 week, followed by pannus overgrowth.

3.3. Subchondral bone

Late changes include total loss of articular cartilage with exposure of underlying bone (eburnation). Osteophytes form at the edges of the articular bone, and cysts form within the subchondral bone. End-stage changes include fibrous anchylosis (at 5 weeks) and bony anchylosis.

Tissi at al. [12] found that the major histopathological changes in the affected joints were the presence of an acute exudative synovitis, starting as early as 48 hrs after infection, and a polymorphonuclear leukocyte-monocyte infiltrate of the subsynovium and periarticular connective tissues. One week later, articular cavities of involved joints were filled with purulent exudate. In mice with persistent articular inflammation, joint destruction progressed rapidly, with loss of cartilage and proliferation of granulation tissue.

4. INFECTIONS OF BONES

Bone infection is characterized microscopically by the presence of inflammatory cells, dead or dying bone, marrow juxtaposition of new bone on dead bone, periosteal new bone, and extensive remodelling of contiguous healthy viable bone.

All bone infections include reactive bone formation and new bone formation.

4.1. Reactive bone formation

Reactive bone formation entails the production of intramembranous bone in response to a stress on bone or soft tissue. Various conditions such as tumors, infections, trauma, or generalized or focal disease can stimulate bone formation. The periosteum may respond with the so-called "sunburst" pattern, as seen with certain tumors, or a progressive layering of the periosteum, which produces an onion-skin pattern of the cortex. The endosteal or the marrow surface may produce new bone, so that on radiological studies, the cortex appears to be thickened, and the coarse cancellous bone appears to be more dense.

Reactive bone may be either woven or lamellar, depending on its rate of deposition. For example, reactive bone around an indolent infection, such as chronic osteomyelitis, may be laid down *de novo* as normally seen with the lamellar bone from the periosteum. In this case, the bone has the time to respond to the persistent stress.

4.2. New bone formation

Early lesions are characterized by an accumulation of polymorphonuclear leucocytes in the marrow. These are mainly of neutrophilic type, with only a few eosinophils being generally observed. Abscesses can sometimes be seen, with collections of lymphocytes located around the small abscesses. An increased occurrence of osteoclasts and signs of bone resorption are often also observed in early lesions.

Chronic lesions often show a predominance of lymphocytes, although plasma cells, histiocytes and some polymorphonuclear leucocytes can also be observed. In some cases, granulomatous foci, rich with neutrophils in the center, may also be observed in the marrow.

Cystic cavities are occasionally found in areas of inflammation, and can be lined by loose connective tissue containing inflammatory cells. Multinucleated giant cells, possibly of foreign-body type, can also be observed diffusely in the inflammatory infiltrates. These cells vary in shape, staining affinity, and in the number and appearance of nuclei. Chronic lesions can show necrotic bone fragments and fibrosis around inflammation foci.

4.3. Osteomyelitis

The term "osteomyelitis" signifies inflammation of the bone and marrow, and the common use of the term almost always implies infection. Osteomyelitis may be complication of any systemic infection, but frequently manifests as a primary solitary focus of disease. All types of organisms, including viruses, parasites, fungi, and bacteria, can produce osteomyelitis, but infections caused by certain pyogenic bacteria and mycobacteria are the most common [13].

Several systems have been used to classify osteomyelitis [14]. In the most common type of osteomyelitis (approximately 50 percent of cases), infection spreads directly from another site, with skin, operative, and posttraumatic infections being the most common sources. It has been estimated that 1 percent of prosthetic joint procedures are complicated by infection. Another large group of osteomyelitis patients (30 percent of cases) have peripheral vascular disease. The least common type of osteomyelitis in clinical practice (20 percent of cases) is thought to result from hematogenous spread by bacteria, often after trauma or medical intervention, such as placement of catheters. Hematogenous osteomyelitis usually begins in the metaphysis of a bone. The metaphysis is thought to be the initial site of infection for anatomic reasons. The branches of the nutrient artery provide an extensive network of vessels to the zones of endochondral ossification in this region.

Chronic recurrent, unifocal or multifocal osteomyelitis is an inflammatory disorder of unknown origin. It can involve various osseous sites and may be associated with palmoplantar pustulosis. Although bacterial cultures, radiological and magnetic resonance imaging (MRI) features of the infection have been described, definite diagnosis relies on histopathologic confirmation

by biopsy. Nonetheless, the histopathologic criteria have not been clearly defined. The spectrum of histopathologic changes in chronic recurrent multifocal osteomyelitis ranges from acute changes to subacute changes, as well as chronic inflammation. Acute histopathologic changes include acute inflammatory infiltration, active bone resorption and necrosis, reactive bone formation, while subacute changes predominantly involves lymphocytic and plasma cell infiltration. Chronic inflammation is characterized in these cases by fibroblastic organization and bony sclerosis [15]. A wide range of reparative changes of bone can often be observed. Immunohistochemistry shows a predominance of CD3(+), and CD45RO(+) T cells, which are mainly CD8(+) [16]. Although these histologic alterations correlate relatively poorly with the clinical features, they correlate well with the radiologic findings.

4.3.1. Acute Infection

In acute infection, the predominant cell type includes the polymorphonuclear leukocytes which efface and obliterate the normal marrow. As these cells break down, their nuclear fragments appear sprinkled throughout the tissue. This is referred to as *karyorrhexis* and *karyolysis*. Necrotic marrow and bone is evident. Usually, extensive bone resorption is seen, with marked osteoclastic activity. Eventually, the infected focus is filled with granulation tissue consisting of organizing hemorrhage, polymorphonuclear leukocytes, lymphocytes, and macrophages. Although resorption is extensive microscopically, pathologic fracture in acute osteomyelitis is rare (Fig. 1).

4.3.2. Chronic Infection

In chronic infection the inflammation is dominated by mononuclear cells, including plasma cells and macrophage/monocyte cells. The osteoclastic resorption, characteristic of both acute and chronic infections, is usually quite extensive, although concomitant attempts at

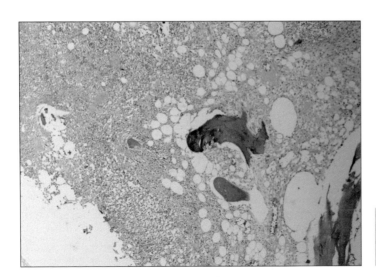

FIGURE 1. Acute osteomyelitis with extensive inflammation with a predominance of polymorphonuclear leukocytes and bone destruction (H-E original magnification x 10).

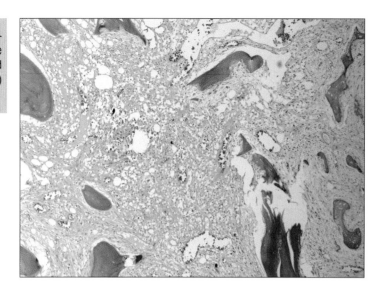

FIGURE 2. Chronic osteomyelitis with diffuse chronic inflammation, fibrosis and bone destruction. In this view, there are foci of necrotic bone (pink areas) where and irregular and poorly cellular, highly calcified bony substance (purple areas) has been despited.

bone repair may obscure, on roentgenograms, the true extent of tissue destruction (Fig. 2).

4.4. Granulomatous Infection

Granulomatous bone infections, are organized inflammatory reactions with a broad differential diagnosis. Excluding foreign bodies, the differential diagnosis of granulomatous disease in bone includes sarcoidosis, tuberculosis (mycobacterial, atypical), histoplasmosis, coccidiomycosis, blastomycosis, sporotrichosis, and salmonellosis. Granulomas are organized inflammatory reactions that may be seen in a wide array of infections and non-infectious conditions. Tuberculosis granulomas show central areas of necrosis (caseation) with surrounding inflammatory reaction consisting mostly of mononuclear cells, epithelioid histiocytes (large macrophages mimicking epithelial cells), and classic Langhans' giant cells, which are large multinucleated cells with abundant cytoplasm and nuclei, organized peripherally in a horseshoe shape or U shape at one end of the cell. These classic features are strongly indicative of tuberculosis, but definitive diagnosis lies on identification by either special stain of the acid-fast bacillus or culture.

5. INFLAMMATION

Inflammation is the reaction of a tissue and its microcirculation to a pathogenic insult, and is characterized by the generation of inflammatory mediators and movement of fluid and leukocytes from the blood into extravascular tissues. The inflammation process is frequently an expression of the host's attempt to localize and eliminate metabolically altered cells, foreign particles, microorganisms, or antigens [17].

The primary purpose of the inflammatory response is to eliminate the pathogenic insult and remove injured tis-

sue components. This process accomplishes either regeneration of the normal tissue architecture and return of physiological function or the formation of scar tissue to replace what cannot be repaired. Depending on persistence of the injury, clinical symptoms, and the nature of the inflammatory response, inflammation can be either acute or chronic. The hallmarks of acute inflammation include accumulation of fluid and plasma components in the affected tissue, intravascular stimulation of platelets, and the presence of polymorphnuclear leukocytes. In contrast, the characteristic cell components of chronic inflammation are lymphocytes, plasma cells, and macrophages [17, 18].

Activation of the inflammatory response can result in resolution, where the source of the tissue injury is eliminated, the inflammatory response resolves, and normal tissue architecture and physiological function are restored. However, the inflammation process can also result in abscess formation, scar formation or persistent inflammation. Abscesses form when the area of acute inflammation is walled off by the inflammatory cells, and destruction of the tissue by products of the neutrophils takes place. Scar formation occurs when the tissue is irreversibly injured. In this case, the normal architecture can be replaced by a scar, even if the initial pathological insult has been eliminated. Persistent inflammation occurs when inflammatory cells fail to eliminate the pathological insult. When inflammatory reaction persists, it may be associated with a cell-mediated immune reaction and may lead to fibrosis and scar formation [17, 18].

5.1. Histologic features

Acute inflammation is characterized by vascular changes, edema, and largely neutrophilic infiltration. The accumulation of neutrophil polymorphs within the extracellular space is the diagnostic histological feature of acute inflammation.

Chronic inflammation is characterized by infiltration

with mononuclear cells, which include macrophages, lymphocytes, and plasma cells, a reflection of a persisted reaction to injury. In case of chronic inflammation tissue destruction is largely induced by the inflammatory cells, and healing through connective tissue replacement of damaged tissue is accomplished by proliferation of small blood vessels (angiogenesis) and, in particular, fibrosis [18].

Granulomatous inflammation is a distinctive pattern of chronic inflammatory reaction in which the predominant cell type is an activated macrophage with a modified epithelial-like (epithelioid) appearance. It is encountered in a relatively few but widespread chronic immune and infectious diseases. Recognition of the granulomatous pattern in a biopsy specimen is important because of the limited number of possible conditions that cause it and the significance of the diagnosis associated with the lesions.

Tuberculosis is the archetype of the granolomatous diseases, but sarcoidosis, cut-scratch disease, lymphogranuloma inguinale, leprosy, brucellosis, syphilis, some mycotic infections, berylliois, and reactions of irritant lipids are also included [17, 18].

6. Conclusions

The upper extremity consists of various potential spaces that can become infected by a wide variety of organisms, which in turn, induce specific and non-specific defense responses. For descriptive purposes, infections can be divided according to the tissue compartment they have infected into three major categories: infections of the soft tissue, infections of the joints and infections of the bone. Despite the growing wealth of information regarding the immune response cascade involved in infections, relatively little information is available on the morphological and histologic changes that accompany infections of the musculoskeletal system. The primary purpose of the inflammatory response is to eliminate the pathogenic insult and remove injured tissue components. This process accomplishes either regeneration of the normal tissue architecture and return of physiological function, or the formation of scar tissue to replace what cannot be repaired. The hallmarks of acute inflammation include accumulation of fluid and plasma components in the affected tissue, intravascular stimulation of platelets, and the presence of polymorphonuclear leukocytes. In contrast, the characteristic cell components of chronic inflammation are lymphocytes, plasma cells, and macrophages.

References

[1] Miyajima A, Miyatake S, Schreurs J, De Vries J, Arai N, Yokota T, Arai K. Coordinate regulation of immune and inflammatory response by T cell-derived lymphokines. FASEB J 1988;2:2462-73.

[2] Cohen S. Cell mediated immunity and the inflammatory system. Hum Pathol 1976;7:249-64.

[3] Wilson D, Berendt A. Bone and joint infection. In: Ed DA, Grainger RG, Adam A, Dixon A, (eds). Grainger and Allison's diagnostic radiology, 4th ed. London: Churchill Livingstone, 2001.

[4] Urschel JD Necrotizing soft tissue infections. Postgraduate Med J 1999;75:645-649.

[5] Fontes RA, Ogilvie CM, Miclau T Necrotizing soft-tissue infections. J Am Acad Orthop Surg 2000;8:151-158.

[6] Safran DB, Sullivan WG. Necrotizing fasciitis of the chest wall. Ann Thorac Surg 2001;72:1362-1364.

[7] Herzberg AJ, Boyd PR, Gutierrez Y. Subcutaneous dirofilariasis in Collier County, Florida, USA. Am J Surg Pathol 1995; 19(8): 934-9.

[8] O'Meara PM, Bartal E. Septic arthritis: process, etiology, treatment outcome. A literature review. Orthopedics 1988;11(4): 623-8.

[9] Ho G Jr, Su EY. Therapy for septic arthritis. JAMA. 1982;247(6): 797-800.

[10] Kono M, Tanaka H, Yayoshi M, Araake M, Yoshioka M, Imai M. Mycoplasma pulmonis arthritis in congenitally athymic (nude) mice. Histopathological features. Microbiol Immunol 1980; 24(5):381-91.

[11] Severijnen AJ, van Kleef R, Grandia AA, van der Kwast TH, Hazenberg MP. Histology of joint inflammation induced in rats by cell wall fragments of the anaerobic intestinal bacterium Eubacterium aerofaciens. Rheumatol Int 1991;11 (4-5):203-8.

[12] Tissi L, Marconi P, Mosci P, Merletti L, Cornacchione P, Rosati E, Recchia S, von Hunolstein C, Orefici G. Experimental model of type IV Streptococcus agalactiae (group B streptococcus) infection in mice with early development of septic arthritis. Infect Immun 1990; 58(9):3093-100.

[13] Lew DP, Waldvogel FA. Osteomyelitis. Lancet 2004; 24-30;364 (9431):369-79.

[14] Esterhai JL. Infection. In: Poss R, at al., editors. Orthopaedic knowledge update 3. home study syllabus. Park Ridge, IL: American Academy of Orthopaedic Surgeons, 1990, p. 150.

[15] Chow LT, Griffith JF, Kumta SM, Leung PC. Chronic recurrent, multifocal osteomyelitis: a great clinical and radiologic mimic in need of recognition by the pathologist. APMIS 1999;107:369-79.

[16] Girschick HJ, Huppertz HI, Harmsen D, Krauspe R, Muller-Hermelink HK, Papadopoulos T. Chronic recurrent multifocal osteomyelitis in children: diagnostic value of histopathology and microbial testing. Hum Pathol 1999;30:59-65.

[17] Fantone JC, Ward PA. Inflammation. In: Rubin E, Farber JL (eds). Pathology, 3rd Ed. Philadelphia: Lippincott-Raven, 1999, pp. 37-75.

[18] Acute and chronic inflammation. In: Robbins SL, Cotran RS, Kumar V (eds). Pathologic Basis of Disease, 6th ed. Philadelphia: WB Saunders Company, 1999, pp. 50-88.

Mimics of Infection in the Hand and Upper Extremity

Milan STEVANOVIC[a]*, **Frances SHARPE**[b]

[a]*Department of Orthopaedic Surgery, Keck School of Medicine,*
University of Southern California, Los Angeles, USA
[b]*Southern California Permanente Medical Group, Fontana, California, USA*

Common pathologic processes that can mimic infection in the upper extremity are reviewed. Key clinical distinguishing features are discussed.

Keywords: mimics; infection; hand; upper extremity.

1. INTRODUCTION

There are a number of reported pathologic processes known to have been initially diagnosed and
treated as infections with the result that the treatment was ineffective. There are probably still more
yet to be reported. Familiarity with non-infectious
inflammatory conditions will aid correct diagnosis
and direct appropriate evaluation and treatment.
As aptly noted by Louis and Jebson: "We have all
been fooled! The hand may be inflamed, but that
does not necessarily mean that it is infected" [1].

Non-specific clinical findings that can be associated with infectious processes can also be seen
with non-infectious inflammatory conditions. Erythema, dactylitis (the sausage-like inflammation of
the fingers), joint effusions, laboratory abnormalities, and radiographic changes can all be found in
both infections and non-infections processes.

The historical, clinical and investigational findings should not be viewed in isolation, but as a
whole. This approach, in combination with a familiarity with a wide variety of conditions and in collaboration with colleagues from rheumatology and
infectious disease, can help lead to the correct
diagnosis and appropriate patient management.

2. INFLAMMATORY ARTHROPATHIES

Inflammatory arthropathies include rheumatoid
arthritis, juvenile rheumatoid arthritis, seronegative
spondyloarthropathies, and crystal induced inflammatory arthritis. Arthropathy and arthritis has also
been described in association with hepatic diseases [2], Crohn's disease, and ulcerative colitis
[3]. Arthralgias may sometimes be accompanied
by joint swelling and effusion. Usually, this can be
distinguished from a septic joint by clinical examination and joint aspiration when the clinical examination is not clear.

Outside of the crystal-induced arthropathies,
rheumatoid arthritis can be the most difficult to distinguish from a septic process, particularly in the
initial presentation both of the juvenile and adult
forms. Confusion with a septic process can occur
when the onset of joint symptoms is acute and
mono-articular. Cell count from joint aspiration
usually demonstrates lower white cell counts
(WBCs) (ranging from 2,000 to 75,000 WBCs per
cc) than with a septic process. Radiographic

*Corresponding Author
Hand and Microsurgery
Department of Orthopedics
2025 Zonal Avenue, GNH Room 3900
Los Angeles, CA 90033
e-mail: stevanov@usc.edu

changes typically occur later in the disease process. Serologic findings are often absent in juvenile forms of rheumatoid arthritis. In adult onset of rheumatoid arthritis, serologic findings remain negative in the first one to two months of the disease, and remain negative in approximately 15% of patients [4].

2.1. Crystal-induced inflammatory arthropathies

2.1.1. Pseudogout

Calcium pyrophosphate deposition disease (CPPD), commonly known as pseudogout, is a crystal arthropathy typically associated with aging. Calcification of the fibrocartilage of the knee (meniscus) and wrist (triangulofibrocartilage complex) seen radiographically is pathognomonic for this diagnosis. Because of this finding, pseudogout has also been termed chondrocalcinosis.

Clinical presentation is usually of mild swelling and joint effusion with decreased range of motion of the affected joint. The symptoms are usually slower in onset and less severe than that seen in gouty arthropathy or in sepsis. In the upper extremity, the wrist is the most commonly affected joint, and pain in particular around the ulnar aspect of the wrist is most typical. Pseudogout affecting the upper extremity is rarely confused with a septic process, since it is not usually accompanied by severe pain or erythema. However, when presenting as an acute process, it can be associated with low-grade fever [5].

The diagnosis of pseudogout can be suspected on radiographic findings, but should be confirmed by aspiration of the affected joint. Joint fluid analysis for crystals will demonstrate rhomboid-shaped weakly positive bi-refringent crystals.

2.1.2. Gout

Of the inflammatory conditions affecting the extremities, gout is the most prevalent disease and the most likely to be misdiagnosed as infection. The term "gout" is derived from the Latin word *gutta,* meaning drop. In the 13th century, it was thought that gout resulted from a drop of evil humor affecting a vulnerable joint [6]. Gout is now recognized to be a crystal deposition disease in which monosodium urate crystals are deposited in the joints and in soft tissues as a result of hyperuricemia. Most patients with hyperuricemia are underexcreters of uric acid, likely as an inherited condition of renal excretion. In addition, increased dietary purines, and myeloproliferative disorders can increase urate production. A decrease in urate excretion can result from renal disease, alcohol intake, and certain medications [6].

The onset of a gouty attack is often marked by the rapid development of warmth, swelling, and pain around an affected joint. The cutaneous erythema associated with the gouty attack may extend beyond the involved joint. Gouty attacks can occur in the joints, resembling septic arthritis or in the soft-tissues, mimicking cellulites.

Systemic symptoms of fever, chills, and malaise may accompany an acute attack, further confounding the diagnosis [6]. Although the disease most commonly presents past the age of forty, early onset gout is that with onset prior to age 25, and strongly suggests a hereditary component or enzyme deficiency [6, 7].

Clinical examination for acute onset gout can be difficult to distinguish from a septic process. A family history of gout or previous episodes of joint pain and inflammation that have spontaneously resolved can suggest a non-infectious process. Clinically, the character of the erythema is not as extensive as cellulitis and somewhat darker in color. There is no clinical finding of distal lymphadenitis. Late clinical findings of tophi clarify the diagnosis of gout. However, tophi usually develop on average of 10 years after the initial attack of gout [7] (Fig. 1). Radiographs are usually normal in early disease or may show soft-tissue swelling. Later findings characteristically include subchondral punched-out lytic lesions with sclerotic margins and over-hanging edges. The joint space is preserved until quite late in the disease process [8]. Serum uric acid levels, either high normal or above the normal range, can suggest a gout attack, but are not diagnostic. In conjunction with a thorough history and physical examination, the hallmark of diagnosis remains the identification of monosodium urate crystals from joint or soft tissue aspiration. Joint aspiration will yield clear to cloudy fluid, with a cell count demonstrating between 25-75,000 WBCs. The diagnosis is confirmed by the

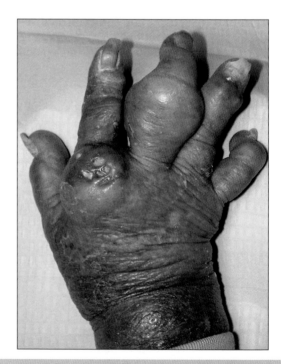

FIGURE 1. This 83-year-old woman with a long-standing history of gout, presents with deformity and drainage from the metacarpophalangeal joint of the index finger.

identification of the needle-like negatively birefringent monosodium urate crystals by polarizing light microscopy [6, 7]. If an inflammatory arthropathy is suspected, but cannot be confirmed by clinical exam and laboratory analysis, antibiotic treatment can be withheld and the patient can be evaluated for response to non-steroidal anti inflammatory medications. In the case of crystal induced arthropathies, patients will also respond to oral colchicine.

3. NEUTROPHILIC DERMATOSES

Neutrophilic dermatoses are a rare collection of diseases histologically characterized as a neutrophilic infiltration of the dermis without findings of infectious agents and/or defined etiology. They are unified by overlapping clinical and histologic features and may be a spectrum of the same disease process. Neutrophilic dermatoses include: neutrophilic dermatosis of the dorsal hands (NDDH), pustular vasculitis, acute febrile neutrophilic dermatosis (Sweet Syndrome) and pyoderma gangrenosum [9, 10]. Although all of these disease entities are rare, pyoderma gangrenosum is the most common.

4. PYODERMA GANGRENOSUM

Pyoderma gangrenosum is a rare idiopathic inflammatory disorder of the skin, characterized histologically as a neutrophillic dermatosis. Although the lesions present more commonly on the lower extremities, the hand and in particular the dorsal surfaces of the hand can also be involved [11]. The initial symptoms can mimic infection, with the presentation of painful and tender folliculocentric pustules or fluctuant nodules with an inflammatory halo. There is subsequent peripheral expansion and ulcer formation. The margins of the ulcer are sharply circumscribed with violaceous raised edges. Necrotic pustles may be present within the raised border. The lesions may be mistaken for acute bacterial infections or indolent mycobacterial or fungal infections [11-13]. Although it can occur at any age, it is most common in young to middleage adults, with a female predominance. There is a strong association with underlying disease, with 50 - 80% of patients having an associated underlying disease [11, 14] and approximately 40% providing a history of antecedent trauma [15, 16]. The most common associated systemic diseases include inflammatory bowel disease and hematologic malignancies, inflammatory arthritis, and immune-system abnormalities [11].

The differential diagnosis includes infection, collagen vascular disease and syndromes with vasculitis such as systemic lupus erythematosus, rheumatoid arthritis, Bechet's disease and Wegener's granulomatosis. Malignant neoplasms, factitious disease, and brown recluse spider bites have also been reported.

One of the hallmarks of this disease is the pathergic response to trauma, and particularly to surgical trauma [12, 14, 15, 17]. That is the, the disease process is rapidly accelerated by surgical trauma. Treatment includes local wound management and systemic and intra-lesional steroids. It should be re-emphasized that surgical treatment other than diagnostic biopsy should not be performed when pyoderma gangrenosum is suspected. If an underlying disease has not been identified, the patient should undergo a thorough diagnostic work-up.

5. CHEMOTHERAPEUTIC EXTRAVASATION

Given an appropriate history, it would be difficult to mistake the findings of chemotherapeutic extravasation with infection. In the absence of this information, the tissue necrosis associated with certain vesicant and irritant agents might be confused with an infectious process. Extravasation injuries are seen more commonly in adults than in children [18]. Some of the most common agents causing tissue necrosis are Doxorubicin, Mitomycin and Vincristine. Acute management usually occurs at the time of infiltration and in centers where chemotherapy is routinely administered. Protocols should be established for the event of an extravasation injury. This includes the immediate cessation of infusion. The intravenous (IV) catheter is left in place to allow for the egress of any residual agent and to attempt to aspirate any residual drug through the IV site [18]. Appropriate doses of antidote therapy (when available) can be delivered through the IV. Topical or subcutaneous injections of antidote care given for up to 24 hours [18, 19]. Surgical intervention is rarely necessary. However, if tissue destruction continues, especially for Doxyoubicin infiltration, early surgical excision may be necessary to stop the progressive destruction of tissue [18].

6. PYOGENIC GRANULOMA

Pyogenic granuloma is a benign tumor of unknown etiology. It has been proposed to originate at a site of trauma. The term "pyogenic" dates back to 1904, when Hartzell identified staphylococci within a lesion. However, pyogenic granulomas are not primarily an infection. Based on the histologic appearance and the absence of trauma in many cases, pyogenic granuloma is thought to be an acquired vascular lesion, in some cases with secondary bacterial contamination, and rarely, infection. Recent studies have suggested that there is upregulation of vascular endothelial growth factor contributing to the pathogenesis of the disease process [20]. The lesion is more common during pregnancy, usually involving the oral mucosa [21]. Outside of this location, the volar surfaces of the hand and forearm are the most common locations [21].

The typical appearance is that of a reddish brown papular mass, with a narrow neck and cauliflower-like cap. The tissue is friable and bleeds easily, and the bleeding is often refractory to pressure application. The size of the lesion varies from a few millimeters up to one centimeter (Fig. 2). Usually, the lesion is solitary, but it has been reported as recurring with multiple satellite lesions, presenting at the site of previous excision. In a report by Warner and Jones, all of these lesions were on the trunk [22].

In addition to distinguishing this tumor from an infection, it should also be distinguished from the amelanotic melanoma. When lesions show rapid growth or recurrence after treatment, the patient may be concerned about malignancy.

Several different treatment methods have been described, with all treatment methods having an incidence of recurrence. The most common method of treatment involves the application of silver nitrate daily for ten days. Excision of the lesion with a one-two millimeter cuff of normal tissue has a relatively low recurrence rate and should be done for those lesions not responding to silver nitrate application [23]. In patients who develop pyogenic granulomas in association with hormonal changes such as pregnancy or use of oral contraceptives, most lesions will spontaneously resolve in 4-8 weeks with completion of pregnancy or discontinuation of oral contraceptives [23].

symptoms of patients with symptomatic retained foreign bodies are pain and swelling. At times, a draining sinus is present. Symptoms may be of either acute or chronic inflammation. Secondary infection may also be present. A high index of suspicion for a retained foreign body should be kept for any patient presenting with unexplained pain, swelling, or inflammation of the hand, as the history of penetrating trauma is frequently forgotten by the patient [25, 26].

The presentation and intensity of the response depends both on the location of the penetration and the retained material. The type of material causing the reaction is also important. Certain materials can produce more than a localized foreign body response, particularly when deposited in or adjacent to a joint. The most reported reactions are those caused by the date palm thorn and the sea urchin spine [24, 27].

The initial examination may reveal a swollen soft tissue mass, mimicking a tumor or an infection. Proximity to a joint can result in synovitis, suggesting joint sepsis or an auto-immune inflammatory arthropathy [24, 25, 28].

Treatment includes the surgical removal of the foreign body. When there is joint involvement, complete synovectomy of all of the inflammatory synovium is recommended [24, 27]. Specimens for both pathologic and microbiologic analysis should be obtained. Microbiologic analysis should include specimens for fungal and mycobacterial organisms. Secondary infections should be treated with a course of appropriately directed antibiotic therapy.

7. Foreign Body Reaction

The hand is susceptible to penetrating trauma from all sorts of objects [24-26]. The most common presenting

8. Primary Tumors

Primary tumors of the hand are less frequently confused with infection. Nevertheless, rare instances of primary

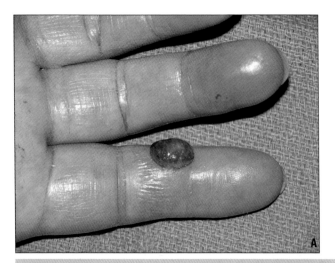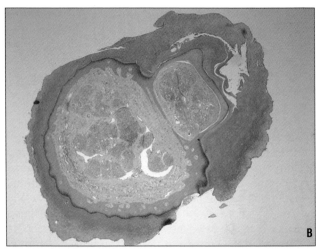

FIGURE 2. (A) The typical pedunculated appearance of a pyogenic granuloma on a pregnant 30 year old woman. **(B)** Histological appearance of a pyogenic granuloma.

skin tumors can present with characteristics of chronic or subacute infection. Malignant tumors that can mimic infection include squamous cell carcinoma, basal cell carcinoma, intradermal squamous cell carcinoma (Bowen's disease), or epitheliod sarcoma. Usually, squamous cell and basal cell carcinoma will mimic infection when the tumors are large and develop ulceration (Fig. 3). Intradermal squamous cell carcinoma (Bowen's disease) is a superficial squamous cell carcinoma in situ, which may resemble a dermatophytic infection [29]. Epitheliod sarcoma usually presents as a painless nodule in the palmar surface of the hand. Ulceration has been reported to occur rarely. With this presentation, there is potential for the misdiagnosis of infection.

9. METASTATIC TUMORS

Acrometastases (distal metastatic lesions) are rare [30, 31]. When present, they almost always involve the bone and most commonly the distal phalanx, but have been seen in the carpals, metacarpals, and phalanges [30, 32]. Cutaneous metastases have also been reported and can be associated with an inflammatory response [33]. The most common presenting symptom is continuous aching. Swelling and erythema may also be present. Untreated, the tumor may erode into the soft-tissues and fungate. Bone involvement shows osteolysis. Individually or in combination, these findings may be mistaken for an infectious process [30, 34, 35]. Presumed infections should be biopsied as well as cultured to reduce chance of misdiagnosis and prevent delayed treatment [30, 34].

The most common sites of primary tumors are lung and kidney. Breast [30, 36], head and neck [30], colon [30, 37], primary bone (chondrosarcoma), and lymphoma [30] have also been reported. Treatment is usually palliative with amputation for finger or metacarpal involvement or local resection for more proximal sites. Adjunctive radiation can be used for sensitive tumors. The prognosis for patients presenting with distal metastatic disease is poor, with more than 50% of patients dead within six months of presentation [30, 37]. Despite this dismal prognosis, there are cases in which wide resection of an isolated metastasis has resulted in long-term disease free periods [30, 36, 38].

10. ACUTE CALCIFIC TENDONITIS

Acute pain around the wrist, edema, erythema, and occasionally low-grade fever is the typical presentation of a patient with acute calcific tendonitis. These symptoms in conjunction with very subtle radiographic findings can lead to the misdiagnosis of an acute infectious process [39-41].

This condition is often seen in middle age patients, but has been reported in children. There is a female predominance [39]. The etiology remains unknown, but it has been suggested that trauma can initiate this process. The most common location for calcification in the hand is within the flexor carpi ulnaris tendon insertion; however, it can also occur in the fingers and dorsal carpal region [41]. The size of the calcific deposit has not been correlated to the level of symptoms [40].

This is a self-limiting condition that normally resolves with or without treatment. Symptoms may persist for three to four weeks and spontaneously resolve [39, 41]. Local anesthetic injection without steroids may change the pH of the lesion and lead to quicker resolution of the symptoms. Splinting and aspirin therapy have also been reported to decrease the duration of symptoms [39, 40].

11. CALCINOSIS

Calcinosis is the soft tissue deposition of calcium phosphate crystals in the soft tissues [42]. The condition can occur as an idiopathic process, but more commonly with associated auto-immune diseases. A wide variety of diseases have been associated with dystrophic calcification. Some of these conditions include connective tissue diseases such as scleroderma, CREST syndrome, myosistis and systemic lupus erythematosis [43]. Uremic tumoral calcinosis is a rare manifestation of renal osteodystrophy [44]. The calcium depositis are firm, irregular and generally non-tender. The lesions may become inflamed, infected or ulcerated and may discharge a chalky white material. When an inflammatory response is associated with the deposition of calcium salts, the clinical findings can be mistaken for an infectious process [44, 45]. Radiographic examination showing soft tissue calcification can differentiate this from an infection (Fig. 4).

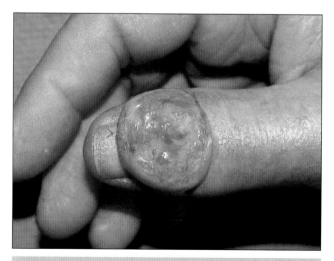

FIGURE 3. Primary squamous cell tumor of the dorsal aspect of the thumb. The patient did not seek treatment for more than six months.

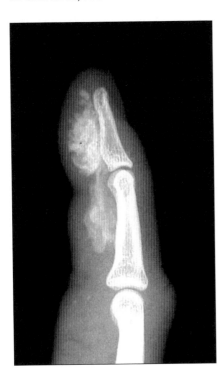

FIGURE 4. Idiopathic calcinosis of the index finger.

12. SARCOIDOSIS

Sarcoidosis is a granulomatous disease of unknown etiology, most frequently presenting as a granulomatous inflammation of the lung. Although involvement of the hands in sarcoidosis is rare, it may rarely preceed systemic disease [46, 47]. Skeletal involvement occurs between 1-15% of the time and is usually associated with chronic progressive disease and associated pulmonary involvement. Rarely, sarcoidosis can present in the hand with isolated osseous and/or soft tissue involvement [48-50]. Swelling, redness and pain are the main local symptoms. Radiographic findings are most commonly seen in the phalanges of the hand and show a combination of lytic lesions and lacy lattice pattern within the diaphysis. MRI findings are present prior to radiographic findings and may show an infiltrative process of the bone and possibly with associated soft-tissue mass [51]. Differentiation between fungal and mycobacterial infections as well as granuloma-like neoplasms can be made through biopsy and culture [50].

13. SPIDER BITE

Much recent attention has been given to the deleterious effects of spider bites. The perceived threat of bites by both the general public and medical community far exceeds the actual risk [52-55]. More than 40,000 species of spiders have been described world-wide; however, very few have significant effects in humans. Many studies have reported cases of dermonecrotic

arachnidism, but most studies are based on presumptive spider bites and unidentified species. Several species have been investigated with respect to their effects in humans, none of which has been found to have significant ones [53, 56, 57].

Brown spiders of the *Loxosceles* species can result in local dermal necrosis with the area of necrosis dependent on the degree of envenomation [58]. This local skin necrosis can be mistaken for infection. Systemic reactions (systemic loxoscelism) are rare but can include hemolytic anemia, renal failure, multi-organ system failure, disseminated intravascular coagulation and death, with the pediatric population at greatest risk [54, 59, 60]. *Loxosceles* species are generally found in the tropical to temperate regions of the Americas, Africa, and Europe. In the United States, the brown recluse *(Loxosceles reclusa)* is found with rare exception within a specific range within the central and southern states. Five additional species are found in the southwestern United States and are more common to the desert regions of the Southwest. Three species are common to Brazil, with *Loxosceles laeta* being the most toxic. *Loxosceles refuscens,* whose venom is reported to be identical to that of the *L. reclusa* is found in the Mediterranean basin [52, 53, 59, 61]. Reports that the brown recluse spider is ubiquitous throughout the United States [23, 62] are unsubstantiated [52, 63]. Attribution of dermonecrotic lesions to spider bites should be made with caution in patients in endemic areas. Brown recluse spider bites outside of endemic areas are improbable. Unless the spider is identified, alternative diagnoses should be considered.

Bites of the brown recluse usually occur at night. The initial area of penetration may be trivial and go unrecognized. Pain varying from mild to severe begins at 2-8 hours. Small punctae and transient erythema with itching may be present. A small bleb or blister appears between 12-24 hours surrounded by a halo of ischemic tissue. The central area may become hemorrhagic. The area of necrosis becomes a dull bluish color, and there is gravitational spread of the local hemorrhage. The central area hardens over the course of days. An eschar may form and drop off leaving an area of ulceration [59]. Systemic symptoms are rare, with the most common symptom being fever. As yet, there is no widely available laboratory test for the identification of *Loxosceles* toxin.

Treatment of loxoscelism remains controversial. Although several different treatments have been described, supportive care including rest, immobilization, local wound care and tetanus prophylaxis seems to be as effective as any other treatment. The two most common medical therapies are dapsone and glucocorticoid therapy. Dapsone inhibits polymorphonuclear cell migration and production of free radicals. In one prospective trial in humans, dapsone in conjunction with supportive treatment and wound care had a lower complication rate than early surgical excision [64]. Systemic glucocorticoids may be valuable in treating systemic symptoms, but does not seem to affect local tissue necrosis. Antivenom has been developed, but is not commercially available, and seems to be useful only if introduced in the first 24 hours after envenomation. Surgical excision with or without skin grafting has been variable advocated without clearly defined benefit [53, 58, 59, 65].

It remains equally important to recognize that most spider bites are often related to either non-pathogenic spiders or other arthropods, or may be other etiologies entirely. Bites from other arthropods can induce a local reaction with secondary infection. Infections caused by methicillin-resistant staphylococcus aureus often produces significant soft-tissue necrosis which can resemble the necrosis associated with brown recluse spider bites [55, 66].

14. FACTITIOUS DISEASE

Factitious disease has been categorized by various authors based on patient characteristics. Other authors have categorized factitious disorders based on the type of self-induced injury. Grunert et al described three groups: 1) wound manipulators; 2) factitious edema; and 3) hand deformity [67]. Al-Quattan further characterized these patients as: 1) wound inducers; 2) foreign body introducers; 3) edema inducers; and 4) passive mutilators [68]. The factitious disorders most commonly misdiagnosed as infection included the post-surgical wound dehiscence, chronic non-healing wounds or recurrent ulcers.

Wound characteristics that suggest this diagnosis include wounds that present in atypical bizarre patterns either with regular borders or with criss-crossing striations, wounds in various stages of healing, ranging from freshly blood-crusted lesions to well-healed scars. Chemically induced injuries may show dependent tails or drip marks.

Patient characteristics may include a nervous patient with lesions associated with unconscious neurotic excoriations, or restlessness. Other patient types are those who are angry, hostile patients, who repeatedly blame either the employer or the situation that resulted in their injury, or previous physicians who were unable to "fix them" [68-70]. Another type of patient is the emotionally dependent and depressed patient. Patients tend to focus on the wound or ulcer despite attempts to gather other aspects of the history. It is usually difficult to observe the patient in the act of self-manipulation. Phelps et al successfully demonstrated self-manipulation in a patient with the use of flourescein labeled tetracycline [71].

These wounds generally respond to protecting the area from patient access, by the placement of a cast or other non-removable dressing. However, in the absence of psychiatric intervention, these wounds often recur [68]. Most authors have recommended a non-confrontational or mildly-confrontational approach to treatment [67, 69, 72-74]. Involvement of psychiatric services has the best chance of disease remission, with better response in the emotionally needy patient rather than in the angry, hostile patient [67, 70].

15. SUMMARY

A wide range of conditions can mimic infection in the hand and upper extremity. Vigilant attention should be given to atypical presentations of lesions of the bone or soft tissues, and the patient's history and physical examination should be considered as a whole, rather than as an isolated wound or lesion. Equally important to recognizing non-infectious processes, is to recognize the atypical infections such as atypical fungal or mycobacterial infections [75-77], viral infections such as congenital syphilis [78], and bacterial supra-infection of non-infectious processes.

REFERENCES

[1] Louis D, Jebson P. Mimickers of Infection. Hand Clin 1998;14(4):519-29.

[2] Chi Z-C, Ma S-Z. Rheumatologic manifestations of hepatic diseases. HBPD Int 2003;2(1):32-7.

[3] McCarty D. Differential diagnosis of arthritis: analysis of signs and symptoms. In: Koopman W, Moreland L, editors. Arthritis and allied conditions: a textbook of rheumatology. 15th ed. Philadelphia: Lippincott Williams & Wilkins; 2005, p. 37-50.

[4] O'Dell J. Rheumatoid arthritis: The clinical picture. In: Koopman W, Moreland L, editors. Arthritis and allied conditions: A textbook of rheumatology. Philadelphia: Lippincott Williams & Wilkins; 2005, p. 1165-94.

[5] Halverson P. Basic calcium phosphate (apatite, octacalcium phosphate, tricapciumphosphate) crystal deposition disease and calcinosis. In: Koopman W, LW M, editors. Arthritis and allied conditions: A textbook of rheumatology. Philadelphia: Lippincott Williams & Wilkins; 2005, p. 2397-416.

[6] Becker M, Jolly M. Clinical gout and the pathogenesis of hyperurecemia. In: Koopman W, Moreland L, editors. Arthritis and Allied Conditions A textbook of Rheumatology. 15th ed. Philadelphia: Lippincott Williams & Wilkins; 2005, p. 2303-39.

[7] Gout EN. Clinical and Laboratory Features. In: Klippel J, editor. Primer on the rheumatic diseases. 12th ed. Atlanta: Arthritis Foundations; 2001, p. 313-9.

[8] Rousseau I, Cardinal E, Raymond-Tremblay D, Beauregard C, Braunstein E, Saint-Pierre A. Gout: Radiographic findings mimicking infections. Skeletal Radiol 2001;30(10):565-9.

[9] Duquia R, Larangeira de Almeida Jr. H, Vettorato G, Souza R, Schwarz J. Neutrophilic dermatosis of the dorsal in the hands: Acral sweet syndrome. Int J Dermatol 2006;45(1):51-2.

[10] Walling H, Snipes C, Gerami P, Piette W. The relationship between neutrophilic dermatosis of the dorsal hands and sweet syndrome. Arch Dermatol 2006;142(1):57-63.

[11] Crowson A, Nuovo G, Ferri C, Magro C. Pyoderma gangrenosum: a review. J Cutan Pathol 2003;30(2):97-107.

[12] Ferlic D. Pyoderma gangrenosum presenting as an acute suppurative hand infections - A case report. J Hand Surg 1983; 8:573-5.

[13] Laurencin C, Shoen S. Pyoderma gangrenosum affecting the hand. J Bone Joint Surg [Br] 1994;76B(6):985-6.

[14] Adam D, Nawroz I, Petrie P. Pyoderma gangrenosum severely affecting both hands. J Hand Surg [Br] 1996;21(6):792-4.

[15] Huish S, de la Paz E, Ellis P, Stern P. Pyoderma gangrenosum of the hand: A case series and review of the literature. J Hand Surg [Am] 2001;26A:679-85.

[16] Youker S, Marks J, Ioffreda M. Occupationally induced pyoderma gangrenosum. J Am Acad Dermatol. 2002;47(2):322-3.

[17] Shands JJ, Flowers F, Hill H, Smith O. Pyoderma gangrenosum in a kindred: Precipitation by surgery of mild physical trauma. J Am Acad Dermatol 1987;16:931-4.

[18] Goolsby T, Lombardo F. Extravasation of Chemotherapeutic Agents: Prevention and Treatment. Semin Oncol 2006;33:139-43.

[19] Dorr R. Antidotes to vesicant chemotherapy extravasations. Blood Rev 1990;4(1):41-60.

[20] Bragado R, Bello E, Requena L, Renedo G, Texeiro E, Alvaraez M, et al. Increased expression of vascular endotherlial growth factor in pyogenic granuloma. Acta Derm Venereol 1999;79(6):422-5.

[21] Witthaut J, Steffens K, Koob E. Reliable treatment of pyogenic granuloma of the hand. J Hand Surg [Br] 1994;19B(6):791-3.

[22] Warner J, Jones E. Pyogenic granuloma recurring with multiple satellites: A report of 11 cases. Br J Derm 1968;80:218-27.

[23] Kann S, Jacquemin J, Stern P. Simulators of hand infections. J Bone Joint Surg [Am] 1996;78A(7):1114-28.

[24] Cracchiolo A, Goldberg L. Local and systemic reactions to puncture injuries by the sea urchin spine and the date palm thorn. Arthritis Rheum 1977;20(6):1206-12.

[25] Morgan W, Leopold T, Evans R. Foreign bodies in the hand. J Hand Surg [Br] 1984;9B(2):194-6.

[26] Peterson J, Bancroft L, Kransdorf M. Wooden Foreign Bodies: Imaging appearance. AJR 2002;178(March):557-62.

[27] Doig S, Cole W. Plant thorn synovitis. J Bone Joint Surg [Br] 1990;72B(3):514-5.

[28] O'Connor C, Reginato A, Delong W. Foreign body reactions simulating acute septic arthritis. J Rheumatol 1988;15(10):1568-71.

[29] Baran R, Dupre A, Sayag J, Letessier S, Robins P, Bureau H. Bowen's disease of the nail apparatus. Report of 5 cases and review of 20 cases of the literature. Abb Dermatol Venereol 1979;106(3):227-33.

[30] Amadio P, Lombardi R. Metastatic tumors of the hand. J Hand Surg [Am] 1987;12A(2):311-6.

[31] Kerin R. Metastatic tumors of the hand: a review of the literature. J Bone Joint Surg [Am] 1983;65A:1331-5.

[32] Wu K, Guise E. Metastatic tumors of the hand: a report of six cases. J Hand Surg 1978;3B:271-6.

[33] Hazelrig J. Inflammatory metastatic carcinoma. Arch Dermatol 1977;113:69-70.

[34] Rose B, Wood F. Metastatic bronchogenic carcinoma masquerading as a felon. J Hand Surg 1983;8(3):325-8.

[35] Tuteja A, Owings M, Pulliam J, Elzinga L. Adenocarcinoma of the colon metastasizing to the foot masquerading as osteomyelitis. J Am Podiatr Med Assoc 1998;88(2):84-6.

[36] Carty H-M, Simons A, Isgar B. Breast carcinoma bone metastasis first presenting to single middle phalanx. Breast 2006;15:127-9.

[37] Buckley N, Brown D. Metastatic tumors in the hand from adenocarcinoma of the colon. Dis Colon Rectum 1987;30:141-3.

[38] Gamblin T, Santos R, Baratz M, Landreneau R. Metastatic colon cancer to the hand. Am Surg 2006;72(1):98-100.

[39] Dilley D, Tonkin M. Acute calcific tendinitis in the hand and wrist. J Hand Surg [Br] 1991;16B(2):215-6.

[40] Moyer R, Bush D, Harrington T. Acute calcific tendinitis if the hand and wrist: a report of 12 cases and a review of th literature. J Rheumatol 1989;16(2):198-202.

[41] Carroll R, Sinton W, Garcia A. Acute calcium deposits in the hand. JAMA 1955;157(5):422-6.

[42] Webb F, Wenley W. Calcinosis. Proc Roy Soc Med 1974; 67(6): 30-2.

[43] Carpenter M. Hydroxyapatitie and other crystalline diseases. In: West S, editor. Rheumatology Secrets. 2nd ed. Philadelphia: Hanley & Belfus, Inc; 2002, p. 338-43.

[44] Asuncion G, Tzarnas C. Uremic tumoral calcinosis: Acute hand presentations mimicking infection. J Hand Surg [Am] 1994; 19A(5):809-12.

[45] Sebesta A, Kamineni S, Dumont C. Idiopathic tumoral calcinosis of the index finger. Scand J Plast Reconstr Hand Surg 2000; 34:405-8.

[46] Kwon B, Bindra R, Liakos P, Gelberman R. Extensive nodular sarcoidosis in the hand. J Hand Surg [Br]1997;22B(5):676-8.

[47] Landi A, Brooks D, DeSantis G. Sarcoidosis of the hand - a report of two cases. J Hand Surg 1983;8:197-200.

[48] Pierson D, Willett E. Sarcoidosis presenting with finger pain. JAMA 1978;239:2023-4.

[49] Rodriguez-Gomes M, Fernandez-Sueiro J, Willisch A, Fernandez-Doningues L, Lopez-Barros G, Vega-Vazquez F. Multifocal dactylitis as the sole clinical expression of sarcoidosis. J Rheumatol 2000;27(1):245-7.

[50] Ugwonali O, Parisien M, Nickerson K, Scully B, Ristic S, Strauch R. Osseous sarcoidosis of the hand: pathologic analysis and review of the literature. J Hand Surg [Am] 2005;30A(4):854-8.

[51] Moore S, Teirstein A, Golimbu C. MRI of sarcoidosis patients with musculoskeletal symptoms. AJR 2005;185(7):154-9.

[52] Vetter R. Arachnids submitted as suspected brown recluse spiders (Araneae Sicariidae): Loxosceles spiders are virtually restriced to their known distributions but are perceived to exist throughout the United States. J Med Entomol 2005;42(4):512-21.

[53] Swanson D, Vetter R. Bites of brown recluse spiders and suspected necrotic arachnidism. N Engl J Med 2005;352(7):700-7.

[54] Elston D. Systemic manifestations and treatment of brown recluse spider bites. Cutis 2004;141(5):336-40.

[55] Vetter R, Pagac B, Reiland R, Bolesh D, Swanson D. Skin lesions in barracks: Consider community-acquired methicillin-resistant Staphylococcus Aureus instead of spider bites. Military Med 2006;171(9):830-2.

[56] Isbister G, Whyte I. Suspected white-tail spider bite and necrotic ulcers. Intern Med J 2004;34(1-2):38-44.

[57] Vetter R, Isbister G. Verified bites by the woodlouse spider, Dysdera crocata. Toxicon 2006;47:826-9.

[58] Rees R, Campbell D, Rieger E, King L. The diagnosis and treatment of brown recluse spider bites. Ann Emerg Med 1987; 16(9):945-9.

[59] da Silva P, da Silveira R, Appel M, Mangili O, Gremski W, Veiga S. Brown spiders and loxocselism. Toxicon 2004;44:693-709.

[60] Lane D, Youse J. Coombs positive hemolytic anemia secondary to brown recluse spider bite: a review of the literature and discussion of treatment. Cutis 2004;74:341-7.

[61] Maretic Z, Russell F. A case of necrotic arachnidism in Yugoslavia. Toxicon 1979;17:412-3.

[62] Glenn J, Lane J, Clark E. Arachnid envenomation from the brown recluse spider. Clin Pediatr 2003;42(4):567-70.

[63] Bennett R, Vetter R. An approach to spider bites: Erroneous attribution of dermonecrotic lesions to brown recluse or hobo spiders in Canada. Can Fam Physician 2004;50:1098-101.

[64] Rees R, Altenbern D, Lynch J, King L. Brown recluse spider bites. A comparison of early surgical excision versus dapsone and delayed surgical excision. Ann Surg 1985;202(5):659-63.

[65] Furbee R, Kao L, Ibrahim D. Brown recluse spider envenomation. Clin Lab Med 2006;26(3):211-26.

[66] Dominguez T. It's not a spider bite, It's community acquired methicillin-resistant Staphylococcus aureus. J Am Board Fam Pract 2004;17:220-6.

[67] Grunert B, Sanger J, Matloub H, Yousif N. Classification system for factitious syndromes in the hand with implications for treatment. J Hand Surg [Am] 1991;16A(6):1027-30.

[68] Al-Quattan M. Factitious disorders of the upper limb in Saudi Arabia. J Hand Surg [Br] 2001;26B(5):414-21.

[69] Agris J, Simmons Jr. C. Factitious (self-inflicted) skin wounds. Plast Reconstr Surg 1978;62(5):686-92.

[70] Kasdan M, Soergel T, Johnson A, Lewis K, White W. Expanded profile of the SHAFT syndrome. J Hand Surg [Am] 1998;23A(1): 26-31.

[71] Phelps D, Buchler U, Boswick J Jr. The diagnosis of factitious ulcer of the hand: a case report. J Hand Surg 1977;2(2):105-8.

[72] Kasdan M, Stutts J. Factitious injuries of the upper extremity. J Hand Surg [Am] 1995;20A(3, Part 2):S57-S60.

[73] Smith R. Factitious Lymphedema of the Hand. J Bone Joint Surg 1975;57A(1):89-94.

[74] Louis D, Lamp M, Greene T. The upper extremity and psychiatric illness. J Hand Surg [Am] 1985;10A:687-93.

[75] Asano Y, Ihn J, Shikada J, Kadono T, Kikuchi K, Tamaki K. Primary cutaneous mucormycosis masquerading as a pyoderma gangrenosum. Br J Derm 2004;150:1212-4.

[76] Chow S, Ip F, Lau J, Collins R, Luk K, So Y, et al. Mycobacterium marinum infection of the hand and wrist. Results of conservative treatment in twenty-four cases. J Bone Joint Surg [Am] 1987; 69A(8):1161-8.

[77] Holder S, Hopson C, Vonkuster L. Tuberculous arthritis of the elbow presenting as a chronic bursitis of the olecranon. A case report. J Bone Joint Surg [Am] 1985;67A(7):1127-9.

[78] Rosenfeld S, Weinert CJ, Kahn B. Congenital syphillis. A case report. J Bone Joint Surg [Am] 1983;65A(1):115-9.

High–Pressure Injection Injuries to the Hand

André GAY[a*], **Dominique CASANOVA**[b], **Régis LEGRÉ**[a], **Guy MAGALON**[c]

[a]*Service de Chirurgie de la Main, Hôpital de la Conception, Marseille, France*
[b]*Service de Chirurgie Plastique, Hôpital Nord Chemin des Bourrely, Marseille, France*
[c]*Service de Chirurgie Plastique, Hôpital de la Conception, Marseille, France*

Subcutaneous fluid or gas insertion into the upper limb is an unusual event whose gravity, by delayed impairment of soft tissue, may reduce limb function and anatomical integrity. Mild toxic injection injuries can involve an extensive soft tissue necrosis with difficulties in management, and sequelae. Such trauma occurs with high-pressure injection as an occupation-related injury and presents an urgent and threatening surgical entity.

Keywords: high–pressure; injection; grease; paint; amputation.

1. Introduction

High-pressure injections injuries were rare prior to introduction of the sophisticated technology of the fast-developing modern industrialization. Hesse described the first case in 1925 [1]. In 1941, Mason and Queen described local tissue modifications caused by injected material at the hand level [2]. High-pressure injuries of the hand represent less than 1% of all hand injuries. A small and harmless puncture may hide the true degree of infection, which most of the time is quite remarkable. This is a real challenge for the surgeon who is involved in its management.

Between 1975 and 1994, we treated 36 patients with high-pressure injection injuries. Reporting our experience, we would like to insist on the need of

*Corresponding Author
Service du Pr Legré, Hopital la Conception
145 Bd Baille, 13385, Marseille cedex, France
Tel: +33 612 907 029
e-mail: andre_gay@hotmail.com

prompt debridement of the injured finger in order that the risk of amputation or finger stiffness is minimized. This could be achieved only by raising treating physicians' awareness of the incidence and severity of those injuries as well as by referring the patient to an experienced surgeon. The open wound technique, followed by intensive rehabilitation, gives the best results.

2. Background

Although high pressure injections are less frequent than other hand injuries, Schoo et al. estimated its frequency as one out of 600 hand injuries [3]. According to our experience, industry workplace hazards increase the risk of injury occurrence. However, implementation of a preventive policy has decreased this frequency in the ten past years.

Various jobs involving the use of pressurized products, mostly airless paintguns, air guns and hydraulic systems, are the causes of most accidents [3]. Other devices involved in high-pressure injuries of the hand are alarm guns, pipe lines, refrigerators, etc. Karcher® can cause hand pressure injections occurring in the domestic environment, which are rather rare [3]. Actually, every device

A. Gay, D. Casanova, R. Legré, G. Magalon

that is able to produce up to 700 kN/m² could cause a high-pressure injection to the hand [4, 5].

3. Clinical Presentations

Clinical findings obtained immediately after injury are often poor, even in the case of injuries which are sometimes completely painless [6]. Locally, a small puncture at the injection site may cause bleeding, or swelling due to the injected material. Presence of acute and severe pain evident a few hours later reveals the severity of the situation. The digit is edematous with diminution of arterial flow, while mobility is decreased due to pain and the edema (Fig. 1). After 24 hours, lesions are irreversible. Without proper surgical management, infection and necrosis can occur within 3 or 4 days.

Mason and Queen established an anatomo-clinical classification of grease-injection lesions [2]. When tissues survive, there is an intense fibrous reaction.

Tissue reaction to the foreign body occurs in presence of a fibrous tumor at the injection site containing oleous material (oleomas). Those tumors may be single or multiple and usually appear ten to fifteen days after the injury. After a quiescent uneventful phase which may last for many years, oleoma evolution can cause severe fibrosis, leading to joint stiffness and loss of function. Ulcerations and fistulae can eventually occur by late oleoma breaching, with possible skin defect. Secondary

infection and scar complications worsen the functional prognosis.

4. Anatomic Considerations

The site of injury determines prognosis [7]. Kaufman injected a cadaveric hand with wax using a high-pressure injection gun [8]. He showed that the degree of penetration of the injected material depends on the encountered tissue strength.

Injection in a less distensible compartment, such as the fingertip, leads more frequently to partial amputations than palm injuries, probably because the palm allows greater material dispersion [9, 10, 11]. Injection over interphalangeal joints meet C-pulleys, which are flexible and thin, allowing penetration of injected material into the sheath and the surrounding tendon. This deteriorates the functional outcome [8, 12, 13]. Injection in the middle segment of the finger encounters the rigid and fibrous A-pulleys, inducing deflection and lateral spread of the material towards the superficial digit tissues and enhancing the chances of cutaneous necrosis occurrence (Fig. 2). Particular risk is involved in injections in the first and

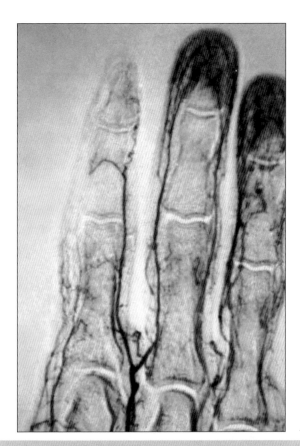

FIGURE 2. Arteriography after paint injection in the distal part of the index finger. Injected-material spread to soft tissues induced a compartment syndrome and altered digit arterial flow.

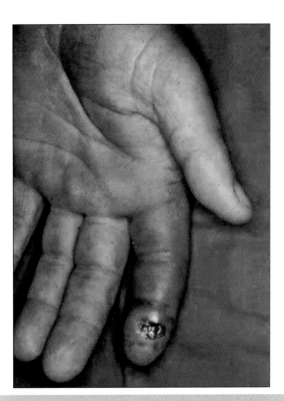

FIGURE 1. Acute grease injection (4 hours after injury).

the fifth finger. Synovial sheaths extend proximally into radial or ulnar bursae and can lead to a compartment syndrome of the forearm or the median nerve entrapment at the carpal tunnel site [13, 14].

Injections typically occur in the fingertip of the non-dominant index finger [11, 15, 16, 17] when the patient tries to wipe a blocked nozzle, or in the palm when he handles a gun with a free hand during equipment testing [16, 18]. The left hand is involved twice as many times as the right one [11, 16]. Other sites likely to be injured are in decreasing order: the thumb, first web space, third digit; the palm is involved in less than 10% of the cases [7, 11, 16].

5. RADIOGRAPHIC EVALUATION

About half of the commercially used grease contains lead as a thickening agent to prevent lubrification film dissolution under high compression load, allowing radiographic depiction of the injected material (Fig. 3). Hand radiography can be helpful in planning surgery. It depicts the injury and delineates spread extent [12, 14, 17]. After air or water injection, it shows distribution of radio-opaque density associated with paint or grease in-

jections and subcutaneous air [11, 15, 17, 18], and therefore, it is useful to guide surgical debridement.

6. GUIDELINES FOR TREATMENT

All high-pressure injection injuries of the hand must be considered emergencies, no matter how benign the clinical presentation may seem, and therefore, they should be referred immediately to a hand surgeon [16, 18] for early surgical management [7, 16, 17, 18].

The aim of surgery is to decompress both neuro-vascular bundles and thus prevent Volkmann syndrome, by removing as much injected material as possible. Local anaesthesia is contraindicated because it increases intra-digital pressure and risk of vascular breach.

The surgical technique is performed under general or loco-regional anesthesia. Peripheral nerve blocks are our choice because of the sympathetic block and vasoparalysis they provide. A tourniquet can be applied after limb elevation. Desmarch bandage use is also contraindicated because it may increase injected material spread along tendon sheaths and neuro-vascular bundles.

The surgical technique involves wide exposure through Brunner or mid-lateral incision. The tendon sheaths have to be examined and a partial to total synovectomy associated with lavage and gentle scrubbing should be performed. All devitalized tissues and injected material should be removed, if necessary, after careful preservation of all the neuro-vascular bundles (Fig. 4) [19]. Solvents should never be used because they may cause a pro-inflammatory effect and ischemic tissue increase in metabolic needs [19]. Dressing must be changed every day to estimate the necessity for iterative debridement [18]. Early physiotherapy (on the 2nd or 3rd postoperative day) is useful to prevent joint stiffness and adherences [20].

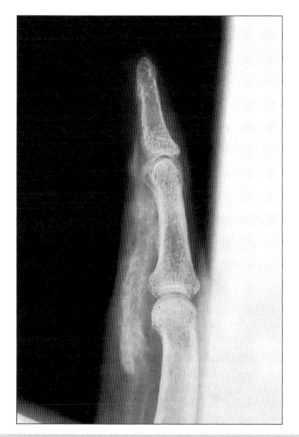

FIGURE 3. Radiography after grease injection. Injected material can be visualized as radio opaque density inside tendon sheath.

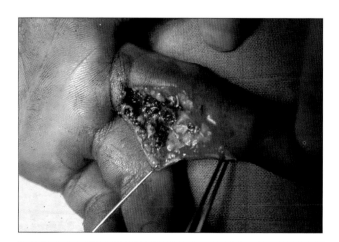

FIGURE 4. Intra-operative view of a high-pressure carbon injection to the finger.

Tetanus toxoid and antibiotics (against Staphylococcus) should be prescribed. There is no consensus on systemic corticosteroids use: Phelps reports their potentially beneficial effect on controlling local tissue reaction and necrosis [21], but Waters maintains that they may favor infection [22]. Our opinion is that their use should be limited to pro-inflammatory injection of the agent. Finger amputation may be the only possible option when surgery is delayed and a stage of necrosis is established. For some authors, destruction of two structures lying among skin, tendon and bundle might justify amputation of all affected fingers except for the thumb [12].

Tenolysis may be considered at a later stage according to classic rules of hand surgery, except for the oleomas that should be removed. A secondary amputation might be decided upon, especially in the case of manual workers with a stiff index finger or a painful non-sensible digit.

7. Prognosis

A functional outcome still remains stable since the first clinical studies. Haufman (1968) reported an amputation rate of 43% in 51 cases [23]. In our experience, the amputation rate was 30.6%. Nevertheless, injections of a non-toxic agent (e.g. water, air, etc.) were also studied in our series, which had not been focused on until the 1960's. Excluding those cases, our amputation rate rises to 40.7% which is similar to Haufman's results.

Several factors have been identified as determinants of the degree of injury severity. Some of them are easy to analyze: type of injected material, injection site, and delay prior to surgery. Others are more difficult to evaluate: amount and spread of injected material, velocity of the injectant and pressure of appliance, temperature of the material, distance between injectant and skin.

7.1. Injection site

Digital injection is the most frequent and the most difficult to establish a prognosis for. In our series, the amputation rate for digital injection was 45% with a 75% rate for pulpal injections (9 out of 12 cases). Palmar injections allow finger preservation, but the functional outcome was often poor in our series (50%).

7.2. Delay prior to surgery

Initial clinical findings are often poor and usually lead to delayed surgical management [6]. The delay prior to surgery is the main prognosis factor we should consider if we are to prevent amputation. In our series, we had a 22% amputation rate when the delay before surgery was of 6 hours or less. After a 12-hour delay, necrosis was evident and amputation was often necessary, which worsened the functional outcome.

7.3. Injected Material

Fuel and paint injections lead to the most severe inflammatory response which induces a high amputation rate (ranging from 60% to 80%). Grease and oil-based compounds are more viscous as they require higher injection pressure than paint or solvents [14, 18]. Moreover, grease causes less inflammatory response and leads to oleomas with chronic fistulae formation. The amputation rate is lower (around 25%) [14, 18] because of their low viscosity that allows easier spread of the injected material [7].

Paint contains 4 components: a binder, solvents, pigments and additives. Some of these compounds are highly irritant, such as soya alkyl, which causes a more intense inflammatory reaction [18]. A binder is the solid part of the paint. It includes various materials such as asphalt or epoxies. The pigments are hard, colored particles containing iron oxide, and black carbon. Binders and pigments constitute the foreign bodies detected in the case of injection. The solvents liquefy the paint and additives are used to give properties such as viscosity, hardness or gloss [10]. These chemicals and the basic pH of paint are probably locally toxic and cause chemical burn [10].

8. Authors' Experience

8.1. Materials and methods

Thirty-nine patients who underwent a high-pressure injection into the hand were treated in the two units of Plastic Surgery of Marseille Academic Hospitals (France) between 1975 and 1994. All patients had a professional high-pressure device for work or domestic use.

Thirty-five men and a woman (mean age: 39.4 years (20-58)) with penetrating injuries were the subjects of the study. Three patients who presented minimal injuries without skin breaching or with only superficial wound were excluded from the series and treated by debridement under local anesthesia and dressing.

8.1.1. Injected material

In most cases, agents for professional use were involved. The injected materials were paint (n=14), oil or grease (n=11), water (n=4), air (n=3), water and sand (n=1), concrete (n=1), water or ashes (n=1) and paint solvent (n=1).

8.1.2. Injection site

In 23 cases (63.8%) injuries involved the non-dominant hand. The most frequent sites were the distal index finger (36.1%), the thenar (22%) and the distal part of the other fingers (14%). Other sites were the volar aspect of the hand (11%), proximal fingers (13%), the hypothenar (3%) and the volar aspect of the wrist (3%). In our series there was no case of dorsal injection.

TABLE 1

Scale used for functional evaluation

Good	Fair	Poor
No painful or functional sequelae	– painful scar – sensitivity loss – stiffness without severe functional problem – oleoma	– disabling pain – digital anaesthesia – severe stiffness – strength loss

8.2. Treatment

Three out of 35 patients who underwent volar injection with a non-toxic agent and without skin or neuro-vascular damage were treated by alcohol dressing and surveillance at surgery departments. In those subjects, we performed a large surgical debridement without consideration of the delay between injury and management, with Brunner incision on the digits, eventually extended depending on the surgical findings. Necrotic tissues and injected material were excised, allowing neurovascular bundles decompression. The procedure was completed by a large synovectomy of the injected digital channels.

In five cases, complementary procedures were necessary: early reintervention for evolutive necrosis (n=3), revascularization due to arterial lesions (n=1), nerve grafting due to substance loss of the median and the ulnar nerves (n=1). Those secondary treatment procedures were performed between 15 days and 25 months after primary treatment, using usual techniques of hand surgery for skin, tendons, neurovascular and C.R.P.S.I.

8.3. Results

Analysis of the results according to etiology, injection site and delay between accident and surgery are presented below. Those results account for subsequent treatment.

Eleven patients (30.6%) underwent digital amputations. Those procedures have been performed either in a state of emergency for necrosis or as important functional sequels that would improve hand

TABLE 2

Results related to the specific type of injected material

Results	Type of injected material			
	Paint n=14	Oil & grease n=11	Other n=11 (2 toxic)	Total
Good	0	1	7	8
Fair	3	2	1	6
Poor	3	2	2	7
Amputations	5	5	1	11
Lost	3	1	–	4

TABLE 3

Results concerning the function of the injected site

Results	Injection site	
	Finger	Volar
Good	3	5
Fair	5	1
Poor	–	6
Amputations	10	1
Lost	4	–

function. The results of the 25 conservatively treated patients have been classified (see Table 1).

8.3.1. Etiology-based results

The lesion intensity varied depending on the type of the injected material (Table 2) and the injection site (Table 3):

Paint: 57% presented poor results and amputations (8 out of 14 cases, including 5 amputations).

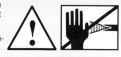

Avertissement!

Les équipements "sans air" produisent des pressions de projection extrêmement élevées.

Ne jamais mettre doigts, mains ou autres parties du corps en contact avec le jet!

Ne pas diriger le jet sur les personnes et les animaux!

①

Attention: danger de blessures par l'injection du produit!

En cas de blessures de la peau par l'injection de peintures ou de solvants, consulter sans retard un médecin. Renseignez le médecine sur la nature de la peinture ou du solvant utilisé.

Avant toute mise en service, respecter les points suivants conformément aux instructions de service:

②
1. verrouiller le pistolet avec le levier de sécurité au pistolet
2. assurer une miss à la terre correcte de l'alimentation électrique
3. respecter et vérifier les pressions admissibles
4. contrôler l'étanchéité de tous le raccords

Respecter sans faute les instructions relatives au nettoyage et à l'entretien réguliers du matériel.
Avant toute intervention sur le matériel et pendant chaque interruption du travail, observer les régles suivantes:

③
1. décharger la pression contenue dans le pistolet et le tuyau
2. verrouiller le pistolet avec le levier de sécurité au pistolet
3. arrêter l'équipment

Pour votre sécurité!

FIGURE 5. Preventive information is the only effective treatment of high-pressure injection to the hand.

Grease: 63.6% presented poor results (7 out of 11 cases, including 4 amputations).

Others: 27% presented poor results (1 amputation for acute necrosis).

Eleven patients out of 27 (40.7%) needed amputation after a toxic injection (with paint, oil, grease, or paint solvent). We noted that 9 patients out of 17 with pulp injection (53%) needed amputation.

9. CONCLUSIONS

The degree of the risk involved in a high-pressure injection to the hand is often hidden behind a tiny skin mark and is not recognized as an emergency. All patients who report a digital high-pressure injection must be considered as potential amputees and must be treated urgently by use of the open-wound technique, which has proven to give the best results. Even with optimal treatment, the amputation rate is still high and the functional result is often poor. The best solution to avoid complications is to prevent these injections by raising awareness (Fig. 5) of the exposed population about the hazards a lot of devices may involve.

REFERENCES

[1] Hesse E. Die chirurgische und gerechtilch-medizinische. Bedeutung der Künstlich hervogerufen Erkrankugen. Arch Klin Chir 1925;136:277.
[2] Mason ML, Queen FB. Grease gun injuries to the hand.pathology and treatment of injuries (oleomas) following injection of grease under high pressure. Quarterly Bullet Northw Univ Med Sch 1941;15:122-132.
[3] Schoo MJ, Scott FA, Boswick JA. High pressure injection of the hand. J Trauma 1980;20:229-237.
[4] Neal NC, Burke FD. High-pressure injection injuries. Injury 1991;22:467-470.
[5] McClinton MA, Wright S. High pressure tool injection injuries. MD Med J 1985;34:289-291.
[6] Hutchinson CH. Hand injuries caused by injection of cement under pressure. J Bone Joint Surg 1968;50-B:131-133.
[7] Harter BT, Harter KC. High Pressure injections injuries. Hand Clin 1986;2:547-552.
[8] Kaufman HD. The clinico-pathological correlation of high pressure injections injuries. Br J Surg 1969;55:214.
[9] Hayes CW, Pan HC. High-pressure injection injuries to the hand. South Med J 1982;75:1491-1498.
[10] Vasilevski D,Noorbergen M, Depierreux M, Lafontaine M. High pressure Injection Injuries to the hand. Am J Emerg Med 2000;18:820-824.
[11] Kartlbauer A, Gasperschitz F. High pressure injection injury : a hand-threatening emergency. J Emerg Med 1987;5:375-379.
[12] Kaufman HD. High-Pressure injection injuries: the problems, pathogenesis and management. Hand 1970;2:63.
[13] Pick RY. The roentgenographic appearance of lead paint as a foreign body. Clin Orthop Rel Res 1980;305-306.
[14] Geller ER, Gursel E. A unique case of high-pressure injection injury to the hand. J Trauma 1986;26:483-485.
[15] Flotre M. High-pressure injection injuries of the hand. Am Fam Phys 1992;45:2230-2234.
[16] Moutet F, Lantuejoul JP, Guinard D, et al. Caractères d'urgence et de gravité des lesions dues aux injections à haute pression au niveau de la main. Ann Chir Main 1991;10:476-481.
[17] Pai CH, Wei DC, Hou SP. High-Pressure Injection injuries of the hand. J Trauma 1991;31:110-112.
[18] Neal NC, Burke FD. High-pressure injection injurie. Injury 1991;22:467-470.
[19] Casanova D, Aubert JP, Legre R et al. Injection sous pression dans le membre supérieur. Arch Mal Prof year;57:26-31.
[20] Palmieri TJ. High-pressure injection injuries to the hand, treatment by early mobilization. Bull Hosp Joint Dis, (NY) 1974;25:18-35.
[21] Phelps DB, Hastings H, Boswick A Jr. Systemic corticosteroid therapy for high-pressure injection injuries to the hand. J Trauma 1976;17:206-210.
[22] Waters WR, Penn I, Ross HM. Airless paintgun injuries of the hand: a clinical and experimentation study. Plastic Reconstr Surg 1967;39:613-618.
[23] Haufman HD. The clinicopathological correlation of high-pressure injection injuries to the hand. Br J Surg 1968;55:214-218.

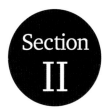

Section
II

ACUTE SOFT TISSUE
INFECTIONS

ACUTE SOFT TISSUE INFECTIONS

Pulp and Paronychial Infections of the Hand

Christian DUMONTIER*, Dominique LE VIET

Institut de la Main, Paris, France

Infections located around and under the nail (paronychia) and in the subcutaneous space of the distal phalanx (felon) are the most frequent hand infections. Clinically, paronychia presents as an acute or a chronic superficial infection or abscess of the paronychial tissues of the hand. Clinical diagnosis is easy. Oral antibiotic therapy can be used in the inflammatory phase, however most patients are seen in the abscess phase and require surgical incision or excision. Acute paronychia should be differentiated from herpetic whitlow for which surgery is contraindicated. Felons are more difficult to diagnose and inadequate treatment may lead to complications, including skin sinus, suppurative flexor synovitis, osteomyelitis, and/or arthritis of the DIP joint. In non-complicated cases, surgical treatment is needed with excision of the necrotic tissues. Antibiotics are useless in most cases and may hide an incomplete excision, but wound samples must be taken and cultured. Antibiotics may be indicated in immuno-compromised patients, in cases of dissemination of infection (lymphangitis, adenopathy) or when suspecting streptococcus infection. At the first dressing, the wound must appear perfectly clean.

Keywords: felon; paronychia; hand infections; surgical treatment; antibiotics; complications.

1. INTRODUCTION

The hand is constantly exposed to the environment, providing a wide variety of pathogens with ample opportunity to invade [1]. Infections of the fingertip region are the most common hand infections accounting for approximately one-third of all hand infections and 2.5 to 5% of all workmen's compensation claims [2–5]. Although most of them are benign, misdiagnosis or inappropriate treatment may lead to prolonged morbidity or even severe complications. Prompt recognition and early initiation of treatment increase the chance of a favorable outcome, while delayed treatment increases the possibility of complications. Knowledge of the anatomy of the fingertip and of the biology of microbial infection is prerequisite to an optimal treatment (Fig. 1).

2. ANATOMY OF THE PULP

Kanavel described the pulp as a "closed sac" of fat formed by vertical septae of connective tissue that attach to the epidermis and the periosteum of the distal phalanx, creating multiple interstitial spaces and compartments [6]. Those compartments contain fat globules and exocrine sweat glands that secret into the epidermis. They have been thought to be a potential cause of "spontaneous" infection [2,5]. The distal interphalangeal joint is surrounded by its capsular structures. The flexor digitorum profundus and its sheath inserts into the volar proximal half of the distal phalanx.

*Corresponding Author
Institut de la Main
6 square Jouvenet, 75016 Paris, France
e-mail: ch.dumontier@gsante.fr
christian.dumontier@sat.aphp.fr

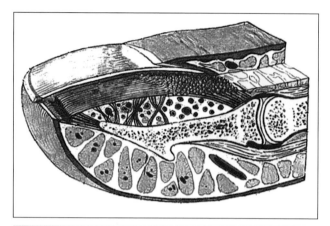

FIGURE 1. Anatomy of the distal phalanx. The pulp is closed by vertical septae (not drawn) creating multiple interstitial spaces and compartments containing fat globules and exocrine sweat glands. Note the proximity of the flexor digitorum profundus. The nail apparatus is firmly fixed onto the phalanx. The cuticle closes the space between the nail plate and nail fold, but once opened, infection will extend along the nail plate and nail folds (drawing by JL Drapé).

3. ANATOMY OF THE NAIL APPARATUS

The germinal matrix and the nail bed insert in the distal phalanx through a tight dermis. They are tightly fixed proximally and distally to the phalanx by ligaments [7]. The nail plate is watertight to the nail bed, but not to the nail matrix. Dorsal to the nail plate, the proximal and lateral nail folds set in the nail plate. The cuticle closes the space between the nail plate and the nail fold. The hyponychium is the mass of keratin between the nail plate and the distal nail bed that is particularly resistant to infection despite frequent bacterial contamination.

4. MICROBIOLOGY OF INFECTION

Bacteria found in a series of 330 whitlows were *S. aureus* in 55% of the cases, *S. epidermidis* in 6%, *Streptococcus* in 12% and polymicrobial cultures in 25% [*Streptococcus+staphylococcus* in 52%, gram (–) bacteriae in 28%, and *enterobacteriae+staphylococcus* or *streptococcus* in 17%) [8]. Another study by the same team found *S. aureus* in 54% out of 454 cases presenting whitlows, *Streptococcus* in 26%, *enterobacteriae* in 6%, and polymicrobial cultures in 21% of the cases [9]. Almost all of these organisms (except for *S. aureus*) come from the oropharyngeal space. Patients appear to be infected by their own germs, the ones they carry on their hands, however, this has not been confirmed [8]. Repeated hand washing is still an efficient and easy measure for preventing hand infections. Recently, attention has been drawn to the increase in the frequency of methicillin-resistant *Staphylococcus aureus,* which is found in up to 40% of Southern Europe inpatients [10].

The risk of developing infection in a patient increases when there is permanent or temporary compromise of immune defenses, such as that of diabetic patients, chronic alcoholics, drug-users or immuno-suppressed patients, i.e. those suffering from corticoid use, AIDS, Rheumatoid Arthritis and other inflammatory diseases [8,11]. Initial clinical examination should focus on those predisposing factors that may determine whether more aggressive treatment is needed. Diabetic patients account for 7 to 58% of hospitalized hand infections [1].

After a penetrating injury, any infection evolves in three phases:

– **the inflammatory phase,** which is characterized by local signs of inflammation, constant pain with attenuation at night, redness, and erythema with minimal swelling. This phase may resolve immediately or after medical treatment. Otherwise, it is followed by abscess formation.

– **the abscess formation phase.** In this phase, the pain becomes intense, pulsatile, and worsens during the night. Clinical exam reveals a red, hot and swollen lesion with pus, sometimes visible through the skin. Regional signs of infection, such as lymphangitis, epitrochlear, or axillary lymphadenitis may be present. The number of white blood cells was found normal and the temperature of the patient up to 38ºC in only 7% of cases [8]. In this phase, the infection may not resolve immediately, and thus it will evolve to the next phase if no treatment is provided.

– **the complication phase,** which may involve skin sinus, suppurative flexor synovitis, osteomyelitis, and/or arthritis of the DIP joint [2, 6]. These complications are rare, i.e. only 5 cases out of 330 have been found [8]. The most frequent complication encountered today is the formation of a non-drained abscess, which is treated only by use of antibiotics. In such a case, clinical signs are scarce, however, the soft tissues become infiltrated and thick. The masked infection continues to progress and will silently destroy the distal phalanx and disseminate to the flexor sheath or to the distal interphalangeal joint.

5. PRINCIPLES AND BASICS OF TREATMENT

5.1. Imaging studies

Plain radiographs should always be obtained in the process of treating a fracture, extirpating a foreign body, and/or ruling out periosteal reaction, or osteomyelitis. Soft tissue shadows, indicative of edema may be detected. Computed tomography and MRI are not recommended, unless unexpected complications occur.

5.2. Laboratory studies

White blood cell count is almost always normal (i.e., <12,000). C-reactive protein and erythrocyte sedimentation rate may increase, especially when complications occur. Even if they are often prescribed, such studies are of no use for diagnosis or an indication for treatment.

6. MANAGEMENT

6.1. Anesthesia

Distal digital nerve block is contraindicated for septic surgery. Instead, proximal nerve block anesthesia should be chosen. Proximal digital blocks should not be applied as "ring blocks" as they may compromise vascularization of the digits. Transthecal digital anesthesia by insertion of anesthetics through the flexor tendon sheath into the core of the digit is an alternative [12]. This technique is indicated for distal anesthesia of the three central digits [13]. Anesthesia is expected to come in 7–8 min [14]. No significant complications have been reported so far, however, this technique should be used with caution in infected fingers. Anesthesia in the first and fifth digits cannot be reliably achieved, and this is a limitation of the technique. More proximal blocks (radial, median, ulnar, axillary) can also be used. Axillary blocks should probably be contraindicated in the case of lymphadenitis. It is now recognized that lidocaine with epinephrine is safe for digital anesthesia [15,16].

6.2. Tourniquet

When the procedure is performed under local digital anesthesia, a digital tourniquet is placed at the base of the finger [5]. It has been shown that the rubber band and Penrose drain deliver high and unpredictable pressure. A sterile rubber glove finger whose tip has been removed may be stretched over the digit, and a rolled rubber glove whose size is the same as the patient's glove size delivers reliable pressure which is under 500 mm Hg [17]. When the patient has distal vascular compromise (atherosclerosis, diabetes or the Raynaud phenomenon), the use of a proximal pneumatic tourniquet is preferred. An awake patient will tolerate a pneumatic tourniquet for about 20 min. The forearm tourniquet is also adequate and may be better tolerated.

6.3. Post-operative dressings

We use a wet non-adherent dressing that keeps the wound wet and provides a good microenvironment for wound healing. The first dressing is made of a sufficient number of large gauzes that absorb bleeding, which is always noticeable. A loose bandage is then wrapped, in an anatomic position, and secured with adhesive tape. The patient is examined after 48 hrs when he gets his second wound dressing. The dressing should be changed at regular intervals according to the progress of healing, usually every other day, which is applied for 2 weeks.

7. ANTIBIOTICS

Any patient presenting with a finger infection should be checked for his tetanus vaccination status. No prophylactic antibiotic should be administered in non-complicated cases. Wound samples for cultures should be taken during surgery. An oral antibiotic should be given only in case of dissemination of the infection (lymphangitis, adenopathy) or when suspecting a *streptococcus* infection. In such a case, the patient should be hospitalized and administered intravenous antibiotics. An oral anti-staphylococcal antibiotic is preferred, however, the final choice depends on the patient's medical history, especially on any allergies that s/he may have, and the results of cultures and antibiograms.

8. FELON

A felon is a subcutaneous abscess in the distal pulp of the fingertip, i.e. an infection developed in the closed space that is formed by multiple vertical fibrous septa [3–5]. The felon represented 12% of a series of 330 finger infections [8]. There is often a history of a penetrating trauma, although some patients find it difficult to recall even minor trauma. Wood splinters, glass slivers, abrasions and minor cuts are the most common causes of such infection [4, 5]. Some felons are iatrogenic, such as the "fingerstick felon", which are diagnosed after multiple finger stick blood tests [18]. After bacterial inoculation, inflammation, and increased pressure within the non-compliant pulp space, local vascular congestion and ischemia are observed. Tissue necrosis ensues and, if it is not surgically treated, the abscess could be decompressed through spontaneous drainage out of the skin by using a sinus tract. The flexor tendon sheath is rarely involved as contiguous to the area, and it is so in case the felon is neglected, or if inappropriate treatment is applied [5]. If antibiotics have been given earlier, that may mask the progression of the infection. Distal phalanx involvement is also rare, except for the case a penetrating trauma has violated the periosteum [2] (Fig. 2).

Clinical diagnosis involves examination of the history of a penetrating trauma, which is followed by rapid onset of throbbing pain, and swelling of the entire pulp that does not extend over the DIP joint unless there is complication (Fig. 3). The pulp has lost its normal ballottement and appears exquisitely tender [5, 8]. In advanced stages of the disease, when fluctuation of the pulp "reappears, the phalanx is dead" [2].

The most common organism causing a felon is S. Aureus, despite the fact that opportunistic bacteriae, usually gram-negative, and polymicrobial infections may be encountered in the immuno-compromised population [3].

The choice of treatment should be based on patient

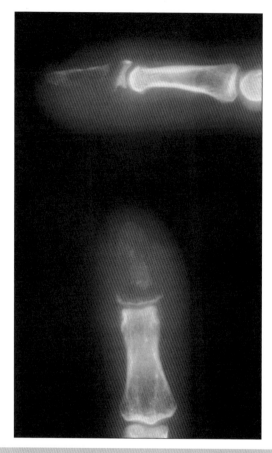

FIGURE 2. X-rays are mandatory in order to avoid complications such as osteomyelitis which may complicate the evolution of a felon.

characteristics, previous management, the stage of infection, and any complications.

The initial phase of cellulitis and inflammation can be treated with antibiotics and soaks. Anti-staphylococcal antibiotics, such as cloaxicillin must be chosen. There are two possible mistakes in this stage: (i) misdiagnosis of cellulitis (mistaking the initial phase with the abscess phase), and (ii) the felon may be caused by another bacterium. In this phase, antibiotics must be administered for 8 to 10 days. If antibiotics are used, all clinical signs should be resolved within 2 days. If there is persistence of any clinical signs, one must consider that infection is progressing and that previous administration of antibiotics may have masked it. In such cases, it is urgent to treat it by surgery.

Most often, patients are examined in the phase of suppuration, when surgical drainage is necessary. Surgery must be carried out in an adapted operating room equipped with appropriate surgical instruments, and under tourniquet use. In the English literature, the type of incision to be applied is still controversial [19]. A transverse incision in the pulp, or a fish-mouth incision (the hockey-stick or J incision is half of a fish-mouth incision) have been recommended [3–5]. However, those incisions sometimes create a painful scar that may deteriorate the ability to pinch. A unilateral longitudinal incision on the non-contact side of the finger may be preferred whenever possible, however, it is regarded insufficient if it is not centered over the pus [2]. When a sinus is present, it should be excised with the incision. A longitudinal incision on the pulp is considered less detrimental to the vascularization of the edges than zig-zag incisions [20].

We mostly recommend, at least in France, excision, not incision. The goal of excision is complete removal of all devitalized tissues, which accelerates the cleaning

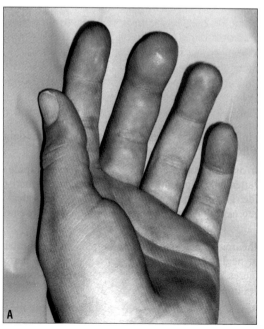

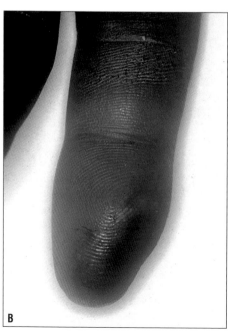

FIGURE 3. (A, B) Clinical presentation of a felon (From Elsevier, Paris, Infections de la main, Monographie du GEM, M. Ebelin ed).

A

B

process, brings oxygen, and leaves only living tissues to the organism. All the skin over the infected tissues is excised and the wound is left open (Fig. 4). Whatever the type of incision, attention must be paid not to harm digital nerves and their branches. All the septa must be opened to allow for complete drainage and the incision must be left open. No gauze or drain should be placed in the wound. Bacteriological wound cultures should be taken. If surgery has been performed properly, the first dressing change should reveal red, healthy, granulating tissue. Once healing has started, patients are instructed to perform desensitization, scar massage and range-of-motion exercises. In the absence of complications, antibiotics should not be given.

Complications: Lymphangitis and axillary or epicondylar adenopathy are treated by use of empiric antistaphylococcal antibiotics administered for about 8 to 10 days. Treatment is adapted to patient characteristics and the results of wound cultures. Clinical signs usually resolve within 48 hrs.

Suppurative flexor tenosynovitis, distal phalanx osteomyelitis and pyogenic arthritis of the DIP joint require large debridement, hospitalization, and intravenous antibiotics. Multiple surgical procedures may be needed, and ultimately, amputation in severe cases, especially in the case of immuno-compromised patients. It is rare, indeed, to treat suppurative flexor tenosynovitis without adapted antibiotic treatment [2]. It is worth considering the fact that 5 out of 115 suppurative flexor tenosynovitis cases have been secondary to a felon [7].

8.1. Differential diagnosis

The felon should be differentiated from a superficial apical infection of the distal finger pulp which usually responds well after a small, simple deroofing incision [1, 3]. Its differential diagnosis may show:

- ORF's disease, which is a viral infection transmitted by sheep. The usual presence of nodules in the hands and the face should make physicians suspicious since pharmaceutical treatment alone should suffice [21].
- Osler nodes, which are oedematous, tender, and take the form of red or purple nodules, are clinical signs of septic emboli most often associated with *Staphylococcus aureus* infective endocarditis [22]. They are usually related to trauma by splinters, or subungueal hemorrhages.
- Acute inflammation of a previously unknown epidermoid cyst may also mimic a felon. There may be a striking X-ray image revealing bone resorption that is usually round and well-demarcated.
- Gout rarely manifests itself by acute pain in the fingertip, although it may mimic a felon. Clinical examination and an X-ray image revealing tophi are usually sufficient for diagnosis.

9. ACUTE PARONYCHIA

Paronychia is the infection in the lateral soft-tissue fold. If

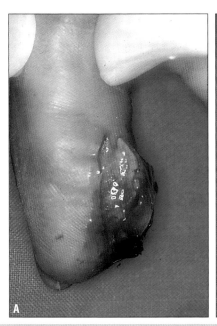 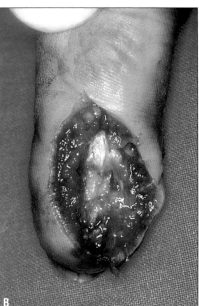 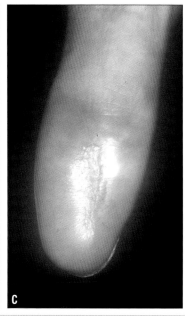

FIGURE 4. (A) Severe felon with significant involvement of the pulp. **(B)** As the patient presented late, complete excision was required to remove all devitalized tissues extending up to the digital sheath. **(C)** Healing was uneventful and patient did not complain of pulp discomfort at 4 months follow-up .

the proximal fold is also involved, it is called "eponychia". If the infection extends to the opposite lateral fold, it is named "run-a-round" infection [5]. These are the most frequent infections of the finger, i.e. 62.8% of a series of 330 finger infections has been reported [8]. Paronychia occurs following disruption of the seal between the nail plate and the lateral fold, with *S. aureus* being the most frequent infecting organism [3, 5, 8]. Penetrating injuries causing paronychia are due to nail biting or sucking, foreign bodies, manicures, or nail hematoma. Constant exposure to a wet or moist environment is a predisposing factor. At an early stage, the fold becomes tender, swollen and erythematous (Fig. 5). If infection persists, diagnosis is easy with the pus often visible through the skin (Fig. 6). Sometimes the pus is not visible, but phlyctenulae appear on the tense skin. The infection extends along the nail walls. Deep extension towards the nail matrix is rare, even in children, but may lead to permanent onychodystrophy.

Treatment depends on the stage of the infection:
- Early infection can be treated with oral anti-staphylococcal antibiotics, warm soaks (with or without antiseptics), and sometimes by the use of a resting splint. Clinical signs should resolve within 2 days.
- In the abscess phase, surgical treatment is required. It involves excision (not incision) of all inflamed tissue, taking care not to injure the nail matrix (Fig. 7). If the pus proceeds below the nail plate, the latter should be removed, otherwise it is left in place. During this surgery, one should look carefully whether the pus proceeds into the pulp. In this case, excision of all the skin over the cavity is necessary. Incision is found in the English literature as a standard technique that involves partial nail removal in order that drainage is facilitated, and placement of a wick in order that early closure of the wound is avoided [1, 5]. In both techniques, the wound is left open for drainage and spontaneous healing. Cultures

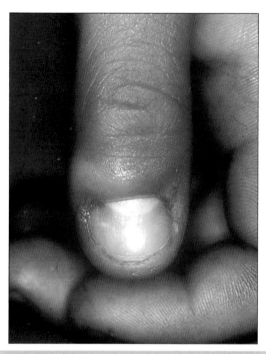

FIGURE 6. Acute paronychia with the pus visible through the skin.

should be obtained during surgery, but we should not use antibiotics except for when we have to deal with complicated cases. Some authors consider that the majority of these infections resolve without leaving permanent sequelae, such as nail dystrophy [1]. In a series of 40 acute bacterial paronychia treated with excision and reviewed after a year, 28 patients were found to have a normal nail, while the others presented with minor sequelaes, such as enlargement of the lunula or irregular proximal nail fold, or major nail dystrophies (7 cases) [7] (Fig. 8).

9.1. Differential diagnosis

Herpetic whitlow is a cytolytic skin infection caused by type 1 or 2 herpes simplex virus. Distinguishing between herpetic whitlow and pyogenic infection is important: incision and drainage for herpetic whitlow are contraindicated for fear of systemic dissemination of the virus, which would potentially mean lethal complications and/or bacterial superinfection [5].

Immuno-compromised patients are more susceptible to infection, as well as health care workers, and especially dentists, who are exposed to contaminated oropharyngeal secretions. Among the population predisposed for infection are adults with genital herpes simplex and patients with gingivostomatitis [23]. Type 1 infections usually occur in patients younger than 20 years of age, whereas type 2 infections occur in patients older than 20 years of age [24].

The onset of infection manifests itself by the appearance of small (1–2 mm), clear vesicles with localized swelling, erythema and intense burning pain, classically

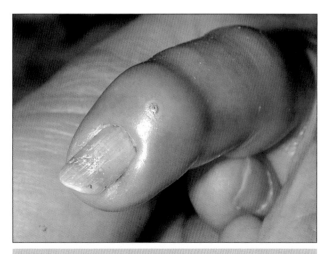

FIGURE 5. Acute paronychia at an early stage with swollen and redness. A drop of pus is already visible.

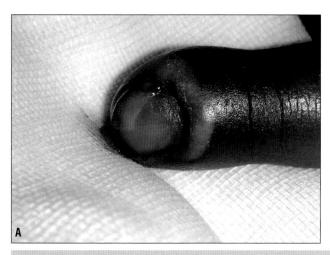
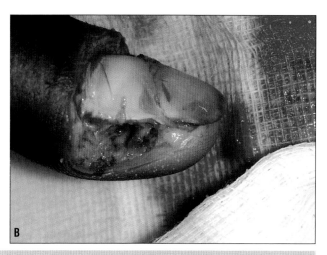

FIGURE 7. (A) and (B). Excision of all the de-vitalized tissues obliged the surgeon to remove almost all of the proximal nail fold, one lateral fold and part of the pulp.

described as out-of-proportion with physical findings. Vesicles may appear turbid (not purulent) and they coalesce within the following 10–14 days before finally ulcerating [5]. Axillary or epitrochlear adenopathy has been found in 15–20% of cases, as well as red streaking of the forearm that may mimic pyogenic cellulites [23]. The pulp space remains soft which is not a characteristic of the felon [25].

Diagnosis may be confirmed by culturing the virus

taken from vesicular fluid, assessing immunofluorescence antibodies titers, or performing a Tzanck smear, which is rarely indicated. The condition resolves within 3 to 4 weeks. No treatment is needed except for that which would relieve pain. Surgery is considered contraindicated. There is, however, one report of surgical decompression (minimal de-roofing of the vesicles) performed in 10 patients who gained pain relief without complications [26]. Surgery may be indicated in the case of bacterial superinfection, where oral or intravenous acyclovir can be used prophylactically [23].

The other differential diagnosis is acute inflammation of chronic paronychia. Multiple finger involvement and clinical examination are usually sufficient for diagnosis. Bacterial superinfection of chronic paronychia may sometimes require surgical debridement.

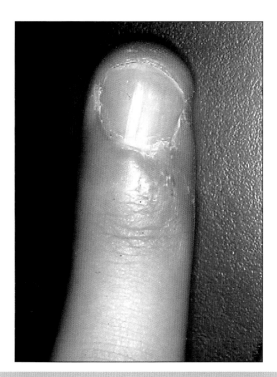

FIGURE 8. Major sequelae of a large acute paronychia with scarring tissue extending from the proximal and lateral fold to the pulp.

10. CHRONIC PARONYCHIA

Chronic paronychia due to infection occurs more commonly in individuals who are constantly exposed to moist environments (mostly females at a 4:1 ratio [27]) and/or immuno-compromised patients). Diabetes, vascular diseases such as arteriopathies or the Raynaud phenomenon, and the Cushing's disease are predisposing factors [7]. Clinically, the proximal fold is erythematous, thick and painful and the cuticle has disappeared. The nail plate may thicken, loose adherence, or present with grooving. There are usually more than one fingers involved. *Candida albicans* is the most frequent offending organism [1]. Evolution may last for years with acute inflammation appearing from time to time.

Prevention from humidity (limitation of hand washing, use of cotton gloves under the usual plastic/rubber gloves, etc.) and control of risk factors are extremely important. Class I dermocorticoids are used to limit chronic inflammation and restore the cuticle that will protect from new inoculation. Broad-spectrum antibiotics (amoxicillin with clavulanic acid) and/or anti-fungus medication (Fluconazole) may be needed in acute phases.

Marsupialization of the nail bed may be needed in the case of chronic paronychia [27, 28]. A crescent of 3 to 5 mm of skin, parallel to the eponychium and extending from the radial to the ulnar border, is excised. In the first publication, surgical technique requires that all tissues are removed. Bednar and Lane [27], on the other hand, suggested that the subcutaneous tissue and fat are left intact, and the nail plate is removed partially or totally, a technique that found to diminish the recurrence rate in their series [27]. After surgery, patients were told to wash their fingers with chlorexhidine gluconate 3 times per day until all drainage stopped. Antibiotics (oral cephalexin) were given for 3 to 5 days, and they were prolonged for 2 weeks if wound cultures were found positive. In that series, 27 out of 28 fingers were cured [27].

10.1. Differential diagnosis

Other organisms may be the cause of chronic paronychia including *dermatophytes, Sporothrix schenckii, Tinea rubrum,* etc. Diagnosis is difficult to make, since the organism should be present into the nail plate to be considered as the cause of infection. The cultures should be taken in specialized laboratories. The decision of which treatment to follow should be made in common with a dermatologist. Rare diseases may mimic chronic paronychia, such as syphilis, tuberculosis and other mycobacterial infections, however, there is no corroborated data concerning the above [25].

11. CONCLUSION

Hand infections are common and acute paronychia is the most common of them. Although complications are rare, misdiagnosis and/or non-adapted treatment may lead to severe complications. In the inflammation phase, conservative treatment may cure patients. At the abcedation phase, surgery is needed and removal of all contaminated tissues to cure the patients. Wound cultures should always be obtained, even if antibiotic treatment is rarely required. The hand surgeon should be suspicious of the potential of complications occurrence in immuno-compromised patients, patients seen late, those being under inadequate antibiotic treatment, or patients with streptococcus infection.

REFERENCES

[1] Lee DH, Ferlic RJ, Neviaser RJ. Hand infections. In: R.A. Berger, A.-P.C. Weiss (Eds.), Hand Surgery, Lippincott, Philadelphia, 2004;2:1177–1803.

[2] Bolton H, Fowler PJ, Jepson RP. Natural history and treatment of pulp space infection and osteomyelitis of the distal phalanx, J. Bone Joint Surg [Br] 1949;31(4):499–504.

[3] Canales FL, Newmeyer WL III, Kilgore ES Jr. The treatment of felons and paronychias, Hand Clin 1989;5(4):515–523.

[4] Hausman MR, Lisser SP. Hand infections, Orthop Clin North Am 1992;23(1):171–185.

[5] Jebson PJ, Infections of the fingertip. Paronychias and felons, Hand Clin 1998;14(4):547–555.

[6] Kanavel AB. Infections of the Hand, Lea & Febiger, Philadelphia, 1921.

[7] Dumontier C L'ongle. Elsevier, Paris, 2004.

[8] Lemerle JP, Panaris et phlegmons de la main. Cahiers Enseignement SOFCOT 1986, pp. 37–46.

[9] Gaillot O, Maruéjouls C. Bactériologie des infections de la main. In: Ebelin M (Ed.), Infections de la main, Elsevier, Paris, 1998, pp. 3–8.

[10] Connolly B et al. Methicillin-resistant *Staphylococcus aureus* in a finger felon. J Hand Surg [Am] 2000;25A(1)356:173–175.

[11] Heinzelmann M, Scott M, Lam T. Factors predisposing to bacterial invasion and infection. Am J Surg 2002;183:179–190.

[12] Chiu DT. Transthecal digital block: flexor tendon sheath used for anesthetic infusion. J Hand Surg [Am] 1990;15(3):471–477.

[13] Chevaleraud E et al. Anesthésie locale des doigts par la gaine des fléchisseurs. Ann Fr Anesth Reanim 1993;12(3):237–240.

[14] Cummings AJ, Tisol WB, Meyer LE. Modified transthecal digital block versus traditional digital block for anesthesia of the finger. J Hand Surg [Am] 2004;29(1):44–48.

[15] Sylaidis P, Logan A. Digital blocks with adrenaline. An old dogma refuted. J Hand Surg [Br] 1998;23(1):17–19.

[16] K. Denkler, A comprehensive review of epinephrine in the finger: to do or not to do. Plast. Reconstr. Surg. 108 (1) (2001) 114–124.

[17] Hixson FP , et al. Digital tourniquets: a pressure study with clinical relevance. J Hand Surg [Am] 1986;11(6):865–868.

[18] Perry AW et al. Fingerstick felons. Ann Plast Surg 1988;20(3):249–251.

[19] Neviaser RJ. Infections. In: Green DP (Ed.), Operative Hand Surgery, Churchill Livingstone, New York, 1982;1:771–791.

[20] Kilgore ESJ et al. Treatment of felons. Am J Surg 1975;130(2):194–198.

[21] Arnaud JP et al. Human ORF disease localized in the hand: a "false felon". A study of eight cases. Ann Chir Main 1986;5(2):129–132.

[22] Cosgrove SE. Cases from the Osler medical service at Johns Hopkins University. Am J Med 2002;113(2)378:158–160.

[23] Hurst LC et al. Herpetic whitlow with bacterial abcess. J Hand Surg [Am] 1991;16A(2):311–314.

[24] Gill MJ, Arlette J, Buchan KA. Herpes simplex virus infection of the hand. A profile of 79 cases. Am J Med 1988;84(1):89–93.

[25] Elhassan BT, Wynn SW, Gonzalez MH. Atypical infections of the hand. J Am Soc Surg Hand 2004;4(1):42–49.

[26] Polayes IM, Arons MS. The treatment of herpetic whitlow — a new surgical concept. Plast Reconstr Surg 1980;65(6):811–817.

[27] Bednar MS, Lane LB. Eponychial marsupialization and nail removal for surgical treatment of chronic paronychia. J Hand Surg [Am] 1991;16A(2):314–317.

[28] Keyser JJ, Eaton RG. Surgical cure of chronic paronychia by eponychial marsupialization. Plast Reconstr Surg 1976;58(1):66–70.

Flexor Tendon Sheath Infections

Frank D. BURKE*, Khalid SALEM

The Pulvertaft Hand Centre, Derbyshire Royal Infirmary , Derby, United Kingdom

Infections involving the flexor tendon sheath threaten one of the hands most prized functions, digital mobility. Any delay in diagnosis or treatment will radically effect outcome.

Keywords: tendon; sheath; infection. ∎

ACUTE FLEXOR TENDON SHEATH INFECTIONS

1. INTRODUCTION

Kanavel [1] described the classic symptoms and signs of flexor tendon sheath infections (FTSI) advising swift diagnosis and treatment. Incision and drainage was the procedure of choice, but late presentation could lead to fulminating infections that were life threatening in the pre antibiotic era, and in such circumstances amputation was often the more appropriate intervention. The introduction of antibiotics radically improved the surgeon's ability to gain control of the situation with improved outcome particularly in those patients presenting early. Kanavel's principles of management remain valid and the use of antibiotics has not displaced the role of incision and drainage except in those cases presenting exceptionally early (where hospitalisation, elevation in the position of optimal func-

tion with intravenous antibiotics may be applied for a trial period of 12 to 24 hours).

2. RELEVANT ANATOMICAL CONSIDERATIONS

Doyle described the anatomy of the flexor tendon sheath and pulley system [2]: the antero-lateral wall of the fibro-osseous tunnel through which the flexor tendons pass is formed by the flexor sheath with the deep transverse metacarpal ligament, the palmer plates, and the palmer surface of the proximal and middle phalanges forming the tunnel's floor. The flexor sheath is composed of two parts: the retinacular and the synovial (membranous). The retinacular part is represented by the cruciate and annular pulleys which overlie the synovial part of the sheath. The latter is a double-walled tube surrounding the tendon in a fashion similar to omental invagination. The walls of the synovial component are termed as visceral and parietal based on their relation to the flexor tendon. The outer synovial wall is a continuous parietal layer reinforced by the denser retinaculer layer externally. The inner visceral wall runs in close proximity to the flexor tendons and is continuous with the parietal layer at the ends of the sheath and through the mesotendon. Between the two synovial layers lies the synovial space containing a thin film of synovial fluid.

The synovial sheaths of the index, middle and ring fingers begin just distal to the distal interphalangeal (DIP) joint and extend into the palm ap-

*Corresponding Author
28 Midland Place, Derby, DE1 2RR
United Kingdom
Tel: +44 1332290480
Fax: +44 1332291425.
e-mail: Frank.burke@virgin.net

proximately a thumb's breadth from the digital web, just proximal to the A1 Pulley at the level of the metacarpal neck. The sheath of the Flexor Pollicis Longus (FPL) is nearly always continuous with the radial bursa (proximal to the metacarpophalangeal joint (MPJ)). The sheath begins distal to the base of the distal phalanx of the thumb and extends proximally over the thenar space terminating in a cul-de-sac which overlies the pronator quadratus. The sheath of the little finger is continuous with the ulnar bursa in about half of cases lying volar to the middle palmer space and the lumbrical canal with which it communicates (Fig. 1). The ulnar bursa extends proximally under the transverse carpal ligament to lie on the pronator quadratus. A connection between the ulnar and radial bursae exists in 50% of cases [1].

Anatomical studies of the vascular supply of the flexor tendons reveals a segmental tendon blood supply with an avascular zone nourished through synovial diffusion [3].

3. ACUTE FLEXOR TENDON SHEATH INFECTIONS

3.1. Differential diagnoses

Herpetic whitlow: a mucocutaneous herpetic infection typically affecting the terminal phalanx characterized by an intense pain in one or more digits. It is usually secondary to unprotected exposure to infected oropharyngeal secretions. Patients present with prodromal viral symptoms followed by an exquisitely tender and oedematous digit and characteristic vesicular lesions containing clear fluid or ulcers with surrounding erythema.

Felon: a closed-space infection of the fingertip pulp, characterized by marked throbbing pain, tension, and edema of the fingertip following a puncture wound.

Paronychia: a superficial infection under the eponicium and in the area of the germinal matrix characterized by oedema, erythema and tenderness proximal to the nail extending into the lateral nail fold.

Pyogenic interphalangeal (IP) joint or metacarpophalangeal (MP) joint infection, caused by a penetrating injury to the digit with signs of swelling, errythema, limitation of movement and localised joint tenderness. The tenderness is localised and increases with finger movement but does not involve the entire flexor tendon sheath.

Gout can present with a swollen errythematous digit, but pain on passive extension of the digit and tenderness over the tendon sheath is less marked, tophaceous crystals are helpful in making a diagnosis.

Rare differentials included acute calcific tendonitis, pyoderma gangrenosa, a flexor tendon sheath haemangioma and in certain geographical areas, brown recluse spider bite.

3.2. Aetiology: possible causative micro-organisms

A study of 68 cases confirmed staphylococcus aureus to be the commonest causative micro-organism in 30% of the sample. In the same sample group A B-Haemolytic streptococcus had a prevalence of 18% and Gram negative micro-organisms 10% [4]. Similar findings have been reported elsewhere in the literature [5-8]. Other organisms implicated as a cause of the condition include Pseudomonas aeruginosa [9], Eikenella corrodens, Pasteurella multocida, Listeria monocytogenes [10], Coliforms and Proteus. These micro-organisms should be considered in the immune-compromised (due to diabetes mellitus, steroids, IV drug abuse or organ transplant). Diphtheroid, Enterococcus, Escherichia Coli and Hemophilus species have also been reported [11, 12]. An acute FTSI on rare occasion can start after an attack of diarrhoea in the hospitalised patient on antibiotics caused by Clostridium difficile or following symptoms and signs of a sexually transmitted disease caused by a gonococcal infection [13]. Despite the small fascial space and the acute nature of the FTSI, the incidence of negative cultures remains as high as 68% in the literature [11]. Those patients with negative cultures are treated with antibiotics usually with surgical exploration and debridement as the consequences of less stringent treatment are often disastrous.

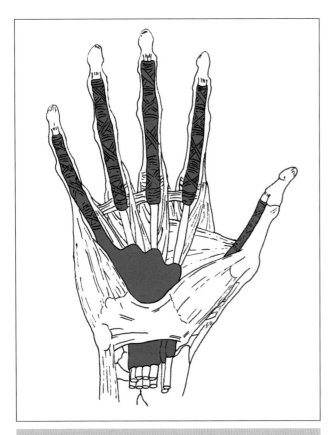

FIGURE 1. The synovial sheaths in the palmer aspect of the hand.

3.3. Mode of transmission

The commonest mechanism of bacterial inoculation in FTSI is by penetrating injury, usually close to the flexion creases of the fingers [6, 9] where the skin lies close to the flexor tendons. On occasion, no obvious source of infection can be identified. Hematogenous spread is rare and should be treated as gonococcal until final cultures are available [14].

3.4. Pathophysiological considerations

The synovial component of the flexor sheath is a closed system with poor blood supply making the host defence mechanisms of limited value and creating an ideal environment for micro-organism proliferation [3].

As the inflammatory process develops the pressure within the flexor tendon, sheath increases exceeding 30 mm Hg and creating a condition similar to a compartment syndrome which compromises the blood supply to the tendon [15]. Tendon survival is further undermined by invading micro-organisms depleting the available nutrient in the synovial fluid. This may lead to tendon or sheath necrosis further complicated by tendon rupture or bowstringing.

3.5. Clinical features

The patient commonly presents with no history of injury or a history of trivial injury with a superficial laceration to the DIP or PIP joint flexion creases a few hours or days previously. Patients may present within 24 to 48 hours of their injury usually with some or all of Kanavel's four cardinal symptoms and signs [1]; (i) exquisite tenderness limited to the course of the flexor sheath, (ii) finger in a semi-flexed position, (iii) exquisite pain on extending the digit, most marked proximally, and (iv) symmetrical swelling of the entire finger (Fig. 2). Generalised swelling of the hand with limitation of movement in the affected finger may also be observed.

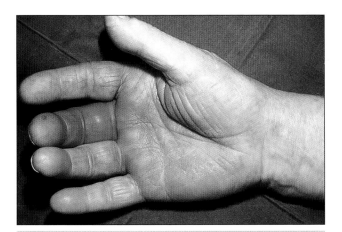

FIGURE 2. FTSI in the right middle digit demonstrating Kanavel's signs.

Opinions on the most specific and important of these signs is varied [1, 6, 10]; the exquisite pain and tenderness over the involved area on the tendon sheath was felt by Kanavel to be the most helpful in the diagnosis. Neviaser felt that pain on passive extension was the most reproducible sign in these patients [9].

Particular vigilance is required when faced with a suspected FTSI of the thumb or little finger; the connection between the flexor sheath in those digits and the radial and ulnar bursa with possible proximal communication (The Space of Parona) allows for delayed presentation with extensive tendon and pulley damage and large palmer soft tissue loss due to the rapid progression of infection with the formation of a horseshoe abscess.

3.6. Investigations

Diagnosis requires basic haematological investigations including a full blood count, ESR and CRP. Although nonspecific, they can advise on the possibility of inflammation or infection. In the absence of a typical history of inoculation, stool analysis for clostridium difficile toxin and a urethral smear for gonococcal infection [13] can be helpful.

A trial aspiration of the tendon sheath to obtain material for culture is helpful. A 20- or 22-gauge needle is used to gain access to the tendon sheath anywhere between the palmo-digital crease and the DIP flexion crease. Lavage with a small amount of saline may be necessary to obtain a sample for culture. Conservative treatment is redundant if pus is observed.

Radiographic imaging of the affected hand is helpful to identify retained foreign bodies or associated pathology for example osteomyelitis and pyoarthrosis.

Ultrasound scanning has been shown to be beneficial in the diagnosis of tenosynovitis; a 25% or greater increase in the diameter of the affected tendon compared to the contra-lateral control was considered diagnostic of tenosynovitis [16]. In chronic cases, identification of the extent of the lesion can be achieved using contrast enhanced MRI imaging [17].

3.7. Management

3.7.1. Non operative

Patients presenting within 24-48 hours after a penetrating injury to the flexor tendon sheath with only one or two of Kanavel's signs and no complicating medical condition or a retained foreign body within the tendon sheath may in the first instance be hospitalised for conservative treatment [18]; broad spectrum intravenous antibiotics elevation and splintage in the position of optimal function with frequent assessment for signs of improvement is crucial if applying expectant treatment for this condition. If there is no apparent improvement in the first 12 to 24 hours, surgical intervention is required. Physiotherapy to regain range of motion is deferred until the signs of inflammation have subsided and the pain is adequately controlled. A course of oral antibiotics based on the culture and sensitivity from the sheath aspirate can then be administered on an out-patient basis. Other indications for exploration include an uncertain history on the time of onset, more than 2 Kanavel signs, complicating medical conditions (i.e. diabetes mellitus or patients on steroid) or when in doubt. Exploration is indicated if imaging reveals gas in the soft tissue (particularly in Escherichia Coli and Clostridial infections) or if there is osteomyelitis or a foreign body.

It is necessary to use a broad spectrum intravenous antibiotic regime to cover both Gram positive and Gram negative micro-organisms until treatment can be modified according to the results of culture and sensitivity (Table 1).

3.7.2. Surgical treatment

The necessity for adequate surgical debridement and copious irrigation of the infection site have not changed with time. A variety of approaches to achieve this have been described; open drainage through a midaxial incision on the ulnar side of the fingers or radially for the thumb and little finger was advocated early in the literature [1]. The incision extends from the web space proximally, running dorsal to the neurovascular bundle which is retained with the volar flap, to terminate slightly distal to the flexion crease of the DIP joint. The proximal sheath is then opened through a transverse incision at the palmer crease. The tenosynovium from the palm to the distal phalanx is excised and the wound is irrigated [1, 19].

Whilst radical, the open method has the disadvantage of wound healing by secondary intention, prolonged rehabilitation and at least 25% of the patients not regaining a full range of motion [18].

A less radical technique has been suggested to improve the postoperative outcome. Irrigation through a proximally inserted cannula with a distal midaxial incision for drainage has been described [20], this also allowed irrigation to continue postoperatively until mobilisation was permitted. Alternatively, through and through irrigation may be used; an incision is created parallel to the DIP flexion crease to visualise the tendon sheath which is then opened, a second transverse incision is made at the region of the A1 pulley - similar to a trigger finger release. A catheter is then fed through the proximal incision and the wound is irrigated, the catheter is secured in place for postoperative irrigation. The distal incision is left open to facilitate drainage.

Neviaser described a closed tendon sheath irrigation procedure, exposing the tendon through a small zigzag incision over the proximal margin of the annular ligament at the metacarpal neck [18] (Fig. 3). The sheath is visualised and incised transversely at the proximal edge of the A1 pulley and the synovial fluid is cultured. A 16-gauge polyethylene catheter with a connector then is inserted under the pulley into the sheath for a distance of approximately 1.5 to 2.0 cm. The distal edge of the sheath is exposed at the level of the distal interphalangeal joint through a short midaxial incision on the ulnar aspect of the digit. The sheath is resected beyond the last pulley and a small rubber drain is inserted into the distal wound.

TABLE 1					
Antimicrobial Treatment Options for FTSI					
	Micro-organism	**Empirical**	**Definitive**	**The allergic patient**	**The immune-compromised**
Acute	Staphylococcus aureus (most common) group A B-Haemolytic streptococcus Pseudomonas Aeruginosa Eikenella Corrodens Pasteurella Multocida Listeria Monocytogenes Coliforms Proteus Diphtheroid Enterococcus Escherichia Coli Hemophilus Clostridium difficile Gonococcus	Regime 1: Flucloxacillin 2 gr. four times daily IV Regime 2: Cefuroxime 1.5 gr. three times daily Special considerations: [a] If a Gram negative Micro-organism is suspected; Metronidazole 500 mg twice daily IV is added to either of the above. [b] If P. Multocida is suspected Augmentin 625 mg orally or 1 gram IV infusion three times daily is given.	According to culture and sensitivity. If cultures are negative, continue with Empirical treatment and observe for clinical improvement.	Vancomycin 1 gram twice daily IV.	Treat similar to the Non-Immune compromised. If the patient is neutropenic consult Microbiologist.
Chronic	Atypical Mycobacterial Species: Marinum, Kansaii, Asiaticum & Bovis.	No role for empirical management in chronic FTSI	Dependent on the culture & sensitivity, consult your Microbiologist.	Dependent on the culture & sensitivity, consult your Microbiologist.	Dependent on the culture & sensitivity, consult your Microbiologist.

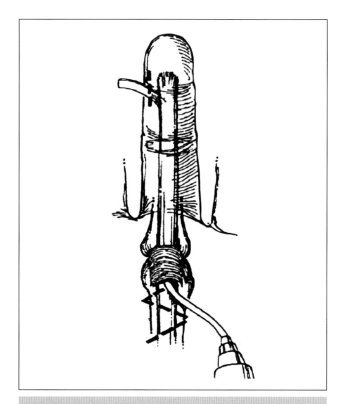

FIGURE 3. Neviaser's Closed Irrigation system for FTSI [18].

The incisions are then closed around the indwelling catheter and drain. The system is tested by flushing saline and dressings are applied allowing for the visualisation of the rubber drain and the catheter. For the thumb, Neviaser suggested that the irrigation catheter is passed through the FPL sheath as it leaves the carpal tunnel. Sheath infections in the little finger requires a second catheter placed through the same transverse incision at the level of the A1 pulley in a retrograde fashion to irrigate the bursa, drainage is facilitated by a rubber drain inserted in the ulnar bursa at the level of the wrist [9]. More recently, Harris and Nanchahal described a similar approach to the sheath using a transverse proximal (at the level of the A1 Pulley) and distal (between the A4 and A5 pulleys) incisions [21]. A 4- French gauge infant feeding catheter is inserted into the sheath via the distal incision. The catheter is passed through the proximal incision and an 8- French gauge tube is placed over the smaller tube and the apparatus is then manoeuvred back into the sheath until all the irrigation holes are within the tendon sheath. The catheters are secured and dressings are applied. In a small series of 12 cases the authors reported good to excellent results in 10 cases [21].

A retrospective observational study on 47 cases of FTSI comparing open drainage (OD) and irrigation to closed catheter irrigation (CCI) concluded that CCI is as effective as OD in the management of FTSI with the advantage of less soft tissue trauma, less complications and a faster rehabilitation. The authors demonstrated no difference in hospital stay between the two groups [22].

A variety of irrigation fluids have been used postoperatively, such as lactated Ringer's solution [11], normal saline [4], various antibiotic preparations [9, 12, 20] and peroxide. Gosain and Markison added lidocaine hydrochloride to the irrigation solution for pain relief [12]. There is no evidence to suggest that the use of antibiotics in the irrigation intraoperatively or postoperatively improves the outcome. As no information on the causative micro-organism is available at the time of the surgery and the choice of antibiotic is empirical, it is likely that the therapeutic effect of the fluid is mechanical rather than chemical. Peroxide can further weaken an already frail tendon.

The hand is rested on a volar slab for the first 48 hours in the position of optimal function with the metacarpo-phalangeal joints flexed no more than 70° to avoid kinking the catheter. The interphalangeal joints are held near full extension. Once the catheter is removed and the infection controlled, physiotherapy is introduced to mobilise the fingers off the splint.

The outcome of surgery relates to the stage of presentation reflected in Michon's classification [23] which is based on the surgical appearance of the synovial fluid, the synovial tissue itself and the flexor tendon; stage one presents with an exudative serous synovial fluid which swells the sheath and is associated with congestion of the synovial tissue while the tendon is normal. Stage two has a cloudy or purulent liquid within the sheath and is associated with a congestive and granulomatous appearance of the synovium; the tendon retains a normal appearance. Stage three presents with a septic necrosis of the tendon sheath and the pulleys. In 28 cases, Juliano and Eglseder [11] demonstrated an excellent outcome in 100% for stage one, 88% for stage two, while all stage three cases underwent amputation. Similar findings were reported by Sokolow et al [4] in a series of 68 cases, where the 14 stage three cases had a poor outcome.

3.8. Complications

Catastrophic complications previously reported after advanced FTSI are rare, nevertheless, a delay in starting active treatment remains the most important factor determining the outcome.

The most commonly reported complication is the loss of normal range of motion [9, 11], this is minimised by early physiotherapy. If the patient develops stiffness postoperatively, tenolysis may be considered once the digit reaches a state of "tissue equilibrium" [10]. Tissue necrosis and tendon rupture occurs most commonly in the immune - compromised, particularly if the ulnar or radial busae are involved [1], necessitating the use of a skin flap or a tendon transfer. Bone and joint involvement with osteomyelitis, septic arthritis and ankylosis has not been reported in recent years, but if encountered, might justify amputation. Other complications include wound dehiscence, and neurovascular damage.

3.9. Virulence and compromised host response

The recent advances in medical practice have allowed many immune- compromised patients the opportunity of a longer and more active life. Hand surgeons are now routinely required to treat infections in this challenging group of patients.

The spectrum of micro-organisms causing infections in the immune-suppressed is similar to that of the general population but the prevalence may be greater because of their diminished defence mechanisms. The infection may develop and spread more rapidly [24] yet the clinical signs described by Kanavel may not be evident. Aggressive early surgical management for those patients is advised. Routine antibiotic regimes are applied till culture and sensitivity results are available. A higher possibility of mixed and atypical infections should be anticipated.

4. Subacute and Chronic Flexor Tendon Sheath Infections

4.1. Clinical features

Patients with subacute and chronic FTSI do not have the classical Kanavel Signs. The history points to a slow insidious onset perhaps after a penetrating injury to the palmer aspect of the digit. Swelling and impaired function are usually the main complaints. There may be no pain or overt signs of infection. The diagnosis may be delayed and there may be remissions and relapses [25].

4.2. Differential diagnosis

A variety of mycobacterium species cause chronic FTSI including M. marinum, M. kansaii, M. asiaticum and M. bovis. Other conditions presenting with a subacute or chronic picture include Gonococcal and Clostridial infections and retained foreign bodies in the flexor sheath.

4.3. Management

Baseline haematological tests are usually not very informative, imaging can help in some of the cases where enhanced MRI scanning of the affected area may show a thickened synovium [17]. The diagnosis is often made at open biopsy; a fibrotic thick synovial sheath containing serous fluid and multiple "rice bodies" is suggestive of mycobacterium infection. Harvested material should be sent for histological and microbiological testing ensuring adequate information is delivered to the microbiologist regarding the suspicion of a "slow" micro-organism that might require a special culture medium and prolonged incubation. More recently 16S rRNA Gene PCR was used to identify microbial presence in sampled tissue and more specifically aid in the identification of the causative strain.

Trial conservative management with anti-inflammatory agents or steroid injection has been described [18] but surgery is advised. The patient requires an extensive tenosynovectomy through a Brunner incision to the finger extending into the palm. The pulley system should be preserved. Post operatively antituberculous medication (Table 1) is empirically started as culture results can take up to 6 weeks. Physiotherapy is started 2-3 days post operatively.

Complications in chronic FTSI are limitation of range of motion, recurrence and amputation.

5. Conclusion

There have been considerable advances in medical practice and health education in the last few decades that have allowed early detection and treatment of FTSI with improved outcomes compared to those described by Kanavel. The micro-organisms responsible for the condition have not changed, but the resistance to antimicrobial agents remains a constant challenge. Methicillin resistant infections are becoming more common [7]. The immune-suppressed patients create a unique additional difficulty for the hand surgeon. Flexor tendon sheath infections were life threatening catastrophes 60 year ago, yet were tamed in the first 20 years of the antibiotic era. Antibiotic resistance and the immune-suppressed are shifting the balance of risk back to that of earlier times.

References

[1] Kanavel AB. Infections of the hand: A guide to the surgical treatment of acute and chronic suppurative processes in the fingers, hand and forearm. 7th Edition ed. 1939, Philadelphia: Lea & Febiger.

[2] Doyle JR. Anatomy of the finger flexor tendon sheath and pulley system. Journal of Hand Surgery - American Volume, 1988; 13(4):473-84.

[3] Lundborg G, Myrhage R, and Rydevik B. The vascularization of human flexor tendons within the digital synovial sheath region-structureal and functional aspects. Journal of Hand Surgery - American Volume 1977;2(6):417-27.

[4] Sokolow C et al. Bacterial flexor tenosynovitis in the hand. A series of 68 cases. Annales de Chirurgie de la Main 1987;6(3): 181-8.

[5] Pinzur MS, et al. Hand infections in the diabetic patient. Journal of Hand Surgery - British Volume 1997;22(1):133-4.

[6] Pollen AG. Acute infection of the tendon sheaths. Hand 1974; 6(1):21-5.

[7] Bell MS. The changing pattern of pyogenic infections of the hand. Hand 1976;8(3): 298-302.

[8] Monstrey SJ et al. Tendon sheath infections of the hand. Netherlands Journal of Surgery 1985;37(6):174-8.

[9] Neviaser RJ. Closed tendon sheath irrigation for pyogenic flexor tenosynovitis. Journal of Hand Surgery - American Volume 1978; 3(5): 462-6.

[10] Boles SD, Schmidt CC. Pyogenic flexor tenosynovitis. Hand Clinics 1998;14(4):567-78.

[11] Juliano PJ, Eglseder WA. Limited open-tendon-sheath irrigation in the treatment of pyogenic flexor tenosynovitis. Orthopaedic Review 1991;20(12):1065-9.

[12] Gosain AK, Markison RE. Catheter irrigation for treatment of pyogenic closed space infections of the hand. British Journal of Plastic Surgery 1991;44(4):270-3.

[13] Rosenfeld N, Kurzer A. Acute flexor tenosynovitis caused by gonococcal infection. A case report. Hand 1978;10(2):213-4.

[14] Levy CS. Treating infections of the hand: identifying the organism and choosing the antibiotic. Instructional Course Lectures 1990; 39:533-7.

[15] Schnall SB et al. Tissue pressures in pyogenic flexor tenosynovitis of the finger. Compartment syndrome and its management. Journal of Bone & Joint Surgery - British Volume 1996;78(5):793-5.

[16] Schecter WP et al. Use of sonography in the early detection of suppurative flexor tenosynovitis. Journal of Hand Surgery - American Volume 1989;14(2 Pt 1):307-10.

[17] Sueyoshi E et al. Tuberculous tenosynovitis of the wrist: MRI findings in three patients. Skeletal Radiology 1996;25(6):569-72.

[18] Neviaser RJ. Tenosynovitis. Hand Clinics 1989;5(4):525-31.

[19] Flynn JE. Hand Surgery. 1966, Baltimore: The Williams & Willkins Co.

[20] Besser MI. Digital flexor tendon irrigation. Hand 1976;8(1):72.

[21] Harris PA, Nanchahal J. Closed continuous irrigation in the treatment of hand infections. Journal of Hand Surgery - British Volume 1999;24(3):328-33.

[22] Gutowski KA, Ochoa O, and Adams WP Jr. Closed-catheter irrigation is as effective as open drainage for treatment of pyogenic flexor tenosynovitis. Annals of Plastic Surgery 2002;49(4):350-4.

[23] Michon J. Phlegmon of the tendon sheaths. Annales de Chirurgie 1974;28(4):277-80.

[24] Kour AK et al. Hand infections in patients with diabetes. Clinical Orthopaedics & Related Research 1996;(331):238-44.

[25] Foulkes GD, Floyd JC, Stephens JL. Flexor tenosynovitis due to Mycobacterium asiaticum. Journal of Hand Surgery - American Volume 1998;23(4):753-6.

Human and Animal Bites Injuries of the Hand

Frank D. BURKE*, Saiidy HASHAM

The Pulvertaft Hand Centre, Derbyshire Royal Infirmary, Derby, United Kingdom

Human and animal bites of the hand remain an important cause of upper limb morbidity and inappropriate management can delay and limit recovery. Prompt diagnosis, appropriate chemotherapy and well timed immobilisation and physiotherapy will ensure minimal long term disability.

Keywords: infection; bite; animal; human; fightbite.

1. INTRODUCTION

Injuries to the hand caused by human and animal bites continue to be a serious problem and are a common cause of hospital admission to a hand service. Wounds from teeth and those contaminated by saliva are well-recognised in having the potential to develop destructive soft tissue, joint and bone infections.

A variety of organisms have been isolated from bite wounds which generally originate from the oral cavity of the biting animal or human or from the patient's skin flora. Many patients unfortunately do not seek immediate treatment, deeming their injuries to be trivial and present late with established signs and symptoms of infection. Delayed presentation is often characterised by a high rate of infection-related complications, prolonged morbidity

*Corresponding Author
28 Midland Place, Derby, DE1 2RR
United Kingdom
Tel: +44 1332290480
Fax: +44 1332291425
e-mail: Frank.burke@virgin.net

and a poor overall functional outcome. The financial ramifications from such injuries are huge with considerable expense to society and the individual.

2. HISTORY

Hand infections and their treatment are recorded in the early writings of the Greeks and Romans [1]. The most famous of these contributors was Hippocrates, who practised around 400 BC and has been considered 'the true father of hand surgery' [2]. The Hippocratic writings cover numerous surgical problems and although these works primarily discuss the treatment of fractures and dislocations, they also describe the treatment of wound infections and many of the principles are still relevant today. Celsus, a cultured Roman, practised medicine in first-century Rome and his treatise De arte medica is the first comprehensive text on the science of medicine. He is best remembered for his description of the four cardinal features of inflammation, *rubor, tumor, calor and dolor* [1]. The Renaissance in Europe throughout the 16th century saw a resurgence of interest in anatomy with dissections of the human body.

Many developments in the centuries that followed arose from experiences gained during European and American wars. However, despite these advances, hand infections remained widespread and potentially life threatening. Surgical treatment amounted to little more than simple incision and drainage with amputation often being performed for fear of death from sepsis [3]. This environment was altered significantly by the pioneering injection studies of Kanavel (1905) [4] and his work in defining the anatomical spaces of the hand and their communications in relation to infection. Based on these findings, he identified the most appropriate location of surgical incisions to drain specific infected fascial spaces which are still used today. This work was later expanded upon by Mason and Koch, who in 1930, described the pattern of extension of a human bite infection of the hand [5]. They simulated a fight bite injury in human cadaveric hands to demonstrate that the flexed position of the fingers, introduced infected material directly into the joint despite an innocuous looking wound. Human bites of the hand had been recognised as a problem even before this time when Hultgen (1910) first described an infection of the index finger in a young girl who had the habit of biting her nails [6]. This article was followed a year later by Peter's [7] (1911) report of a hand infection resulting from a fight bite injury.

The greatest advance in the management of hand infections was the discovery of antibiotic agents. Since the work of Alexander Fleming (1929) [8], the evolution of antibiotic agents has been rapid with the development of newer drugs to combat the increasing problem of antibiotic resistance. Although the use of broad spectrum antibiotics can prevent the progression and improve the clinical outcome of hand infections, they are seen as an adjunct to treatment and there is no substitute for surgical decompression and debridement in established cases.

3. FACTORS AFFECTING HOST RESPONSE TO INFECTION

There are a number of factors that contribute to the development of a hand infection. The site and the anatomical space that it occupies can have a significant effect on the clinical outcome. The infecting organism, its virulence, and susceptibility to antibiotics will also play a role in a patient's recovery. Equally important are the host defences against infection. Immunosuppression can result from malnutrition, corticosteroid use, systemic disease, HIV infection, chronic alcohol excess and malignancy. Patients suffering from diabetes mellitus have an altered host defence with the propensity to develop infection. The diabetic process creates systemic and local factors which favour the establishment and development of infections [9]. Laboratory studies have demonstrated a reduced cell-mediated response in diabetic patients with impaired white cell phagocytosis, fibroblast

function and bacteriocidal activity [9]. In addition, local ischaemia will impair wound healing and in turn, make those wounds more susceptible to bacterial infection. Clinicians need to recognise the seriousness of hand infections in such patients for their response is quite unique.

4. HUMAN BITES

4.1. Epidemiology

Human bites are the third most common mammalian bite, but have the highest complication and infection rate. The true incidence of human bites to the hand is unknown since they are a group of patients that often fail to seek medical attention following such injuries. Bites may be categorised according to the mechanism of injury as either occlusal or through the use of a clenched fist. The occlusal injury results from the biting process and occurs accidentally or in anger during sporting events, sexual activity, or assaults by second parties [10]. Clenched fist injuries are the result of striking another individual in the mouth, often during a fight (hence the term "fight bite").

Most of the epidemiological studies on human bite injuries to the hand come from the United States. One study from New York City determined the incidence to be 11.8 per 100 000 population/year [11]. Mann et al. (1977) summarised the literature on human bite injuries and found that men predominated (4:1) with injuries occurring mainly in the third decade [12]. A study by Chuinard et al. (1977) reported similar findings and demonstrated that the right hand was more commonly involved and that the most common cause of hand infection was the result of a fist blow to the mouth [13]. Approximately 60 - 75% of all bite wounds are to the hand and upper extremity [14]. The overall infection rate for human bites is estimated to be between 10 and 30% [15, 16].

4.2. Pathophysiology

The location and the depth of the wound should be taken into consideration because of the complex anatomy and the various closed spaces of the hand. These spaces can provide routes for extension of infection to a deeper or distant location if not treated early. This is best illustrated by the clenched fist injury. These injuries usually occur over the dorsal aspect of the 3rd, 4th and 5th metacarpophalangeal (MCP) joints. With the hand held in a clenched fist position at the time of injury, the tooth can penetrate the skin but can also violate the dorsal subcutaneous space, extensor tendon, subtendinous space (between the tendon and capsule) and the joint. As a result, bacteria from a victim's mouth may be inoculated directly into these 3 spaces or indeed introduced into the metacarpal head. It is important to note the site of penetration through the skin surface relative to the position of the hand. In the flexed position (Fig. 1a), the defects in the skin, dorsal subcutaneous space, tendon, subtendinous space and capsule, lie in a line. However, in the extended position (Fig. 1b), the site of penetration of the skin is proximal to the metacarpal head. As the fingers are extended, the extensor hood and skin retract, and in doing so, drag bacteria proximally into the dorsum of the hand. The skin wound may be small and innocuous and one can wrongly assume that the capsule and joint space have not been breached because undamaged tendon is seen in the wound. For this reason, many patients unfortunately do not seek medical advice early, deeming their injuries to be trivial. Other factors which make these injuries prone to infection include the relatively avascular nature of both the extensor tendon and joint capsule, the lack of protection offered by the overlying skin and the high concentration of pathogenic organisms in the human mouth [12, 15, 17]. Thus, it is imperative that when presented with a clenched fist injury, or if suspected from the history, that the hand is examined in both flexed and extended positions.

4.3. Diagnostic difficulties

The signs and symptoms of human bite wounds to the hand will vary and are dependent on factors such as the time from injury to treatment, the degree of contamination, the severity of the wound and associated complications, e.g. fracture. Patients who present early (within 18-24 hours) may not have any signs of infection apart from the wound inflicted by the bite. However, those who present later (24-48 hours), typically have an infected wound, swelling, erythema, pain and a reduced range of motion in the hand (Fig. 2). Often they are reluctant to flex the MCP joint through its full range. In the more established infections (>48 hours), patients may present with local abscess formation, tendon rupture or evidence of septic arthritis. Fever, lymphadenopathy and even signs of systemic toxicity (raised white cell count

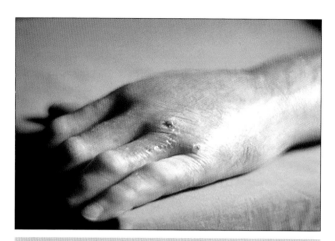

FIGURE 2. A four-day old fight bite injury.

and/or inflammatory markers, e.g. C-reactive protein) may also be present. Such patients should not pose diagnostic dilemmas to the examining clinician, though difficulties may be encountered in cases when the presentation is more subtle or patients lie about the circumstances of injury. Extension within the subcutaneous or fascial planes of the dorsum is easily recognised as it lies superficially. However, infection may extend to locations in the hand that are not obvious at first consideration. Bacteria may spread along the plane deep to the extensor tendon and proximally into the palm around the lumbricals and interosseous muscles.

Bacterial extension from a clench fist injury may spread proximally from the MCP joint. The capsule is thin and extension may occur at specific areas of inherent capsular weakness. This may occur dorsally, where the capsule attaches to the metacarpal head, or laterally, between the accessory collateral and collateral ligaments [12]. Infections can then easily extend to any or all of the deep spaces of the hand and fingers and even proximally into the forearm.

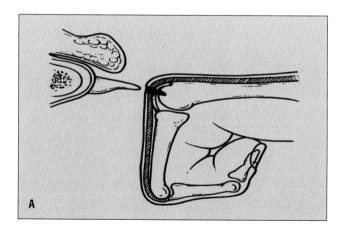

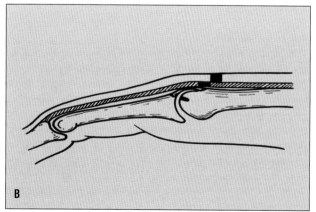

FIGURE 1. Fightbite injury (after Lister). **(A)** Flexed position. **(B)** Extended position.

4.4. Microbiology

The human mouth has a high concentration of pathogenic organisms with human saliva containing up to 108 million bacteria per millilitre and representing as many as 42 species [17]. A multicentre prospective study of 50 patients with infected human bite injuries was conducted by Talan et al. (2003) [18]. Of the injuries, 56% were clenched fist injuries and the remaining 44% were occlusal. The median number of isolates per wound culture was 4 (3 aerobes and 1 anaerobe). Aerobes alone were isolated from 44% of wounds and anaerobes only from 2%; both groups were isolated in 54% of wounds. Isolates included Streptococcus anginosus (52%), *Staphylococcus aureus* (30%), *Eikenella corrodens* (30%), *Fusobacterium nucleatum* (32%) and *Prevotella melaninogenica* (22%). Candida species were found in 8%. Many strains of *Prevotella* and *S. aureus* were β-lactamase producers [18].

The mixed variety of organisms found in the oral cavity represents a symbiotic relationship since not all are pathogenic and few can survive outside their normal environment. These bacteria are well tolerated within the undamaged oral cavity and are prevented from becoming virulent by the combined effect of saliva and competition from non-virulent organisms. However, infection of the hand may result when bacteria are directly inoculated into traumatised or damaged tissue [19]. The devitalised tissue potentiates the colonisation of both aerobic and anaerobic bacteria that may lead to clinical infection. In the same fashion, the type of organisms found in the oral cavity may evolve with the quality of the host's dentition and oral hygiene. In the well kept mouth, the dominant flora is either aerobes or facultative anaerobes. In contrast, in the neglected or diseased mouth, the bacterial types are mainly anaerobic [12]. For this reason, clinicians should treat all hand infections as polymicrobial in nature (Table 1).

In addition to bacterial infection, human bites have been reported to transmit hepatitis B and C, HIV, tuberculosis, syphilis, herpes and tetanus [20, 21].

4.5. Treatment

4.5.1. Evaluation

The mechanism and the time from injury to presentation are all important determinants of outcome. Present and past medical illnesses should be documented to highlight any potential altered host response to infection. The tetanus status of all patients should be checked and prophylaxis administered to those who are in need. Physical examination should document the location of the wound, depth and the range of motion. **A wound over the dorsum of the hand, especially over the MCP joint, should be treated as a clenched fist injury and must be formally explored.**

Plain radiographs of the hand should strongly be considered especially in 'fight bite' wounds to exclude

TABLE 1		
Organisms identified in human bite infections (adapted from Talan DA et al. 2003) [22]		
Aerobes		**Anaerobes**

Streptococcus:
  – S. anginosus
  – S. oralis
  – S. viridans group
		Prevotella:
		  – P. melaninogenica
		  – P. buccae

Staphylococcus:
  – S. aureus
  – S. epidermidis
		Fusobacterium:
		  – F. nucleatum
		
		Peptostreptococcus:
		  – P. micros

Eikenella corrodens Corynebacterium Haemophilus Candida		Veillonella Campylobacter Eubacterium

bony injury and to detect any tooth fragments remaining within the wound or joint. Infections that have progressed for some time without treatment may show radiographic signs of septic arthritis (Fig. 3). Baseline blood tests (full blood count, urea and electrolytes, liver function and inflammatory markers) as well as cultures should be sent where there are signs of systemic infection. Wound swabs (for culture and Gram stain) are mandatory in such cases.

4.5.2. Wound management

Basic principles of wound care are directed towards irrigation, open drainage and debridement of devitalised tissue. Patients who present with established signs of in-

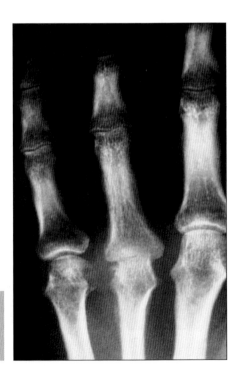

FIGURE 3.
Septic arthritis arising from a fight bite.

fection should be admitted into hospital for elevation and intravenous (IV) antibiotics under hand surgery supervision. Copious irrigation with normal saline should be performed prior to admission. Exploration of the wound under local anaesthesia may also be performed to document any damage to underlying structures and deep spaces. The wound should be examined in both flexion and extension.

Formal exploration is required if there is a localised collection, devitalised tissue, foreign body or joint penetration. Any structures that are damaged, e.g. extensor tendon, should not be repaired until infection is controlled. The wound should be left open, the hand splinted in the position of function and elevated. The wound should be re-examined 24-48 hours later with the view to further toilet and debridement if necessary. If the infection has resolved secondary suture can be considered, or the wound left to close by secondary intention.

Controversy still exists as to whether wounds which present for treatment early should be primarily closed. Clinically non-infected wounds presenting less than 8 hours after injury may be considered for primary closure [10]. This is only after thorough irrigation, debridement and careful wound exploration to exclude tendon or joint involvement. Upon discharge, patients continue on oral antibiotics, are splinted, and instructed to elevate the limb.

4.5.3. Antimicrobial therapy
Prophylactic antibiotics are recommended for all bite injuries. There are numerous recommended antibiotic regimes but selection is based on the knowledge of expected organisms. As no single agent will eradicate all major pathogens responsible for human bite infection, emphasis should be placed on covering the most common pathogens initially. Subsequent sensitivities based on wound swabs or Gram staining will allow clinicians to adjust therapy accordingly.

Empirical broad spectrum antibiotic cover should be directed *against S. anginosus, S. aureus, Eikenella* corrodens and oral anaerobic organisms. Penicillin has historically been used as the first line antimicrobial agent in the management of human bite injuries. Although effective against *Streptococcus* species, increasing rates of resistance to this drug, especially with *S. aureus* and certain oral anaerobes has been demonstrated and relates directly to β-lactamase production [18]. It is therefore recommended to use β-lactam/β-lactamase-inhibitor combination antibiotics, such as amoxicillin-clavulanic acid (Augmentin®) or the newer quinolones with enhanced anaerobic activity, such as moxifloxacin, which are highly active against the major aerobic and anaerobic pathogens isolated from human bite wounds [10, 16, 18].

Second generation cephalosporins, e.g. cefotaxime, may offer adequate coverage but are less active against anaerobes than the aforementioned agents. Doxycycline may be used for patients who are penicillin allergic. Clindamycin is well concentrated in bone and for this reason is recommended for staphylococcal joint and bone infec-

tions such as osteomyelitis. Alternatively, a combination of antibiotics can be used, though advice from a microbiologist should be sought prior to commencing treatment.

Specific attention should be paid to *E. correndens*. This organism is part of the normal oral flora and may be isolated from 30% of human bite wounds [18]. It is resistant to a number of antibiotics including clindamycin, first generation cephalosporins and anti-staphylococcal penicillins such as flucloxacillin. Therefore, these antibiotics should be used in combination rather than as single agents if this organism is suspected.

There are no standard guidelines for duration of antibiotic therapy. In general, prophylactic antibiotics may be given up to 5 days and 7-14 days in established infections. For wounds complicated by septic arthritis or osteomyelitis, up to 6 weeks treatment may be required. Parenteral antibiotics may be switched to oral only when there are signs of resolving infection.

Viral pathogens may be transmitted by human bites, of which HIV and hepatitis B and C viruses are the most important. Prophylaxis is not routinely provided for bite injuries from an unknown source but should be considered if the source is high risk.

5. COMPLICATIONS

Complications of human bite wounds to the hand are frequent and are usually the result of delayed presentation or failure to diagnose such injuries. Stiffness, particularly of the fingers, and pain are common features. Loss of articular cartilage frequently occurs if treatment is delayed, leaving a stiff MCP joint with reduced grip. Intensive physiotherapy to mobilise the distal joints will reduce long-term disability, with splintage of the MCP joint in mild flexion, ensuring the joint settles into an acceptable functional position as it stiffens. Other complications include tendon rupture, tendon adhesions, septic arthritis, osteomyelitis, toxic shock syndrome and even death [12, 23]. Amputation at any level may be considered necessary to control infection but this has become rare over recent years.

Most complications can be eliminated or reduced by maintaining a high index of suspicion and engaging in early wound debridement with antibiotic therapy.

6. DOMESTIC ANIMAL BITES

6.1. Dogs

Dogs are responsible for approximately 80 - 90% of animal bite wounds and about 2% of patients require hospital admission as a result [24]. The majority of injuries are to the upper limb and occur by direct interaction with their own pet or a dog known to them. Wounds are often multiple with areas of crushed tissue and deep punctures. Their victims are typically young with a peak incidence between 5 and 9 years of age.

An estimated 4 - 25% of dog bite wounds become infected [10]. Mixed organisms, both aerobic and anaerobic, have been cultured. The most common aerobic isolates include *Pasteurella* species (canis, multocida), *Streptococci, Staphylococci, Moraxella* and *Neisseria.* Common anaerobes include *Fusobacterium, Bacteroides, Porphyromonas* and *Prevotella species* [22].

6.2. Cats

Cat bite injuries account for only 5 - 15% of all animal bites. Although cats have a weaker biting force than dogs, the infection rate may be more than double (up to 50%) and the median time from bite to appearance of first symptoms of infection is much shorter [10, 23]. This predominately relates to their sharp slender teeth which can easily penetrate joint capsule or bone [24]. Bacteria are driven deeper into the tissues and as a result, complications such as septic arthritis and osteomyelitis, are more common than in dog bite injuries. As with dogs, most bites are to the upper limb.

The organisms causing infection are very similar to those in dogs but *Pasteurella multocida* is the causative pathogen in the majority of infections [22, 25].

Treatment of animal bites is the same as for any hand bite: copious irrigation, appropriate antibiotic therapy and exploration and debridement where indicated. Tetanus prophylaxis should be updated and rabies immunization status of the animal should be evaluated (see below). Antibiotics should be administered in all cases and should be directed against the most common pathogens. The use of B-lactam/B-lactamase-inhibitor combination antibiotics, such as amoxicillin-clavulanic acid (Augmentin®) is recommended but second-generation cephalosporins with anaerobic activity are also effective [22].

6.3. Rabies

Rabies is the result of a neurotropic virus that is transmitted to humans through an animal bite, skin, mucosa or inhalation contact. The likelihood of human exposure to a rabid domestic animal has greatly decreased since the 1950s and is in part credited to urban vaccination programmes. In contrast, rabies among wildlife (bats in particular) has increased and therefore any skin wound inflicted by a wild animal (in some countries) must be considered rabid until proven otherwise [10].

The decision to administer rabies prophylaxis is dependent on a number of factors. These include the type of animal involved, the type of exposure, the local epidemiology of rabies and the availability of the animal for observation and testing. If a bite was caused by a healthy dog or cat, the animal can be confined and observed for 10 days. Prophylaxis is not required if the animal remains healthy although any illness during the designated period requires evaluation by a veterinary sur-

geon. Treatment for bite victims in animals that are not available for testing or the rabies immunization status of the animal is not known, includes aggressive wound cleansing, administration of human rabies immunoglobulin and a five dose course of rabies vaccine.

7. Summarising Key Points

(1) All bite wounds are potentially serious injuries and patients are at risk for significant complications.
(2) A detailed history and examination of the bite injury is critical. Particular attention should be paid to clenched fist injuries and potential deep space infections.
(3) The cornerstone of management in established hand bite injuries is thorough toilet, elevation and IV antibiotics. Wound exploration and debridement may also be necessary.
(4) Antibiotic therapy should be directed against the most common pathogens initially and altered accordingly with culture and sensitivities.
(5) Clinicians should have a low threshold for surgical intervention particularly in those patients that fail to respond to earlier measures.

References

[1] Sournia JC. The Illustrated History of Medicine. London: Harold Starke, 1992: 59- 94.
[2] Gahhos FN, Ariyan S. Hippocrates, the true father of hand surgery. Surg Gynecol Obstet 1985;160:178-184.
[3] Kanavel AB. Infections of the hand. A guide to the surgical treatment of acute and chronic suppurative processes in the fingers, hand, and forearm. 7th ed. Philadelphia: Lea and Febiger, 1939.
[4] Kanavel AB. An anatomical, experimental, and clinical study of acute phlegmons of the hand. Surg Gynecol Obstet 1905;1:221-260.
[5] Mason ML, Koch SL. Human bite infections of the hand. Surg Gynecol Obstet 1930;51:591-625.
[6] Hultgen JF. Partial gangrene of the left index finger caused by the symbiosis of the fusiform Bacillus and the spirochaeta Denticola. JAMA 1910;10:857.
[7] Peters WH. Hand Infection apparently due to Bacillus fusiformis. J Infect Dis 1911;8:455-462.
[8] Fleming A. On antibacterial action of cultures of penicillium, with special reference to their use in isolation of B. influenzae. British Journal of Experimental Pathology 1929;10:226-236.
[9] Gauchi PA, Eriksson E. Diabetes mellitus and wound healing. In Kahn CR, Weir GC (eds): Joslin's Diabetes Mellitus. 14th ed. Philadelphia: Lippincott Williams and Wilkins, 2005:1133-1144.
[10] Taplitz RA. Managing bite wounds. Postgraduate Medicine 2004; 116:49-52.
[11] Marr JS, Beck AM, Lugo JA. An epidemiological study of the human bite. Public Health Rep 1979;94:514-521.
[12] Mann RJ, Hoffeld TA, Farmer CB. Human bites of the hand: Twenty years of experience. J Hand Surg Am 1977;2:97-104.

[13] Chuinard RG, D'Ambrosia RD. Human bite infections of the hand. J Bone Joint Surg Am 1977;59:416-418.

[14] Epstein JB, Scully C. Mammalian bites: Risk and management. Am J Dentistry 1992;5:161-167.

[15] Bunzli WF, Wright DH, Hoang AT, Dahms RD et al. Current management of human bites. Pharmacotherapy 1998;18:227-234.

[16] Brook I. Management of human and animal bite wounds: An overview. Advances in Skin & Wound Care 2005;18:197-203.

[17] Shields C, Patzakis MJ, Myers MH, Harvey JP Jr: Hand infections secondary to human bites. J Trauma 1975;15:235-236.

[18] Talan DA, Abrahamian FM, Moran GJ, Citron DM et al. Clinical presentation and bacteriologic analysis of infected human bites in patients presenting to emergency departments. Clin Infect Dis 2003;37:1481-1489.

[19] Barnes MN, Bibby BF. A summary of reports and a bacteriologic study of infections caused by human tooth wounds. J Am Dent Assoc 1939;26:1163-x.

[20] Riggs L. Medical-legal problems in the emergency department related to hand injuries. Emerg med Clin NA 1985; 3: 415-418.

[21] Vidmar L, Poljak M, Tomazic J, Seme K et al. Tranmission of HIV-1 by human bite. Lancet 1996;347:1762-1763.

[22] Talan DA, Citron DM, Abrahamian FM, Moran GJ et al. Bacteriologic analysis of infected dog and cat bites. N Eng J Med 1999;340:85-92.

[23] Long WT, Filler BC, Cox E II, Stark HH. Toxic shock syndrome after a human bite to the hand. J Hand Surg Am 1988;13:957-959.

[24] Benson LS, Edwards SL, Schiff AP, Williams CS et al. Dog and cat bites to the hand: Treatment and cost assessment. J Hand Surg Am 2006;31:468-473.

[25] Arons MS, Fernando L, Polayes IM. Pasteurella multocida - The major cause of hand infections following domestic animal bites. J Hand Surg Am 1982;7:47-51.

Deep Space Infections of the Hand and Wrist

Zoe H. DAILIANA*, Nikolaos RIGOPOULOS, Sokratis E. VARITIMIDIS, Konstantinos N. MALIZOS

Department of Orthopaedic Surgery and Musculoskeletal Trauma,
University of Thessalia, Larissa, Greece

Suppurative conditions of the closed spaces and compartments of the hand and wrist result in a "vicious circle", where the septic inflammatory reaction leads to pressure elevation that decreases soft tissue perfusion and facilitates expansion of the infection. The functional outcome of deep space hand and wrist infections is directly related to i) the virulence of the infecting pathogen, ii) the competence of the immune defense of the host, iii) the delay in diagnosis and initiation of treatment, and iv) the effectiveness of the applied treatment. When therapeutic intervention is delayed, the infection contiguously extends to the adjacent compartments, and the function of the hand becomes permanently impaired if the involved deep spaces are inadequately drained.

Keywords: closed deep space; compartment; dissemination; hand; infection; purulent.

1. INTRODUCTION

The ability to perform the activities of daily living is based on the complex organization of the anatomical structures of the hand and wrist. An apparent or even occult breakage of the protective mechanical barriers of the hand against bacteria during the daily activities, may subsequently lead to infection. The delicate arrangement of the anatomical elements of the hand and wrist in closed spaces and compartments predisposes to rapid dissemination of the infection and the inflammatory reaction. From the early 20th century the anatomy of the hand has been related to the patterns of hand infections [1].

Infections in closed deep spaces, cavities and compartments of the hand, although well recognized, are often misdiagnosed. In case of delayed

*Corresponding Author
Department of Orthopaedic Surgery and Musculoskeletal Trauma,
School of Health Sciences, University of Thessalia
22 Papakiriazi St., Larissa 41222, Greece
Tel: + 30 2410 682722
Fax: + 30 2410 670107
e-mail: dailiana@med.uth.gr

diagnosis and inadequate management, deep space infections may result in significant loss of hand function. A detailed knowledge of the anatomy and the particular communications between hand and wrist compartments is crucial for the early diagnosis, assessment of the severity and prompt treatment of every infectious condition [1, 2].

2. COMPARTMENTS AND DEEP SPACES OF THE HAND AND WRIST

The retinaculum cutis delineates fibrous compartments for vessels, nerves and tendons and consists of the palmar fascia, the natatory ligament and the dorsal paratendinous cutaneous system. These fibrous structures divide the hand and the wrist into closed cavities known as compartments.

In the digits the tendons are enclosed in fibro-osseous tunnels. The **tendon sheaths** consist of two layers: the inner synovial layer, surrounding the tendon as a "glove" and the outer layer, enclosing the former one. Between these two layers, there is a narrow space containing a small volume of serous fluid, which promotes nutrition and gliding of the tendon. The thumb and little finger sheaths are very frequently in continuity with the radial and ulnar bursae that extend proximally in the palm, the carpal tunnel and the distal forearm. The ***fingertip pulps*** are separated by vertical septae (from the periosteum to the skin) in small noncompliant compartments containing sweat glands and fat globules.

In the hand the compartments have been classically grouped into the ***thenar, hypothenar, adductor*** and the ***4 interossei compartments.*** However, in the aforementioned description, subcompartmentalization of the muscle groups is often observed [2]. Apart from the compartments containing muscles, several spaces (tunnels or cavities) are enclosed in fibrous sheaths and are separated by vertical septae, that anchor the dermis to the underlying palmar fascia, muscle and bone and act as barriers to the horizontal spread of an infectious condition. Thus, between the thenar and hypothenar compartments and overlying respective spaces, the ***midpalmar space*** is located deep to the palmar aponeurosis and the flexor tendons of the long, ring and little fingers and superficial to the 3rd-5th metacarpals. On the dorsum of the hand, the ***subaponeurotic extensor tendon space*** is located between the metacarpals-interossei and the extensor tendons with their interconnections. Finally, the ***web spaces*** (2nd, 3rd, 4th) are also semi-closed spaces of the hand, delineated by the dorsal fascia and skin, the extensor mechanisms and the MCP joint capsules, proximally limited by the vertical septae of the palmar aponeurosis.

In the wrist and the proximal forearm, two more spaces are recognized: the ***carpal tunnel*** and the ***space of Parona.*** The latter is located between the pronator quadratus muscle and the flexor digitorum profundus tendons.

3. The Double Mechanism: Compartment Syndrome and Infection

The communications between the closed spaces and compartments of the hand facilitate the spread of infections. In the palmar aspect of the hand vertical septae not only anchor the dermis to the underlying tissues, but also act as barriers to the horizontal spread of infections. Thus, expanding infections follow the path of least resistance into the adjacent spaces.

A fingertip infection [***felon***] may spread proximally into the tendon sheath. The same is true for the tendon sheath infections [***pululent flexor tenosynovitis***] that may expand proximally to the hand and the wrist. Purulent tenosynovitis of the index finger may also spread into the ***thenar space,*** whereas tenosynovitis of the middle and ring finger may involve the ***midpalmar space*** and more proximally the ***carpal tunnel*** and the ***space of Parona.*** Finally, tenosynovitis of the thumb and the little finger may extend to the radial and ulnar bursae and the space of Parona [3, 4].

Infections into closed cavities or tunnels result in the accumulation of exudates or pus and the establishment of high pressures within the compartments. This may subsequently lead to reduction of blood flow, regional anoxia and tissue hypo-perfusion with a deficient immune response and failure of the antibiotics to concentrate in tissues contained. A double pathophysiologic pathway is established: i) the "vicious circle" of infection within the closed space: infection compromises the soft tissue perfusion and subsequently, ischemia inhibits the local immune response; and ii) the elevation of tissue pressure within the compartment/closed space leads to expansion of the ischemic zone which facilitates infection dissemination, and further enhances its catastrophic result [1-3, 5].

Schnall et al. [6] associated the compartment syndrome with infection in the upper extremity and reported four such cases in 1994, although only sporadic cases of infections mimicking a compartment syndrome have been reported since 1984 [7]. In 1996, the tissue pressure was recorded in a series of 14 patients suffering from pyogenic flexor tenosynovitis and found to range between 20 and 73 mm Hg [5]. According to Matsen, increased pressure within any closed space (not necessarily a compartment surrounded by fascia) may be as detrimental as a compartment syndrome [8]. The application of these observations to the closed spaces of the hand must alert physicians to the escalating risk of a "vicious circle" initiating from a closed space infection. The elevated pressure and the infectious exudates lead to deficiency of the microcirculation and local immune response, which aggravates and further expands the initial compartmental infection, with catastrophic consequences on the hand anatomy [1-3, 5]. Delay in diagnosis and therapeutic intervention of an initially local infection leads to dissemination, facilitated by the unrestricted motion of the adjacent anatomical structures and a limited capacity of the involved anatomical spaces.

4. Sites

The most common site of trauma and subsequent infection is the distal phalange of the index and of the middle finger of the dominant hand, followed by the thumb, which indicates that the most vulnerable fingers are those contributing to good motor activity [9, 10]. Usually, the initial injuries of the fingers and the palm are minor and thus, underestimated by the patients and the primary care physicians, leading to considerable delay in seeking medical advice and referring these patients.

5. Clinical Signs and Symptoms

Due to the deep location of closed space infections of the hand, the typical signs of an infection are often absent, while hand edema may camouflage the presence

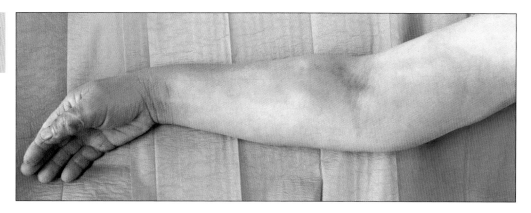

FIGURE 1. Thumb infection with signs of proximal extension (lymphangiitis).

of an abscess. In general, patients present with throbbing pain, swelling and restricted finger motion. Lymphangiitis may be noted occasionally, but systemic signs of infection are usually absent (Fig. 1). It has been shown that neither the severity of infection nor the response to treatment is related to the initial temperature or the WBC count [11].

5.1. Felon

This abscess of the fingertip pulp results in a painful, swollen, red and tense pulp (Fig. 2) that may rapidly become necrotic (Fig. 3). Patients present with rapid onset of severe, throbbing pain. These infections may expand to the distal phalange or to the flexor tendon sheaths (Fig. 4).

5.2. Pyogenic flexor tenosynovitis

Infections inside the osteo-fibrous tunnels of the flexor tendons rapidly expand along the tunnel and often include proximal regions, such as the radial or ulnar bursae, the thenar, midpalmar or Parona's spaces. These

infections are usually the result of direct penetration of the sheath, but expansion from a felon of the distal phalange is also possible. Patients usually present with 2 or more of the 4 typical clinical signs of Kanavel: tenderness

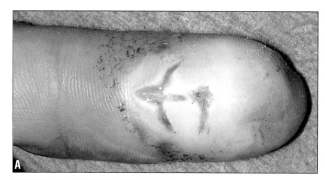

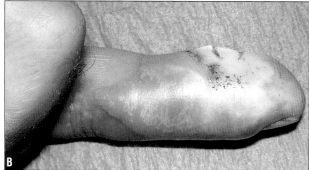

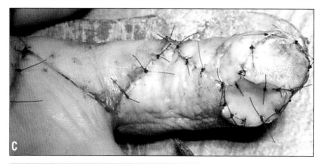

FIGURE 3. Inadequately treated felon with a cross-type incision in a general practitioner's office **(A, B)** resulting in distal phalange amputation and necessitating coverage with an homodigital flap **(C)**.

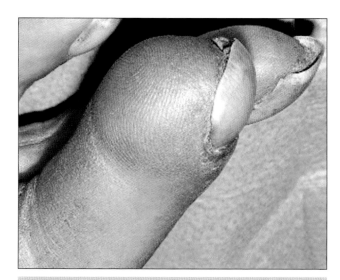

FIGURE 2. Middle finger felon in a farmer.

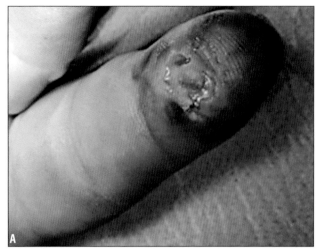

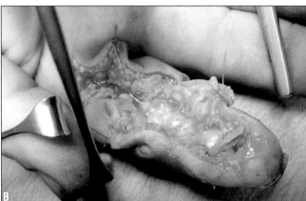

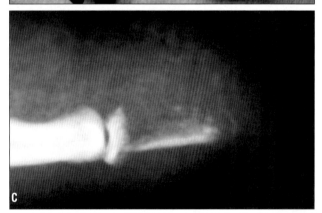

FIGURE 4. Felon after a neglected crush injury of the index finger **(A)** extending to the flexor tendon sheath **(B)** and causing osteomyelitis of the distal phalange **(C).**

along the tendon sheath, finger swelling, semi-flexed position of the finger and painful extension (Fig. 5).

5.3. Thenar space and compartment infections

Infections of the thenar space are often the result of expansion from the adjacent spaces, such as the midpalmar space, and the thumb or index tenosynovial sheath. Apart from painful swelling of the thenar region (Fig. 6) and sometimes the first web space, thumb motion is painful and limited.

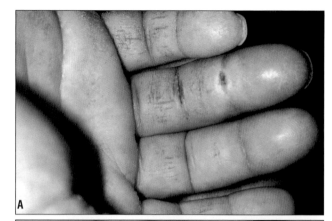

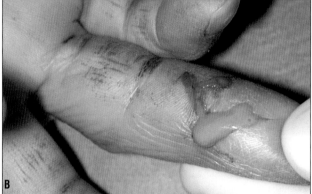

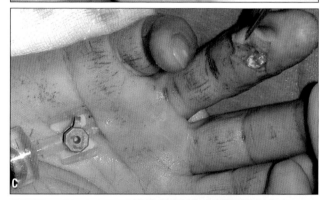

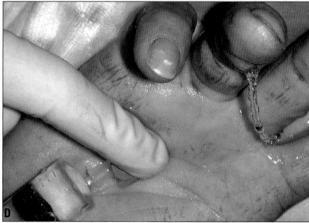

FIGURE 5. Purulent flexor tenosynovitis of the ring finger in a farmer **(A).** Mini-open approach and drainage through incisions at the level of the A1 and A5 pulleys **(B)** and intraoperative irrigation **(C, D).**

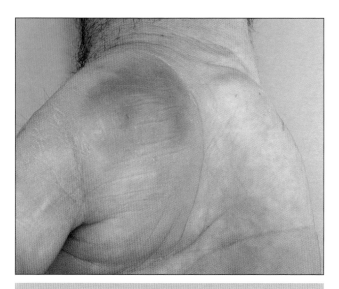

FIGURE 6. Thenar space infection.

5.4. Adductor compartment infections

Although the adductor pollicis muscle may be part of the thenar compartment, it is reported to be a separate compartment in 71% of the dissections performed in an anatomic study of the compartments of the hand [3]. These infections may extend to the thenar compartment and space and also to the dorsum of the hand and the first web space (Fig. 7).

5.5. Midpalmar space infections

The midpalmar space is often infected as a result of pyogenic tenosynovitis of the long and ring fingers. The swelling and erythema is usually located in the palm, whereas painful motion of the long and ring fingers is the most prominent clinical finding.

5.6. Hypothenar space and compartment infections

These infections present with painful swelling of the hypothenar eminence and inability to abduct and oppose the small finger (Fig. 8).

5.7. Web space infections

Infections classically spread dorsally into the dorsal subcutaneous web space resulting in collar-button (hour-glass) abscesses (Fig. 9). Patients present with painful swelling of the web space and distal palmar region. The web space is extremely tender, and in the case of large accumulations, the neighbouring fingers are abducted.

5.8. Subaponeurotic extensor tendon space infections

Infections in the closed space between the metacarpals-interossei and the extensor tendons usually present with swelling and erythema of the dorsum of the hand. Pal-

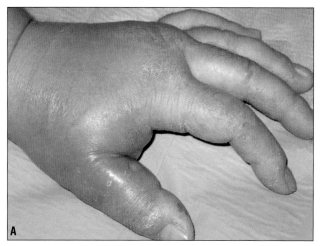

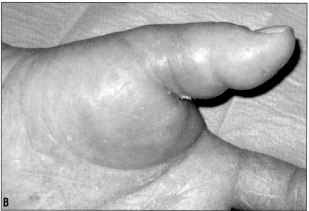

FIGURE 7. Neglected purulent flexor tenosynovitis of the thumb extending to the thenar **(A)** and adductor compartments **(B)**.

pation reveals tenderness and warmth, while finger extension is limited and painful.

5.9. Carpal tunnel and Parona's space infections

These infections are usually the result of a proximal extension of a midpalmar space or a radial or ulnar bursa infection. Swelling, tenderness, warmth and erythema are usually obvious at the distal palmar aspect of the forearm, while wrist and digital flexion is painful or even absent.

6. UNDERLYING CONDITIONS AND AGGRAVATING FACTORS

Apart from the type of injury (penetration, human or animal bite, injection injury) and the causative micro-organism (e.g. organisms that cause necrotizing fasciitis), several factors may have a negative impact on the clinical course of deep space infections and may aggravate its course and worsen the prognosis [1, 4]:

Patients with **diabetes mellitus** are susceptible to

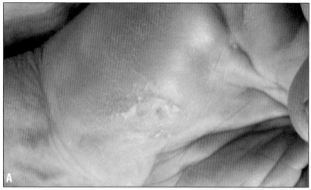

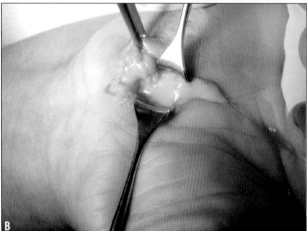

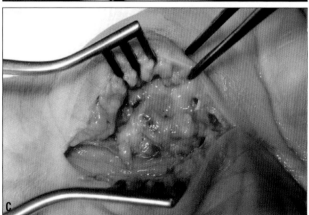

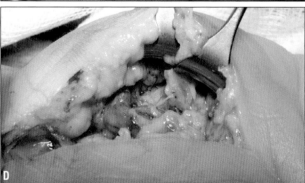

FIGURE 8. Hypothenar space infection **(A)**, was treated with drainage **(B)** and debridement of the hypothenar space **(C, D)**. Debridement was performed with respect to the neighbouring ulnar artery and nerve **(C)**.

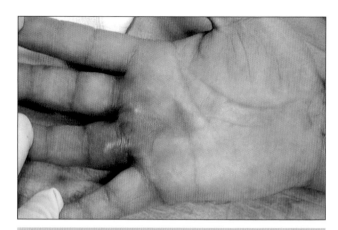

FIGURE 9. Web spaces infection.

more severe infections, usually polymicrobial (involving gram-positive, gram-negative and anaerobic bacteria), most often requiring surgical debridement [12]. *Immunocompromised patients* are susceptible to opportunistic infections [3]. *Intravenous drug users* usually suffer from severe polymicrobial infections, with most of the organisms being common oral or skin flora [13]. *Exposure to tropical fish and acquaria* may predispose to mycobacterium marinum infections [14]. *Special occupational groups* (e.g. meat and poultry handlers) are more exposed to and vulnerable to streptococcal or staphylococcal infections [15-17]. *Exposure to sexually transmitted diseases* (e.g. *Neisseria gonorrheae*) may also lead to deep space infections [3, 18]. Failure to acknowledge the polymicrobial or specific nature of the aforementioned hand infections is a frequent cause of a poor outcome. Finally, *delayed treatment,* as a result of patients' negligence or inadequate initial assessment of the severity and extent of infection from the primary care physicians and *inadequate management* are factors compromising the prognosis [19]. Several authors reported an average delay of 8 days after apparent inoculation resulting in complication rates as high as 50% [11, 19, 20].

7. Diagnostic Approach

The diagnostic approach includes a complete laboratory testing (complete blood count, ESR, CRP) and imaging studies. Radiographs will rule out skeletal involvement or foreign bodies (see Fig. 4c), while ultrasound is very helpful for the detection of deep space collections and changes of the dimensions of the tendons [21, 22].

Multiple culture samples (for common bacteria, mycobacteria and fungi) must be obtained before the administration of antibiotics and should be directed to the Microbiology laboratory without delay, for Gram staining, antibiotic resistance phenotypes, detection of the mec A gene, and molecular typing of the isolates.

8. CAUSATIVE MICRO-ORGANISMS

Multiple organisms have been isolated in the majority of cases, in several series of hand infections reported in the literature. Polymicrobial infections and mixed aerobic and anaerobic flora is the rule rather than the exception. Infections with two or more bacteria may occur in more than 50% of cases, whereas anaerobic infections, alone or in combination with aerobic bacteria have been reported to occur in almost 30% of patients [20].

Polymicrobial and mixed infections must be suspected in immunocompromised patients, patients with diabetes mellitus, intravenous use of drugs [3] and in human bite injuries, which present the highest incidence of polymicrobial flora [11]. It must be underscored that the presence of either anaerobes or *Eikenella corrodens* or both has been significantly associated with poor results [11].

Staphylococcus aureus and beta-hemolytic streptococci grew in 50-78% of infection cultures reported in the literature [1, 10, 11, 19]. In general, Gram-positive aerobes were the most common organisms cultured, followed by Gram-negative anaerobes, Gram-negative enterics, Gram-positive anaerobes and Gram-negative aerobes [19]. Atypical infections (fungal, mycobacterial, viral and *Neisseria gonorrheae*) requiring special cultures must be also considered, especially in the immunocompromised patients [4].

Relatively high rates of false negative cultures of 20-30% and up to 55% [9] have been reported in most series. Negative cultures can be partially attributed to the empirical antibiotic oral therapy that many patients receive prior to their admission and culture sampling, to the failure to request specific cultures, and to the poor handling of samples.

9. DIFFERENTIAL DIAGNOSIS

Several non-infectious conditions may mimic a closed space infection of the hand: foreign body reactions, crystalline deposition disease (gout, pseudogout) (Fig. 10), pyogenic granuloma, acute calcium deposition, acute non-specific flexor tenosynovitis, injection injuries, calcific tendinitis, and even tumors [3].

10. TREATMENT

A hand infection diagnosed early can initially be treated conservatively, with rest, elevation of the hand and iv broad-spectrum antibiotics, taking into account the pathway of inoculation, the degree of environmental contamination where the initial injury occurred and the underlying general health status of the host. However, in deep space hand infections, apart from

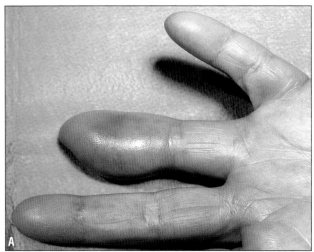
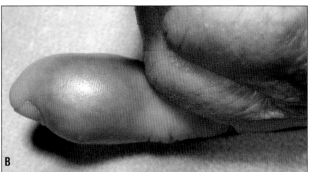
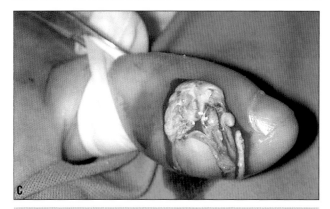

FIGURE 10. In contrast to the clinical signs of a ring finger infection **(A, B),** the intraoperative findings revealed a crystalline deposition disease **(C).**

antibiotic coverage and immobilization with hand elevation, surgical incision and drainage of all potentially communicating spaces and compartments is the cornerstone of successful treatment.

10.1. Antibiotics

The chemotherapeutic agents initially selected should be at least effective against a wide spectrum of Gram-positive cocci, whereas antibiotics acting against Gram-negative or anaerobic bacteria are necessary in crush injuries and wounds occurring in heavily contaminated environments suspicious for anaerobic flora (soil, human bite injuries), as well as in special patient groups, including immunocompromised patients, those suffering from diabetes mellitus or intravenous drug users [3, 4, 12, 13, 19, 23]. Inappropriate antibiotic selection is one cause of failure in the treatment of hand infections. Failure to definitively treat all offending organisms may leave a residual infection that results in recrudescence, further tissue destruction, and subsequent permanent disability [20].

Empirical therapy with broad-spectrum intravenous antibiotics must be administered immediately after obtaining three or more culture samples in the operating room (for common bacteria, mycobacteria and fungi). According to relevant data published in the last two decades, staphylococci are emerging once again as a serious problem, especially in the community. Thus, the choice of the appropriate antimicrobial agent is of great importance for the defense against community acquired staphylococcal infections [19, 24-28]. The usual choice for single antibiotic coverage is a ***penicillinase-resistant penicillin derivative,*** which is, however, ineffective for many anaerobes (*Eikenella corrodens* and *Pasteurella multocida*) and other "uncommon" organisms. In addition, the PVL-positive staphylococci contain genetic elements encoding resistance to different antibiotics (oxacillin, fucidic acid, tetracycline, kanamycin) and produce the Panton-Valentine leucocidin that destroys neutrophils, resulting in characteristic purulent ulcers [29]. ***Penicillin G*** is the drug of choice for human oral flora and anaerobic infection [20]. The 1st generation ***cephalosporins*** are the ideal choice as they provide coverage for Gram-positive aerobic and Gram-negative enteric bacteria. In many countries, however, 1st generation cephalosporins are not available and hterefore, 2nd generation cephalosporins are used. Finally, ***clindamycin,*** a common choice for anaerobes and gram-positive cocci (including PVL-positive staphylococci), is ineffective for *Eikenella corrodens* and is also bacteriostatic rather than bacteriocidal [20].

Thus, empirical therapy should include penicillin G or clindamycin and either an antistaphylococcal penicillin or a 2nd generation cephalosporin, until sensitivities are obtained. Coverage for gram-negative and anaerobes is recommended for infection occurring in immunocompromised patients, patients with diabetes mellitus, intravenous drug users and individuals with a history of human bite [3, 19, 30].

The antibiotic regimen is modified according to the wound culture results. The duration of antibiotic administration is based on the intensity of the inflammatory reaction of the wound, the resolution of the infection and the underlying conditions of the host. In general, appropriate parenteral antibiotic therapy (according to susceptibility tests) should be continued for at least 24-48 hours, followed by comparable oral antibiotic therapy for 5 to14 days [3].

10.2. Surgical treatment

The formation of an abscess, which may subsequently evolve in a compartment syndrome, needs surgical drainage of all infected hand/wrist compartments by trained hand surgeons, supplemented by copious intraoperative and adequate postoperative irrigation. Intraoperative inspection of neighbouring compartments for insidious signs of infection and administration of the appropriate antibiotics according to the special characteristics of the infecting pathogens are of critical importance to obtain a satisfactory functional outcome. Failure to acknowledge the polymicrobial nature of hand infections, as well as inadequate surgical debridement, are the factors most frequently correlated with poor outcomes [20]. In patients with diabetes mellitus or the immunocompromised ones, delay in surgical management may be catastrophic for their hands and even threatening to their lives.

Surgical drainage must be performed under regional anaesthesia in the operating room for optimal conditions instead of a limited procedure in the emergency room [20]. Incision and drainage may be performed through either a limited approach (see Fig. 5b, c) or a wide zigzag approach, allowing recognition and protection of the neurovascular bundles [30], and thorough surgical exploration to ensure drainage of the infected spaces and debridement of all necrotic tissues (see Fig. 8b-d). All nonviable necrotic tissue, slough and purulence must be removed and granulations must be curetted, so as to leave well-perfused tissues, with normal humoral and cellular immune response that antibiotics may penetrate adequately [20]. Multiple culture samples must be obtained intraoperatively, as the definitive operating room cultures usually have the greatest number of organisms recovered [11].

Extensive intraoperative irrigation is indicated in all deep space infections followed by postoperative continuous sheath irrigation, necessary in cases of purulent tenosynovitis and other closed space infections [31, 32] (see Fig. 5b-d). The irrigation system must be flashed every 6 hours postoperatively and must be continuously observed by experienced nursing staff.

Postoperatively, a soft dressing is applied and the hand is splinted in a resting position. Early active mobilization of fingers, after removal of the irrigating catheters leads to superior functional results [5, 31, 32]. Although supervised rehabilitation and hand therapy contributes to a better outcome, certain population groups may have limitations or difficulties in accessing rehabilitation services after discharge from the Hand Unit.

11. Authors' Experience

The authors have assessed the outcome of compartmental hand and wrist infections in relation to the infecting pathogen, the delay in diagnosis and the method of treatment. During a period of 5 years, in a rural region with approximately 1,500,000 inhabitants, 668 patients with hand/wrist infections presented in the Emergency Care Unit (ECU was on duty 125 full days per year). Fifty-eight patients (38 males, 20 females) suffering from 59 compartmental infections were admitted for surgical treatment. Most infections (n=49) were limited in one compartment, whereas in 10 cases, 2 or more compartments were involved. The majority of these infections originated from or extended to the flexor tendon sheath (see Figs. 4 & 7).

Two patients had diabetes mellitus, while two other patients were under immunosuppression. The majority of patients (30) had a minor trauma in a contaminated environment (agricultural and animal care workers etc). Thirty of the 58 patients were on antibiotics with empiric coverage, and were referred to our centre with a delay of more than 10 days. All patients were treated with drainage, debridement of necrotic tissues and intra-operative irrigation. Post-operative continuous sheath irrigation was performed in cases of purulent tenosynovitis. Appropriate antibiotics were administered after 3 or more culture samples had been obtained intraoperatively. The initial empirical treatment with intravenous (iv) antibiotics (second generation cephalosporin or clindamycin in combination with aminoglycosides and addition of penicillin in selected cases) were modified later according to culture and susceptibility tests. After the initial intravenous antibiotic administration (minimum of 2 days), and according to the initial response, antimicrobial agents were administered orally for a mean period of 5 more days (range: 4-7 days). Passive motion exercises were initiated on the third postoperative day, at patient's tolerance, after removal of the irrigation catheters.

The eradication of the infection, the final ROM, the restoration of strength and sensation of the hand, and the DASH score determined the outcome and were correlated with factors such as the infecting pathogen, the delay in diagnosis and the method of treatment [33, 34]. The mean hospitalization period was 7.2 days (range: 3-18 days). Intra-operative cultures were false negative in one third of the cases (n=20), and in the majority of positive cultures, *Staphylococcus aureus* was detected (29 of 39 positive cultures). In 11 cases, Methicillin-Resistant Staphylococcus aureus isolates (MRSA) were positive for the PVL gene [24-26]. Proximal extension of the infection was observed in 17% of patients. Re-operation and/or re-admission were necessary in 16 out of 58 patients (27.5%). Twelve of these 16 patients with recurrence had received the initial treatment with a mean delay of 14 days from the onset of symptoms.

The mean follow-up period was 30.2 months (range: 6-58 months); at their latest examination (and after re-operations) results were excellent in the majority of cases (n=49). Poor results included 2 arthrodeses, 2 amputations at the level of the distal phalange (see Fig. 3c) and limited ROM due to adhesions in 2 hands. The DASH score was 10.55 (range: 0.0-44.44) and all patients returned to their previous occupations and activities after 6-12 weeks. There was a significant association between the DASH score and the type of infecting bacteria (p=0.04), which was worse in the case of PVL(+) staphylococci. Also, there was a significant association among hand and wrist active ROM and the multiple compartmental involvement (p=0.01), as well as the infection with PVL(+) staphylococcus (p=0.03).

12. CONCLUSIONS

Infections in closed deep spaces, cavities and compartments of the hand are often initially misdiagnosed. Knowledge of the anatomy and particular communications of hand and wrist compartments as the *fingertip pulps, tendon sheaths, thenar and hypothenar compartments and spaces, midpalmar space, adductor compartment, interossei compartments, web spaces, subaponeurotic extensor tendon space, carpal tunnel,* and the *Parona's space,* is crucial for early diagnosis and prompt treatment of these rapidly expanding conditions. In the palmar aspect of the hand, vertical septae act as barriers to the horizontal spread of infections and thus, expanding infections follow the path of least resistance.

Infections in closed cavities or tunnels result in the accumulation of exudates or pus and the establishment of high pressures within the compartments, and may lead to reduction of blood flow, regional anoxia, tissue hypo-perfusion, deficient immune response and failure of antibiotics to concentrate to target tissues. Due to the deep location of closed space infections of the hand, the typical signs of infections are often absent while the hand edema may camouflage the presence of an abscess. In general, patients present with throbbing pain, swelling and restricted finger motion. Prognosis is aggravated in several groups of patients, such as immunocompromised patients, intravenous drug users, those suffering from diabetes mellitus, and patients receiving inadequate or delayed treatment. In some of the aforementioned groups of patients, polymicrobial and mixed aerobic and anaerobic infections must be suspected. Surgical drainage of all infected compartments, supplemented by intraoperative and adequate postoperative irrigation, and administration of antibiotics appropriate for the special characteristics of the infecting pathogens are key steps towards obtaining a satisfactory functional outcome and preventing further tissue damage.

The selected antibiotics must at least be effective against a wide spectrum of Gram-positive cocci, whereas antibiotics acting against Gram-negative or anaerobic bacteria may be necessary in crush injuries, heavily contaminated wounds occurring in environments suspicious for anaerobic flora, immunocompromised patients, those suffering from diabetes mellitus and intravenous drug users. Empirical therapy with broad-spectrum intravenous antibiotics should be administered immediately after obtaining three or more samples for culture. Negligence or delayed management may lead to permanent loss of function of the hand.

REFERENCES

[1] Kanavel AB. Infections of the hand: a guide to the surgical treatment of acute and chronic suppurative processes in the fingers, hand and forearm. Philadelphia New York, Lea & Febiger, 1912.

[2] DiFelice A, Seiler JG III, Whitesides TE. The compartments of the hand: an anatomic Study. J Hand Surg 1998;23A:689-96.

[3] Clark DC. Common acute hand infections. Amer Family Physician 2003;68:2167-76.

[4] Spann M, Talmor M, Nolan W.B. Hand infections: Basic principles and management. Surg Inf 2004; 5:210-220.

[5] Schnall SB, Vu-Rose T, Holtom PD, Doyle B, Stevanovic M. Tissue pressures in pyogenic flexor tenosynovitis of the finger. J Bone Joint Surg 1996;78B:793-5.

[6] Schnall SB, Holtom PD, Silva E. Compartment syndrome associated with infection of the upper extremity. Clin Orthop 1994;306:128-131.

[7] Bohn WW, Coleman CR. Streptococcal gangrene mimicking a compartment syndrome. A case report. J Bone Joint Surg 1985;67A:1125-26.

[8] Gaspard DJ, Kohl RD Jr. Compartmental syndromes in which the skin is the limiting boundary. Clin Orthop 1975;113:65-8.

[9] Phipps AR, Blanshard J. A review of in-patient hand infections. Arch Emerg Med 1992;9(3):299-305.

[10] Stevenson J, Anderson IW. Hand infections: an audit of 160 infections treated in an accident and emergency department. J Hand Surg [Br] 1993;18 (1):115-8.

[11] Dellinger EP, Wertz MJ, Miller SD, Coyle MB. Hand infections. Bacteriology and treatment: a prospective study. Arch Surg 1988;123 (6):745-50.

[12] Kour AK, Looi KP, Phone MH, Pho RW. Hand infections in patients with diabetes. Clin Orthop 1996;331:238-44.

[13] Gonzalez MH, Garst J, Nourbash P, Pulvirenti J, Hall RF Jr. Abscesses of the upper extremity from drug abuse by injection. J Hand Surg [Am] 1993;18 (5):868-70.

[14] Bhatty MA, Turner DP, Chamberlain ST. Mycobacterium marinum hand infection: case reports and review of literature. Br J Plast Surg 2000;53(2):161-5.

[15] Barnham M, Kerby J. A profile of skin sepsis in meat handlers. J Infect 1984;9(1):43-50.

[16] Fehrs LJ et al. Group A beta-hemolytic streptococcal skin infections in a US meat-packing plant. JAMA 1987;258:3131-4.

[17] McCarthy GM, Britton JE, John MA. Occupational injuries and infection control. Acad Med 1999;74:464-5.

[18] Gomperts BN, White LK. Gonococcal hand abscess. Pediatr Infect Dis J 2000;19:671-2.

[19] Weinzweig N, Gonzalez M. Surgical infections of the Hand and Upper Extremity: A County Hospital Experience. Ann Plast Surg 2002; 49:621-7.

[20] Spiegel JD, Szabo RM. A protocol for the treatment of severe infections of the hand. J Hand Surg [Am] 1988;13(2):254-9.

[21] Schecter WP, Markison RE, Jeffrey RB, Barton RM, Laing F. Use of sonography in the early detection of suppurative flexor tenosynovitis. J Hand Surg [Am] 1989;14:307-10.

[22] Chau CL, Griffith JF. Musculoskeletal infections: ultrasound appearances. Clin Radiol 2005;60(2):149-59.

[23] Brook I. Management of human and animal bite wounds: an overview. Adv Skin Wound Care 2005;18:197-203.

[24] Deresinski D. Methicillin Resistant Staphylococcus Aureus: An Evolutionary, Epidemiologic and Therapeutic Odyssey. Clin Infect Dis 2005;40:562-73.

[25] Petinaki E, Kontos F, Miriagou V, Maniati M, Hatzi F, Maniatis AN. Survey of methicillin-resistant coagulase-negative staphylococci in the hospitals of central Greece. Int J Antimicrob Agents 2001;18:563-6.

[26] Karanas YL, Bogdan MA, Chang J. Community acquired methicillin-resistant Staphylococcus aureus hand infections: Case reports and clinical implications. J Hand Surg 2000;25A:760-3.

[27] Connoly B, Johnstone F, Gerlinger T, Puttler E. Methicillin-resistant Staphylococcus aureus in a finger felon. J Hand Surg 2000;25A:173-5.

[28] Maltezou HC, Giamarellou H. Community-acquired methicillin-resistant Staphylococcus aureus infections. Int J Antimicrob Agents 2006;27:87-96.

[29] Chini V, Petinaki E, Foka A, Paratiras S, Dimitracopoulos G, Spiliopoulou I. Spread of Staphylococcus aureus clinical isolates carrying Panton-Valentine leukocidin genes during a three-year period in Greece. Clin Microb Infect 2006;12:29-34.

[30] Jebson PJ. Deep subfascial space infections. Hand Clin 1998;14:557-66.

[31] Harris PA, Nanchahal J. Closed continuous irrigation in the treatment of hand infections. J Hand Surg 1999;24B:328-333.

[32] Gutowski KA, Ochoa O, Adams WP Jr. Closed catheter irrigation is as effective as open drainage for treatment of pyogenic flexor tenosynovitis. Ann Plast Surg 2002;49:350-4.

[33] Strickland JW, Glogovac SV. Digital function following flexor tendon repair in zone II: a comparison of immobilization and controlled passive motion techniques. J Hand Surg 1980;5A:537-4.

[34] Hudak PL, Amadio PC, Bombardier C. Development of an upper extremity outcome measure: the DASH. Am J Ind Med 1996;29:602-8.

Septic Trauma of the Extensor Apparatus

Ioannis X. TSIONOS*, Nikolaos E. GEROSTATHOPOULOS, Ioannis A. IGNATIADIS,
Sarantis G. SPYRIDONOS, Paraskevi A. TZORTZI, Alexandros S. KYRIAKOS

Hand and Upper Extremity Surgery– Microsurgery Unit, KAT General Hospital, Athens, Greece

The bacterial load delivered to the wound during an extensor apparatus traumatism varies among traumas occurring in different environments. Tissue quality, delay in presentation and patient immune competence may influence morbidity from such traumas. Debridement and irrigation are the cornerstones of treatment. Simple trauma to the extensor apparatus does not need prophylactic antibiotic prescription. More complex trauma with fractures of the underlying skeleton and joint penetration may profit from such prophylaxis. Repair of tendon lesions may be undertaken primarily or in a staged fashion. Trauma to the extensor tendons of the hand caused by bites needs special attention, due to its particular anatomy and microbiology. Prophylactic antibiotic prescription is preferred by many physicians. Joint penetration should not be missed, as this increases morbidity. Trauma inflicted in an aquatic environment can be infected by particular germs and this should be considered when the patient's history is suggestive. Finally, atypical infections may result from inoculation of mycobacteria, fungi and some bacterial species widespread in nature. They are characterized by an indolent course and non-responsiveness to classic antibiotic treatment. The initial inoculation incident may have been trivial. These infections should be part of the differential diagnosis in the above setting.

Keywords: extensor tendon; tendon laceration; infection; bites; sepsis.

1. ANATOMIC CONSIDERATIONS

In the dorsum of the hand soft tissues are arranged in thin parallel layers. The extensor tendons are covered on their dorsal aspect by a thin multi-layer semitransparent film called "paratendon" [1]. Beneath the tendon a loose connective tissue space exists, which is called mesotendon. At the meta-carpophalangeal (MCP) joint level, a subtendinous bursa is located between the dorsal joint capsule and the extensor apparatus [2].

The MCP joint is a crossroad of fascial planes. Pus accumulated inside the joint may extend to other spaces in the hand, following routes where the least resistance is encountered. Dorsal extension is possible, as well as palmar, through either the capsule between main and accessory lateral collateral ligaments or through the proximal border of the volar plate [3].

At the finger level, bacterial inoculation superficial to the extensor apparatus can generate an infection with the potential of spreading dorsally, as well as towards the palmar spaces, along the palmar neurovascular bundles or the lumbrical and interosseous tendons [2, 3]. In contrast, infection located under the extensor tendon is more space-limited by the extensor tendon attachments to the side of the phalanges [2].

*Corresponding Author
39 Thyssou Str.
111 42 Athens, Greece
Tel: +30 210 2132248
Mob: +30 6945 132989
e-mail: jtsionos@yahoo.com

2. Mechanism of Contamination, Epidemiology, Microbiology

2.1. General principles

Lesions of the extensor apparatus can be produced by different mechanisms. They range from trivial puncture-type wounds (e.g. by splinters, thorns etc) (Fig. 1), to simple sharp lacerations (e.g. simple knife wounds), to severe trauma with soft tissue and tendon defects and open fractures of the underlying skeleton (e.g. lawn-mower injuries, or crush/gunshot injuries). The bacterial load delivered to tissues originates from the patient's own skin flora and the environment. Local factors (such as tissue quality, vascular perfusion, closed space inoculation), as well as systemic (such as the competence of immune response) also have a great impact on the outcome of such traumas.

The level of contamination of simple hand lacerations, after antiseptic cleansing, is considered very low, approaching the levels reached in elective hand surgery [4].

In complex hand trauma, isolated germs include a variety of gram-positive and gram-negative bacteria (including anaerobes), and occasionally fungi. In injuries occurring during agricultural activities, hand wounds are colonized by gram-negative or mixed gram-positive and gram-negative bacteria and anaerobes, while wounds which occur in a household or in an industrial setting yield mainly gram-positive strains. Fungi and mycobacteria may occasionally contaminate wounds having come in contact with elements of nature. In farm or stable injuries, fecal contamination may result in inoculation of the wound with enterococci and anaerobes, such as clostridia. Anaerobes may also be important contributors when a concomitant vascular injury or extensive devitalization causes inadequate blood perfusion [4-10].

Nevertheless, infection rates after complex hand traumatisms are rather low compared to those of open long bone fractures [8].

2.2. Bite wounds

Bite wounds in the hand show a predilection towards its dorsal aspect (Fig. 2) [3]. Microorganisms implicated in resulting infections come from the skin flora of the victim and the mouth of the aggressor.

2.2.1. Dog bites

Dog bites account for more than 80% of animal bite wounds [11, 12] and frequently occur in young victims, predominantly males [13], while playing with an animal known to them or getting involved with fighting dogs. Roughly speaking, half of them concern the hand and the forearm [11].

Wounds due to a dog bite may be punctures, lacerations, or a combination. Large dogs exert enormous pressures with their jaws, and therefore crushing, avulsion and devitalization of tissues may increase morbidity. An estimated 4% to 25% of dog bites cause infection [12]. Polymicrobial aerobic (42%) and mixed aerobic-anaerobic (48%) infections are commonplace [13].

Pasteurella species (gram-negative aerobic and facultative anaerobic bacteria [14]) are found to participate in 50% of dog bite infections [13, 14]. Streptococcus (46%) and staphylococcus (46%) species follow in close proximity [13]. Other aerobic bacteria include neisseria (16%), corynebacterium (12%), moraxella 10%), enterococcus (10%), EF-4b (10%), bacillus, pseudomonas, actinomyces, escherichia coli, eikenella corrodens, capnocytophaga, and NO-1 [12, 13].

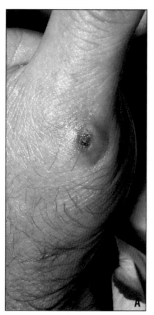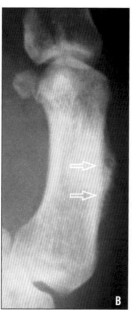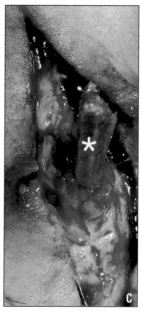

FIGURE 1. (A) Chronic infection (B) with periostitis (arrows) of the 1st metacarpal, caused by a palm thorn. Methicillin-resistant staph. aureus was isolated. (C) Note the intense tissue reaction in the extensor apparatus due to the presence of the thorn.

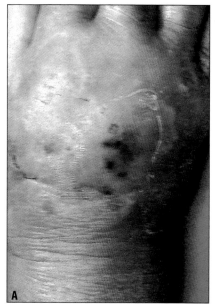
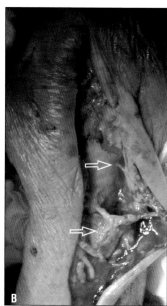

FIGURE 2. **(A)** Infection of the dorsum of the hand following a cat bite. Note the extensive infiltration and necrosis of the subcutaneous tissues [**(B)**-arrows)]. The infection extended superficial to the extensor tendons.

Anaerobic bacteria, such as fusobacterium (32%), bacteroides (30%), porphyromonas (28%), prevotella (28%), propionibacterium (20%), peptostreptococcus (16%) and eubacterium are more frequently isolated from purulent wounds and abscesses [13].

2.2.2. Cat bites
Cats cause 5% of all animal bites in humans [11]. They mostly occur in the elderly, unlike to dog bites, and predominantly in females [13]. Cat bites are considered to be more prone to infection than dog bites (30% - 75% versus 4% - 25%) [12, 15, 16] because the sharp teeth of a cat are usually the cause of puncture wounds, through which bacteria are injected deeply into closed s-paces, even into a joint. Polymicrobial aerobic (32%) or mixed aerobic and anaerobic infections (63%) are a routine [13].

Pasteurella species are very frequently identified (75%) [13]. Streptococcus species come second among aerobes (46%), followed by staphylococcus (35%) and moraxella (35%). Other strains include corynebacterium (28%), neisseria (19%), EF-4b (16%), enterococcus (12%), bacillus (11%), weeksella, capnocytophaga, acinetobacter, NO-1 and pseudomonas [12, 13].

Anaerobes, such as fusobacterium (33%), porphyromonas (30%), bacteroides (28%), prevotella (19%), propionibacterium (18%), peptostreptococcus and fili-factor villosus are among the species cultured [13].

2.2.3. Other animal bites
The animals implicated may be domestic, zoo animals, or animals of the wild nature. The microbiology of such bites is similar to that of cat and dog bites [17]. To the threat of sepsis is sometimes added the destructive nature of bites by animals, such as bears or sharks, the danger of systemic envenomization and toxic effects the

bites of some reptiles, the scorpion or the spider have, or the probability of systemic allergic reactions caused by bee or wasp stings.

2.2.4. Human bites
Human bites may be on the dorsum of the hand, causing "clenched fist injuries", which occur when a person with his hand in clenched-fist position strikes the mouth of another person. Most patients are young males [18], although women of lower social classes may be involved, too [19].

A dreadful reputation has been built up as to the risk of infection from human bites, which may be partly due to selection bias [3, 19-21]. Nevertheless, clenched-fist injuries seem particularly prone to infection, due to their particular anatomy, not microbiology [2, 20]. Most clenched fist injuries are located over the MCP joints of the middle, ring and little finger and some over the MCP joint of the index finger and the proximal interphalangeal (PIP) joints [22]. Lesions produced by teeth in successive soft tissue layers are aligned when the MCP is in flexion, but their relative position is different in extension, sealing the inoculated spaces.

The frequency of deep involvement in such injuries is high. About 16% of injuries situated over the MCP joints and 33% over the PIP joints show extensor tendon lacerations [22]. The frequency of dorsal capsular violation is found to be about 70% in MCP and PIP joints [22]. The invading tooth may cause bony or cartilaginous lesions [22]. Occasionally, a fragmented tooth is found in the joint.

Human bite infections are also polymicrobial with aerobic (44%) or mixed aerobic and anaerobic microorganisms (54%) routinely isolated [18].

In a well-conducted study, it was found that among aerobic isolates streptococcus species prevailed (84%

of cases), followed by staphylococcus species (54%). *Eikenella corrodens* (a facultative anaerobic human mouth flora bacillus) followed with 30%, *haemophilus* with 22% and then *corynobacterium* (12%), *gemella* (12%), *candida, enterobactec cloacae, neisseria, enterococcus, klebsiella* and other [18]. *Prevotella* (36%) and *fusobacterium* (34%) species prevailed among anaerobic isolates, followed by *veillonella* (24%), *peptostreptococcus* (22%), *campulobacter* (16%), *eubacterium* (16%), *actinomyces, lactobacillus, bacteroides* and others.

2.3. Infections caused by marine organisms or occurring in an aquatic environment

Fish spines and bones can cause puncture-type wounds on the dorsum of the hand during fishing or fish handling. A spine may penetrate into deep tissues and even inoculate a joint [11]. Infections may also occur in an aquatic environment (including aquariums) by contamination through a skin break or an overt wound.

Inoculated bacteria reflect the flora of the environment and the patient's skin. *Streptococcus, staphylococcus, pseudomonas* and *enterobacter* species have been isolated from such infected wounds [17]. *Aeromonas* species are aerobic gram-negative bacilli whose natural habitat is fresh water and seawater. Their virulence is augmented by immunosuppression and tissue necrosis. Aeromonas also resides the gut of medicinal leeches and can infect tissues which they are applied to [14]. *Vibrio vulnificus* (a gram-negative bacillus) can infect wounds exposed to contaminated seawater (or sometimes freshwater) or caused by a fish bone or spine [14, 23, 24].

Mycobacterium marinum is a pathogen found in inadequately chlorinated freshwater or saltwater, known for its tendency to produce destructive tenosynovitis of the flexor and less usually of the extensor tendons, as well as osteomyelitis, arthritis and bursitis [6, 7, 14]. It usually causes chronic persistent infections and grows optimally at 30-32°C.

2.4. Atypical infections

Some unusual microorganisms may be traumatically inoculated in the vicinity of the extensor apparatus of the hand and cause infections of the subcutaneous tissue, the tenosynovium or an underlying bone or joint. In this category are included mycobacteria other than tuberculosis (such as the above mentioned *m. marinum,* and the mycobacteria *avium, terrae, malmoense, fortuitum, chelonei, kansasii*), the *nocardia* species and several fungi [6, 7].

Inoculation is usually produced by a trivial traumatism during an occupational activity, or a hobby which brings the victim in contact with elements of the nature, such as plants, thorns, wood splinters, soil, dust, beach sand or water. These infections are generally chronic. Although immunodeficiency favors such infections, some of these microorganisms are also pathogens for healthy subjects.

Although chronic atypical infections are treated elsewhere in this book, it should be noted that they must be part of the differential diagnosis of extensor apparatus infections, on the basis of the clinical presentation and the patient's immune profile.

3. Clinical Presentation

Before signs of infection develop, the main element of the clinical presentation is the trauma itself, being anything from a puncture-type wound to a complex trauma, with fractures and possibly, soft tissue defects. Subjects who suffered seemingly trivial wounds (such as clenched fist injuries, puncture-type cat bites, scratches or punctures from fish spines, thorns etc.) will usually seek care when and if infection develops. Occasionally, the subject may not recall a minor incident of inoculation.

Presence of a foreign body (tooth fragment, fish spine, thorn or wood splinter) (Fig. 1) should be suspected and sought out by appropriate imaging modalities. Osteochondral lesions of the metacarpal head may be visualized by a skyline view [25].

The latency period of a developing infection depends on the local anatomy and the virulence of the offending microorganism(s). For example, in bite wounds it seems to range from 12 to 24 hrs, with infection evolving more rapidly in cat than dog or human bites [13]; it averages 22 hrs in infected human bites, but is shorter in clenched fist injuries. However, *eik. corrodens* grows slowly [26] and inoculated patients may not manifest evidence of infection for more than a week [12].

The infection may present as cellulitis +/- lymphangitis-lymphadenitis, purulent drainage or abscess formation. Pain, swelling and limitation of motion are observed. It can spread via tissue contiguity, through lymph vessels, or hematogenously. It may reach underlying bones (Fig. 1) and also extend to the palmar spaces of the hand. It may follow the fascial planes of the upper extremity (Fig. 2), sometimes resembling necrotizing fasciitis [17].

Systemic signs, such as fever, malaise, and an elevated white blood count and erythrocyte sedimentation rate may be noted. Septicemia and remote inoculation are most often the result of suppression of the immune response or of the presence of artificial implants [14], although it occasionally affects otherwise healthy individuals.

Atypical infections involving the extensor apparatus have a chronic and indolent course, with longer latency periods. Depending on the etiology, special signs may be identified [7]. In mycobacterial infections, masses may be palpated, representing infected subcutaneous tissues and tenosynovium; skin ulceration may develop. Actinomycetomas and eumycetomas show destructive granulomas, with abscess formation, sinuses and fistulas draining granules of the infecting organism. Some fungal infections, such as sporotrichosis, show characteristic patterns of lymphocutaneous spread. Involvement of an underlying bone or joint is a probability. Disobedience to classic antimicrobial schemas, as well as immunodeficiency should also orient the diagnostic process.

4. TREATMENT

4.1. Treatment of patients presenting early with contaminated wounds

Cleansing, thorough irrigation and tissue debridement are the cornerstones of treatment of any contaminated hand trauma involving the extensor apparatus. Checking the status of tetanus immunization should not be omitted.

Simple lacerations in the vicinity of the extensor apparatus without involvement of bones, tendons, joints, nerves or vessels do not seem to benefit from antibiotic prophylaxis, provided a thorough cleansing and debridement has been performed [8]. A loose skin closure should be chosen in case of heavy contamination.

Questions also arise as to the usefulness of prophylactic antibiotic coverage in complex hand trauma (i.e. bone, joint, tendon and/or neurovascular injury); although such an attitude is well established in the case of open long bone fractures [9], its application to hand trauma is not statistically established, probably because of lower infection rates in this anatomic area [8, 27]. To date, it seems that the use of antibiotics in this clinical setting is at the surgeon's discretion and should not constitute a substitute for debridement [8]. Factors such as degree of contamination, crushing and devascularization, delay in presentation and co-existence of systemic illness may have to be taken into account [28]. Use of a single agent (such as flucloxacillin or erythromycin) has been proposed [28]. A combination of 1st or 2nd generation cephalosporin with an aminoglycoside is reasonable, with the addition of penicillin or clindamycin where anaerobic strains are suspected. Combining a fluoroquinolone with vancomycin is an alternative [8, 9]. The duration of prophylactic coverage should not exceed 5 days [8, 9].

Extensor tendon lacerations can be primarily repaired when soft tissue coverage is adequate or provided by flaps. Flaps may be applied immediately or after repeated debridements, depending on local conditions [29, 30]. In case of coexistent tendon substance defects, extensor tendon reconstruction can be performed secondarily or at the time of flap coverage in selected cases [29].

Early treatment of bite wounds is a somewhat con-troversial issue. The transmission of rabies through animal bites, as well as human immunodeficiency, hepatitis B and hepatitis C viruses through human bites are some of the risks involved [31-33]. Measures should be taken, when available, according to existing guidelines. The practice of performing debridement in all bite wounds has been challenged [3, 20], as selection bias may have led to falsely high estimates of morbidity. However, at least for bites on the dorsum of the hand, dilemmas are minor. As (i) tendon lesions may be underestimated by clinical examination and (ii) joint inoculation may have occurred, any such bite should be explored and debrided. Cultures are considered of little value, as they are not predictive of the causative pathogen(s) of a future infection [34]. Tendon lesions can be repaired and the wound be closed loosely on the following conditions: (i) the patient is seen at less than 8-12 hrs after the bite [12], (ii) there is no sign of infection, (iii) a proper tissue bed has been arranged, and (iv) the tendon lesion, if repaired, does not seal a contaminated space, such as the MCP joint or the dorsal subtendinous space over the phalanges. Otherwise, tendon repair and wound closure are performed when infection has been ruled out (on average, 72 hrs later). Nylon monofilament suture is preferred for such early skin or tendon repair, in order to minimize bacterial colonization. In case of tendon substance defects, any reconstructive procedures should be undertaken secondarily.

When inoculation of an MCP or PIP joint has occurred or is suspected, the joints are explored, debrided and irrigated [2, 8, 17, 21, 22, 26, 33]. The wound is left open. Successive dressing changes and irrigations follow. Tendon repair and skin closure are performed when infection outbreak has become remote, usually 48-72 hrs later.

The prophylactic use of antibiotics in mammalian or human bite wounds is controversial, with only scarce supportive literature [8, 35-38]. Although confirmatory research is needed, a prophylactic 3-5 day course of oral antibiotics seems reasonable in patients with animal or human bite wounds to the hand [8, 12, 34, 38]. Coverage should mainly be provided against pasteurella, eik. corrodens, streptococcus, staphylococcus and anaerobic bacteria [12, 13, 18].

Penicillin is generally active against *past. multocida* and *eik. corrodens,* as well as against many anaerobic bacteria, but resistance to its action may exist or arise [14, 17, 39]. Resistance to penicillin is commonplace for some strains, such as staphylococci. Amoxicillin plus clavulanate per os is thus a reasonable choice [12, 18]. Alternatives to penicillins may be second-generation cephalosporins (especially with enhanced anaerobic activity) or fluoroquinolones (especially with enhanced anaerobic activity, such as moxifloxacin) [13, 18], the latter being suitable for penicillin-allergic adult individuals.

For bites with bone or joint contamination, hospital admission and intravenous antibiotic therapy seems to be the best choice [33]. A combination of amoxicillin plus clavulanate or ampicillin plus sulbactam can be used for this purpose [12].

4.2. Treatment of patients presenting late with infected wounds

Here, collection of biologic material for culture, meticulous surgical debridement, as well as patient admission and intravenous prescription of antibiotics are essential prerequisites. Antimicrobial treatment without debridement may only be attempted in superficial cellulitis-type infections with no collection of pus, where the inoculation site has been trivial and no skin break is present at the moment of examination. Medical treatment alone may also cure some atypical infections (e.g. extensor tenosynovitis caused by *myc. marinum* in immunocompetent subjects, actinomycetomas) [7], but incision, debridement and synovectomy are routinely needed for diagnosis.

Tissue or fluid specimens are obtained after preparation of the skin surrounding the wound with alcohol or povidone-iodine solution [13, 18] and before irrigation and debridement [17]. Tissue samples are preferred over swabs or liquid from the wound in chronic infections, as they may contain more living microorganisms [7]. Specimens are obtained for smears and staining as well as for culture, preferably from the deep aspects of the lesion. In chronic infections and when an atypical or fastidious pathogen is suspected, 3 samples are needed for staining (each for gram, acid-fast bacillus and fungal stains) and 5 for cultures (each for aerobic and anaerobic bacteria, tuberculous and non-tuberculous mycobacteria and fungi), the so-called "eight pack" culture [7]. Samples may also be sent for histopathologic examination. The incubation period may be long [7, 13, 18]. It is useful that prior to laboratory testing the origin of the samples, any clinical suspicion as to the cause of the infection, as well as any antibiotic coverage be mentioned.

During exploration, particular attention must be paid on dissecting and evacuating collections of pus from different depths of the wound, as these may have developed in multiple potential spaces separated by natural tissue layers [40].

The rules of debridement are the same as for early presenting patients. All devitalized tissues should be excised to viable ones and debridement should extend to bone and cartilage, should the infection involve bones or joints. No attempt is made to repair extensor tendon injuries at this point. Whenever there is evidence of extension of the wound into palmar spaces of the hand, the appropriate treatment should be applied. Wounds are left open, covered with moist gauzes, and repeat debridement may be needed. Immobilization is helpful in reducing pain and hindering infectious biologic material from being squeezed along tissue pathways. Range of motion exercises are introduced when sepsis settles. Reconstruction of any soft tissue defects and loose closure of skin gaps may be undertaken when the clini-

cal setting shows that the infection has subsided [17], generally not earlier than 48-72 hrs after the debridement. A repeat culture may help in such decision-making. When signs and symptoms persist despite apparently adequate debridement, repeat x-ray control should check for bone involvement [17].

Antibiotic treatment must start immediately after taking specimens for culture. The skin flora should be covered, as well as particular strains, depending on the etiology (and hence the microbiology) of each wound. Principles given in section 4.1 as to the choice of antibiotics are applicable.

In infected bite wounds, anaerobes, staphylococci, streptococci, as well as pasteurella and/or eik. corrodens species must be covered. If a single antibiotic is desirable, amoxicillin-clavulanate or ampicillin-sulbactam is a good choice [8, 12, 13, 18, 34]. When a combination is deemed appropriate, penicillin plus dicloxacillin, penicillin plus clindamycin, a 2nd or 3rd generation cephalosporin plus clindamycin, or a fluoroquinolone plus clindamycin can be used [8, 13, 18]. Any choice should be reconsidered according to culture results and the responsiveness of the infection. Inpatient intravenous antibiotic treatment must be continued until the clinical appearance of the patient is improving, generally for no less than 5 days in moderately severe infections. Outpatient per os coverage should then be considered for compliant patients. The length of treatment is substantially increased when there is bone involvement.

In acute infections acquired in an aquatic environment, aeromonas and vibrio vulnificus should be suspected and initial empiric therapy should be directed against these pathogens (as well as common strains of skin flora), especially when similar cases have recently been reported in the same geographic area. Doxycycline i.v. as well as cephalosporins (such as ceftriaxone) are suitable for *v. vulnificus* [23, 24]. Broad-spectrum antibiotics, such as a second- (e.g. cefoxitin) or third- (e.g. cefotaxime) generation cephalosporin, an aminoglycoside or ciprofloxacin, are appropriate against aeromonas species [41, 42].

The reader could refer to other chapters of this book for the treatment of chronic atypical infections, such as those caused by mycobacteria and fungi.

5. Complications

Complications after septic trauma to the extensor apparatus are local and systemic. Local complications, such as septic arthritis, osteomyelitis, joint stiffness, extensive tissue necrosis and amputation may result from delayed or inadequate treatment. Systemic complications such as generalized sepsis with remote abscess formation, and even death, may be the result of immune deficiency of the host, but they may occasionally appear in immunocompetent patients. Reconstructive procedures may vary from delayed primary repair of the extensor apparatus to secondary extensor tendon reconstruction, to soft tissue coverage with local, island or free flaps, and to bone reconstruction.

6. CONCLUSION

Trauma to the extensor apparatus of the hand potentially inoculates deep tissues with microorganisms from the environment as well as from the patient's own skin flora. The risk of infection depends on tissue damage as well as on the particular microbiologic profile of the traumatism.

For wounds potentially implicating the extensor apparatus, surgical exploration and debridement is mandatory. Prophylactic antibiotic coverage is a controversial issue and should better be preserved for complex lesions (such as combined tendon and skeletal lesions), lesions with heavy contamination and/or extensive devascularization, and for special types of extensor tendon lacerations, i.e. the ones produced by human and animal bites. In exploring bite wounds, deep tissue and especially joint involvement should not be missed and early tendon repair should not be undertaken if this creates a closed inoculated cavity, e.g. over the MCP and PIP joints.

Treatment of patients with infected wounds should comprise evacuation of any collection, extensive debridement, and sampling of biologic material for histopathologic examination and culture. The choice of intravenous antibiotic coverage is initially based on the etiology of the traumatism, to be later updated according to clinical responsiveness and laboratory results. Any tendon reconstruction should be performed in a delayed primary or secondary stage, when the infection has subsided and viable soft tissue coverage is ensured.

Finally, any chronic infection with indolent course and/or resistance to usually prescribed antibiotics should raise the suspicion of an atypical microorganism, probably inoculated during a previous minor traumatic incident.

REFERENCES

[1] Smith JW, Bellinger CG. La vascularisation des tendons. In: Toubiana R (ed), Traite de chirurgie de la main. Paris: Masson, 1980;1:375-80.
[2] Faciszewski T, Coleman DA. Human bite infections of the hand. Hand Clin 1998;14 (4):683-90.
[3] Peeples E, Boswick JA Jr, Scott FA. Wounds of the hand contaminated by human or animal saliva. J Trauma 1980;20 (5):383-8.
[4] Marshall KA, Edgerton MT, Rodeheaver GT, Magee CM, Edlich RF. Quantitative microbiology: Its application to hand injuries. Am J Surg 1976;131:730-3.
[5] Fitzgerald RH Jr, Cooney WP 3rd, Washington JA 2nd, Van Scoy RE, Linscheid RL, Dobyns JH. Bacterial colonization of mutilating hand injuries and its treatment. J Hand Surg 1977;2A:85-9.
[6] Hoyen HA, Lacey SH, Graham TJ. Atypical hand infections. Hand Clin 1998;14(4):613-34.
[7] Patel MR, Malaviya GN, Sugar AM. Chronic infections. In: Green DP, Hotchkiss RN, Pederson WC, Wolfe SW (eds), Green's operative hand surgery. Philadelphia: Elsevier, 2005. pp. 94-158.
[8] Hoffman RD, Adams BD. The role of antibiotics in the management of elective and post-traumatic hand surgery. Hand Clin 1998; 14(4):657-66.
[9] Wilkins J, Patzakis M. Choice and duration of antibiotics in open fractures. Orthop Clin North Am 1991;22(3):433-7.
[10] Cooney WP 3rd, Fitzgerald RH Jr, Dobyns JH, Washington JA 2nd. Quantitative wound cultures in upper extremity trauma. J Trauma 1982;22(2):112-7.
[11] Snyder CC. Animal bite infections of the hand. Hand Clin 1998;14 (4):691-711.
[12] Taplitz RA. Managing bite wounds. Currently recommended antibiotics for treatment and prophylaxis. Postgrad Med 2004;116(2):49-59.
[13] Talan DA, Citron DM, Abrahamian FM, Moran GJ, Goldstein EJ. Bacteriologic analysis of infected dog and cat bites. N Engl J Med 1999;340(2):85-92.
[14] Winn W Jr, Allen S, Janda W, et al. Koneman's color atlas and textbook of diagnostic microbiology. 6th ed. Baltimore: Lippincott Williams & Wilkins, 2006.
[15] Smith P, Meadowcroft A, May D. Treating mammalian bite wounds. J Clin Pharm Ther 2000;25:85-99.
[16] Garcia V. Animal bites and pasteurella infections. Pediatr Rev 1997;18:127-30.
[17] Stevanovic MV, Sharpe F. Acute infections in the hand. In: Green DP, Hotchkiss RN, Pederson WC, Wolfe SW (eds), Green's operative hand surgery. Philadelphia: Elsevier, 2005, pp. 55-93.
[18] Talan DA, Abrahamian FM, Moran GJ, Citron DM, Tan JO, Goldstein EJ. Clinical presentation and bacteriologic analysis of infected human bites in patients presenting to emergency departments. Clin Infect Dis 2003;37:1481-9.
[19] Dreyfuss UY, Singer M. Human bites of the hand: A study of one hundred-six patients. J Hand Surg 1985;10A (6):884-9.
[20] Lindsey D, Christopher M, Hollenbach J, Boyd JH, Lindsey WE. Natural course of the human bite wound: Incidence of the infection and complications in 434 bites and 803 lacerations in the same group of patients. J Trauma 1987;27(1):45-8.
[21] Lindsey D. Wounds of the hand contaminated by human or animal saliva. Discussion. J Trauma 1980;20(5):389.
[22] Patzakis MJ, Wilkins J, Bassett RL. Surgical findings in clenched-fist injuries. Clin Orthop 1987;220:237-40.
[23] Kaye JJ. Vibrio vulnificus infections of the hand. J Bone Joint Surg 1990;72A(2):283-5.
[24] Said R, Volpin G, Grimberg B, Friedenstrom SR, Lefler E, Stahl S. Hand infections due to non-cholera vibrio after injuries form St Peter's fish (Tilapia Zillii). J Hand Surg 1998;23B(6):808-10.
[25] Eyres KS, Allen TR. Skyline view of the metacarpal head in the assessment of the human fight-bite injuries. J Hand Surg 1993;18B(1):43-4.
[26] Schmidt DR, Heckman JD. Eikenella corrodens in human bite infections of the hand. J Trauma 1983;23(6):478-81.
[27] Whittaker JP, Nancarrow JD, Sterne GD. The role of antibiotic prophylaxis in clean incised hand injuries: a prospective randomized placebo controlled double blind trial. J Hand Surg 2005;30B(2):162-7.

[28] Platt AJ, Page RE. Post-operative infection following hand surgery. Guidelines for antibiotic use. J Hand Surg 1995;20B(5):685-90.

[29] Scheker LR, Langley SJ, Martin DL, Julliard KN. Primary extensor tendon reconstruction in dorsal hand defects requiring free flaps. J Hand Surg 1993;18B(5):568-75.

[30] Melissinos EG, Parks DH. Post-trauma reconstruction with free tissue transfer - Analysis of 442 consecutive cases. J Trauma 1989; 29(8):1095-103.

[31] Richman KM, Rickman LS. The potential for transmission of human immunodeficiency virus through human bites. J Acquir Immun Defic Syndr 1993;6:402-6.

[32] Bartholomew CF, Jones AV. Human bites: a rare risk factor for HIV transmission (corresp). AIDS 2006;20:631-2.

[33] Kelly IP, Cunney RJ, Smyth EG, Colville J. The management of human bite injuries of the hand. Injury 1996;27(7):481-4.

[34] Fleisher GR. The management of bite wounds. N Engl J Med 1999; 340(2):138-40.

[35] Cummings P. Antibiotic to prevent infection in patients with dog bite wounds: a meta-analysis of randomized trials. Ann Emerg Med 1994;23:535-40.

[36] Elenbaas RM, McNabney WK, Robinson WA. Evaluation of prophylactic oxacillin in cat bite wounds. Ann Emerg Med 1984;13: 155-7.

[37] Zubowicz VN, Gravier M. Management of early human bites of the hand: A prospective randomized study. Plast Reconstr Surg 1991; 88:111-4.

[38] Medeiros I, Saconato H. Antibiotic prophylaxis for mammalian bites. The Cochrane Database of Systematic Reviews 2001, Issue 2. Art. No.: CD001738. DOI: 10.1002/14651858.CD001738.

[39] Rayan GM, Putnam JL, Cahill SL. Eikenella corrodens in human mouth flora. J Hand Surg 1988;13A:953-6.

[40] Lister G. Inflammation. In Lister G (ed), The hand: Diagnosis and indications. 3rd ed. Edinburgh: Churchill Livingstone 1993. pp. 323-353.

[41] Hermansdorfer J, Lineaweaver W, Follansbee S, Valauri FA, Buncke HJ. Antibiotic sensitivities of aeromonas hydrophila cultured from medicinal leeches. Br J Plast Surg 1988;41(6):649-51.

[42] Sanger JR, Yousif NJ, Matloub HS. Aeromonas hydrophila upper extremity infection. J Hand Surg 1989;14A (4):719-21.

Staphylococcal Infections of the Soft Tissues in the Upper Extremity

Sokratis E. VARITIMIDIS[a*], Zoe H. DAILIANA[a], Nikolaos RIGOPOULOS[a],
Antonios MANIATIS[b], Konstantinos N. MALIZOS[a]

[a]Department of Orthopaedic Surgery and Musculoskeletal Trauma, University of Thessalia, Larissa, Greece
[b]Department of Microbiology, University of Thessalia, Larissa, Greece

The upper extremity, as the most exposed region of the body, is the limb most vulnerable to infections. Staphylococci are the most commonly encountered pathogens. If not recognized early and treated properly, staphylococcal infections of the soft tissues in the upper extremity may cause significant morbidity and disability. When diagnosed early, conservative treatment with the administration of appropriate antibiotics may manage the infection adequately. In infections with pus formation, immediate surgical drainage is indicated, supplemented by debridement of the infected tissues and adequate coverage of the wound. Tissue samples should be obtained for cultures, in order to identify the infecting agent and its susceptibility to chemotherapy. Panton-Valentine leukocidin (PVL) positive *Staphylococcus aureus* is emerging as an important pathogen in staphylococcal soft tissue infections. It is acquired not only in health service institutes, but also in the community. Clindamycin, fluoroquinolones, aminoglycosides, vancomycin, teicoplanin, linezolid and rifampicin are the most commonly administered antibiotics. A multidisciplinary approach, with the collaboration of several specialties including, orthopaedic surgeons, microbiologists, and infectious diseases specialists, is required for an optimal outcome.

Keywords: staphylococcal infections; *Staphylococcus aureus;* MRSA; PVL; soft tissues; upper extremity; surgical drainage.

1. INTRODUCTION

The hand, the forearm and even the elbow, are the most exposed anatomical regions of the upper extremity in daily living, thus making them vulnerable to inoculation by bacteria from the environment. The protective barrier provided by the intact skin is able to restrain most environmental pathogens. However, this "appendage" of the dermis, where the normal skin bacterial flora is found, is suscepti-ble to invasion by pathogens, as they form gaps in the protective stratum corneum. Furthermore, the organization of the hand and wrist structures in anatomical compartments, although functionally essential, may enhance the expansion of infections, thus increasing their catastrophic sequelae.

2. EPIDEMIOLOGY

Staphylococci are the most commonly encountered pathogens in upper extremity infections. *Staphylococcus aureus* is responsible for the majority of nosocomial infections caused by Gram-positive cocci, especially in the intensive care unit. Methicillin-resistant *Staphylococcus aureus* (MRSA) is an emerging pathogen around the globe. It was first recognized in 1961 after the introduction of methicillin, [1] and since then, has been associated with many outbreaks in almost every country of the world.

*Corresponding Author
Lecturer, Department of Orthopaedic Surgery and
Musculoskeletal Trauma
University of Thessalia, School of Medicine
22 Papakiriazi Street, 41222 Larissa, Greece
Tel: +30 2410 682723
Fax: +30 2410 670107
e-mail: svaritimidis@ortho-uth.org

The β-lactam resistance of MRSA is determined by the function of penicillin binding protein 2a (PBP2a) encoded by the methicillin resistance gene *mecA*. PBP2a of MRSA binds to b-lactam antibiotics at a much lower affinity than that of the intrinsic set of PBPs of *S. aureus*. By nucleotide sequence determination of a MRSA-specific chromosomal region, it was found that the *mecA* gene is carried by a novel genetic element, designated staphylococcal cassette chromosome *mec* (SCC*mec*), which is inserted into the chromosome. Sequence analyses have defined three major SCC*mec* types (SCC*mec* types I, II, and III) among nosocomial MRSA strains. These are distinguished on the basis of their size, which ranges from 26 to 67 kb, and genetic composition, in which recombinases and antibiotic resistance genes are included in the genomes [2].

Community-acquired MRSA (CA-MRSA) has been reported worldwide. This emerging pathogen has distinct genetic and clinical characteristics, as well as the ability to infect young and healthy individuals [3-6]. These MRSA strains differ from nosocomial MRSA strains on the basis of their genetic background and antibiogram. CA-MRSA strains typically demonstrate resistance to fewer antimicrobials than do strains acquired within hospitals. CA-MRSA strains harbour the recently described SCC*mec* type IV element in their genomes. Compared with other SCC*mec* types, the SCC*mec* type IV element is distinguished by its small size, the absence of antibiotic resistance markers and the presence of genes encoding several superantigens (exotoxins), such as the Panton-Valentine leukocidin (PVL) [7]. Rare SCC*mec* types V and VT carrying PVL have also been described [8].

The pathogenicity of *S. aureus* infections is related to various bacterial surface components (e.g., capsular polysaccharide and protein A), including those that recognize adhesive matrix molecules (e.g., clumping factor and fibronectin binding protein), and extracellular proteins (e.g., coagulase, hemolysins, enterotoxins, toxic-shock syndrome [TSS] toxin, exfoliatins, and Panton-Valentine leukocidin [PVL]) [9]. In general, the precise roles of individual staphylococcal toxic factors in invasive infections are difficult to assess, but PVL production has been preferentially linked to furuncles, cutaneous abscesses, and severe necrotic skin infections [10-12]. The PVL exotoxin destroys neutrophils, resulting in purulent ulcers, necrotic musculoskeletal infections, and recently, in necrotizing pneumonia. Infections caused by PVL-producing CA-MRSA are an emerging public health issue worldwide. Outbreaks have recently been described in Australia, Europe and the United States [12-14].

3. Diagnosis

Diagnosis for staphylococcal infections is based on clinical signs and symptoms, and on laboratory tests which include blood tests and cultures of blood and tissue samples.

3.1. Clinical signs and symptoms

The patient's general health status is assessed and a complete medical history is taken. Information about work, hobbies and habits of the patient is of paramount importance. Fever, if present, is a sign, but not a prerequisite for the diagnosis of infection. The affected area usually appears swollen, tender and erythematous, and in case the diagnosis is delayed, this is indicative of pus accumulation. Infection can be secondary to a negligible wound or hematogenous. A portal of entry may or may not be noticeable (a small incision, a scratch or a bite wound) [15]. Pain is elicited with contraction of the arm and hand muscles, and when a joint is involved (septic arthritis), the range of motion is very limited. There is no difficulty in diagnosing the infection when a draining wound is present. However, draining wounds can lead to the spread of infection among individuals with close contact (family members, colleagues, team-mates) and other patients during hospitalization. Therefore, wound dressing and simple preventive measures in personal hygiene (daily showers, hand washing, avoiding sharing personal items, avoiding physical contact, and use of gloves) of both patients and caregivers are useful first steps towards controlling the spread of the infection.

Infections caused by PVL producing *S. aureus* strains should be considered in the diagnosis of skin and soft tissue infections (mainly in patients suffering from purulent ulcers or necrotic lesions) for the choice of the most efficient empiric antibiotic therapy and elimination of inappropriate use of antimicrobials.

3.2. Susceptibility testing

Identification of microorganisms such as *S. aureus* is made by Gram-stain, catalase, coagulase and API Staph system (BioMerieux, La Balme les Grottes, France). Susceptibility to various antimicrobial agents (penicillin, oxacillin, cefoxitin, erythromycin, clindamycin, gentamicin, tobramycin, kanamycin, ciprofloxacin, cotrimoxazole, rifampicin, vancomycin, teicoplanin, and linezolid) was tested by the disk diffusion method, according to NCCLS (National Committee for Clinical Laboratory Standards) guidelines [16].

3.3. Detection of mecA and PVL -genes

Polymerase Chain Reaction (PCR) is used to detect mecA and Panton Valentine Leukocidin (PVL) genes of Staphylococcus, while molecular typing of the isolates is performed by pulsed-field gel electrophoresis (PFGE). *Staphylococcus aureus* ATCC 49775 serves as the reference strain for PVL.

4. Treatment

Any delay in the initiation of treatment after diagnosis of a soft tissue infection could have serious consequences. Treatment, either non operative or surgical, should start

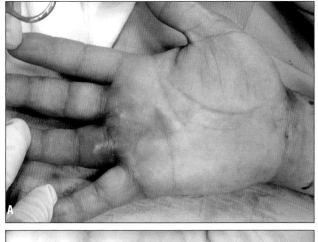

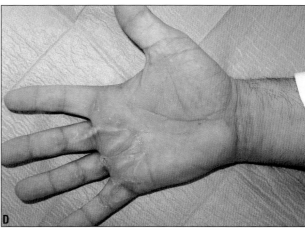

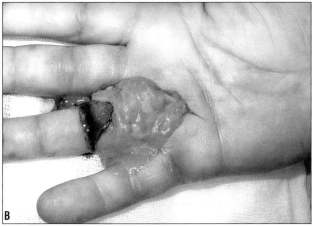

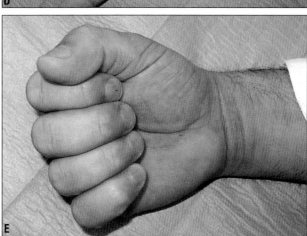

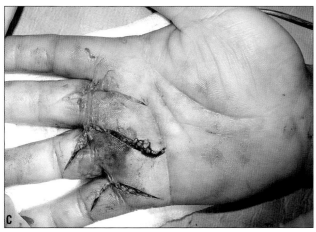

FIGURE 1. (A) Severe staphylococcal infection of the palm. **(B)** Infection was drained through Bruner's incisions and a Panton Valentine leukocidin positive *Staphylococcus aureus* was identified as the infecting organism. **(C)** After surgical drainage, irrigation and debridement the wound was left to heal without primary closure. **(D & E)** Appearance of the hand three months after surgery. No relapse of the infection occurred and function of the hand returned completely.

immediately. Non operative management of the infection is indicated only if the infection is recognized at very early stages and includes administration of antibiotics and analgesics, splinting of the extremity in a functional position and hydration of the patient [17]. Definitive antimicrobial therapy should be a combination of various agents including, vancomycin, fluoroquinolones, clindamycin, linezolid, and rifampicin. Antibiotics should be administered intravenously at the beginning of the treatment and can continue orally once the infection is under control. For MRSA strains that produce toxins, such as PVL, antimicrobial agents acting to inhibit protein synthesis, such as linezolid or clindamycin, may be a more appropriate selection. It must be emphasized that vancomycin and teicoplanin do not inhibit toxin production [18]. Protection for tetanus should be provided if the patient is not regularly vaccinated, i.e. every five years.

Surgical treatment is indicated for draining infections or when pus is present. It includes immediate drainage of the accumulated fluid and debridement through incisions adequate to allow exposure of the entire infected area. This is performed through an extensile incision or through a Bruner approach when the infection involves the fingers. All necrotic or suspected tissues are removed and the wound is irrigated copiously. Tissue samples are acquired for microbiologic and pathologic evaluation, and frozen sections will provide valuable information. Delays in initiating treatment or incomplete debridement are recognized as factors contributing to the failure to eradicate staphylococcal (especially PVL infections) of the upper extremity. It is important that after debridement, the wound should be left open. In cases where a joint is infected (septic arthritis), a drain must be inserted into that joint after debridement. In most cases, unless flap coverage or skin grafting is considered necessary, the wounds should be left open to heal by secondary intention (Fig. 1). Flap coverage of the wound or application of skin grafts can be performed if there is no sign that the infection persists [19, 20].

Antibiotics should be administered based on tissue cultures taken from the site of infection, and should not be given before tissue samples are taken. Immediately after tissue samples are taken, clindamycin combined with an aminoglycocide should be administered. Once the tissue culture results are available, then a more appropriate regimen may be chosen. If no causal agent is identified from the cultures, the antibiotic regimen should continue empirically, targeting the most common bacteria. The choice should be based on their incidence, clinical signs (appearance and odor of pus) and the environment where the infection occurred [21]. A common reason for the inability to identify a pathogen from the culture is related to the administration of antibiotics before the culture was acquired. In addition,

when cultures are taken from patients after an extended period of antibiotic administration, an increased number of co-existing micro-organisms, including, anaerobes, mycobacteria and fungi, are observed. In these cases, chemotherapy needs to be modified with an appropriate regimen in order to eradicate these additional micro-organisms.

After debridement the extremity is placed in a splint for both pain relief and maintaining the limb in a functional position. Range-of-motion exercises should be initiated during splinting to avoid stiffness of the joints that is possible after long immobilization. The presence of an experienced physical therapist is of paramount importance for functional recovery of the upper extremity.

Radiographic evaluation should always be performed, especially when the infection is out of control despite treatment. A foreign body (wood, glass, fish bone) that has not been detected or active osteomyelitis in the involved anatomical sites are potential reasons for persistence of the infection.

5. Authors' Experience

In the last three years, 146 patients were treated for staphylococcal soft tissue infections of the upper extremity in our unit. The age of the patients ranged from 8 days (neonate) (Fig. 2) to 86 years. In 51 patients, a PVL(+) S. aureus was isolated. The majority of PVL(+) upper

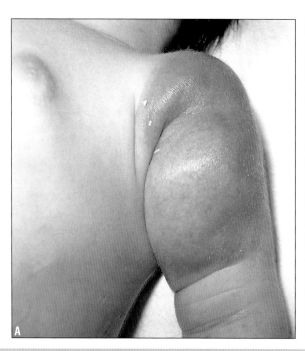 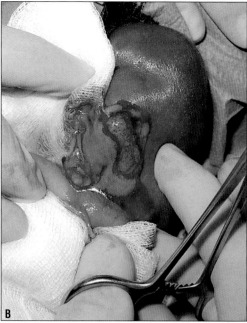

FIGURE 2. (A) Severe staphylococcal soft tissue infection of the left proximal humerus in a 8-day-old neonate with sepsis symptoms and pus accumulation. **(B)** Surgical drainage of the abscess was absolutely indicated as a first step to eradicate the infection.

extremity infections were located in the hand/wrist (Fig. 3). The remaining were in more proximal sites: 6 in the forearm/elbow and 2 in the humerus/shoulder. The vast majority (96%) of PVL(+) MRSAs belonged to the MLST-80 clone. This is the predominant clone in Europe that expresses resistance to fucidic acid and tetracyclines. The remaining 4% belonged to a newly emerging clone that expresses resistance to aminoglycocides (gentamicin, tobramycin). Upper extremity infections due to PVL(+) MRSA were more common in young or middle-aged men, especially those working in a highly contaminated environment (e.g., carpenters, farmers, or meat processing workers). It is interesting that the majority of PVL(+) upper extremity infections were encountered during spring and summer. The majority of these infections were community-acquired and to a lesser extent health-care-unit associated or hospital-acquired.

For the management of these infections, we have employed surgical drainage, continuous irrigation of the wound, flap coverage, splinting of the extremity, and physical therapy. Antibiotics were selected either empirically or after susceptibility testing. Of the patients suffering from PVL(+) upper extremity infections, 17.5% required at least one re-operation, while 12% were readmitted. In contrast, of the patients suffering from all other upper extremity musculoskeletal infections, the rate of re-operation and re-admissions was 12% and 4%, respectively. The mean hospitalization period was 6 days for PVL(+) upper extremity infections and 4.5 days for the remaining soft tissue staphylococcal infections.

6. PREVENTION

S. aureus outbreaks originate from the community (community acquired) or from health care institutions. Appropriate measures are very important in order to minimize the risk of infection originating from either of these

sources. *S. aureus* can colonize in the host for long periods of time before causing the infection. This is more important in patients that have been hospitalized in the past and have come in contact with the organism [14, 22]. Education of health care personnel, patients, accompanying persons, high risk populations and adherence to infection control guidelines are very important to prevent spreading of *S. aureus* [23]. Frequent washing of hands, use of sanitation gels, avoiding contact with the infected wounds and covering the wound with clean dressing are very simple and easy-to-follow measures that should be followed by health care providers. Appropriate use of antibiotics and early recognition of the infection by the physicians are also key factors in limiting the spread of infection. Patients should not share personal items such as towels, blankets and clothing. Prophylactic administration of antibiotics to persons related to patients with staphylococcal infections is not generally accepted.

7. CONCLUSION

In the last decade, staphylococcal infections are re-emerging as a serious problem in the community, affecting patients of all ages [24]. PVL-positive MRSA is a pathogen that can cause significant morbidity and mortality. Prompt and appropriate management is of great importance for the treatment of staphylococcal soft tissue infections in the upper extremity. When treated early and appropriately, a functional limb with no deficit can be anticipated. In neglected cases or when appropriate treatment is not provided, the infection may have serious consequences. It can compromise the function of the upper limb and it may be limb- or even, life-threatening. A collaborative effort of various specialists is required to eradicate the infection and for full recovery of the patient. Orthopaedic surgeons, internists, microbiologists, pathologists, radiologists, infectious diseases specialists, and physical therapists need to work together in order to optimize the final outcome.

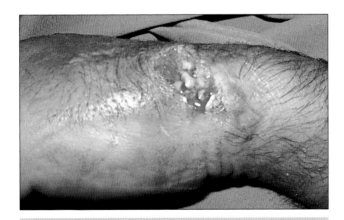

FIGURE 3. Infection of the left wrist caused by PVL (+) *Staphylococcus aureus*. Emergent intervention is required as the necrotic lesion may risk the entire extremity's function if left untreated.

REFERENCES

[1] Jevons MP. Celbenin-resistant staphylococci. Br Med J 1961;i: 124-5.

[2] Ito T, Katayama Y, Asada K, Mori N, Tsutsumimoto K, Tiensasitorn C, Hiramatsu K. Structural comparison of three types of staphylococcal cassette chromosome *mec* integrated in the chromosome in methicillin-resistant *Staphylococcus aureus*. Antimicrob. Agents Chemother 2001;45:1323-1336.

[3] Maltezou HC, Giamarellou H. Community-acquired methicillin-resistant *Staphylococcus aureus* infections. Int J Antimicrob Agents Feb 2006;27(2):87-96.

[4] Loveday HP, Pellowe CM, Jones SR, Pratt RJ. A systematic review of the evidence for interventions for the prevent and control

of methicillin-resistant *Staphylococcus aureus* (1996-2004): report to the Joint MRSA Working Party (Subgroup A). J Hosp Infect May 2006;63 Suppl 1:S45-70.

[5] Vandenesch F, Naimi T, Enright MC, et al. Community-acquired methicillin-resistant *Staphylococcus aureus* carrying Panton-Valentine leukocidin genes: worldwide emergence. Emerg Infect Dis 2003;9:978-984.

[6] Chini V, Petinaki E, Foka A, Paratiras S, Dimitracopoulos G, Spiliopoulou I. Spread of *Staphylococcus aureus* clinical isolates carrying Panton-Valentine leukocidin genes during a three-year period in Greece. Clin Microb Infect 2006;12:29-34.

[7] Said-Salim B, Mathema B, Braughton K, Davis S, Sinsimer D, Eisner W, Lickhosvay Y, Deleo FR, Kreiswirth BN. Differential distribution and expression of Panton-Valentine leukocidin among community-acquired methicillin-resistant *Staphylococcus aureus* strains. J Clin Microbiol Jul 2005;43 (7):3373-9.

[8] Gerogianni I, Mpatavanis G, Gourgoulianis K, Maniatis A, Spiliopoulou I, Petinaki E. Combination of staphylococcal chromosome cassette SCC*mec* type V and Panton-Valentine leukocidin genes in a methicillin-resistant *Staphylococcus aureus* that caused necrotizing pneumonia in Greece. Diagn Microbiol Infect Dis 2006;56:213-216.

[9] Clark DC. Common acute hand infections. Amer Family Physician. 2003;68:2167-76.

[10] Schnall SB, Vu-Rose T, Holtom PD, et al. Tissue pressures in pyogenic flexor tenosynovitis of the finger. J Bone Joint Surg [Br] 1996;78:793-5.

[11] DiFelice A, Seiler JG III, Whitesides TE. The compartments of the hand: an anatomic Study. J Hand Surg [Am] 1998;23:689-96.

[12] Chang MC, Huang YL, Liu Y, Lo WH. Infectious Complications Associated With Toothpick Injuries of the Hand. J Hand Surg 2003; 28A:327-331.

[13] Deresinski S. Methicillin-Resistant *Staphylococcus aureus:* An evolutionary, Epidemiologic, and Therapeutic Odyssey. Clin Infect Dis 2005;40:562-73.

[14] Kowalski TJ, Berbari EF, Osmon DR. Epidemiology, Treatment, and Prevention of Community-Acquired Methicillin-Resistant *Staphylococcus aureus* Infections. Mayo Clin Proc Sep 2005;80(9): 1201-1208.

[15] Weinzweig N, Gonzalez M. Surgical infections of the Hand and Upper Extremity: A County Hospital Experience. Ann Plast Surg 2002; 49:621-7.

[16] National Committee for Clinical Laboratory Standards. (2000a) Performance standards for antimicrobial disk susceptibility tests (7th ed). Approved standard M2-A7. Wayne, PA: NCCLS.

[17] Spann M, Talmor M, Nolan WB. Hand infections: Basic principles and management. Surgical infections 2004;5:210-220.

[18] Ohlsen K, Ziebuhr W, Koller KP, Hell W, Wichelhaus TA, Hacker J. Effects of subinhibitory concentrations of antibiotics on a-toxin (hla) gene expression of methicillin-sensitive and methicillin-resistant *Staphylococcus aureus* isolates. Antimicrob Agents Chemother 1998;42:2817-2823.

[19] Koschnick M, Bruener S, Guenter G. Free tissue transfer: an advanced strategy for post-infection soft tissue defects in the upper extremity. Ann Plast Surg 2003;51:147-154.

[20] Schnall S, Thommen V, Holtom P et al. Delayed primary closure of infections. Clin Orthop Rel Res 1997;335:286-290.

[21] Schnall SB, Waller S. Hand Infections. In Orthopaedics, Mosby Inc. 2002:738-748.

[22] Sanford MD, Widmer AF, Bale MJ, Jones RN, Wenzel RP. Efficient detection and long term persistence of the carriage of methicillin-resistant *Staphylococcus aureus*. Clin Infect Dis 1994;19:1123-28.

[23] Zinderman CE, Conner B, Malakooti MA, LaMar JE, Armstrong A, Bohnker BK. Community-acquired methicillin-resistant *Staphylococcus aureus* among military recruits. Emerg Infect Dis. 2004;10:941-944.

[24] Lu D, Holtom P. Community-acquired Methicillin-resistant *Staphylococcus aureus,* a new player in sports medicine. Curr Sports Med Rep 2005;4:265-270.

chapter 21

Gangrenous and Necrotizing Soft Tissue Infections in Upper Limb Surgery

Efthymia GIANNITSIOTI, Helen GIAMARELLOU*

4th University Department of Internal Medicine, ATTIKON University Hospital, Athens, Greece

Although rare, necrotizing and gangrenous soft tissue infections of the upper limb are very often associated with severe limb dysfunction, partial or total limb amputation and death. Diagnosis is difficult and a delay of 24 hours from the onset of symptoms to surgical intervention proved to be independently associated with death. Mortality rates range from 40-60% and amputation of the affected limb is essential in 50% of cases. Adverse outcome is frequent in patients with underlying diabetes mellitus, chronic renal failure and malignancies. Necrotizing fasciitis type I caused by aerobes (Staphylococcus aureus, Streptococci, Enterobacteriaceae) and anaerobes, necrotizing fasciitis type II caused by group A β-hemolytic Streptococcus, anaerobic clostridial gangrene and mucosal necrotizing infections emerging in immunocompromised hosts, are the most recognizable clinical issues. The hallmark of gas gangrene is the presence of crepitus on examination. Tissue cultures and gram staining and histopathology of intraoperative specimen must be always performed. Antimicrobial treatment with clindamycin plus penicillin is the choice for streptococcal and anaerobic infections, whereas antistaphylococcal agents are indicated for S.aureus and b-lactams, carbapenems or quinolones for gram negative bacteria. Hyperbaric oxygen may be an adjunct to the classical therapy. However, a high index of clinical suspicion for early diagnosis and immediate radical surgical intervention are mandatory to save the patient's life.

Keywords: necrotizing fasciitis; clostridial gangrene; upper limb; necrotizing soft tissue infections. ∎

1. INTRODUCTION

Necrotizing infections of the soft tissues and the skin are relatively uncommon in orthopaedic surgery [1]. Only 13 cases of skin and fascia necrosis were detected at a 9-year follow-up at an Orthopaedic Department [1]. However, these in-fections very often lead to amputation of the limb. Moreover, even after appropriate antimicrobial treatment and adequate surgical intervention, mortality rates are very high, i.e. ranging from 30 to 60% [1]. The spectrum of the infections of the deep soft tissue ranges from localized bacterial, viral and parasitic lesions to rapidly spreading tissue-destructive infections associated with systematic toxicity [2, 3]. A few areas of infectious diseases have a more confusing nomenclature because diagnosis is usually based on clinical findings, whereas surgical exploration and pathology definitely set the diagnosis of necrotizing infections of the skin and subcutaneous areas [2, 3]. In an attempt to present as clearly as possible this issue, clinical syndromes related to necrotizing and gangrenous diseases of the soft tissues are categorized as follows: a) necrotizing fasciitis; b) gas gangrene (clostridial myonecrosis) and anaerobic cel-

*Corresponding Author
4th Department of Internal Medicine,
Attikon University Hospital
Rimini 1, 12462, Chaidari, Athens, Greece
Tel: +30 210 5326426
Fax: +30 210 5326446
e-mail: hgiama@ath.forthnet.gr

lulitis; c) progressive bacterial synergistic gangrene; d) synergistic necrotizing cellulitis; e) gangrenous cellulitis in immunocompromised patients; f) very localized areas of skin necrosis complicating conventional cellulitis [4].

2. EPIDEMIOLOGY

Until the middle of the 20th century, soft tissue gangrene was considered as a wartime injury since it massively affected soldiers who sustained gunshot wounds. Gas gangrene was common during the First World War as the European soil was rich in animal feces containing large numbers of vegetative spores of clostridia. In contrast, gunshots in North Africa causing gangrene were less common, as soil there is sandy containing few clostridia spores.

In the modern world, even at the theatre of the battle, such infections are rare because wounded soldiers are usually rapidly transferred to hospitals for immediate surgical reconstruction and concomitant antimicrobial treatment [2]. Sporadic cases of soft tissue gangrene have been reported. However, the emergence of immunocompromised hosts, the increased number of patients with underlying conditions such as diabetes mellitus, malignancies or chronic renal failure, have transformed the physical history of necrotizing and gangrenous infections of the skin and soft tissues [2, 3].

Trauma has been the most common portal of entry (45%) while spread from another location may also occur [5]. However, in about 20% of cases there was not identified trauma or other presumed portal of entry [2, 6].

3. PATHOGENESIS

Infectious gangrene is a form of cellulitis that rapidly progresses, producing extensive necrosis of the subcutaneous tissues and the overlying skin. The anatomic location, the causative pathogen and host predisposing factors account for distinguishable clinical conditions. Such clinical entities include a) necrotizing fasciitis type I, which is a mixed infection caused by anaerobes (usually *Bacteroides fragilis*) and aerobes *(Enterobacteriaceae)* [5], and b) necrotizing fasciitis type II caused by *Streptococcus pyogenes.* Less often group B or C streptococci may have also been involved [5, 7, 8]. In most types of gangrenous cellulitis an abundant polymorphonuclear leukocytic exudates is present. On the contrary, in clostridial myonecrosis the exudates is thin containing fluid, fibrin and gas but few leukocytes. In streptococcal gangrene, fibrin thrombi are present in the small veins of the dermis and subcutaneous fat [2-4]. In most cases, soft tissue necrosis has developed secondarily to inoculation of the causative agent at the site of infection. Sometimes, it may result from extension of an infection involving deeper sites to the subcutaneous areas. Occa-

sionally, gangrenous cellulitis begins at the site of a metastatic infection in the course of bacteremia [4].

Streptococcal fasciitis is characterized by rapidly distracted tissues and systematic toxicity. Expression of protein M (especially type 1, 3) which acts as super antigen, induces an acute systematic inflammatory cascade and toxic shock [4, 7]. Clostridial toxins induce tissue distraction and shock in gangrenous cellulitis [2].

4. CLINICAL FEATURES

Clinical presentation of necrotizing and gangrenous infections of the skin and soft tissues is heterogenous and requires a high index of clinical suspicion [7-8]. Outpatient empirical administration of antibiotics prior to the patient's hospitalization may transform the initial clinical picture, leading to an underestimation of the severity of the underlying infection. Thus, physicians must be alert in any case of soft tissue infection in order to carefully assess any clinical sign and symptom related to the disease [9]. Polymicrobial synergistic infection was the most common cause described (54-83%) [6, 10-11], mainly caused by *Streptococcus pyogenes* and *Enterobacteriaceae,* whereas monomicrobial infection was more often caused by *Streptococcus pyogenes* [3-4].

Advanced age (>60 years old), the presence of more than two comorbidities, anemia and thrombocytopenia and a more-than-24-hours delay from the onset of symptoms to surgery were identified as independently associated with death in two large cohort series [5, 9]. Another case series confirmed these results and further demonstrated that female gender, malignancies and diabetes mellitus were independently associated with death [6, 10]. Mortality rates were high (>30%) and influenced also the young patients especially in cases of streptococcal toxic shock syndrome (50%) [11].

Severe necrotizing soft tissue infections are characterized by the following signs and symptoms: a) pain disproportionate to skin lesions especially in streptococcal infections, b) violaceous bullae, c) cutaneous hemorrhage, d) skin sloughing, d) skin anesthesia, e) rapid progression of the lesions, e) gas in the tissues, f) systematic toxicity (fever, tachycardia, tachypnea hypotension, shock, organ failure) [3, 7, 12]. Mortality is very high. Pain, either localized or generalized, is the most important clue in severe soft tissue infections. A portal of entry is detectable in the majority of cases.

Early in the course of deep skin and soft tissue infection, local signs of inflammation such as swelling, pain, redness, warmth and tenderness are prominent. At the early course, the disease usually resembles uncomplicated cellulitis. Gas may be detected on physical examination (crepitus) or/and by imaging (computerized tomography, MRI or ultrasonography scanning). Later, erythema is superceded by violaceous bullus lesions, massive local swelling and symptoms and signs of systemic toxicity which rapidly develop [2, 3, 8, 9].

4.1. Necrotizing fasciitis

Necrotizing fasciitis is a deep-seated infection of the subcutaneous tissues. It is characterized by extensive tissue destruction, thrombosis of the blood vessels, abundant bacteria rapidly spreading along the fascial planes and the relatively few acute inflammatory cells, although micro abscesses have been described. Skin may be spared. There are two distinguishable forms of the disease [2, 3]:

4.1.1. Necrotizing fasciitis type I

This is a mixed infection caused by aerobes and anaerobes that predominate in patients with diabetes mellitus and peripheral vascular disease [2]. In a large series [9], two third of patients presented with mixed infection. The predominant isolates were *S. aureus,* enterococci, other streptococci, *Escherichia coli, B. fragilis, Peptostreptococcus* spp, *Prevotella* and *Porphyromonas* spp. There was an average of 4-6 isolates per specimen. A monomicrobial form of the disease may also exist involving *S. aureus,* group A β-hemolytic *Streptococcus, Aeromonas hydrophila* and *Vibrio vulnificus* [12, 13].

Regarding necrotizing fasciitis of the upper limb, *S. aureus* and group A *b-hemolytic Streptococcus* are the predominant pathogens [12-14]. Only in 7% of cases necrotizing fasciitis is situated in the upper limbs compared to 65% where lesions are localized in the lower limb [5].

Non-clostridial anaerobic cellulitis and synergistic necrotizing cellulitis are both variants of the same syndrome. A distinguishable sign is that in cellulitis lesions from subcutaneous tissues are well detectable, whereas in necrotizing fasciitis the initial lesion may be trivial (abrasion, insect bite or injection site). In about 20% of cases, there was not visible lesion that could be considered as the portal of entry for the skin and soft tissue infection [6, 12].

4.1.2. Necrotizing fasciitis type II

According to the Center for Diseases Control (CDC), 10-15,000 cases of invasive group A streptococcal infections have been annually reported. Among them, 5-10% were identified as necrotizing fasciitis cases [13]. This clinical issue is caused by group A β-hemolytic Streptococcus (and sometimes by group C and G streptococci) and was previously called "streptococcal gangrene" or flesh-eating disease" [4]. In contrast to type I fasciitis, type II may occur at any age group, in patients without underlying diseases while the portal of entry is often unknown [2]. Predisposing factors include: a) a history of blunt trauma, b) muscle strain, c) childbirth, d) chickenpox, e) intravenous drug use, f) non-steroid anti-inflammatory drugs (NSAID), and g) penetrating injury from surgical procedure or laceration [15]. The administration of NSAID aims to the patient's relief from the inflammatory signs and symptoms. However, NSAIDs may mask the real clinical picture which probably has an impact on the early diagnosis of necrotizing soft tissue infection [15]. In penetrating injuries, the skin is the main portal of entry for streptococci. Hematogenous translocation to the site of blunt trauma or muscle strain may also be possible [13, 16]. It should be considered that group A streptococci is a contiguous pathogen that may spread by skin contact and cause epidemics. This issue is important for the families of the patients and health care workers. Regarding pathogenesis of streptococcal gangrene, streptococcal exotoxin acts as super-antigen that can provoke rapid proliferation of T-lymphocytes leading to production of cytokines [Interleukin 6 (IL-6), Tumor necrosis-α (TNFα-), Interleukin-1 (IL-1), Tumor necrosis-β (TNFβ) that precipitate shock, tissue destruction and organ failure [17, 18]. Clinically unexplained localized pain, disproportional to the observed primary lesion, is the most characteristic symptom that must alert physicians. In post-surgical wounds, pain may be attributed to the whole procedure and this may lead to delay in diagnosis of the proliferating skin infection [2, 9, 13]. Diffuse or local erythema is present. Within 24-48 hours, erythema changes into a reddish-purple lesion, frequently blisters and bulla, first presenting with clear fluid and rapidly turning to a blue-maroon color with subsequent rupture. The lesion evolves into a sharply demarcated area covered by necrotic eschar and surrounded by a border of erythema. Lymphangitis is rarely present [4]. Additionally, fever, malaise, anorexia, myalgias and even diarrheas may develop during the first 24 hours. Systemic toxicity previously described appears as skin and soft tissue lesion proliferate. Streptococcal strains containing M protein type 1 and 3 can produce pyogenic exotoxins A, B, C and therefore, they have been associated with streptococcal fasciitis and toxic shock syndrome [17,18].

The histopathologic findings concerning early fascial disease revealed superficial epidermal necrosis, edema and hemorrhage with few inflammatory cells, whereas clinically advanced, necrotic skin lesions and thrombosis, neutrophilia infiltrates and gram positive diplococci were detected [3, 17].

Progressive synergistic bacterial gangrene predominantly involves the abdominal area, following surgical operations and thus, it is beyond the scope of the present chapter [4].

Necrotizing fasciitis of the upper limb is a very rare condition that is illustrated by case studies reported in the literature. In order to highlight the most important issues, a short summary of several interesting case reports is presented. A case report of group G streptococcal gangrene described the evolution of toxic shock and cellulitis of the hand in a woman. Group G Streptococcus was isolated from intraoperative tissue and blood cultures. Despite two radical debridements and radiological evidence of reduced fluid retention in the fascia layers, amputation of the wrist was necessary to restrict invading infection and save the patient's life [19]. The authors indicated the unfamiliarity of physicians with the antimicrobial treatment of the diseases because of its rarity [19]. A fatal case of group A streptococcal gangrene following axillary branchial plexus block for carpal tunnel decompression in a diabetic woman was described to indicate the delay in diagnosis and surgical debridement [20]. Another case report referred to a 69-year-old diabetic man who underwent hemodialysis and died of methicillin-resistant *S.aureus* (MRSA) fasciitis despite radical debridement and excision of the cephalic vein [21]. Even less acute forms of necrotizing soft tissue infections have been described. A sub-acute form of the disease was detected due to the high index of suspicion of surgeons who regularly explored primary hand lesion. Necrotizing fasciitis from *Proteus* spp and *E. coli* was diagnosed by intraoperative tissue cultures and the patient adjusted well to her carpal amputation [22]. An acuter streptococcal necrotizing fasciitis of both hands after minimal cut with knife was also reported [23]. Radical amputation in a case of necrotizing infection of the upper limb preceded survival while in other cases, refusal of amputation led to death [24].

Regarding patients with necrotizing fasciitis in case series, it has been demonstrated that survival rates were better if the infection was situated in the extremities than in the abdomen [10, 11]. However, a 24-hour delay in surgical debridement significantly aggravated prognosis and increased the probability of death [9, 10].

4.1.3. Clostridial cellulitis and gas gangrene
Clostridium perfringens is the most common pathogen implicated in clostridial cellulitis. This is an infection usually preceded by local trauma or recent surgical incision. Gas production detected in the skin is the hallmark of clostridial cellulitis. Gas is detected clinically (crepitus) and by ultrasonography and MRI scanning. Early surgical exploration of the skin lesions is required [2, 25].

Clostridial gas gangrene includes three types of soft tissue infection: a) simple wound contamination, b) anaerobic cellulitis, and c) clostridial gas gangrene [25]. The first type is a very common issue which is not accompanied by a real infection process. The second type, anaerobic cellulitis, is marked by devitalized tissue in a wound and although gas production is detected, neither expansion to the contiguous tissues nor bacteremia and systemic toxicity are present [2]. The third type is the so-called "clostridial gas gangrene" or "myonecrosis". This includes traumatic gas gangrene, spontaneous non-traumatic gas gangrene and recurrent gangrene. The initial trauma introduces organisms producing an anaerobic environment with an acid PH which initiates the necrotizing process within hours [25]. Recent studies suggest that clostridial s-toxin diffuses to the surrounding tissues and invades systemic circulation. S-toxin promotes disregulation between polymorhonuclear and endothelial cells and urges leukocytes for increased respiratory activity. These actions lead to vascular leykostasis, edothelial damage and tissue hypoxia which promote the anaerobic infection pro-

cess. Shock associated with gas gangrene is attributed to the effect of toxins. Alpha toxin is considered to directly suppress myocardial contractility leading to decreased cardiac output hypotension. This is a differentiation from the shock of gram negative bacteria where cardiac output is increased. Moreover, another clostridial toxin, theta toxin is believed to indirectly suppress the normal vascular tone via indirect inhibition of platelet activating factor and prostacyclines [2].

The first symptom of gas gangrene is the sudden onset of localized pain within 6 hours that may last for several days after the initial skin incision. The skin quickly becomes red, then bronze and purple. Crepitus is the clinical characteristic most frequently found. Radiology reveals gas production in the subcutaneous tissues. Bacteremia may occur in 15% of patients sometimes with intravascular hemolysis. Shock is present in 50% of patients at the time of hospital admission. Multi-organ failure is consequently developed [2, 4, 13]. Clostridial infection was independently associated with limb loss in a large series of necrotizing soft tissue infections [26].

Spontaneous non traumatic gas gangrene is usually observed in immuno-compromised patients with colonic carcinoma, hematological malignancies, AIDS, neutropenia with Clostridium septicum being the most frequent pathogen. Other clostridia are implicated in post-surgical complication especially at the abdomen and will not be further analyzed in this chapter [2].

4.1.4. Pyomyositis
This infection involves the subcutaneous tissues and the muscles and it is more often situated in the extremities, although psoas and trunk can be also affected. Ultrasonography and CT may be helpful to early diagnosis. Extensive surgical excision is required for the subcutaneous tissues but not for the muscles. The most common causative agent is *S. aureus,* but *Streptococcus pneumoniae* and gram negative bacteria may be also involved. Blood cultures are positive in 5-30% of cases [2, 12].

4.1.5. Anaerobic streptococcal myositis
Unlike other streptococcal invasive infections, anaerobic streptococcal myositis complicates surgical wounds after incision. Radical debridement sparing the muscle is strongly recommended [12].

---

5. DIAGNOSTIC EVALUATION

The first goal in diagnosis of necrotizing and gangrenous soft tissue infections is to determine the depth and extent of the infection. Clinical examination as already mentioned may help, although giving a name to the infection is not easy and many times not evident [7, 23]. Ultrasonography, CT or MRI scans are useful to distinguish whether the infection is localized on the skin or spread along the fascial planes, although no method has proven to be specific. Thus, clinical judgment is the most important diagnostic tool [7-8]. Statistical models with good negative prognostic value (NPV 95%) and positive prognostic value (PPV 95%) have been also developed in an attempt to elucidate necrotizing fasciitis cases. This score is named LRINEC: Laboratory Risk Indicator for Necrotizing Fasciitis [27]. The second goal in diagnosis is to reveal the responsible pathogen. For this purpose, immediate surgical exploration and debridement must be always accompanied by tissue and fluid cultures with multiple specimens taken from the infected area. Frozen section is required for histopathology in every case of infection. Gram staining is a quick reliable and cheap method of initial identification of the responsible pathogen and can distinguish among streptococci, staphylococci and gram negative bacteria, clostridia and mycoses as well. Susceptibility tests of the isolated bacteria must be performed [9, 13]. Direct microscopy of the specimen with potassium-hydrocloride solution may reveal fungi. [28]. Fungal cultures must be also obtained. It is strongly recommended that we should send immediately drainage for gram's staining, culture and susceptibility tests, preferably before the initiation of any antimicrobial treatment [17]. Besides, examination of frozen section and paraffin embedded specimens may result in prompt diagnosis of a fatal disease [23].

6. NECROTIZING SOFT TISSUES INFECTIONS IN SPECIAL POPULATIONS

Non-clostridial anaerobic cellulitis, synergistic necrotizing cellulitis, type I fasciitis occur more often in diabetic patients. Systematic toxicity marked by tachycardia, tachypnea, fever, leukocytosis, hyperglycemia and acidosis may be life-threatening, if immediate and accurate treatment is neglected, and is related to patients with diabetes mellitus and invasive soft tissue infections. Moreover, the occasional absence of pain in streptococcal fasciitis in these patients may be attributed to the underlying diabetic neuropathy [2, 13]. Mycoses (Mucor, Absidia and Rhizopus spp) are pathogenic for the rapidly expanded necrotic infections of the soft tissue in uncontrolled hyperglycemia in patients with diabetes mellitus and chronic renal failure [4, 29]. However, mucormycosis of the upper extremities has been also described to affect immunocompetent patients who had motor vehicle collision and trauma, as well as to follow injuries that occur during agricultural activities [29].

Invasive fungal infections have emerged as a significant problem in patients with malignancies with and without chemotherapy-associated neutropenia. *Aspergillus* spp, *Fusarium* spp, *Candida* spp, *Mucor* spp, and *Rhizopus* spp were the most frequently detected pathogens in a large survey conducted at an Oncology Hospital [28]. Clinically, it is difficult to distinguish between bacterial and fungal etiology of cutaneous and soft tissue infections. A high index of suspicion for a fungal etiology must be maintained particularly whenever cutaneous and soft tissue lesions do not respond to appropriate antimicrobial treatment [28].

Regarding intravenous drug users, who are extremely affected by cutaneous and soft tissue pathogens, the following issues must be taken into consideration: an upsurge in skin infections, primary abscesses and more invasive community-acquired MRSA infections have occurred within the last years [30]. It should be also pointed out that *C. perfringens* and *C. novyi* have been reported as causative agents in heroine abusers who undergo subcutaneous injection of black tar heroin [12]. Moreover, *Pseudomonas aeruginosa* affects more frequently injection drug users than general population [30].

7. TREATMENT OF INVASIVE SOFT TISSUE INFECTIONS

Treatment of severe, necrotizing and gangrenous soft tissue infections consists of antimicrobial chemotherapy and surgical intervention. There is no doubt that the second one is vital for the survival of patients suffering from those infections. Regarding antimicrobial therapy, Table 1 summarizes the recent guidelines of the Infectious Diseases Society of America [12].

Necrotizing fasciitis due to streptococci must be treated with penicillin plus clindamycin [12]. Clindamycin reduces exotoxin production and TNFα expression as it has been demonstrated in *in vivo* studies [12]. Penicillin should be added because streptococci present an increasing resistance of clindamycin and macrolides. Antimicrobial treatment should follow surgical debridement and specimen isolation but it should be initiated immediately, and not be postponed until the microbiological results of cultures are obtained [1]. Intravenous γ-globulin (IVGG) is recommended in case of streptococcal toxic shock syndrome, although systematic evidence is limited [12]. In clostridial gangrene, clindamycin plus penicillin is recommended because 5% of clostridia strains are resistant to penicillin [12]. Clindamycin is not strongly recommended in cases of erythromycin-resistant or methicillin-resistant *S. aureus* strains because of inducible cross-resistance phenomena [12]. Piperacillin/tazobactam is considered for nosocomial soft tissue infections caused by Enterobacteriaceae or for mixed aerobic plus anaerobic infections [31]. Newer fluoroquinolones like moxifloxacin and levofloxacin may be efficacious especially in patients with penicillin-induced allergic reactions, however, more data are necessary [32]. Antistaphylococcal penicillins and penicillin is the first choice for staphylococcal and streptococcal skin infection in the community although the emergence of community-acquired MRSA infections raise questions. Vancomycin must be the choice in those cases [31, 32].

TABLE 1

Treatment of necrotizing infections of the skin, fascia and muscles (modified from the IDSA guidelines) [12]

Antimicrobial agents of 1st line[a]	Adult dosage
Mixed infections- aerobes + anaerobes	
– Ampicillin/sulbactam or	1.5-3.0g every 6-8 h IV
– Piperacillin/tazobactam +	4.45 g every 6 h IV
Clindamycin[b]	600-900 mg/Kg every 8 h IV
– Imipenem/cilastatin	1g every 6-8 h IV
– Meropenem	2g every 6-8h IV
– Ertapenem	1g every day IV
– Cefotaxime +	2g every 6 h
metronidazole or	500 mg every 6 h IV
clindamycin[b]	600 mg/kg every 8 h IV
Streptococcal infections	
– Penicillin +	2-4 MU every 4-6 h IV
Clindamycin[b]	600-900 mg/kg every 8 h IV
S.aureus infections	
– Oxacillin	1-2 g every 4 h IV
– Vancomycin	30 mg/kg/day in 2 divided doses
– Clindamycin[b]	600-900 mg/kg every 8 h IV
Clostridium spp infections	
– Clindamycin[b] +	600-900 mg/kg every 8 h IV
– Penicillin	2-4 MU every 4-6 h IV

[a] In cases of severe hypersensitivity to penicillin, clindamycin or metronidazole plus an aminoglycoside or quinolone is an alternative treatment. For staphylococcal infections, vancomycin 1g every 12 hours, or linezolid 600 mg every 12 hours or quinupristin/dalfopristin 7 mg/kg/24 h, or daptomycin 6mg/kg/24 h are the alternative proposed treatment.
[b] Clindamycin (IV) requires an infusion time of 30 minutes

Despite the initiation of adequate antimicrobial treatment, patients are condemned to die without having undergone early and radical surgical procedures. Surgical debribement remains the cornerstone of therapy [2, 4, 10]. Surgical reconstitution is by all means a difficult process. Almost half of the patients who were hospitalized because of necrotizing skin infections consequent to burnt wounds, required skin grafting. Hospitalization at ICU is a usual phenomenon after surgical procedure for these infections [33]. Amputation may reach even half (41%) of cases of necrotizing infection of the limbs [34]. Even in cases that amputation is spared, the post-infection functional status of the upper limb, especially of the hand, is problematic.

Regarding hand infections, the immobilization and elevation are necessary to decrease edema in the dorsum of the hand and prevent edema extension. Controlled mobilization is possible after the acute infection and is also required to prevent from post-infection joint contractures and stiffness [35]. Local transposition flaps, free muscle flaps and skin grafts have been used in the healing of post-infectious lesions of the upper arm. In a series of 24 patients with severe necrotizing infections of the upper limb, free tissue transfer with muscle, musculocutaneous or himeric flaps, proved efficacious in covering the significant defect space (average 10 x 14 cm) with success [36]. Soft tissue coverage is important to consider when planning the incision or deciding if the wound should be left open. Once the infection is controlled, wound closure and early range of motion therapy yields the best functional results [35]. To achieve these goals, early, radical, aggressive and repetitive debridement to remove all skin and subcutaneous tissues that are undermined by the infection must always be performed [35].

Case reports consider treatment with hyperbaric oxygen (HBO) to improve healing of wounds after severe necrotizing soft tissue infections of the limbs [37]. However, complications in case of such therapy have been described and should be taken into consideration. Air embolism, combustion, ear or sinus pain, generalized tonic-clonic seizures, pneumothorax, transient myopia and tympanic membrane rupture may occasionally occur [2]. Hyperbaric oxygenation has given satisfactory results in tissue non-surgical reconstruction, always applied as an adjuant in antimicrobial and surgical treatment. The role of hyperbaric oxygen therapy along with radical surgical debridement and antibiotic administration needs further elucidation. More trials are needed to establish the already reported encouraging results [38].

8. CONCLUSIONS

In conclusion, necrotizing and gangrenous skin and soft tissue infections require a high suspicion index by the clinicians. The combination of early diagnosis with both early radical and repeated surgical debridement and adequate antimicrobial treatment is the only way to succeed salvage not only of a functional limb, but also of the patient's life. Aggressive soft tissue procedures are often required along with appropriate, based on intraoperative cultures, antimicrobial treatment. Although rare, those infections are always life-threatening and must keep alert all the physicians involved.

REFERENCES

[1] Theis JC, Rietveld J, Danesh-Clough T. Severe necrotizing soft tissue infections in orthopaedic surgery. J Orthop Surg 2002;10(2): 108-113.
[2] Stevens DL. Necrotizing fasciitis, gas gangrene, myositis and myonecrosis. In Infectious Diseases Cohen J, Powderly WG eds, 2nd ed Edinburgh Elsevier, 2004.
[3] Lesaffer J, van Holder C, Haeck L. Necrotizing fasciitis of the first ray caused by group A Streptococcus. J Hand Surg [British and European volume], 2006;31B:3:317-319.

[4] Swartz MN, Pasternack MS. Skin and soft tissue infections. In: Principles and practice of infectious diseases. 6th ed. Mandel GL, Bennett JE, Dolin R eds, Philadelphia USA, 2004.

[5] Yuang Meng Liu, Chih-Yu Chi, Mao-Wong HO, Chin Ming Chen, Wei-Chih Liao, Cheng-Mao HO, Po-Chang Lin, Jen-Hsein Wong. Microbiology and factors affecting mortality in necrotizing fasciitis. J Microbiol Immunol Infect 2005;38:430-435.

[6] Childers BJ, Potyondy LD, Nachreiner R, Rogers FR, Cilders ER, Oberg KC, Hendricks DL, Hardesty RA. Necrotizing fasciitis: A fourteen year retrospective study of 163 consecutive patients. Am Surg 2002;68 (2):109-116.

[7] Fontes Ra Jr, Ogilvie CM, Miclau T. Necrotizing soft tissue infections. J Am Acad Orthop Surg 2000;8(3):151-158.

[8] Headley AJ. Necrotizing soft tissue infections: a primary care review. Am Fam Physician 2003;68(2):323-328.

[9] Chin-Ho Wong, Haw- Chong Chamg, Shanker Pasupathy, Lay-Wai Khin, Jee-Lim Tan, Cheng-Ooi Low. Necrotizing fasciitis: clinical presentation, microbiology and determinants of mortality. J Bone Joint Surg [Am] 2003;85:1454-1460.

[10] Taviloglu K, Cabioglu N, Cagatay A, Yanar H, Ertekin C, Baspinar I, Ozsut H, Gulogly R. Idiopathic necrotizing fasciitis: risk factors and strategies for management. Am Surg 2005;71(4):315-320.

[11] Heitmann C, Pelzer M, Bickert B, Menke H, Germann G. Surgical concepts and results in necrotizing fasciitis. Chirurg 2001;72(2): 168-173.

[12] Stevens DL, Bisno AL, Chambers HF, Everett D, Dellinger P, Goldstein EJC, Gorbach SL, Hirschmann JV, Kaplan EL, Montoya JG, Wade JC. Practice guidelines for the diagnosis and management of skin and soft tissue infections. Clin Infect Dis 2005;41:1376-1406.

[13] Chapnick EK, Abter El. Necrotizing soft tissue infections. Infect Dis Clin North Am 1996;10:835-855.

[14] Bluman EM, Mechrefe AP, Fadale PD. Idiopathic staphylococcus aureus necrotizing fascitis of the upper extremities. J Should Elbow Surg 2005;14(2):227-230.

[15] Stevens DL. Could non steroidal ani-inflammatory drugs (NSAIDs) enhance the progression of bacterial infections to toxic shock syndrome? Clin Infect Dis 1995; 21: 977-980.

[16] Stevens D. Streptococcal toxic shock syndrome: spectrum of disease, pathogenesis and new concepts in treatment. Emerg Infect Dis 1995;1:69-78.

[17] Bisno AL, Stevens DL. Streptococcal infections of the skin and soft tissues. N Engl J Med 1996;334:240-245.

[18] Dahl PR, Perniciaro C, Holmkvist KA, O' Conor MJ, Gibson LE. Fulminant group A Streptococcus necrotizing fasciitis: Clinical and pathological findings in 7 patients. J Am Acad Dermatol 2002;47: 489-492.

[19] Mac Donald J, Lennox PA. Unusual etiology of simultaneous deep space hand infection and necrotiziing fasciitis of the foot. Plastic and Reconstructive Surgery 2005;116(1):10e-13e.

[20] Nseir S, Pronnier P, Soubrier S, Onimus T, Saulnier F, Mathieu D, Durocher A. Fatal streptococcal necrotizing fasciitis as a complication of axilliary branchial plexus block. Br J Anaesth. 2004 March; 92 (3): 427-9.

[21] Verman DJ, Rao ARN, Johnson JR, Sheil AGR. A patient on haemodialysis with necrotizing fasciitis of the left arm. Nephrol Dial Transplant 1998;(13):781-783.

[22] Wong CH, Tan H. Subacute necrotizing fasciitis. Lancet 2004; 364:1376.

[23] Shroeder JL, Steinke EE. Necrotizing fasciitis-The importance of early diagnosis and debridement. AORN 2005;82(6):1031-1040.

[24] Lim YJ, Yong FC, Wong CH. Necrotizing fasciitis and traditional medical therapy- a dangerous liaison. Ann Acad Med Singapore 2006;35:270-273.

[25] Perry BN, Floyd WE 3rd. Gas gangrene and necrotizing fasciitis in the upper extremity. J Surg Orthop Adv 2004 Summer; 13(2):57-68.

[26] Anaya DA, McMahon K, Nathens AB, Sullivan SR, Foy H, Bulger E. Predictors of mortality and limb loss in necrotizing soft tissue infections. Arch Surg 2005;140 (2):151-157.

[27] Wong CH, Khin LW, Heng KS, Tan KC, Low CO. The LRINEC (Laboratory risk indication for necrotizing fasciitis) score: a total for distinguishing necrotizing fasciitis from other soft tissue infections. Crit Care Med 2004;32 (7):1535-1541.

[28] Radhakrishnan R, Donato M, Prieto VG, Mays S, raad, I, Kuerer HM. Invasive cutaneous fungal infections requiring radical resection in cancer patients undergoing chemotherapy. J Surg Oncol 2004;88:21-26.

[29] Moran SL, Strickland J, Shin A. Upper-extremity mucormycosis infections in immunocompetent patients. J Hand Surg 2006;31A: 1201-1205.

[30] Gordon RJ, Lowy FD. Bacterial infections in drug users. N Engl J Med 2005;353:1945-1954.

[31] Fung HB, Chang LY, Kuczynzki S. A practical guide to the treatment of complicated skin and soft tissue infections. Drugs 2003; 63 (14):1459-1480.

[32] Miller L, Perdream-Remington F, Rieg G, Mehdi S, Perlroth J, Bayer A, Tany A, Phung T, Spellberg B. Necrotizing fasciitis caused by community associated methicillin resistant Staphylococcus aureus in Los Angeles. N Engl J Med 2005;352:1445-1453.

[33] Endorf FW, Supple KG, Gamelli RL. The evolving characteristics and care of necrotizing soft tissue infections. Burns 2005;31:269-273.

[34] Ozalay M, Ozkoc G, Akpinar S, Hersekli MA, Tandogan RN. Necrotizing soft tissue infection of a limb: clinical presentation and factors related to mortality. Foot Ankle Int 2006;27 (8):598-605.

[35] Spann M, Talmor M, Nolan W. Hand infections: Basic principles and management. Surgical Infections 2004;5(2):210-220.

[36] Koschnick M, Bruener S, Guenter G. Free tissue transfer: an advanced strategy for postinfection soft-tissue defects in the upper extremity. Ann Plast Surg 2003;51(2):147-154.

[37] Yuen JC, Feng Z. Salvage of limb and function in necrotizing fasciitis of the hand: the role of hyperbaric oxygen treatment and free muscle flap coverage. South med J 2002;95(2):255-257.

[38] Jallali N, Withey S, Butler PE. Hyperbaric oxygen as adjuvant therapy in the management of necrotizing fasciitis. Am J Surg 2005; 189(4):467-468.

Life Threatening Infections of the Upper Limb

chapter
22

Antonio LANDI[a*], Andrea LETI ACCIARO[a], Mauro CODELUPPI[b],
Emanuele NASOLE[c], Maria Concetta GAGLIANO[a]

[a]Department of Emergency, Unit of Hand Surgery and Microsurgery,
Policlinico of Modena, Italy
[b]Department of Medicine and Medical Specialities, Infectious Diseases Clinic,
University of Modena and Reggio Emilia, Modena, Italy
[c]Hyperbaric Center, GyneProMedical, Bologna, Italy

The authors report their experience in managing life threatening infections of the upper limb. The proposed classification ranges from necrotizing fasciitis and gas gangrene to toxic shock syndrome and various infective diseases, and underlines the peculiar aspects of infections in the immunocompromised population. The cornerstone of treating these severe infections is based on a multidisciplinary effort with the collaboration of the intensive care unit and infectious diseases service in the acute phase, in addition to the physiotherapist in the following phases. The authors propose common guidelines for the prompt diagnosis and treatment of potentially life threatening infections. The first-line medical therapy is based on the general health and age of the patient (newborn or elderly). Improvements in life-saving procedures have extended the goals of the treatment towards achieving maximal preservation of function, highlighting the relevant role of a rehabilitation program and the treatment of early and late sequelae of life threatening infections of the upper limb, such as skin defects, stiffness, and tendon and nerve disruption.

Keywords: infection; upper limb; necrotizing fasciitis; HBO; sequelae.

1. INTRODUCTION

Infections in the upper extremity induce a variety of problems, including severe life-and limb-threatening complications. They can progress rapidly and spread to the other areas of the body, even under antibiotic therapy and life-supporting measures. Not uncommonly, minor medical interventions, such as injection, are associated with the risk of a life-threatening infection. Medical personnel must strictly follow the guidelines for hand hygiene, asepsis, and proper skin disinfection [1]. On this basis, strict attention must be paid to the observation of common guidelines for prevention, prompt diagnosis and treatment of the potential life-threatening infections.

2. CLASSIFICATION

Infections that can result in severe suffering and systemic life-threatening disorders include: gas gangrene, necrotizing fasciitis, septic thrombophlebitis, acute osteomyelitis, toxic shock syndrome, infective diseases (tetanus, rabies, botulism and vibrio vulnificus), and infections in the immunocompromised population.

*Corresponding Author
Unit of Hand Surgery and Microsurgery,
Policlinico of Modena, L. go del Pozzo, 71
41100 Modena, Italy
Tel: +39 (0)59 4224494
Fax: +39 (0)59 4222818
e-mail: chirurgiamano@policlinico.mo.it

The mortality rate following infection by Gram negative bacilli appears to be stable during the last decades (25%). The incidence is higher in immunocompromised patients [2, 3] affected by co-morbidities, such as HIV disease, leukaemia, lymphomas, cytotoxic therapies, diabetes, liver cirrhosis, chronic hepatitis, haemochromatosis, and drug or alcohol abuse.

Improved life-support measures, antiretroviral therapies and the increase of allogenic transplantation [4] (also in the case of non-life-threatening conditions, such as hand and facial transplantations) have dramatically increased patient longevity. For the immuno-compromised population, this gives rise to the problem of living with a chronic disease, as life expectancy has been extended considerably.

3. Infections in the Immunocompromised Population

A wide variety of agents can cause or involve soft tissue infection in patients with immune impairment. They include nosocomial (frequently multi-resistant) strains of bacteria, like Pseudomonas aeruginosa, Acinetobacter and methicillin-resistant Staphylococcus aureus, fungi (namely Aspergillus, Candida, Fusarium and many other moulds and yeasts), and viruses (Herpesvirus, in particular). In addition, more unusual organisms, particularly the so-called "endemic" fungi, such as Penicillium, Cryptococcus or Hystoplasma can cause infections in patients suffering from cell-mediated impairment of the immune system.

In neutropenic patients, dermatologic manifestations of gram negative bacteraemia include erythematous maculopapular lesions, cellulitis, nodules, ecthyma gangrenosum, painful necrotic lesions secondary to dissemination, and vasculitis. Indwelling vascular access devices predispose to Gram positive infections (mainly Staphylococcus). Toxic-like syndromes, sometimes related to Streptococci viridians, can be associated with diffuse erythrodermia. Nodules (Candida) and necrotic lesions (Fusarium and Aspergillus) need to be evaluated as being related to fungal infection in patients with neutropenia. In immunocompromised patients, histology and all possible diagnostic procedures, such as cultures, protein chain reactions, and antigen detection are required for correct diagnosis.

In the elderly, infections are a common cause of increased morbidity and mortality. They are quite different from the infections affecting the young population, because of the age-related changes regarding immunology, epidemiology and bacteriology, as well as the different clinical presentations and predisposing co-morbidities [5]. Delayed diagnosis may lead to serious local and systemic complications.

Hospitalization and the frequent use of urinary or venous catheters are the most important risk factors related to life-threatening nosocomial infections. On the other hand, affections that predispose to infections or those that deteriorate existing infections, such as jaundice, boils, childhood leukaemia, urinary dysfunctions or obstructions, malnutrition, high factor VIII serum level etc. [6-8] can also be found in the newborn and children.

4. Guidelines in Antibiotic Therapy

The main prerequisite for application of appropriate therapy is comprehension of the aetiology of the infection. In patients with neutropenia and fever, a first-line antimicrobial therapy usually involves anti-Pseudomonas agents, (ceftazidim or piperacillin/tazobactam, plus an aminoglycoside or a monotherapy with carbapenems). An antifungal agent (amphotericin B-desoxicolate, its lipid- associated derivatives, or caspofungin) is added to antimicrobial agents administered to patients with persistent fever, because they are at high risk of developing deep-seated mycosis.

In non-neutropenic patients, the management and treatment depend on predisposing factors (since the relative incidence of pathogens differs according to the underlying conditions) and the pathogen; for instance, amphotericin B or new azoles are generally administered as medical treatment in the case of fungal infections (e.g. those due to Cryptococcus, Candida, Histoplasma), while acyclovir or ganciclovir are administered for Herpesvirus and Cytomegalovirus, respectively.

5. Physiopathology and Clinical Manifestations of Tissue Damage

Usually, the major life-threatening infections in the limbs follow traumatic skin lesions, –requiring surgical intervention or invasive procedures– and are due to Gram positive bacilli. The incidence of Gram positive infections in septic shock increased from 10% in the 1970s to 30% in the current years [9].

These infections can develop in various anatomical locations following direct trauma, and spread "in contiguity" from nearby infected areas, or via metastatic dissemination through the lymphatic and the vascular system. The location and the clinical signs may reveal the aetiology prior to obtaining culture results. Staphylococcus mainly affects the skin, rapidly inducing local suppuration and necrosis. The beta-hemolytic streptococcus rapidly extends to the surrounding tissues activating a more intense inflammatory process, while the anaerobic germs induce severe necrosis.

6. Cellulitis and Lymphedema

Clinical appearance of the soft tissue infection commonly starts with acute cellulitis and lymphedema (Fig. 1a).

Blood cultures have positive results in less than 5% of cases, while needle aspiration has positive results at a variable percentage, ranging between 5 and 40%. Studies have indicated that Streptococcus is the most commonly isolated bacteria, while Staphylococcus is rarer. Less usual pathogens, such as Peptostreptococci, Capnocytophaga canimorsus, Pasteurella multocida, Aeromonas hydrophila can also appear. For patients in immunosuppressive conditions, or those exposed to risk factors of unusual aetiology, injuries, animal bites, and malignancy, microbiological examination is mandatory. In some cases, this may need to be followed by needle aspiration or biopsies.

By delaying diagnosis, the pathogenic micro-organisms induce progressive and aggressive liquefaction and necrosis of the superficial and deep structures, dissecting the limb along the soft tissue planes [10] (Fig. 1b). The process can become self-perpetuating and culminate in the release of increasing quantities of systemically acting toxins. Direct invasion "in contiguity" through the vascular and lymphatic systems contributes to the bacterial dissemination and may result in septic thrombophlebitis, septic emboli and/or distant metastatic infections.

6.1. Medical and surgical guidelines

Prompt surgical drainage and debridement of the involved tissues (Fig. 1c, d) must be performed in combination with antibiotic therapy (Table 1). For patients who do not run the risk of being affected by unusual pathogens, intravenous Oxacillin (2 gr/4 hours) is the primary regimen, while Cefazolin (1 gr/8 hours) can be an alternative for less severe cases. Another alternative option is ampicillin/sulbactam. For patients with severe clinical infection and hypersensitivity to penicillin, alternatives include Vancomycin, Clindamycin, Cotrimoxazole, or a new generation fluoroquinolone that has anti-staphylococcal action (like levofloxacin). Macrolide can be an alternative option for less severe forms, although rapid increase in Strept. pyogenes resistance to macrolide and clindamycin has been reported, in Italy at least. In the presence of diabetes, the possible pathogens are Enterobacteriaceae, and therefore, the primary choice can be a third generation cefalosporin or ampicillin/sulbactam, plus an aminoglycoside.

---

7. GAS GANGRENE

Progression of the infection due to contamination of the wound by Clostridial spores (e.g. C. perfringens, C. septicum, C. hystoliticum, or C. novyi) can rapidly lead to gas gangrene. In presence of deep wound infections of the limb, with necrotic tissues and local hypoxia due to lack of communication with the external environment, Clostridium (mainly C. perfrigens) germinates and pro-

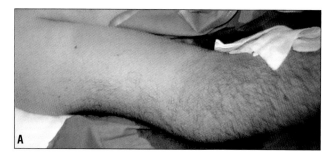
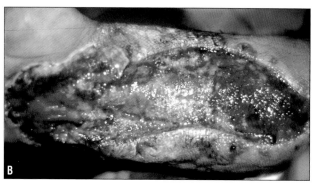
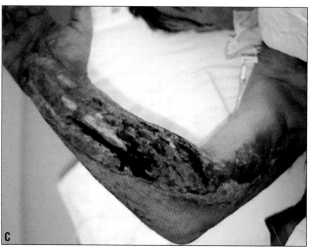
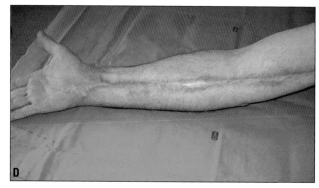

FIGURE 1. (A) Severe lymphedema of the entire upper limb following a CTS surgical procedure. **(B)** NF of the wrist and forearm rapidly develop after the infection and lymphedema. **(C)** Appearance, 10 days after the fasciotomy and surgical debridement which was up to the arm. **(D)** Appearance at 10 months follow-up, showing healing by secondary intention with the use of a collagen medical device.

TABLE 1

Treatment Guidelines

Condition	Etiologies	Primary treatment	Alternative	Hypersensitivity to penicillin
Extremity cellulitis, not associated with venous catheter	Streptococci (group A, B, C, G), Staph aureus (less common)	*Severe Cases:* Oxacillin 2 gr/4 hr *Mild Cases:* Cefaxazolin 1-2 gr/8 hr	Ampicillin/sulbactam	Vancomycin or Clindamycin + aminoglycoside
Diabetes	Streptococci (group A, B, C, G), Staph aureus, Enterobacteriaceae; clostridia (rare)	*Severe Cases:* Imipenem/meropenem + Vancomycin *Mild Cases:* Third generation Cephalosporin or Ampicillin/sulbactam 3 gr/8 hr +/-Clindamycin		

duces enzymes and exotoxins inducing liquefaction and massive necrosis of the subcutaneous fat, the fascia and the muscles [9]. Biopsies of the necrotic tissues can show gram positive, large spore-forming bacilli. Oedema can rapidly occur, which may greatly extend within hours, involving the entire limb. The hydrogen sulphide and carbon dioxide diffuse into the limb along the soft tissue planes. The gas quickly becomes apparent in the fascia and the muscle, producing crepitation that can be detected by palpation [9, 11]. Myonecrosis develops within a few days from the beginning of the infection, and the progression and systemization of the infection may lead to septic shock and multiple organ dysfunction [11]. The deep wounds appear to be contaminated by Clostridium in 30% of the cases, and the differential diagnosis is mainly clinical, distinguishing the gas gangrene from the gas produced by simple anaerobic germs.

Gangrene without arterial vascular occlusive disease or traumatic lesion is uncommon, however, in children spontaneous gangrene involving multiple limbs may be associated with gastro-enteritis, hyperosmolarity and hypenatraemia following maternal diabetes mellitus or malpractice in milk formula feeds [12]. The causes of those events are often parent illiteracy, or the difficulty they find in following instructions for food preparation if they are in a foreign language.

In less developed countries a new facet has emerged concerning severe diffused gangrene associated with herbal enemas [12] that follows severe dehydration and affects paediatric patients. Purgation and enemas are often used in tribal folklore. The cytotoxic effects on the liver and the kidney together with the veno-occlusive and vasoconstrictive nature of some herbal medicines used by tribal people are well-known. Perineal and distal colon mucous membrane necrosis may be a characteristic sign. In such cases, an aggressive fluid therapy and correction of the metabolic disturbance comprise the main therapeutic goals. Surgery in the acute phase

is indeed a rare tactic, but once gangrene is established, it should be radical. It may be delayed for as long as it is necessary for the lesions to demarcate.

---

8. NECROTIZING FASCIITIS

Hippocrates [13] first described Necrotizing Fasciitis (NF) in the 5th century B.C. Necrotizing soft tissue infection results in massive necrosis of the skin, subcutaneous fat, fascia and muscles. The incidence of NF has been reported to be 0.4 cases out of 100,000 adults, and 0.08 cases out of the same number of children [10]. The mortality rate ranges from 43.5% to 73%, varying with age (increases in the elderly) and in association with predisposing factors.

According to the microorganisms involved, two types of NF are recognized: (i) a polymicrobial, involving mixed and synergic infection caused by aerobic and anaerobic bacteria (Bacterioides or Peptostreptococcus in combination with E. Coli, Enterobacter, Klebsiella or Proteus), which occurs mainly after surgery or in decubitus ulcers, perianal abscesses, drug injection and immunosuppressive conditions, and (ii) a monomicrobial, involving Group A Streptococcus (S. pyogenes) with or without staphylococcus co-infection [10, 14], or rather frequently, Vibrio vulnificus, Aeromonas hydrophila or methicillin-resistant Staphylococcus aureus (MRSA). According to the progression of the disease, NF is also divided into three categories: (i) fulminant, lasting several hours with few blisters on a small skin area, (ii) acute, lasting several days with large skin areas involved, and (iii) sub-acute, lasting several weeks with localized skin involvement [13].

During childhood, the secondary streptococcal super-infection following Varicella is one of the most common causes of NF [14]. In adults the extremities are most commonly affected, whereas the trunk is usually affected in very young children, which means higher mortality rate because critical underlying structures are affected [13].

Early differential diagnosis of acute severe cellulitis can be life saving. It is based on the presence of severe pain, bullae related to deep vessel occlusion, ecchymosis, skin necrosis, anaesthesia, rapidly spreading lesions and toxic and systemic signs. Cultures and microscopic examinations of biopsies and drainage fluids can help differentiate staphylococcal from streptococcal aetiology, least in the case of monomicrobic fasciitis.

In its acute form, NF spreads within 2-3 days, rapidly devastating the tissues of the limb. The necrosis extends into the fat and then into the fascia below, followed by the muscles. Direct invasion to the vascular system increases local disruption and systemic dissemination of the disease. In the fulminant type the multiorgan system failure can also occur within a few hours. Spread of the infection and the general health of the patient at the time of admission must be immediately considered for therapeutic planning and timing of surgery (Fig. 2). Among the factors favourable for prognosis are creatinine and lactate serum levels, as well as the following coagulation parameters: platelet counts, prothrombin time (PT) and partial thromboplastin time (PTT). In the presence of prolonged PT, the mortality rate significantly increases. Alteration of all three coagulation parameters increases the mortality rate up to 75%. No significant differences between medical treatment and surgical intervention exist [16]. The cornerstone of necrotizing fasciitis management is early diagnosis, while prompt radical debridement in combination with the administration of broad spectrum antibiotics (Table 2) is essential for saving the patient's life. At the level of the hand (Fig. 3, 4) and fingers, this infection can also induce necrotizing cellulitis, with acute compartmental syndrome and fingertip ischemia (Fig. 5). This can be treated only by prompt fasciotomy and drainage.

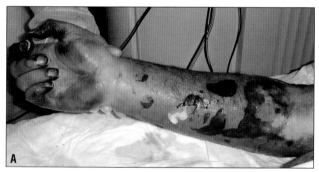

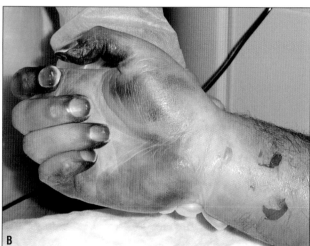

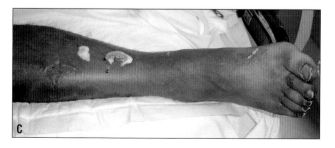

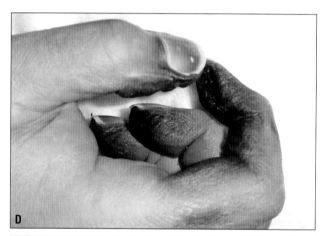

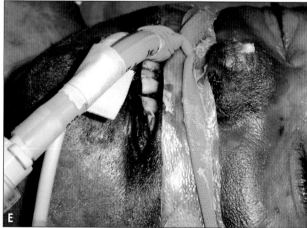

FIGURE 2. (A, B) Septicaemia sustained by streptococcal (pneumoniae) and enterococcal infection in a transplanted and immunocompromised 57-year-old patient in the upper extremity, (C) as well as the lower limb. (D) Severe ischemia of the hand with necrosis of the fingertip, and (E) facial necrosis, as a result of multiple septic emboli.

TABLE 2

Management of Necrotizing Fasciitis

Type of Infection	Antimicrobial Agent	Adult Dosage	Alternatives/Penicillin Hypersensitivity
Mixed infection	Ampicillin/sulbactam or Piperacillin/tazobactam + Clindamycin + Ciprofloxacin	1.5-3.0 gr/6-8 h, iv 4.5 gr/8 h, iv 600 - 900 mg/8 h, iv 400 mg/12 h, iv	Clindamycin + Aminoglycoside or + Fluoroquinolone or: Metronidazole + Aminoglycoside or Fluoroquinolone
Mixed infection	Cefotaxime +Metronidazole or Clindamycin	2 gr/8 h, iv 500 mg/6 h, iv 600 - 900 mg/8 h, iv	
Streptococcus	Penicillin G + Clindamycin	2-4 MU/4-6 h, iv 600 - 900 mg/8 h, iv	Vancomycin Linezolid
Staphylococcus No risk of Methicillin resistant strains	Oxacillin or Cefazolin	2 gr/4 h, iv 1 gr/8 h, iv	Vancomycin Linezolid
Methicillin resistant strains (MRSA)	Vancomycin	500 mg/6 h, iv	Linezolid if intolerant to vanco
Clostridium infections (gas gangrene)	Penicillin G +Clindamycin	2-4 MU/4-6 h, iv 600 - 900 mg/8 h, iv	

8.1. Medical and Surgical Guidelines

Medical treatment of polymicrobial necrotizing fasciitis must include agents which effectively act against both aerobes and anaerobes. For the therapeutic treatment, a combination of ampicillin/sulbactam or piperacillin/tazobactam plus clincamycin and ciprofloxacin, or alternatively, a third generation cephalosporin plus metronidazole or clindamycin should be administered. Monotherapy requires use of carbapenems, such as imipenem, meropenem, or ertapenem, which have a wide range of action against anaerobes and Enterobacteriaceae. Streptococcal fasciitis is usually treated with a combination of penicillin plus clindamycin. Recently, the

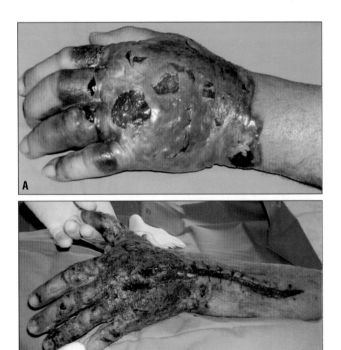

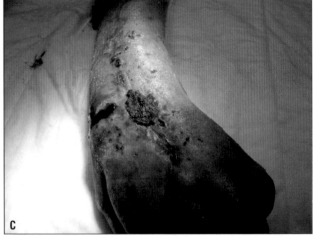

FIGURE 3. (A) Localized NF involving the dorsal tissues of the hand. **(B)** View showing the fasciotomy and surgical debridement of the necrotic tissues which extended to the wrist. **(C)** Appearance at follow-up.

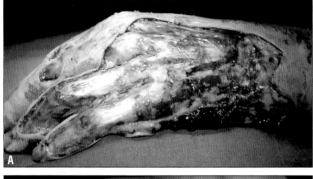

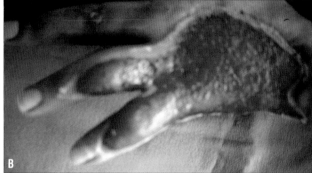

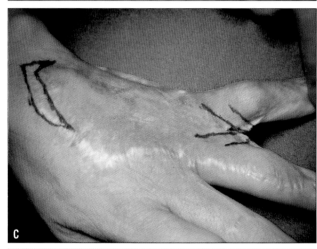

FIGURE 4. (A) Radical excision of necrotic tissues was performed for the treatment of NF of the ulnar digits and hand. **(B)** View showing the progression of soft tissues and skin repair. **(C)** A local flap was drawn at follow-up in order to correct skin retraction and the defect of the hand at the 4th interdigital space.

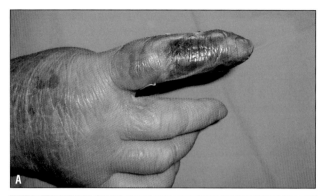

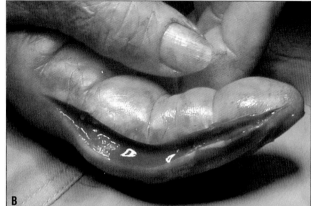

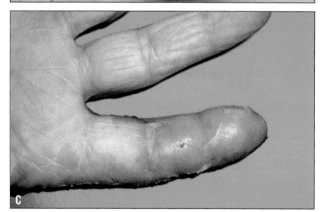

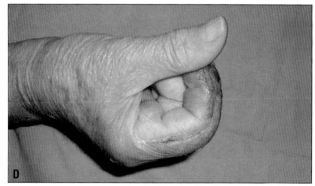

FIGURE 5. (A) Necrotizing cellulitis of the index finger with fingertip ischemia following a needle injury to the distal interphalangeal joint. **(B)** Digital fasciotomy was performed. **(C)** The fingertip was salvaged, and **(D)** good functional results with good pinching was observed at follow-up.

greater efficacy of clindamycin over that of b-lactam antibiotics has been underlined. Penicillin should be added because increasing resistance of Streptococcus to macrolides and Clindamycin has been reported. Staphylococcal fasciitis treatment requires oxacillin, however, for patients with predisposition or recent hospitalization (risks of Methicillin-resistant strains), vancomycin or teicoplanin seems to be more appropriate. Clostridial infections are generally treated with penicillin plus clindamycin.

Surgical treatment requires prompt, radical and complete removal of the necrotic tissues, and it is necessary to extend excisions beyond the visible margin of the infection until the subcutaneous tissue can no longer be separated from the deep fascia.

During the acute phase of the management, supportive care in the intensive care unit (ICU) is often necessary, where mechanical ventilation, fluid supply, cardiac monitoring and adequate nutritional support can be provided. Hyperbaric oxygen (HBO) treatment is very useful as an adjunctive to surgery and antibiotics, especially in presence of Clostridial and anaerobic microorganisms [17]. This procedure provides the tissues with increased oxygen supply and facilitates oxygen penetration into the hypoxic areas. This increases leukocyte and fibroblast function, reduces tissue oedema and ischemia, enhances the local action of antibiotics, and promotes angiogenesis and granulation.

A mean oxygen tension of 250 mmHg is necessary to stop the alpha toxin production [18], considering that the Clostridium perfrigens may grow even in presence of oxygen tensions of up to 70 mmHg [19]. However, the acute problem in the case of gas gangrene is mainly the high rapidity in progression, and therefore, it is mandatory to stop the alpha toxin production as soon as possible. Three to four HBO treatments minimum are necessary in order to get a response. In the case of necrotizing fasciitis, adjunctive HBO treatment is recommended both for understanding the anaerobic aetiology and for stopping the necrotizing progression that is due to anaerobic co-infection [20].

An aggressive and proper treatment when there is suspicion for infections remains the priority, while it is essential at the planning stage of HBO treatment to estimate the massive systemic effects related to progression of the infection, which can rapidly lead to haemolytic anaemia, septic shock and multiple organ failure. For a more accurate diagnosis of CPK increase and hypoca-

leomia, it is essential to perform a repeated follow-up as well as hourly monitoring of diuresis, blood pressure, cardiac output and respiratory frequency. The absence of gas in tissues does not exclude anaerobic infection, and it is not an exclusion criterion for treatment with HBO.

It is our opinion that in presence of gas gangrene, the recommended treatment protocol should include the application of oxygen at 3 atmospheres absolute (ATA) pressure for 90 min, three times during the first 24 hrs, and then twice daily for the next 4-5 days (Fig. 6a). The continuation in treatment depends on the patient's response to HBO therapy (Fig. 6b). In our experience, no deaths occurred after the fourth session.

In presence of necrotizing fasciitis, it is recommended to apply the initial treatments at a pressure of 2.5-2.8 ATA for 90 to 120 minutes, twice a day. Once the patient's condition is stabilized, treatments may be applied on a daily basis only. Because of the nature and the general progression of this disease, it may be necessary to extend the treatment to 10-15 days.

HBO is recommended as an adjunct procedure only when high mortality and morbidity rates are excepted, despite an aggressive standard treatment application. In selected cases, after the initial fasciotomy, more extensive surgical procedures can usually be postponed, with the application of HBO treatment; only segmental debridement of necrotic tissue is required during the course of HBO treatment.

The process should last until clear demarcation between dead and viable tissues is evident. Complications stemming from HBO treatment –and thus, contraindications for its application– could be avoided or reduced if pressures remain three times below normal atmospheric pressure and sessions last no longer than two hours. Major complications include myopia, lasting for weeks or months, ear trauma and lung damage. Severe complication may result in respiratory failure. If congestive heart failure occurs, the symptoms may be even

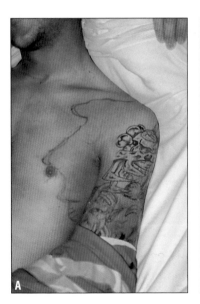
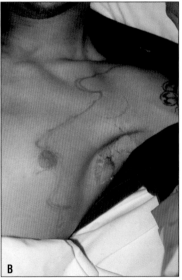

FIGURE 6. (A) Infection of the entire upper limb that spans to the thorax is seen as the result of gas gangrene of the forearm. **(B)** Regression of the infection at the thoracic and arm level was observed following the HBO therapy and radical surgical debridement of the forearm.

worse, while patients with lung disease may be at higher risk of embolism [21].

Although there are no randomized trials of HBO available, the reported meta-analysis of clinical series strongly supports its use [22] in patients with gas gangrene and necrotizing fasciitis. HBO greatly decreases the amputation rate (from 50-55% to 17%) [23]. The early use of a combination of HBO treatment, surgery, and antibiotic therapy, can decrease the mortality rate even more [17, 23-25]. However, in presence of severe septicaemia with multiple and widely extended NF, amputation of the involved segments remains the only reasonable procedure to be followed because the disease incurs high mortality rates and no expectations for a functional outcome.

The effects of the infection can last beyond the acute life-threatening episode and it is necessary to assess them for fear of late sequelae appearing as interrelated or global stiffness, severe skin defect and retraction, and muscle and/or tendon disruption. In the case of growing patients, the long-term follow-up must be assessed for fear of angular deformities and length inequalities between the limbs.

Dressing the wound, following surgical removal of the necrotic tissues, should promote granulation tissue formation and speed up healing by secondary intention. Advanced wound dressing and medical devices, such as collagen or hyaluronic derivatives may improve granulation, leading to definitive treatment or preparing a healthy wound bed for split-thickness skin grafting (Fig. 1d), but in presence of exposed bone, joint or tendon, it is necessary to provide a later coverage by harvesting local or free flaps.

8.1.1. Flaps
Frequently, the first choice concerning the upper limb is the use of local flaps, such as the pedicled flap, or mainly, adipofascial or fasciocutaneous flaps that guarantee sufficient coverage of the elbow, forearm and hand. However, it is the harvest of free perforator flaps that has largely expanded flap use, even though in both adults and children the donor sites for free flaps is particularly scarce. Perforator flaps are valuable alternatives to the traditional muscle or myocutaneous free flaps, as they have the advantage of minimizing donor-site morbidity and improving the result from an aesthetic, functional and psychological perspective [26]. However, the final choice should take into account: (i) the need for a reliable vascular pedicle of sufficient size, and (ii) the necessity to have a good vascular supply of the harvested flap. It is recommended that you avoid randomized or adipofascial flaps that do not have a vascular axis, since such an axis guarantees a good blood supply.

In presence of muscular, tendon and bone defects, it is possible to reconstruct the lost tissues during the same operative procedure. To restore the flexors of the forearm, we use composite flaps for localized defect, or neuromuscular flaps (e.g. the gracilis muscle free flap)

for severe disruption. To restore the extensors of the hand, we use the extensor digitorum brevis free flap.

Tendon transfer is the first choice in restoring the muscular function, following coverage of tissue damage with a previous non-functioning neuromuscular flap. Effort is required for the repair of a nerve defect when there are no possibilities for nerve grafting. In presence of severe segmental loss of both the median and the ulnar nerves in the arm or forearm, a possible salvage procedure is that of St. Clair Srange, i.e. the transfer of a pedicled ulnar nerve followed by termino-lateral suture of the distal stump of the median nerve to the reconstructed ulnar nerve. This technique may give protective sensibility to the hand; however, intrinsic motor functional results are less convincing [27]. The termino-lateral suture to a neighbouring functioning nerve may be applied in cases with single nerve loss.

At the joint level, it is necessary to distinguish between deformity from tissue contracture and intrinsic stiffness, while planning the treatment of both, because the upper extremity requires mobility and agility to function properly, and any loss of movement at any level is a problem for the entire limb. Considering the upper limb as an interrelated kinematics chain, it is useful to treat the stiffness starting from the proximal joints and moving distally. Stiffness of the first ray is particularly invalidating [28]. Treatment should include the first dorsal interosseous muscle detachment, the adductor muscle "Z" lengthening, and further syndesmotomies to release the intrinsic stiffness of the trapezio-metacarpal joint.

ROM always needs to be assessed on a regular basis until a "plateau" is reached. It is worth considering surgery when ROM is not satisfactory for the realization of particular hand functions, i.e. when it is below 70°. On the other hand, good function and range of movement (ROM) of the shoulder and the elbow are prerequisites for successful surgery of the hand, because the surgeon is able to place the limb in appropriate position.

8.1.2. Tenoarthrolyses
Tenoarthrolysis [29] of the dorsal apparatus (TADA) is a very useful technique to correct stiffness of the fingers in extension (Fig. 7). On the other hand, severe stiffness of the fingers in flexion may be corrected with total anterior tenoarthrolysis (TATA) [30]. The periosteum is dissected from the phalanges in order to achieve complete lifting of the flexor apparatus, the volar plates and the neurovascular bundles (Fig. 8). This technique allows tenolysis, arthrolysis and skin repair at the same operation, avoiding combinations of different surgical procedures which may add iatrogenic injuries and fibrosis. The TATA also permits selection of the same lateral incision of an eventually previous finger fasciotomy.

9. GUIDELINES IN REHABILITATION PLANNING

Improvements in life-saving procedures extended the goals of treatment of necrotizing fasciitis towards

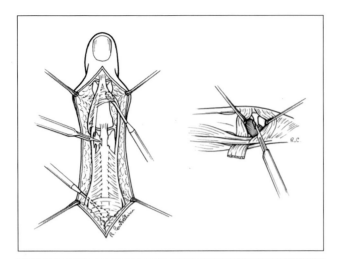

FIGURE 7. Diagram showing the TADA technique for each of the metacarpophalangeal and interphalangeal joints of the finger.

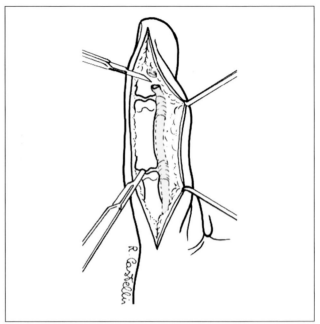

FIGURE 8. Diagram showing the dissection of the entire flexor apparatus from the phalanges in TATA.

achieving maximal preservation of function. Thus, an adequate and early rehabilitation program and a psychological adjuvant therapy to be applied during the prolonged hospitalization have been additionally included in the treatment course. Unattended joints of the hand that do not undergo an appropriate rehabilitation program frequently develop either interrelated stiffness that involves all the small joints of the same ray, or global stiffness [28].

On this basis, the rehabilitation program must be initiated immediately after haemodynamic stabilization and radical surgical debridement in order that the stiffness that follows the longstanding immobilization of the unattended joints is avoided. The treatment plan includes: (i) monitoring of fluid volume depletion (evaluating the serum level of creatinine) to avoid renal insufficiency, (ii) administration of low-dose heparin to avoid deep vein thrombosis, (iii) nutritional status care to avoid gastrocolitis or infection recurrences, and (iv) intravenous pain control systems to achieve pain relief, since the patient is not able to take oral analgesic.

Early therapeutic intervention is of utmost importance when infections of the fingers and the hand induce the onset of severe stagnant oedema in the hand. The oedema triggers off a vicious cycle of decreased arterial, venous, and lymphatic flow, which results in minimal hand movement due to pain, and the eventual onset of the permanent intrinsic and extrinsic fibrotic tissue scarring, leading to long-term loss of hand function.

The role of the therapist during the initial phase of the acute infection is to splint the hand and wrist in a functional position (distal interphalangeal joints at 5° in flexion, proximal interphalangeal joints at 10° in flexion, metacarpophalangeal joints at 60° in flexion, and wrist placed at 15°-25° in extension). The thumb should be in alignment with the forearm and abducted away from the palm. The entire arm should be elevated.

The splint is usually placed volarly and is used to protect the affected area, minimize oedema and reduce pain from overstretched ligaments and articular capsules, thus helping to avoid finger flexion contractures. In cases of severe infection, lymphatic drainage massage is initially contraindicated; however, if the infection manifests copious irrigation, it should be performed following surgical debridement and/or administration of appropriate antibiotics. The therapist should not manually activate lymph drainage in the acute phase of the infection, because then there might be the risk of infection infiltration into more proximal uninfected fascial tissue.

Once the physician indicates that the infection is responding to antibiotics, the role of the therapist is to reduce, as much as possible, local oedema by performing elevation and retrograde drainage massage of the entire arm, and to educate the patient on performing both passive and active assistive range of motion exercises for both the involved and the uninvolved joints. It is in the patient's best interest to begin performing various tendon gliding exercises (hook fist, full fist and straight fist exercises) at least 5 minutes every hour in order to create a distal muscle pump which would help in activating efficient venous return from the hand and also in preventing the formation of tendon adhesions due to fibrotic scarring. Frequently, among dressing changes it is quite advantageous for the patient to immerse the hand and the forearm in sterile water contrast baths. The contrast bath temperature should be at 38°-44°C in order to provoke vasodilatation and at 10°-18°C to provoke vasoconstriction. The patient should place the involved hand in the warm basin for at least 10 minutes and perform gentle fisting exercises, and then immerse it hand/forearm in the cold water for one minute and return to the warm bath for 4 minutes. This cycle should be continued for 30 minutes. The cyclical vasodilatation - vasoconstriction aids in increasing circulation to the area and stimulating lymph drainage. Only in cases of severe tenacious oedema the patient should end the contrast bath treatment in the cold water basin. If the patient starts physical therapy with the hand already in a rigid posture, the therapy course should be changed, focusing on specific joint mobilization exercises and manipulations that will be followed by dynamic hand splinting to gradually stretch tendon and capsular contractions and restore to normal the range of motion and strength.

10. PERIPHERAL SEPTIC THROMBOPHLEBITIS

Peripheral Septic Thrombophlebitis can occur not only by spread of neighbouring infections, but also spontaneously, by direct colonization following break injuries of the skin, or invasive procedures [31]. *Staphylococcus aureus* is the causative agent in 65-78% of the cases reported before 1968. More recently, the importance of nosocomial microorganisms such as *Enterobacteriaceae, Pseudomonas, Enterococci, Candida* and *Malassenzia furfur* has progressively increased.

In presence of a skin portal of entry (cannulation, injection, bites, wounds etc.) the superficial venous system of the limb is mainly involved. Therefore, the "simple" superficial thrombophlebitis may be first thought of when differential diagnosis is to be made. The septic emboli following the involvement of the vein system can also result in metastatic infections and in the newborns in particular, in thromboembolic acral ischemia (Fig. 9). An initial combination of anti-pseudomonas penicillin (like piperacillin +/-tazobactam) or third/fourth generation cephalosporin (ceftadime or cefipime plus vancomycin) should be initiated, until culture results become available.

11. OSTEOMYELITIS

In presence of a persistent fistula in the infected area, Osteomyelitis must always be suspected. Staphylococcus aureus and the group B Streptococcus are the most common causative agents. The bone can be involved by an invasion "in contiguity" where a chronic form is quickly established; or Osteomyelitis can be an acute one that is due to haematogenous dissemination of the microorganisms, mainly occurring during childhood [6, 32].

Bone infections occurring before the individual completes his first year of life are globally classified as osteoarthritic infections. They occur because of the vascular communication between the articular space and the meta-diaphysis, easily allowing germs to pass. After the first year of life, acute haematogenous osteomyelitis

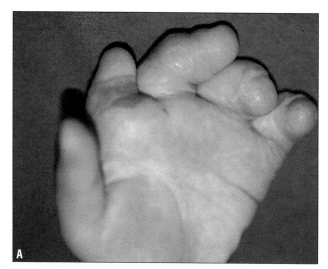

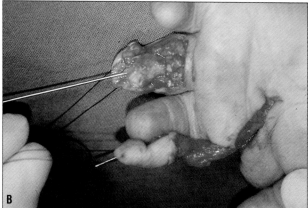

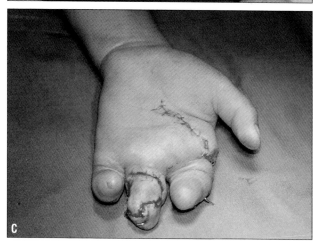

FIGURE 9. (A) Sequelae in the forearm and long fingers following an intrauterine septic thromboembolia. **(B)** The 2nd ray was amputated, and a pedicle volar flap was harvested to cover the skin defect following the surgical extension of the severely flexed ring finger. **(C)** Postoperative findings after surgical correction of the deformities at the long fingers.

or arthritis of the epiphysis may occur [32]. In the newborn, direct invasion of infection into the bone from neighbouring infected areas is a very rare event, which becomes more frequent at later ages in the form of a chronic or sub-acute osteomyelitis. In young patients, a-cute bone infection must be suspected in presence of fever, localized pain and leukocytosis.

The x-ray features are often inconclusive within the first fifteen days. In presence of suppurating arthritis, drainage of the joint must be performed to decrease the bacterial load and the endo-articular pressure, and detect the microorganism [32]. The drainage should be in combination with prompt antibiotic therapy (Table 3).

12. Toxic Shock Syndrome

The infection that is due to particular types of Staphylo-coccus aureus and Streptococcus pyogenes, which produce toxins, can also result in a toxic shock syndrome (TSS). This life-threatening infection was first detected in 1978 in children presenting with group I Staphylococcus aureus [6]. The syndrome results from toxaemia, not septicaemia, and as a result of cutaneous infections, skin lesion and traumatic or surgical wounds [33]. It is thought to be a superantigen-mediated disease, where the toxins activate the immune system, bypassing the usual immuno-response sequence. TSS develops within two days from the lesion contamination, leading to severe hypotension, diffused intravascular coagulation and acute respiratory distress syndrome [33]. In paediatric patients, TSS occurs most commonly due to non-steroidal anti-inflammatory drug abuse, complications due to Varicella, arthritis, osteomyelitis, or wound super-infections. However, in children, the mortality rate is 3-10%, which is much lower than adult mortality rate that ranges from 30% to 70% according to host-pathogen interaction, virulence factors, and host immunity capacity [15, 33, 34].

Clinical criteria for the diagnosis of TSS include fever, profound and refractory hypotension, erythematous rash with subsequent desquamation, and involvement of three or more of the following organ systems: gastrointestinal (vomiting, diarrhoea), muscular (severe myalgia or increase in CPK), mucous membranes (hyperaemia), renal (insufficiency), liver (hepatitis), central nervous system (disorientation), blood (thrombocytopenia). Blood cultures are exceptionally positive, but Staphylococcus aureus can be isolated from focal skin lesions. An anti-staphylococcal agent like oxacillin should be administered intravenously. Intravenous γ-globulin (IVIG) is usually recommended, however, evidence supporting its use is still absent.

13. Contaminated wounds and bites

Among the infections life-threatening diseases following contaminated wounds or bites, tetanus and rabies play a significant role, whereas in exceptional cases, Vibrio Vulnificus and botulism. Vibrio Vulnificus [35] in the upper limb occurs in rare cases of rapidly progressing infections with a history of saltwater contact. On the other hand, botulism [36] can occasionally contaminate traumatic injuries. Botulinum toxin inhibits acetylcholine release, blocking peripheral synapses, including neuro-muscular junctions. The infection presents the typical manifestations of descending cranial nerves and generalized motor paralysis, with dysphagia and further ventilatory failure disproportional to the wound severity. Supportive therapy, especially ventilatory support, is the most important part of the treatment. Antitoxin therapy is carried out by use of trivalent serum, but reported hypersensitivity rate ranges from 9% to 20%. Wound debridement and Penicillin G or metronidazole therapy are generally recommended, but the role of antibiotics has never been extensively tested.

Tetanus and rabies are related to the Clostridium

TABLE 3			
Management of Osteomyelitis			
	Microorganisms	Therapy	Dosage
Newborn	Streptococcus Staphylococcus aureus	Ampicillin-Sulbactam + Cefotaxime	50 mg/Kg/8 h iv 33 mg/Kg/8 h iv
< 5 years	Streptococcus Staphylococcus aureus Haemophilus infl. Type B	Ampicillin-Sulbactam + Riphampycin	50 mg/Kg/8 h iv 10 mg/Kg/12 h po
> 5 years	Streptococcus Staphylococcus aureus	Ampicillin-Sulbactam + Riphampycin	50 mg/Kg/8 h iv 10 mg/Kg/12 h po
Surgery & Traumatic injuries	Streptococcus Staphylococcus aureus Staphylococcus epiderm. Gram negative	Ampicillin-Sulbactam + Cefotaxime +/- Metronidazole	50 mg/Kg/8 h iv 33 mg/Kg/8 h iv 10 mg/Kg/8 h iv

tetani and Rhabdovirus infections. The wide policy of vaccination and IG-prophylaxis, both in the human population and in the animal host, has significantly reduced the incidence of these diseases. Tetanus in Italy decreased from 700 cases/year to 100-200 during the last three decades [37, 38], and rabies in Europe has been reported only in 278 cases from 1978 to the present (mainly in the Eastern Europe, due to the great number of wild foxes and bats inhabiting there) [39, 40]. However, the reported cases of Tetanus in the less developed countries are significantly more, resulting in up to 800,000 deaths, mainly of newborns and children. The worldwide recorded data of the Rabies are quite similar, i.e. 1,000 deaths/year and 30,000 new cases/year [38, 40]. The treatment provides neutralization of unbound toxin (3-6000 units of toxin intra-muscular injection) and removal of the source of infection (wound surgical debridement). Antibiotics should be administered in order to interrupt toxin production. Penicillin, which has been used for many years, has been found to work as a GABA antagonist favouring convulsions, and therefore, metronidazole is now considered the drug of choice. Control of spasm and rigidity, and supportive intensive care treatment are considered the cornerstone of therapy. Sedation, and administration of benzodiazepines or/and other drugs (eg. Propofol) are always the mainstay of treatment.

The rabies virus is highly neurotropic with a prolonged incubation period, usually between 20 and 90 days. During this incubation period, immunization can halt infection. No tests are currently available to diagnose rabies in humans before the clinical onset of the disease. Immunofluorescent antibody detection on skin biopsies performed early in the course of illness is the most reliable test. Anyway, once symptoms occur, rabies is almost always fatal, so prevention is essential. Wounds due to animal bites at risk of developing rabies need to be considered as post- exposure prophylaxis. All wounds should be cleaned with soap and water because this practice has proved to protect against experimental rabies at 90%. Administration of human rabies immune globulins and vaccine is recommended mainly in the presence of bites by skunks, racoons, bats, or foxes. Bites by dogs, cats, or ferrets should be prophylactically examined after observation of the animal for 10 days.

14. CONCLUSION

Strict attention must be paid to the observation of common guidelines for prevention, prompt diagnosis, and treatment of the potential life-threatening infections.

The multidisciplinary approach to these pathologies plays the most significant role in life saving efforts. The main cornerstone in managing life threatening infections is early diagnosis, while prompt fasciotomy and radical deridement in combination with the administration of broad-spectrum antibiotics are essential for saving the patient's life. During the acute phase, supportive care in the Intensive Unit is necessary to provide ventilation, fluid and cardiac support, mainly for patients undergoing major surgerical procedures.

HBO is useful as an adjunctive procedure both in stopping the progression of the infection and improving the oxygenation of the surrounding necrotizing tissues.

Following the acute phase, the effects of the infection can last beyond the emergency treatment and it is necessary to assess them for fear of the late sequelae. An early rehabilitation program and wound dressing, reducing significantly the incidence of skin defect or retraction, and stiffness requiring further surgery, must play a relevant role.

On this basis, a tight collaboration among the orthopaedist, intensive care service, the internist with a specific skill in infectious diseases and the physiatrist, must lead to common guidelines in order to minimize the time towards achieving a prompt diagnosis and immediately initiating a first line of medical, surgical and life-supporting treatment.

REFERENCES

[1] Bader L, Maydl G, Gieseke K, Heesemann J. Bacterial infections following injections and infusion caused by errors of hygiene. MMW Fortschr Med 2005;147(4):28-32.
[2] Tomono K. Etiology of sepsis occurring in the immunocompromised host and its prevention. Kansenshogaku Zasshi. 1989; 63(5):479-488.
[3] Seltzer DG, McAuliffe J, Campbell DR, Burkhalter WE. AIDS in the hand patient, the team approach. Hand Clin. 1991; 7(3):433-445.
[4] Baumeister S, Kleist C, Dohler B, Bickert B, Germann G, Opelz G. Risk of allogenic hand transplantation. Microsurgery. 2004; 24(2):98-103.
[5] Werner H, Kuntsche J. Infection in the elderly, what is different?. Z Gerontol Geriatr. 2000; 33(5):350-356.
[6] Aldin AS, Kinzl L, Eisele R. Severe complications of staphylococcus aureus infection in the child. Unfallchirurg. 2001; 104(1):85-90.
[7] Hirotsu T, Akatsuka J. Infectious complications in childhood leukaemia. Acta Perdiatr Jpn 1991; 33(4):564-572.
[8] McCarthy JJ, Dormans JP, Kozin SH, Pizzutello PD. Muscoloskeletal infections in children: basic treatment principles and recent advancement. Inst Course Lect 2005;54:515-528.
[9] Lewis RT. Soft tissue infections. World J Surg 1998;22:146-151.
[10] Wilkerson R, Paull W, Coville FV. Necrotizing fasciitis, review of the literature and case report. Clin Orhtop Relat Res 1987; 216:187-192.
[11] Stevens DL, Bryant AE. The role of clostridial toxins in the pathogenesis of gas gangrene. Clin Infect Dis 2004;35:93-100.
[12] Mokoena T, Hadley GP. Surgical management of multiple limb gangrene following dehydratation in children. S Afr Med J 1991; 80:185-188.
[13] Descamps V, Aitken J, Lee MG. Hippocrates on necrotizing fasciitis. Lancet 1994;344:556.

[14] Trent JT, Kirsner RS. Necrotizing fasciitis. Wounds. 2002; 14(8):284-292.

[15] Floret D. Clinical aspects of streptococcal and staphylococcal toxinic diseases. Arch Pediatr 2001;4:762-768.

[16] Hsiao GH, Chang CH, Hsiao CW, Fanchiang JH, Jee SH. Necrotizing soft tissue infections. Surgical or conservative treatment? Dermatol Surg 1998;24(2):243-247.

[17] Yuen JC, Feng Z. Salvage of limb and function in necrotizing fasciitis of the hand: role of hyperbaric oxygen treatment and free muscle flap. South Med J 2002;95(2):255-257.

[18] Van Unnik AJM. Inhibition of toxin production in clostridium perfringens in vitro by hyperbaric oxygen. Leeuwenhoek Microbiol 1965;131:181-186.

[19] McLeod JW. Variation in the periods of exposure to air and oxygen necessary to kill anaerobia bacteria. Acta Pathol Microbiol Scand 1930;3(Suppl):225.

[20] Headley AJ. Necrotizing soft tissue infections: a primary care review. Am Fam Physician 2003;68(2):323-8.

[21] Brummelkamp WH. Consideration on hyperbaric oxygen therapy at three atmosphere absolute for clostridial infection type welchii. Ann NY Acad Sci 1965;117:688-699.

[22] Clark LA, Moon RE. Hyperbaric oxygen in the treatment of life-threatening soft-tissue infections. Respir Care Clin North Am 1999;5(2):203-19

[23] Escobar SJ, Slade JB Jr, Hunt TK, Cianci P. Adjuvant hyperbaric oxygen therapy for treatment of necrotizing fasciitis reduces mortality and amputation rate. Undersea Hyperb Med 2005; 32(6):437-43.

[24] Riseman JA, Zamboni WA, Curtis A, Graham DR, Konrad HR, Ross DS. Hyperbaric oxygen therapy for necrotizing fasciitis reduces mortality and the need for debridements. Surgery 1990; 108(5):847-50.

[25] Desola J, Escola E, Moreno E, Munoz MA, Sanchez U, Murillo F. Combined treatment of gaseous gangrene with hyperbaric oxygen therapy, surgery and antibiotics. A national cooperative multicenter study. Med Clin (Barc) 1990;94(17):641-50

[26] Van Landuyt K, Hamdi M, Blondeel P, Tonnard P, Verpaele A, Monstrey S. Free perforator flaps in children. Plast Reconstr Surg 2005;116:159-169.

[27] Greenberg BM, Cuadros CL, Panda M, May JW. St. Clair Strange procedure: indications, technique and long term evaluation. J Hand Surg 1988;13:928-935.

[28] Landi A, Caserta G, Saracino A, Facchini MC. Stiffness of the thumb. In: Joint stiffness of the upper limb. Landi A et al (eds). Martin Dunitz London. 1997. pg. 277-287.

[29] Saffar P. Treatment of stiffness of the proximal interphalangeal joint. In: Joint stiffness of the upper limb. Landi A et al (eds). Martin Dunitz London. 1997. pg. 265-272.

[30] Saffar P. La tenoarthrolyse totale anterieur. Ann Chir Maine 1983; 4:345-350.

[31] Feided C. Thrombophlebitis septic. www.emedicine.com/emerg/topic581.htm, 2004.

[32] Senes FM, Campus R, Mantero E. Patologia infettiva perinatale dell'arto superiore. In: L'arto superiore nell'ambito della patologia perinatale. Landi A, Bernasconi (eds). Mattioli1885. Fidenza. 2003. pg.150-162.

[33] Long WT, Filler BC, Cox E, Stark HH. Toxic shock syndrome after a human bite to the hand. 1988;13(6):957-959.

[34] Chuang YY, Huang YC, Lin TY. Toxic shock syndrome in children: epidemiology, pathogenesis, and management. Paediatric drugs. 2005;7(1):11-25.

[35] Shah MA, Pettit AM, Viegas SF. Vibrio vulnificus infection of the upper extremities. Am J Orthop 2004;33(11):568-571.

[36] Thorne FL, Kropp RJ. Wound botulism: a life threatening complication of hand injuries. Plast reconstr Surg 1983;71(4):548-551.

[37] Bardenheier B, Prevots DR, Khetsuriani N. MMWR 1998; 47(ss2):1-13.

[38] Mandolini D, Ciofi degli Atti M, Pedalino B, Bella A, De Mei B, Parrocini S, Salmaso S. Epidemiologia del tetano in Italia. BEN-Notiziario ISS 2002;Vol.15 (3).

[39] WHO. Regional Office for Europe. Health for all statistical database. www.who.dk/country.htm.

[40] WHO. Rabies Bulletin. www.who-rabies-bulletin.org.

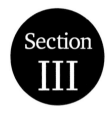

Section III

INFECTIONS IN CHILDREN AND CHRONIC OSTEOMYELITIS

Infections in Children and Chronic Osteomyelitis

Upper Extremity Infections in Children

Shalom STAHL*, Edward CALIF

Hand Surgery Unit, Rambam Medical Center, Haifa, Israel

Upper extremity infections in children range from superficial infections to severe surgical emergencies. Patients may present with non-specific symptoms and deceptively "mild" appearance. Misdiagnosis or mistreatment often results in long-term morbidity and considerable residual disability. Solid knowledge of the anatomy, etiology and pathogenesis of these infections, coupled with timely intervention are the key for effective management and avoidance long-term functional impairment.

Keywords: hand; upper extremity; infection; children.

1. INTRODUCTION

Musculoskeletal infections usually occur during childhood and constitute a considerable cause of morbidity. Since the hand has many compartments and delicate structures, morbidity is usually associated with a protracted healing course and substantial disabling sequelae. Accurate diagnosis, and prompt and adequate treatment are essential for ensuring a good long-term outcome.

Hand infections in children range from superficial and mild infections to severe emergencies that require prompt surgical treatment. Most superficial infections are easily diagnosed and readily treated effectively, while some suppurative infections, especially those involving bony and articular struc-

tures, still are both therapeutic and surgical challenges [1]. Neglected and mistreated deep infections often result in significant functional impairment that might affect the child's hand.

While adults usually disclose their medical histories and complaints in detail, children usually express their complaints poorly. Predisposition or previous injuries that have incited infection are not reported most of the time, while clinical presentation of infection may not be specific. Infants may merely present with lethargy, restlessness, or irritability. Therefore, a vigilant and thorough physical examination is mandatory.

The etiology of hand infections is diverse. Infection in children may occur following nail biting (onychophagia) and finger/thumb sucking. These phenomena are common in the pediatric age group and represent the earliest form of habitual manipulation of the body. Thumb sucking is usually associated with oral pleasure and self-comforting behavior. It occurs mainly among children up to five years of age [2]. In addition to orthodontic complications and finger deformities, finger sucking may cause fingertip infections. Nail biting may cause damage to the cuticles and the nails, dental problems, and secondary bacterial infections.

Severe infections in pediatric population should be managed by a multidisciplinary team consisting

*Corresponding Author
The Unit of Hand Surgery, Rambam Medical Center
P.O. Box 9602, Haifa 31096, Israel
Tel: 972 4 8542619
Fax: 972 4 8542750
e-mail: s_stahl@rambam.health.gov.il

of a pediatrician, an infectious-diseases specialist, a hand surgeon, nursing staff and rehabilitating therapists.

The management of hand infections in children requires solid knowledge of the local anatomy, etiology and pathogenesis of these infections. Surgical interventions should be performed in an operating room setting and under general anaesthesia in order that pain is adequately managed and violation of delicate anatomic structures is avoided.

This chapter provides an overview of the clinical course, natural history, microbiology, and management of these often uneventful, but occasionally life-threatening infections.

2. CELLULITIS AND ABSCESS

This is a common skin affliction, usually following a minor penetrating trauma through which there is direct inoculation, or a pre-existing skin abrasion complicated by secondary infection. It manifests itself as diffuse local hyperemia, edema, tenderness, and fever. The disease-causing pathogen is usually *Staphylococcus aureus* or *Streptococcus pyogenes.* A careful evaluation is prerequisite to ruling out deeper infection. Treatment includes a trial of oral antibiotics, while severe cases necessitate intravenous antibiotics. If an abscess forms, surgical drainage is indicated for immediate application.

3. DEEP SPACE INFECTIONS

The hand has three anatomically defined potential spaces that lie between the muscle fascial planes, and include the thenar, midpalmar, and hypothenar spaces

[3]. Deep space infections are caused either by direct inoculation through penetrating injuries, or by contiguous spread from untreated flexor tenosynovitis. The causative pathogen is usually *Staphylococcus aureus* or *Streptococcus.* The clinical presentation includes tender swelling, principally on the dorsum of the hand. Dorsally placed loose connective tissue facilitates greater expansion. Pus from the thenar or midpalmar spaces may rupture the Parona's space. Deep space infections require immediate surgical treatment. Incision, drainage and irrigations are essential, and parenteral antibiotics with anti-staphylococcal action should be administered preferably after obtaining a culture (Fig. 1).

The subaponeurotic space lies dorsally in the hand, deep to the extensor tendons, above the periosteum of the metacarpals and the fascia of the dorsal interosseous muscles. Infection in this space manifests itself as tender swelling, erythema, and often fluctuation on the dorsum of the hand, which may be difficult to differentiate from cellulitis symptoms. The abscess is decompressed through a small single incision.

The space infection which spreads towards both the palmar and the dorsal sides is known as collar-button abscess. As the space palmarly is limited, infection spreads to the dorsal subcutaneous tissues. The treatment requires palmar and dorsal incision.

4. PURULENT FLEXOR TENOSYNOVITIS

This is a suppurative infection of the flexor tendon sheath, which usually results from direct puncture or spread of deep space infection or a felon. The patient typically presents the Kanavel's classic signs: a flexed digital posture, tenderness over the flexor sheath, diffuse swelling, and painful passive stretching. Kanavel's signs

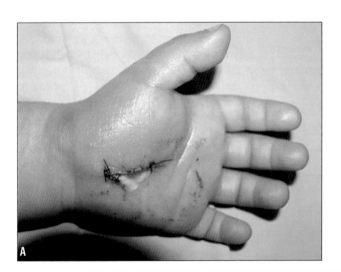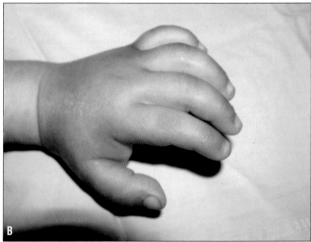

FIGURE 1. A penetrating injury complicated by deep space infection. The child has been treated elsewhere by drainage and irrigation through the wound in skin. Note the swelling on both palmar **(A)** and dorsal **(B)** aspects of the hand, as well as the draining pus due to the persisting deep space infection.

are of great clinical importance in evaluating purulent tenosynovitis in the pediatric population, since they are easy to elicit, regardless of the child's compliance and cooperation.

Purulent flexor tenosynovitis of the thumb or the little finger may ascend though the radial and the ulnar bursae, respectively, and eventually rupture the Parona's subtendinous potential space. This may result in "horseshoe" tenosynovitis.

In the majority of cases, staphylococci are the causative agent of this pyogenic infection. Therefore, administration of empiric anti-staphylococcal intravenous antibiotics should be introduced, after obtaining cultures from a draining wound whenever present, and adapted thereafter when culture results are available. Developing infections, if diagnosed early, can be amenable to intravenous antibiotics and close observation. Infection progressing despite treatment or established infection necessitates urgent incision, drainage, and irrigation in order that tendon scarring or necrosis with subsequent finger function impairment is prevented.

5. PARONYCHIA

This infection involves the space arround the nail fold. Any disruption of the seal between the proximal nail fold and the nail plate may provide access to bacteria and cause infection within the eponychial space. While in adults hangnails, manicures, and identifiable penetrating injuries incite infection, in children, usually, this is not the case. Instead, habits of oral manipulation such as nail-biting and finger sucking are often reported. The offensive pathogen, as in most other hand infections, is usually *Staphylococcus.* However, in our clinical practice we noticed an emerging mixed-organism pattern of infection, featuring mainly *Staphylococci,* but also *Streptococci,* and gram-positive and gram-negative anaerobes. This pattern of infection is similar to infection occurring when there are human bites and clenched-fist injuries. In such a case, broad-spectrum antibiotics are necessary in addition to surgical debridement, drainage and irrigation. Neglected paronychia may result in spreading of the pus under the nail sulcus to the opposite eponychial side, producing a "run-around" abscess [4].

Early infection may be successfully treated by anti-staphylococcal agents. When a fluctuant abscess is present, drainage should be applied. The fold is incised away from the nail bed, the pus is drained, and the space is irrigated. This is followed by wide-spectrum antibiotics and local wound care until complete secondary healing is attained.

6. FELON

The felon is a palmar closed-space infection of the pulp of the distal phalanx. The patient typically presents with tender swelling and erythema of the pulp, and complains of marked throbbing pain. A history of a penetrating injury is commonly reported, however, in our practice we have repeatedly encountered children with felons who had a history of onychophagia or finger sucking, and a polymicrobial culture originating from the oral cavity. The most commonly isolated pathogen in felons is *Staphylococcus aureus.* Antimicrobial treatment should essentially involve a wide-spectrum agent. Incision and drainage should be applied. We recommend the unilateral high longitudinal incision performed over the non-opposing aspect of the finger. This approach maintains the volar fat pad as a unit, preventing the development of an unstable tip when pinching or tapping [5]. Meticulous discharge of the pus without violating the adjacent flexor tendon, the digital neurovascular structures and the nail matrix, is more likely to be successful when performed in an operating room setting and when the patient is under general anaesthesia. After surgical drainage the wound is dressed and soaks are applied 24 hours later.

The osseous blood supply in children is unique. The digital arteries provide the epiphysis with a nutrient supply before entering the closed compartment. This guarantees intact blood perfusion to the epiphysis despite the compromised tissue perfusion within the pulp space caused by the rising pressure. Growth disturbances are therefore unlikely to occur, and viable bone remains available for osseous regeneration, in case the distal portion of the phalanx is destroyed by osteomyelitis. Therefore, bone that appears in surgical exploration to be necrotic but not sequestrated should not be excised, since bones of children have a remarkable reparative potential.

7. BITE-WOUND INFECTIONS

This is a common kind of infection affecting the pediatric age group, especially those children who have household pets.

7.1. Human bite-wound infections

Approximately 40% of human bite injuries of children involve the upper extremity [6]. The human saliva is a rich culture medium. One milliliter of saliva may contain up to 100 million organisms and up to forty-two different strains of bacteria [7]. Therefore, these infections are typically polymicrobial. Isolated pathogens mostly are *Streptococci, Staphylococcus aureus, Eikenella corrodens,* and anaerobes. Initial presentation may be deceptively mild, while the true severity of the injury may be hidden. Surgical exploration, irrigation and debridement are often needed, and the wound is left open for healing by secondary intention. Anti-tetanus prophylaxis, local wound care and wide-spectrum antibiotic administration are essential.

7.2. Animal bite-wound infections

Children are the most frequently reported victims of animal bites [6] mainly by dogs and cats. Similarly, this is a mixed aerobic-anaerobic infection. *Pasteurella multocida* is isolated in up to 50% of dog-bite infections and 80% of cat-bite infections [8]. Usually these injuries manifest themselves with signs of local cellulitis. Purulent discharge may be observed. Local infection may be complicated by flexor tenosynovitis, deep-space infection, collar-button abscess consisting of a web space infection that involves both the palmar and the dorsal sides, septic arthritis and osteomyelitis. Uncomplicated wounds should be treated by a wide-spectrum antibiotic agent, such as Amoxycillin-clavulanate, and local wound care. Primary wound closure is contraindicated. Complicated wounds need to be aggressively treated by irrigation and debridement. Involved joints should be explored and irrigated. Empiric wide-spectrum antibiotics should be introduced while waiting for culture results. Anti-tetanus prophylaxis is essential and the possibility of rabies development should be considered.

8. Viral Infections

Those infections are usually caused by *herpes simplex virus.* Herpetic Whitlow is a herpetic infection of the nail bed and the pulp. Typically, children with herpetic stomatitis infect their fingers during finger sucking. They present with painful vesicular lesions of the fingers. Surgical drainage is contraindicated since it may induce a secondary purulent infection and spread the initial. The infection is self-limited even without anti-viral therapy; however, infection development including local erosions may be rather destructive. Antiviral therapy reduces the duration of the clinical signs appearance. Acyclovir is a safe and effective therapeutic choice.

Varicella infection in the upper extremity in young children can be complicated by secondary bacterial infection, which may require hospitalization and antibiotic treatment.

Enteroviral infection usually manifests itself as a mild febrile disease, occasionally accompanying papular or papulovesicular lesions of the palm and the sole. This infection is self-limited and no special treatment is suggested.

9. Osteomyelitis and Septic Arthritis

It is difficult to estimate the exact incidence of childhood osteomyelitis and septic arthritis. Nelson [9] estimated that one in 5000 children under the age of thirteen years suffer from osteomyelitis, and about twice as many suffer from septic arthritis. Approximately 50% of osteomyelitis cases are children up to 5 years old. Most cases of septic arthritis are children three years old or younger. Boys have higher predisposition than girls to both osteomyelitis and septic arthritis [10].

Osteomyelitis and septic arthritis in the hand usually occur by direct inoculation, or contiguously by direct spread of soft-tissue infection, rather than via a hematogenous route. Causative agents are accordingly the same pathogens that are encountered in soft tissue infections following penetrating injuries or bite-wounds. Due to the unique osseous blood supply young infants have, and the presence of perforating capillaries that communicate between the metaphysis and the joint space, adjacent osteomyelitis and septic arthritis may coexist.

Diagnosis of osteomyelitis is often difficult to make, and persistence of a non-healing wound despite standard treatment should raise the index of suspicion for osteomyelitis. Technetium bone scans, and radiographs at a later stage, may be helpful. The diagnosis of septic arthritis is confirmed by finding purulent fluid in the joint.

The treatment of osteomyelitis includes empiric intravenous antibiotic administration while waiting for culture results and susceptibility patterns. Intravenous therapy may be substituted by oral therapy according to the clinical course and laboratory markers. Provided that the isolated pathogens are susceptible to oral antibiotics, the duration of the antibiotic therapy should be 4 weeks at least in the case of acute osteomyelitis. Septic arthritis is treated by intravenous antibiotics. Surgical drainage is indicated if symptoms and signs do not resolve rapidly following conservative treatment.

10. Neonatal Infections

Infectious diseases are a major cause of morbidity and occasional mortality in neonates. Prematurity, low gestational age, very low birth weight, and longer hospital stay are significant risk factors. The maternal and the nursery environment are the two principal sources of newborn infection. Clinical presentation is often non-specific, and irritability, poor feeding, and impoverished movement may be present [11].

Cutaneous infections in neonates are mostly caused by *Staphylococcus aureus.* They include localized infections and local manifestation of symptoms of a widespread infection such as those of the scalded skin syndrome. Neonatal fungal skin infections are either local such as onychomycosis, or part of a generalized candidal skin affliction. Viral infections such as neonatal varicella may appear on the skin of the upper limbs. Local infection may accompany focal ischemia caused by septic emboli particularly in the case of meningococcal infections.

SUMMARY

Hand infections in children may present with non-specific symptoms and have deceptively "mild" appearance. Inconsequential preceding trauma is often reported in such cases. If misdiagnosed or improperly treated, those infections may result in long-term morbidity and significant residual disability. Prevention, adequate knowledge of the local anatomy and natural history, precise diagnosis and rapid intervention are the key principles for effective management.

REFERENCES

[1] McCarthy JJ, Dormans JP, Kozin SH, Pizzutillo PD. Musculoskeletal infections in children: basic treatment principles and recent advancements. J Bone Joint Surg Am 2004;86:850-63.

[2] Figueiredo GC, Figueoredo EC. Dystrophic calcinosis in a child with a thumb sucking habit: case report. Rev Hosp Clin Fac Med Sao Paulo 2000;55(5):177-80.

[3] Stevanovic MV, Sharpe F. Acute infections in the hand. In Green DP, editor. Green's Operative Hand Surgery, 5th edition. Philadelphia: Elsevier Churchill Livingstone, 2005, p. 55-93.

[4] Jebson PJ. Infections of the fingertip. Paronychias and felons. Hand Clin 1998;14(4):547-55.

[5] Canales FL, Newmeyer WL 3rd, Kilgore ES Jr. The treatment of felons and paronychias. Hand Clin 1989;5(4):515-23.

[6] Edward MS. Infections due to human and animal bites. In: Feigin R, Cherry J, editors. Textbook of pediatric infectious diseases. Philadelphia: WB Saunders Co, 1992. p. 2334-2345.

[7] Faciszewski T, Coleman DA. Human bite wounds. Hand Clinic 1989;5:561-9.

[8] Rabalais GP. Hand infections in children. In: Gupta A, Kay S, Scheker LR, editors. The Growing Hand. Diagnosis and Management of the Upper Extremity in Children. London: Mosby, 2000. p. 941-948.

[9] Nelson JD. Skeletal infections in children. Adv Pediatr Infect Dis 1991;6:59-78.

[10] Gutierrez K. Bone and joint infections in children. Pediatr Clin North Am 2005;52(3):779-94.

[11] Schelonka RL, Freij BJ, McCracken GH Jr. Bacterial and fungal infections. In MacDonald MG, Seshia MM, Mullett MD (eds). Avery's Neonatology. Pathophysiology & management of the newborn. 5th edition. Philadelphia, Lippincott Williams & Wilkins 2005:1235.

Specific Bacterial Immunotherapy in Treating Chronic Osteomyelitis

Ferdinando DA RIN*, Mauro CIOTTI

Department of Bone Infection, Codivilla-Putti Institute, Cortina d'Ampezzo, Italy

The authors analyze their experience in treating chronic bone infections with Specific Bacterial Immunotherapy (S.B.I.T.). This therapy is based on the subcutaneous injection of a staphylococci pool (type 5 and 8) that was collected from patients with bone infections caused by the same germ, using a protocol initiated in our hospital in 1963. Approximately 150 patients of different ages and etiologies (hematogenic, post-traumatic and iatrogenic) were evaluated according to the opsonisation activity and stimulation of complement (C3), before and after the use of the S.B.I.T. The best results were obtained from young patients with hematogenous infection. Overall, although SBIT was found to provide favourable results, it does not exclude the need for antibiotic therapy or surgery.

Keywords: chronic osteomyelitis; immunotherapy; opsonisation.

1. INTRODUCTION

Istituto Codivilla-Putti, established especially for treating chronic infections, was the product of the efforts of Professor Vittorio Putti in 1930. As with most sanatoriums built in those years to treat septic diseases, the Institute is located in a famous winter sport resort. The abundance of "good air" and sun were the only therapeutic treatments available to medical science at that time.

In the new era of infectious diseases, we are now facing growing obstacles in modern therapeutic management of chronic osteomyelitis. Today, resistance, particularly to staphylococci, often confounds the use of antibiotics. Staphylococci are the major pathogens responsible for bone infections. As a result, clinicians treating these diseases require not only solid surgical knowledge and skills, but also an awareness of the most recent advances in the field of antibiotic therapy. In addition, the physician should be aware of the immunoresponses of the body that are triggered in special circumstances. An unsuccessful treatment protocol is some cases, has led scientists to reevaluate the immune system in search of possible deficiencies.

Immunodeficiency may manifest with a reduced inflammatory reaction and an increased frequency of multifocal processes and an increased tendency towards chronicity [1]. Although the use of "immunotherapy" was initiated at the beginning of the 20th century, it is still a field of investigation and advancement (Table 1) [2-4].

2. DEFINITION OF OSTEOMYELITIS

Osteomyelitis refers to infections in bone. It is accepted by most, that osteomyelitis may be acute or chronic. Chronic osteomyelitis, as all types of inflammatory bone lesions sustained by pyogenic germs, may involve the bone marrow and intertrabecular spaces. This may induce suppuration which will impede the healing process. Moreover, foci may be engendered in the internal aspect of the bones.

*Corresponding Author
Department Bone Infection
Istituti Codivilla-Putti, Cortina d' Ampezzo
32043 Cortina d' Ampezzo, Italy
Tel: +39 043 688 3111
e-mail: darin.ferdinando@iol.it
         darin.ferdinando@libero.it

TABLE 1

Chronological Milestones in the Field of Immunotherapy [2-4]

Year	Finding	Author(s)
1884	Leucotoxin	Van de Velde
1901	Anti-Staphylolysin	Neisser, Wechsberg
1925	Anti-Staphylococcus-Sera	Baker, Shands
1936	Anatoxin-Therapy	Ramon
1938	Exp. Allergic Osteomyelitis	Derizanov
1939	Autovaccination	Schoolfield
1953	Sensitisation and Osteomyelitis	Grundmann
1968	Opsonin Activity	Williams
1971	Prophylactic Immunisation	Weber
1972	Anti-Staphylolysin-titre	Queneau, Bertoye
1973	Anti-Nuclear Factors	Hierholzer
1973	Wound-Specific Antibodies	Ring, Seifert
1976	The Staphylococci	Cohen

Chronic osteomyelits may be related to several factors. Chronicity may be the result of initially acute osteomyelitis (hematogenous, post-traumatic, iatrogenous), that passes gradually into the chronic phase. This is attributed to a diminished host immune response. Chronicity may be also induced by rapid evolution of the acute type. This sometimes can result from inadequate antibiotic administration. Finally, chronicity may occur *ab initio* without an initial acute phase or generalized immune response.

3. CHARACTERISTICS OF THE STAPHYLOCOCCUS

Staphylococci are the most important micro-organisms in the Microccaceae family. This is attributed to the findings of Ogston [5, 6], who found that microscopically, their elements appeared in clusters. They have a spherical form and are asporigenic and normally non-capsulated, gram-positive, aerobic and optionally anaerobic bacteria. Staphylococci are easily cultured on common culture media at an optimal temperature of 37°C. They are among the most resistant germs to heat and disinfectants. According to their colony colours they are classified into aureus, albus, citreus and aurantiacus categories.

More recently, they have been divided into aureus and epidermidis, based on the production of coagulase by the former. By phagic typisation 4 groups have been identified, whose major representatives in chronic bone pathologies are types 5 and 8 [7].

Staphylococcus produces many extracellular substances that show almost all antigenic properties [8]. The most interesting is coagulase that fosters a fibrin barrier around the staphylococcus that might oppose the action of phagocytes and opsonins [9]. It can also induce in the host a form of "allergy" that further reduces his defenses [10-14].

Moreover, it seems that the bacterial resistance develops proportionally to its capacity to produce para-aminobenzoic acid that is necessary to its metabolism, or its precursor, folic acid. It is supposed that para-aminobenzensulfonamide removes para-aminobenzoic acid from the bacterial body. Due to the antibiotic action the bacterial bodies may lose their strong cellular wall, and transform to spheroblasts with a weak antigenic function or absent antigenic capacity, which are responsible for some infections with a chronic evolution.

4. SPECIFIC BACTERIAL IMMUNOTHERAPY (S.B.I.T.)

Our immunological experience in treating chronic forms of osteomyelitis at the Istituto Putti in Cortina started in 1963 [15-19]. Immunotherapy was introduced by applying progressive administration of increasing doses to a staphylococci pool, that had been collected from patients with bone infections attributed to the same germ and then inactivated in an aqueous solution suspension. Simultaneously, an autologous immunostimulation was also carried out, in which therapy was based on isolating the responsible bacterial agent directly in the patient's exudate. Pseudomonas aeruginosa autologous immunotherapy was also performed, although this method was abandoned when it became clear that this bacterium was not the principal pathogenic agent that provoked bone infection.

Today, only Staphylococcus strains 5 and 8 are isolated, as these two strains alone appear responsible for 98% of bone infections [20]. This was demonstrated in a joint research study with the Institute Pasteur in Paris. As mentioned above, antibiotics are administrated in gradually increasing doses. Antibiotics are injected subcutaneously with the main treatment protocol lasting about three months. After cesation of treatment for one month, it may be necessary to be repeated. The protocol is shown in Table 2.

4.1. Mechanism of Action

Before mechanisms of action can be discussed, some general information regarding the resistance to infection is required. The host's defense against bacterial infections is initiated through two classical mechanisms: 1) a natural **non-specific** immunoresistance (attributed to humoral and cellular factors and mainly related to phagocyte reactions), and 2) an acquired **specific** immunity (attributed to specific antibody production and Ag-Ab reaction).

We shall focus mainly on the former mechanism, as its deficiency is considered to be the major cause of chronic septic forms of osteomyelitis. It comprises the fastest immune response and it is activated through hu-

TABLE 2

Treatment protocol

1st injection	.0.10 cc
After 3-4 days	
2nd injection	.0.20 cc
3rd injection	.0.40 cc
4th injection	.0.40 cc
5th injection	.0.60 cc
6th injection	.0.80 cc
7th injection	.1 cc
8th injection	.1 cc
9th injection	.1 cc
10th injection	.1 cc
Starting doses for children and adults	
Adults (over 16 years):	
After one month	.2 cc
After 20 days	.2 cc
Children (under 16):	.1 cc
(3-4 injections every 5-6 days)	

moral and cellular factors. Briefly, humoral factors may be divided principally into three types.

- **Complement (C)** is a biological entity that shows itself through the concomitant action of several constituents, some of which are thermolabile. It recognizes a group of known substances that are present in fresh serum and is able to interact, in clearly defined sequence, with all possible Ag-Ab combinations. Compliment does not show antibody activity and there is no evidence that its blood levels increase as a consequence of the immunisation processes. Lepow [21] and Beker [22, 23] have reported that at least some C components have enzymatic activity against bacterial cellular walls, which are opsonised and become weaker to phagocytic action.

The bacteriocidines are produced mainly by leukocytes, and the majority are thermostable. They are principally active against Gram+.

Fleming discovered the enzyme, **Lysozime,** in 1922. It is present in several body fluids and tissues, as well as in the internal parts of neutrophile granulocytes. It consists of a protein that is able to depolymerise some polysaccharides contained in many bacterial species. Moreover, it stimulates phagocytosis, bacterial suspensions agglutinations, and inhibits inflammatory processes [24, 25].

Opsonins act on micro-organisms by making them more vulnerable to phagocytosis. Generally, neutrophiles are able to phagocytate aggressive micro-organisms only after a specific opsonin has attached to the micro-organisms (opsonisation). Their action also fosters the elimination of micro-organisms from the blood by means of the reticuloendothelial system.

Non-specific cellular immunity is mainly related to phagocytosis, i.e. the capacity of some cells to take up

corpuscular matter of a different nature and origin. These cells comprise part of the so-called "reticulohistocytic" system (R.H.S). Metchnikoff [26] considers that cells with the capacity for phagocytosis are essentially macrophages and microphages. **Macrophages** are classified into fixed and mobile, and include (i) the reticular cells in the spleen and in the lymphonodules, (ii) the Kupfer cells in the liver, (iii) the fixed osteoclasts, and (iv) the mobile histiocytes, which pass from the tissues into blood circulation (Fig 1 shows the origin of macrophages). **Microphages** are represented by the blood polymorphonucleic leukocytes, essentially by neutrophiles.

Acquired specific immunity is attributed to specific antibody production and Ag-Ab reaction. For the most part, it does not appear that staphylococcal infections have such characteristics. A study by Ring and colleagues found that only 26 cases with post-traumatic osteomyelitis out of 112 had an increased antistaphylolysinic level [27].

It has been observed that the staphylococci pathogenicity appears on one hand as an increased resistance to the defensive powers of the patient, and on the other hand, as a capacity to establish a kind of allergy that further reduces body defenses. The production of toxins might have only a minor role in the pathogenicity [28]; as a matter of fact, there is no parallelism between germ virulence and the seriousness of the illness. It has been observed that the two factors provoking allergy (hypersensitivity against the germ or its products and increased reaction capacity) do not always evolve in parallel, but seperately. Sensitivity to the microorganism and its antigens, without variation of the host reactivity, may be observed and such a mechanism induces a very dangerous condition, called by immunologists "specific hyperreceptivity". Such a mechanism could account for how this state may result from inappropriate use of antibiotics.

An insufficient immune system, predisposition to germ invasion, inadequate microbial sterilisation (inappropriate antibiotics, dosage, or choice), bacterial persistence, can result in hyper receptivity. In this regard, we examined whether there was some immunological deficit among chronic osteomyelitis patients. Patients with acute forms of the disease were not evaluated, as they show different characteristics from what is considered normal reactivity.

Giedrys and Galand examined phogcytosis and intracellular killing of homologous and heterologous staphylococci by determining the colony-forming units according to the methods Maloe and Solberg after immunisation and auto vaccination [29, 30]. In another study from Bari, the immunological effects of SBIT were assessed in 22 patients with chronic osteomyelitis at a follow-up of 20 months [31]. The authors evaluated the phagocyticity of polymorphonucleates and monocytes of bacteria that were isolated from at least two or three samples; together with the dosage required to inhibit

F. DA RIN, M. CIOTTI

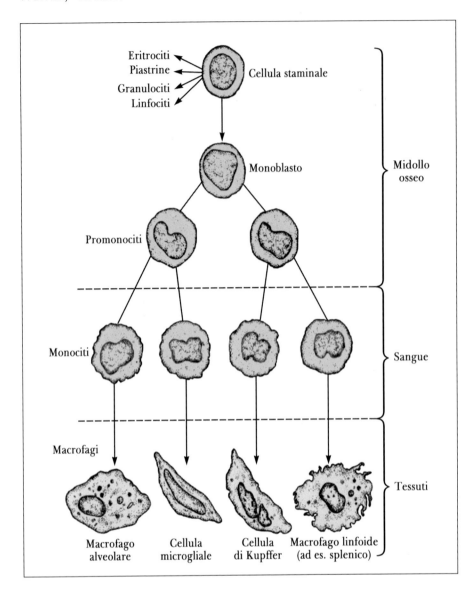

Eritrociti
Piastrine
Granulociti
Linfociti

Cellula staminale

Monoblasto

Promonociti

Monociti

Macrofagi

Macrofago
alveolare

Cellula
microgliale

Cellula
di Kupffer

Macrofago linfoide
(ad es. splenico)

Midollo
osseo

Sangue

Tessuti

FIGURE 1. Differentiation of monolytic cells from stem cells. The first changes from stem cells into monoblasts and then in promonocytes happen in the bone marrow. Later on, the promonocytes differentiate themselves into blood monocytes that pass into different tissues, where their transformation is completed into macrophages with specific functions depending on the tissue where they are localized.

leukocyte migration (LIF). In this study, the patients were divided into two categories (responders (n=3) who had almost normal parameters and non-responders (n=19) who were immuno-compromised) and were compared to 40 normal volunteers. The results showed that chronic osteomyelitis is associated with significant immunological compromises (Table 3). Evaluation after the administration of SBIT showed a significant improvement of the results. (Table 4 shows phagocytosis and LIF before and after SPIT treatment).

150 cases with various etiologies, including hematogenic, post-traumatical and iatrogenous, were assessed according to the following parameters: antibody titre, complement (fraction 3), phagocytic activity, opsonisation capacity, bactericidal reaction, bacterial agglutinins and "T" lymphocyte count [32]. The results indicated a reduction in the phagocytic activity as a whole, and especially in the opsonisation activity. Specifically, the opsonisation capacity deficit was 62%, the antibody

activity deficit was 34% and the "T" lymphocytes decreased by 4%.

It has been thought that in immunotherapy, more fac-

TABLE 3			
The immunological condition of patients before SBIT treatment			
	Phagocytosis*		
Patients	PMN	Monocyte	LIF**
19 non-responders	60.6±19.1^	52.6±11.7^	30.5±9.3^
3 responders	87.0±3.2	87.6±5.3	54.3±12.4
40 (control)	86.9±4.45	87.1±4.2	48.3±6.9

* phagocytosis = percentage of cells that engulf the specific bacteria
** LIF = percent inhibition of leukocyte migration
^ = Statistically significant

TABLE 4

The results before and after SBIT treatment

| Patients | Phagocytosis* | | | | LIF** | |
| | PMN | | Monocyte | | | |
	before	after	before	after	before	after
19 Non-resp onders	65.7±19.1	72.4±12.4^	30.6±8.9	70.4±8.9^	25.8±8.1	30.6±8.9
3 Responders	87.0±3.1	85.3±6.1	87.3±5.3	85.2±4.7	54.3±12.4	60.3±11.2

* phagocytosis = percentage of cells that engulf the specific bacteria
** LIF = percent inhibition of leukocyte migration
^ = Statistically significant

tors could be involved. Their principal activity is to reduce the allergising effect, and therefore, to desensitise against the germ proteins and to increase the phagocytic activity. Neither the entity nor the duration of osteomyelitis can be defined, although it does not appear to be limitless. Desensitisation can be achieved by the correct antibiotic choice, particularly for acute forms that may develop bactericidal properties, and sterilising the infected site. In chronic forms, it is possible to provoke this mechanism by carrying out surgical debridement that restores the vascularization, and conditions that are necessary in order to have the desired antibiotic action. Upon termination of the immuno-stimulation treatment in our study, the overall laboratory and clinical findings were improved. The results were as follows:

Laboratory

Parameter normalization	35%
Minor increases	34%
No variations	25%

Clinical

Good	50%
Reduced	28%
Bad	22%

4.2. Clinical evaluation

We clinically evaluated the results obtained with immunotherapy in about 7,500 cases treated since 1963. Among these findings were: spontaneous elimination of sequestra, demarcation or resorption, output colour change, trend to fistula healing, reduction of congestive facts, less frequent recurrence, reduced articular rigidity, stimulation of bone reparation, and reduction of soft tissues calcification. Some of these effects (sequestrum resorption or demarcation reduced articular rigidity, and increased repairing capacity) may be explained in part by hypothesizing that reticuloendothelial cells are able to differentiate in different tissues once stimulated accordingly [33].

We also examined for differences between children, who are known for their receptive immune potential, and adults. In this comparison of 100 adults (10 females, 90 males) and 100 children (20 females and 80 males), the type of infection was not considered. Table 5 shows the etiology of the infection and the time in which stabilization or healing was achieved.

Healing is considered when the patient does not show any recurrence at least after 1 year from stabilization. Stabilization is considered when the patient does not show any clinical, radiographic or bio-humoral sign of inflammation. As chronic infections may recur, even after more than 1 year after stabilization, the term "healing" has been adopted only for assessment purposes of this study [34].

Another study was designed to define the potential efficiency of Immunotherapy concerning both hematogenic and post-traumatic infections. In this study we examined 50 patients with hematogenous osteomyelitis, all less than 16 years old, and 117 patients with post-traumatic infected pseudoarthrosis. The latter showed non-union at 6 months after trauma. The distinction between hematogenic and post-traumatic etiologies was

TABLE 5

Differences in the Outcome Between Children and Adults

Etiology of Infection	Children	Adults
Hematogenous	66	19
Post-traumatic	30	40
Iatrogenic	4	41
Stabilization Time		
1-6 months	36	15
6-12 months	30	26
>1 year	31	37
non attained	3	22
Healing of the infection		
Obtained	90	73
Not obtained	10	27

chapter 24

made in this study, as the ratio between bacterial count versus host responses differs significantly between the two etiologies.

In our hematogenic cases, all patients were infected by a coagulase positive *Staphylococcus aureus.* Males were infected most often (78%), and the prevailing ages were between 10 and 16 years. Lower limbs were involved three times more than arms, while there was no difference between proximal diaphyseal and distal diaphyseal localization (Fig. 2). In 30% of cases, the lesion involved the whole bone segment (panosteatis), while the remaining 70% showed a localization in the diaphysis (42%) or meta-epiphysis (28%). In males, diffused forms were more frequent, while in females, localized forms.

The follow-up took place from 1 to 10 years following healing, as defined above. Healing was obtained in 86% of the cases (88.5% when considering localization). Of these, 74% was achieved from the first treatment, and only in 12% after possible recurrences. Of these relapses, only half involved bony tissue, while the other cases involved periodical opening of abscesses and fistulae, without any bone involvement (Fig. 3). Half of the patients (50%) healed with immunotherapy alone; in 38% immunotherapy was supplemented by surgical intervention, while the remaining 11.5% did not heal. The time elapsed from the initiation of treatment to healing varied. In this study, 46% of the cases healed within 6 months, 30% between 6 months and 1

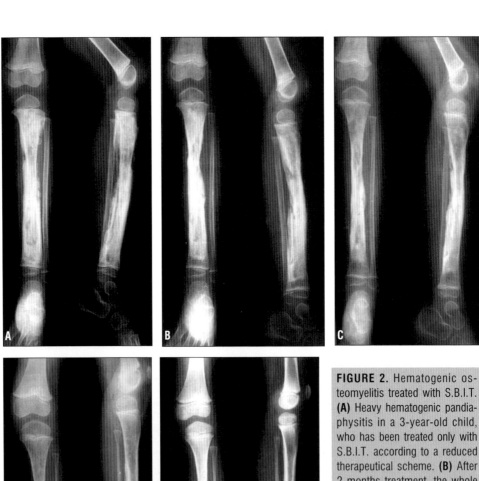

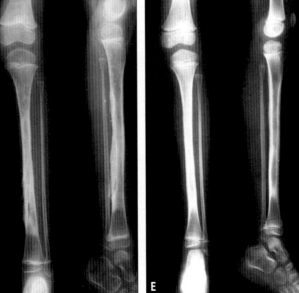

FIGURE 2. Hematogenic osteomyelitis treated with S.B.I.T. **(A)** Heavy hematogenic pandiaphysitis in a 3-year-old child, who has been treated only with S.B.I.T. according to a reduced therapeutical scheme. **(B)** After 2 months treatment, the whole diaphysis partially recovers; there are still sequestra, of which one is posterocortical. Fistulae are closed. **(C)** Two months later the important sequester has also recovered. **(D)** 15 months from the beginning of the therapy. **(E)** One year later after the preceding view, the limb has fully recovered, without any clinical or laboratory inflammation evidence.

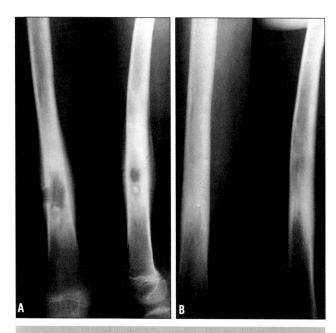

FIGURE 3. (A) A case of osteomyelitis in a 16-year-old boy with dia-physis, who had already undergone surgical debridement. He shows minimal sequestrum in the diaphysis. S.B.I.T. without antibiotics has been administered. There was a fistula on the side of an old surgical scar. **(B)** Rx control after 8 months; the focus fully recovered. After 2 months from the immunological treatment, it spontaneously eliminated the sequestrum and the fistula closed.

riostal reaction or osteolysis). In 7 cases there were still traces of active infection.

In 3 cases, growth disturbances greater than 2.5 cm were observed at later follow-up (in 2 cases short-ening was attributed to growth cartilage lesions and in 1 case there was lengthening). In 5 other cases, limb lengthening was initially observed, which disappeared later. At a later follow-up, 5 cases showed some limi-tation in the range of movement in the articulations near the infection foci. In 4 of these cases, the limi-tation had been observed at the first follow-up and did not improve with casting. Three patients showed de-formities of the bone segments (coxa varia, femur procurvatum).

In this study, we also examined 147 cases of post-traumatic infective pseudoarthrosis. Of these, 75.5% were related to pseudoarthrosis subsequent to osteosynthesis. This cohort included 118 males (83.3%) and 29 female patients (19.7%), with a mean age of 32 years and 5 months (range: 18 - 68 years). The most fre-quently involved bone was the tibia (99 cases), followed by the femur (35 cases). Twenty-five cases involved two-bone fractures (19 tibia - fibula and 6 radius - ulna frac-tures).

Seven cases involved the radius and ulna, 3 cases the clavicle, 1 case the humerus and 1 case the hand. The mean time elapsed between trauma and the begin-ning of the infection in males was 30 days (7 days - 5 months) (Fig. 4). The time lapse between the beginning of infection and initiation of therapy averaged 8 months (range: 6 months - 4 years). This treatment almost always allowed protective weight bearing (only the most serious cases had to wait 6 months before being able to use the infected limb). At the first hospitalization, 89% of the patients showed a fistula defect.

year, and 24% between 1 and 5 years with an average time elapsed of 9.6 months. Radiographic examination showed that the damaged bone segments had fully healed in 20 patients, whereas 33 patients showed bone remodelling (residual osteosclerosis without pe-

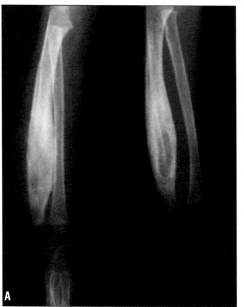

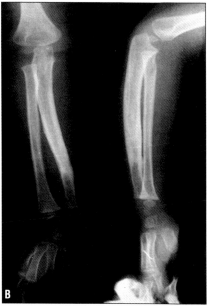

FIGURE 4. (A) Pandiaphysites of ulna bone in an 11-year-old, treated only with a cycle of therapy with S.B.I.T. and antibiotic therapy. **(B)** Radiograph taken one year later, where you can see the complete reconstruction of the ulna.

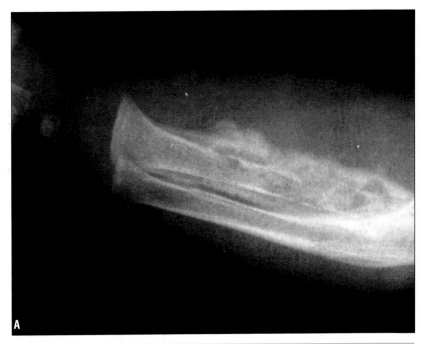
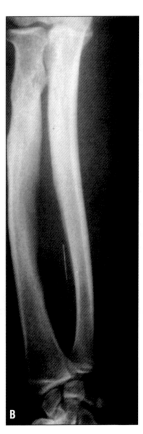

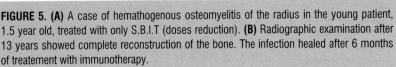

FIGURE 5. (A) A case of hemathogenous osteomyelitis of the radius in the young patient, 1.5 year old, treated with only S.B.I.T (doses reduction). **(B)** Radiographic examination after 13 years showed complete reconstruction of the bone. The infection healed after 6 months of treatement with immunotherapy.

In all cases, therapy consisted of immunotherapy plus antibiotic therapy. In 112 cases immunotherapy was repeated and in 5 cases it was administered 3 times. Surgical debridement was performed in 98 cases, and in 22 cases it was required more than once. Paltrinieri parafocal osteotomy (all tibial) was performed in 4 cases [35]. In 45 cases, the Ilizarov system was applied after resection of the defect. Amputation was required in only one case. The timing of bone union varied according to the involved bone. Bony union was achieved in tibia on an average of 9.9 months (range: 3 - 36 months).

Most cases healed (76.8%) within 1 year from the beginning of the therapy, 26 cases (26%) did not achieve union, of which 18 cases are still receiving treatment (Fig. 5). Similar rates were observed with femurs, with bony union achieved on an average of 9.2 months (range: 3-35 months). 84% of cases involving femurs healed after a 12-month therapy, whereas the non-consolidated cases were 10 (28.6%). Of the later, 6 cases are still under treatment. The forearm did not show substantial differences between the ulna and radius. In 2 out of 7 cases, we observed bony nonunion with bone tissue loss preoperatively. The fistulae closed fairly rapidly after 6 months in 53.48% of cases. The average follow-up was after 15 months (range: 4 months - 7 years).

Delayed consequences included:

Articular stiffness. Patients who were treated with immunotherapy, plaster casts (either cylinder or valve casts), and protective walking showed significant articular functional limitations in 26 cases only (17.6%). Fourteen cases involved the ankle joint, 8 cases the knee, and 4 cases out of 7, the elbow.

Shortenings. Significant shortening (more than 4 cm) was observed in only 2% of the cases, whereas shortening less than 4 cm was observed in 30.5% of the cases. In total, 102 cases showed shortenings that did not have a negative impact on the function of the infected limb.

Axial deviations was observed in 18.3% of the cases: varus deformity in 15 cases, valgus deformity in 12, recurvatum in 17, and procurvatum in 10.

Calcification of soft tissues occurred at a percentage of only 3.4%. Calcification was very frequent in cases where there was no systematic introduction of immunotherapy.

Relapses took place in 26.5% of our patients (39 cases). In 15 cases (10.2%) there was a simple reopening of the fistula that healed soon, in 13 cases the recurrence of the infection was associated with new nonunion of the fracture. Afterwards, 9 cases healed and these have been considered early relapses (within 1 year from healing), while the late ones were 11 cases (7.5%), of which10 healed.

5. FINAL CONSIDERATIONS

The efficacy of immunotherapy is certainly higher in children. This is confirmed by the need for fewer surgical interventions, and by the overall stabilization and healing results. We analyzed 50 cases of hematogenous osteomyelitis in order to consider which factors might have influenced prognosis. Among these factors we found:

1. Age was not correlated with poor prognosis.
2. The same applied to gender, though males showed major lesions [36]. Some may consider that females have a more favorable prognosis.
3. Prognosis is poorer when the lesion is on the femur. (21% of the cases did not heal, while no healing is observed in only 5-6% when the lesion is located in other areas).
4. The extension of the lesion, (pandiaphysitis) and the deep localization (diaphysis) of the infection adversely influence the illness evolution.
5. Finally, prognosis depends on the chronicity of the lesion. Healing frequency is adversely proportional to the duration of osteomyelitis. Failures were observed only when symptoms lasted more than 1 year. It is clear that immunotherapy has to be initiated as soon as possible.

An analysis of 147 cases of infected pseudoarthroses provides similar results:

1. Healing is significantly influenced by the fistula healing. Healing was achieved in 86% of the cases, when fistula closed within 6 months. The frequency of healing was lower when the fistula remained open for longer periods of time.
2. In contrast, recovery is not influenced by the time elapsed from the trauma to the onset of infection.
3. The presence of a fistula upon hospitalization did not affect healing.
4. The time elapsed from the onset of the infection to the immunological treatment is of great importance. With time periods that last less than 6 months, recovery is achieved at satisfactory rates. These rates are reduced significantly (to 50.6%) when the time elapsed is greater than 1 year.
5. Localization of the infection influences results. Hand Infections tend to recover quickly, whereas the average recovery time for tibial infections is longer, and for femoral infections, the longest.
6. Septic pseudoarthroses are more common in male patients than women (118 cases vs 29 cases).

6. CONCLUSIONS

The comparison of the results obtained from the treatment of hematogenous and post-traumatic osteomyelitis allows for several conclusions to be made. These include:

1. Immunotherapy (associated with surgical therapy) ensures high recovery rates (among the highest mentioned in the scientific literature) [37].
2. Such therapy notably reduces recurrences (12% instead of 40% mentioned in the literature), as it fortifies natural defenses.
3. Immunological therapy is more efficacious (and certainly less toxic) than antibiotic therapy. The two approaches have to be associated, as immunotherapy does not substitute antibiotic therapy (only 15% of patients affected by chronic osteomyelitis fully recover by antibiotic administration only).
4. Immunotherapy remarkably reduces surgical interventions.

We may conclude that Specific Bacterial Immunotherapy (S.B.I.T.) has to be considered an important defense, which does not exclude, but should be associated with antibiotic therapy, and even more, with surgery. The positive results obtained should be studied with sophisticated research methods, as the concept "immunity messenger" broadens the range of therapeutical approaches, which are still difficult to evaluate.

REFERENCES

[1] Eisen H. Immunologia. Piccin Editore, Padova
[2] Ring J. History and classification of anaphylaxis. Novartis Found Symp 2004;257:6-16.
[3] Seifert J, Ring J, Lob G. Humoral and cell-bound immune reactions in chronic bone infections. Verth Dtsch Ges Inn Med 1975;81:1185-7.
[4] Stranger Jones YK, Bae T, Schneewind O. Vaccine assembly from surface proteins of staphylococcus aureus. Proc Natl Acad Sci USA 2006;103 (45):16942-7.
[5] Ogston A. On Abscesses Classics in infectious diseases. Rev Infect Dis 1984;6(1):122-128.
[6] Giunchi G, Sorice F Malattie infettive, Casa Editrice, 1973, Vallardi-Roma
[7] Fournier JM, Hannon K, Moreau M, Karakawa WW, Vann WF. Isolation of type 5 capsular polysaccharide from *Staphylococcus aureus*. Ann Inst Pasteur Microbiol 1987;138:561-567.
[8] Verdier I, Durand G, Bes M, Taylor KL, Lina G, Vandenesch F, Fattom AI, Etienne J. Identification by PCR and agglutination test of the capsular polysaccharides in staphylococcus aureus clinical isolates J Clin Microbiol 2007;45:725-9.
[9] Tager M, Drumond MC. Staphylocoagulase Ann NY Acad Sci 1965;128:92-111.
[10] Sorice F, Ortona L. L'infezione Stafilococcica. Ed. Scient, 1955, Napoli, Italy.
[11] Zironi A.: "Characteristics of immune tollerance (relationship between para-immune and not immune tollerance) Boll Ist Sieroter Milan 1960 Mar-Apr.;39:89-96.
[12] Zironi A. The basic characteristics of the immune state. Boll Ist Sieroter 1960;39:189-203.
[13] Zironi A. On specific states of the organism (immunita paraim-

munity, immune tollerance, adaptation). Boll Ist Sieroter Milan 1960; 39: 385-96.

[14] Zironi A. L'allergia nelle malattie infettive. Ed Ist Sieroter Milan, Italy, 1951.

[15] Savoini E. L'autovaccino antistafilococcico nella cura della osteomielite ematogena cronica, Clin Ortop Vol XVII magg.-giu, 1965 Fasc. III.

[16] Savoini E. Moderne Richtungen in der Behandlung der Chronischen Osteomielitis. Z Orthop 1975;113:344-356.

[17] Savoini E, Capanna R, Gherlinzoni F. Immunita umorale ed osteomielite cronica. COM 1980;66 (4):511-515.

[18] Savoini E, Capanna R, Mercuri M, Stilli S. Risultati nel trattamento immunoterapico e chirurgico nelle osteomieliti croniche dell' infanzia. COM 1981;67(4):397-404.

[19] Ciotti M, Argazzi M, Bergami PL. La vaccinoterapia nell'osteomielite cronica. Atti SERTOT 1992;XXXIV (2)

[20] Fattom A, Schneerson R, Szu SC, Vann WF, Shiloach J, Karakawa WW, Robbins J.B. Synthesis and Immunologic properties in mice of vaccines composed of Staphylococcus aureus type 5 and type 8 cpasular polysaccharides conjugated to Pseudomonas aeruginosa exotoxin A. Infection and Immunity July 1990, p. 2367-2374.

[21] Lepow M, Hughes PA. Meningococcal Immunology. Immunol Allergy Clin North Am 2003;23 (4):769-86.

[22] Beker ME. Study of the physiological state of microorganismus under examination. Mikrobiologica 1980;49(6):1016-7.

[23] Beker ME. Some aspects of the microbial synthesis of biologically active substances. Mikrobiol Zh 1973;35(1):83-7.

[24] Ferrina F. Current trends of scientific concepts on antibodies. Progr Med (Napoli) 1961;17:550-64.

[25] Matracia S, Brusca A. Lysozyme activity in fatigue and experimental staphylococcal septicaemia" G. Batteriol. Immunol 1956;49(9-10):402-10.

[26] Metchnikoff E. Immunity in Infective Diseases. Cambridge University Press, Boston, 1905. Reprinted by Johnson Reprint Corp, New York-London, 1968.

[27] Ring J. Immunological aspects of chronic post-traumatic osteomyelitis. Kongr Fur Ski traumatologie Val D'Isere, 1974.

[28] Zironi A. Isoimmunity generic specificita of reactive processes. G Mal Infett Parassit 1967;19(12):925-9.

[29] Giedrys-Galant S, Halasa J. Phagocytosis and Intracellular Killing of Various Strains of Staphylococcus aureus in Rabbits Immunized by S. aureus. In: J. Jelijaszewicz (Ed.) The Staphylococci, Zbl. Bakt Suppl 14 Gustav Fischer Verlag, Stuttgart, 1985.

[30] Halasa J, Giedrys-Galant S, Podkowinska I, Braun J, Strzelecka G, Dabrowski W. Evaluation of certain immunological parameters in the course of autovaccine treatement in patients with chronic ostitis and carbunculosis. Arch Immunol Ter Exp 1978;26:589-593.

[31] Mastrorillo G, Minoia L, Jirillo E. De Vito D. Il vaccino autogeno antistafilococcico nel trattamento delle osteomieliti croniche: basi scientifiche. Quad Inf Osteoart 2001;23-30 Ed Masson.

[32] Da Rin F, Salfi C. Italian Experience with use of SBIT in the treatement of osteomyelitis. International Congress Italian-Japan Of Hand Surgery, Osaka, 2004.

[33] Snyderman R, Mergenhagen S. Chemotaxis of macrofages. In: Nelson DS (Ed) - Immunobiology of the Macrophage. New York, Academic Pres, s p. 323 - 1976.

[34] Morrey BF. Hematogenus osteomyelitis at uncommon sites in children. Mayo Clin Proc 1978;53:707.

[35] Paltrinieri M. Parafocal osteotomy in the treatement of consolidation delays and pseudoarthrosis of the long bones of the lower limbs Chir Organi Mov 1966;55(1):15-39.

[36] Daoud A, Martin M. Treatement of chronic osteitis of the calcaneum with calcanectomy. Rev Chir Orthop Reparatrice Appar Mot.1971;57(5):415-9.

[37] Shinefield HR, Black S. Prospect for active and passive immunization against staphylococcus aureus. Pediatr Infect Dis I 2006;25(2):167-8.

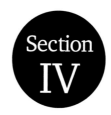

Section
IV

INFECTIONS OF THE MAJOR JOINTS

Infections of the Major Joints

Septic Arthritis of the Shoulder, Elbow and Wrist

chapter
25

Charalampos G. ZALAVRAS*, Stephen B. SCHNALL, John M. ITAMURA

*Department of Orthopaedic Surgery, University of Southern California,
Keck School of Medicine, LAC + USC Medical Center, Los Angeles, CA, USA*

Septic arthritis of the shoulder, elbow, or wrist is uncommon. Staphylococcus aureus is the most prevalent organism. A high index of suspicion for septic arthritis is necessary for all patients with upper extremity joint complaints, irrespective of age and medical status. The joint aspirate differential white blood cell count may be helpful in the diagnosis. Prompt treatment with joint drainage and antibiotics acting against Staphylococcus aureus is necessary.

Keywords: septic arthritis; shoulder; elbow; wrist; microbiology.

1. INTRODUCTION

Bacterial septic arthritis is a serious health problem, associated with considerable morbidity [1, 2]. Septic arthritis usually involves the large joints of the lower extremity [3]. Involvement of the upper extremity joints occurs less frequently, and the literature on septic arthritis of these joints is limited [4-11]. This chapter will summarize the current knowledge on the diagnosis, microbiology, management, and outcome of septic arthritis of the shoulder, elbow, and wrist in adult patients.

*Corresponding Author
Department of Orthopaedic Surgery, LAC + USC
Medical Center, 1200 N. State Street, GNH 3900,
Los Angeles, CA 90033, USA
Tel: +323 226 7346
Fax: +323 226 4501
e-mail: zalavras@usc.edu

2. INCIDENCE

Septic arthritis of a large joint of the upper extremity is an uncommon clinical entity. Series of septic arthritis of the shoulder include 7 to 23 patients treated over periods of several years [4, 6-8, 10]. Leslie et al [6] reported 18 patients over a period of 18 years in two institutions. We treated 17 patients with septic arthritis of the shoulder over an 11-year period at the musculoskeletal infection ward of our institution [11].

The large joints of the upper extremity were involved in 18 of 89 (20%) patients with septic arthritis in the series by Kelly et al. [3], and in 39 of 214 (18%) patients in the series by Kaandorp et al. [12]. Specifically, the shoulder was involved in 4% to 12% of patients with septic arthritis in these series, the elbow in 6% to 8% of patients, and the wrist in 2% to 6% of patients [3,12].

3. RISK FACTORS

3.1. Patient status

The age and medical status of the patient have been reported as major factors for the development of septic arthritis of the glenohumeral joint by several authors [4-7, 10]. In these series the mean age of patients ranged from 57 to 65 years and co-morbidities, such as diabetes mellitus, chronic liver disease, malignancy, or immunosuppression, were present in 87% to 100% of patients. Leslie et al. concluded that septic arthritis of the shoulder is associated with aging of the population and increased survival of elderly patients with chronic, debilitating disease; the authors stated that this infection rarely develops in young adults and healthy individuals of any age [6].

A recent study, summarizing our experience with septic arthritis of the upper extremity, reported a mean age of 44 years and presence of at least one serious medical condition in 33% (17 of the 52) of patients [11]. The most common co-morbidities were diabetes mellitus (8 patients, 15%), infection with the human immunodeficiency virus (3 patients, 6%), and liver disease (3 patients). Fourteen of 52 patients (27%) reported a history of intravenous drug abuse; eleven of these IVDA patients were otherwise healthy, whereas three had medical co-morbidities. Overall, compromised host status was present in 54% (28 of 52) of patients [11]. This represents a younger and healthier cohort compared to previous studies, but still underscores the importance of patient factors.

3.2. Joint trauma

Penetration of the joint has been reported as a predisposing factor for development of infection. Injection or aspiration of the shoulder prior to infection had been performed in 44% (8 of 18) of patients in the series by Leslie et al. [6]. Trauma to the wrist area was reported in 61% (17 of 28) of patients with septic wrist [9]. Blunt trauma to the affected joint within the month before admission was reported by 12 of 52 patients (23%) in the series by Mehta et al.[11].

3.3. Remote infection site

Infection at another site has been reported as a risk factor for a septic arthritis because the joint may be seeded during episodes of bacteremia [4, 10]. A remote extra-articular infection was present in 50% (8 of 16) of patients in the series by Gelberman et al. [4]. In 7 of these 8 patients both infections were caused by the same pathogen.

4. Clinical Picture

The clinical picture is characterized by pain and limited motion of the affected joint. Although these symptoms appear to be invariably present [6, 9, 11], the diagnosis of septic arthritis is often not considered upon patient presentation and a considerable delay in treatment may occur [4, 6]. Gelberman et al. reported delayed diagno-

sis of shoulder septic arthritis in 6 of 16 patients and attributed the delay to the low index of suspicion of the treating physicians [4]. Leslie et al. reported that the diagnosis of septic shoulder was not considered upon admission in 14 of 18 patients in their series. Subtle clinical findings, especially in the presence of preexisting joint disease, may be dismissed by the treating physician, and presence of a serious associated medical condition may divert the physician's attention away from the involved joint. Therefore, the key to diagnosing septic arthritis is having a high index of suspicion for the possibility of joint infection and proceeding without delay in joint aspiration and synovial fluid analysis and culture.

5. Diagnostic Modalities

Diagnosis of septic arthritis is often delayed [4-6], therefore attention should be paid to diagnostic modalities that may confirm the diagnosis.

5.1. Peripheral blood laboratory exams

The erythrocyte sedimentation rate (ESR) and the C-reactive protein (CRP) appear to be sensitive tests for the diagnosis of septic arthritis of the upper extremity. In four series elevated ESR values were present in all 70 patients that were tested [6, 7, 9, 11]. Gelberman et al. reported elevated ESR in 15 of 16 tested patients [4]. The mean ESR value in patients treated at our institution was 76 mm/hour, ranging from 28-140 mm/hour [11]. In our series the CRP was available for 40 patients and was elevated in 38 (95%) with a mean value of 15.2 mg/dL, ranging from 0.2-54.4 mg/dL [11]. The ESR and the CRP values are highly sensitive for septic arthritis of upper extremity joint. However, both are indicators of acute inflammation, and, as such, they are nonspecific.

The peripheral white blood cell (WBC) count may be normal even in the presence of infection. Leslie et al. reported a normal peripheral WBC count in 38% of patients with septic shoulders [6]. Our experience was similar with a WBC count of 10 x 109/l in 42% (20 of 48) of patients [11].

5.2. Joint fluid analysis

The WBC count in the joint aspirate in septic arthritis usually exceeds 50,000/mm^3, but is not a very sensitive diagnostic tool [13-15]. Interestingly, previous studies on septic arthritis of the large upper extremity joints did not focus on the diagnostic usefulness of the joint aspirate. Leslie et al. [6] did not report any joint aspirate data in their series of septic shoulders and other studies reported considerable variability in the WBC count of the joint fluid [4, 9, 11]. Rashkoff et al. [9] reported that the absolute WBC count ranged from 20,000-150,000/mm^3 in patients with septic wrists, but did not provide any data on the differential. Gelberman et al. [4] reported a

WBC count ranging from 35,000 to 259,000/mm^3; the authors mentioned that patients with septic arthritis of the shoulder had a joint fluid WBC differential with a strong predominance of polymorphonuclear leukocytes but did not provide any quantitative data.

In the recently reported series of patients from our institution [11], the WBC count ranged from 10,450 to 880,000/mm^3 with a mean value of 136,300/mm^3. The WBC count was greater than 50,000 per mm^3 in 76% (35 of 46) of aspirates. This study was the first to provide details on the WBC differential count of the joint aspirate. The average value of polymorphonuclear leukocytes was 91% (range: 72-100%). All aspirates had greater than 70% polymorphonuclear leukocytes and 91% of aspirates (42 of 46 aspirates) had greater than 85% polymorphonuclear leukocytes. Assessment of the subgroup of aspirates with positive cultures demonstrated that 96% of aspirates had greater than 85% polymorphonuclear leukocytes. Elevation of polymorphonuclear leukocytes in the joint fluid may be a useful diagnostic feature.

5.3. Imaging studies

Plain radiographs are noncontributory at early stages. Radiographs were normal initially in series of patients with septic shoulders [6, 16]. Soft tissue swelling over the dorsum of the wrist and hand was reported in patients with septic wrist arthritis [9].

Imaging studies may be useful to exclude other pathological processes but it should be remembered that septic arthritis may develop in the presence of underlying joint pathology. Therefore, infection should always be considered in the differential diagnosis.

6. MICROBIOLOGY

Staphylococcus aureus is the most common pathogen in septic arthritis of the upper extremity, identified in 41-87% of cases [4, 6, 7, 9, 11]. Staphylococcus aureus was the most frequent pathogen in our series, present in 76% (19/25) of aspirates with positive cultures [11]. It should be noted that cultures may be negative if empirical antibiotic therapy is initiated before joint fluid aspiration and culture [11].

Oxacillin-resistant Staphylococcus aureus (ORSA) is gradually emerging as a pathogen, and community-acquired ORSA septic arthritis has been reported [17]. Ross [13] reported that in the last 5 years, 25% of septic arthritis cases treated in two medical centers were caused by ORSA, and a recent study of septic arthritis of the shoulder reported an ORSA prevalence of 17% [10]. In our series, ORSA was identified in two of 25 culture-positive cases, resulting in an 8% (2/25) prevalence of this resistant pathogen [11].

Gram negative organisms have been identified in 8-22% of cases [4, 6, 7, 9, 11], and anaerobic infections have also been reported [18]. Although gonococcal infection is the most common cause of septic arthritis in patients younger than 30 years [19], in our series and in previous studies [4-9, 11] there were no patients with septic arthritis of the shoulder, elbow, or wrist from Neisseria gonorrhoeae.

7. TREATMENT

Treatment consists of antibiotic administration and evacuation of intra-articular pus with drainage and decompression of the involved joint. Proposed drainage techniques include joint aspiration, arthroscopic lavage, and arthrotomy.

7.1. Antibiotic therapy

Empiric antibiotic therapy should provide coverage for Staphylococcus aureus because of its preponderance. The increasing prevalence of ORSA raises the question regarding empiric coverage for this resistant pathogen. The specific antibiotic may be chosen based on the antibiogram of the treating institution. Vancomycin may be considered, especially if risk factors for an ORSA infection are present, such as intravenous drug use [20]. Concomitant coverage against Gram-negative rods, including Pseudomonas aeruginosa, has been proposed for elderly or immunocompromised patients with signs of sepsis [7].

There are no comparative studies in the literature regarding the optimal duration of antibiotic therapy. Systemic antibiotic therapy followed by oral therapy is usually administered for a total of 3 to 4 weeks.

7.2. Joint drainage

Drainage can be provided by closed needle aspiration, arthroscopy, or open arthrotomy. No randomized controlled studies are available on the treatment of septic arthritis, and in all published series the decision to perform recurrent aspirations or operative arthrotomy was determined by the admitting physician.

Glenohumeral joint aspiration gave satisfactory results in the study by Master et al. [8], despite the advanced age of the patients, the presence of multiple risk factors in each patient, and the presence of gram-negative organisms. However, the authors emphasized that early diagnosis with prompt institution of antibiotics and drainage occurred. In contrast, Leslie et al. [6] reported disappointing results in 10 patients treated by frequent joint aspiration; one patient died, seven patients had persistence of infection, and two patients had no motion at the glenohumeral joint. However, the diagnosis was initially missed in the majority of patients and treatment was delayed.

The shoulder joint is difficult to drain adequately with needle aspiration and repeat aspirations should be performed until no effusion is present. It is important to remember that open surgical drainage will be necessary if the patient is not clinically improving and there is evidence of persistence of infection. Long duration of symptoms before treatment, previous joint pathology, and suspicion of adjacent osteomyelitis warrant early consideration of open surgical drainage.

8. OUTCOME

Early diagnosis is imperative for optimal treatment results [4, 6, 9, 21]. Studies have shown persistent pain and limitation of motion after delayed diagnosis [4-6]. It should also be remembered that septic arthritis may also result in death of the patient [5, 6, 18].

In summary, Staphylococcus aureus is the most common pathogen isolated in septic arthritis of the shoulder, elbow, or wrist, and should be targeted by empiric antibiotic therapy. A high index of suspicion is necessary for the diagnosis of septic arthritis in a large joint of the upper extremity, irrespective of patient age and medical status. The joint aspirate WBC count differential may be a useful diagnostic feature, especially if greater than 85%. Prompt treatment with antibiotics and joint drainage is necessary.

REFERENCES

[1] Weston VC, Jones AC, Bradbury N, Fawthrop F, Doherty M. Clinical features and outcome of septic arthritis in a single UK Health District 1982-1991. Ann Rheum Dis 1999;58(4):214-219.

[2] Kaandorp CJ, Krijnen P, Moens HJ, Habbema JD, van Schaardenburg D. The outcome of bacterial arthritis: a prospective community-based study. Arthritis Rheum 1997;40(5):884-892.

[3] Kelly PJ, Martin WJ, Coventry MB. Bacterial (suppurative) arthritis in the adult. J Bone Joint Surg [Am] 1970;52(8):1595-1602.

[4] Gelberman RH, Menon J, Austerlitz MS, Weisman MH. Pyogenic arthritis of the shoulder in adults. J Bone Joint Surg [Am] 1980;62(4):550-553.

[5] Kelly PJ, Coventry MB, Martin WJ. Bacterial Arthritis of the Shoulder. Mayo Clin Proc 1965;40:695-699.

[6] Leslie BM, Harris JM, 3rd, Driscoll D. Septic arthritis of the shoulder in adults. J Bone Joint Surg [Am] 1989;71(10):1516-1522.

[7] Lossos IS, Yossepowitch O, Kandel L, Yardeni D, Arber N. Septic arthritis of the glenohumeral joint. A report of 11 cases and review of the literature. Medicine (Baltimore) 1998;77(3):177-187.

[8] Master R, Weisman MH, Armbuster TG et al. Septic arthritis of the glenohumeral joint. Unique clinical and radiographic features and a favorable outcome. Arthritis Rheum 1977;20(8):1500-1506.

[9] Rashkoff ES, Burkhalter WE, Mann RJ. Septic arthritis of the wrist. J Bone Joint Surg [Am] 1983;65(6):824-828.

[10] Cleeman E, Auerbach JD, Klingenstein GG, Flatow EL. Septic arthritis of the glenohumeral joint: a review of 23 cases. J Surg Orthop Adv 2005;14(2):102-107.

[11] Mehta P, Schnall SB, Zalavras CG. Septic arthritis of the shoulder, elbow, and wrist. Clin Orthop Relat Res 2006;451:42-45.

[12] Kaandorp CJ, Dinant HJ, van de Laar MA, et al. Incidence and sources of native and prosthetic joint infection: a community based prospective survey. Ann Rheum Dis 1997;56(8):470-475.

[13] Ross JJ. Septic arthritis. Infect Dis Clin North Am 2005;19(4):799-817.

[14] Li SF, Henderson J, Dickman E, Darzynkiewicz R. Laboratory tests in adults with monoarticular arthritis: can they rule out a septic joint? Acad Emerg Med 2004;11(3):276-280.

[15] McCutchan HJ, Fisher RC. Synovial leukocytosis in infectious arthritis. Clin Orthop Relat Res 1990;(257):226-230.

[16] Armbuster TG, Slivka J, Resnick D, et al. Extaarticular manifestations of septic arthritis of the glenohumeral joint. AJR Am J Roentgenol 1977;129(4):667-672.

[17] Fridkin SK, Hageman JC, Morrison M, et al. Methicillin-resistant Staphylococcus aureus disease in three communities. N Engl J Med 2005;352(14):1436-1444.

[18] Goon PK, O'Brien M, Titley OG. Spontaneous Clostridium septicum septic arthritis of the shoulder and gas gangrene. A case report. J Bone Joint Surg [Am] 2005;87(4):874-877.

[19] Cucurull E, Espinoza LR. Gonococcal arthritis. Rheum Dis Clin North Am 1998;24(2):305-322.

[20] Brumfitt W, Hamilton-Miller J. Methicillin-resistant Staphylococcus aureus. N Engl J Med 1989;320(18):1188-1196.

[21] Ward WG, Goldner RD. Shoulder pyarthrosis: a concomitant process. Orthopedics 1994;17(7):591-595.

Infected Total Elbow Arthroplasty

Pierre MANSAT

Service d' Orthopedie - Traumatologie

Centre Hospitalier Universitaire Toulouse, Purpan, France

Despite multiple improvements in total elbow arthroplasty, infection has remained a relatively common and potentially catastrophic complication. Once the diagnosis of an infected total elbow arthroplasty is suspected or confirmed, treatment is focused on surgical intervention. Several options are possible: irrigation and debridement with retention of the components, staged exchange arthroplasty, immediate exchange arthroplasty, and resection arthroplasty. Decision must take into consideration: the duration of symptoms, the component fixation, bacteriology, and the patient's general health status.

Keywords: septic arthritis; infection; total elbow arthroplasty; resection.

1. INTRODUCTION

Deep peri-prosthetic infection following total joint arthroplasty is a major complication resulting in substantial morbidity and a decline in functional outcome. Initially limited to excisional arthroplasty, treatment options have moved towards either prosthetic retention or reimplantation for eradication of the infection [1-4].

2. INCIDENCE AND ETIOLOGY

2.1. Incidence

Despite multiple improvements in total elbow arthroplasty, infection has remained relatively com-

mon with reported rates of around 5% [5]. The rate of deep infection has remained reasonably stable over time despite improvement of surgical techniques. Before 1979, the rate was 6.9%; from 1979 to 1983, the rate was 5.4%, and between 1984 and 1989 it was 7.7%. When considering papers published since 1989, one can find that the rate has remained at around 4% for the periods 1989 to 1993 and 1994 to 1998, and 3.9% and 4.5% for the period 1999 to 2003 [5]. The French Orthopedic Society recently reviewed a series of 321 total elbow arthroplasties for rheumatoid arthritis [6]. After 5 years, in the average infection rate at follow-up was 1.3%. There were no acute infections and only 4 late infections were reported. The same results have been recently reported by Gille and co-authors [7].

2.2. Etiology

With a complication rate of 5% [5], the rate of infections for elbow arthroplasties remains well above that for the lower extremities arthroplasties, in part because of the high prevalence of severe rheumatoid arthritis or posttraumatic arthritis [1-3, 8-10]. The elbow joint is subcutaneous with relatively little soft-tissue envelope, and disruption of the skin may easily lead to joint sepsis. In addition to being immunocompro-

*Corresponding Author

Service d'Orthopedie-Traumatologie

Centre Hospitalier Universitaire Toulouse, Purpan

Place du Dr Baylac, 31059, Toulouse, France

Tel: +33 5 61 77 21 39

Fax: +33 5 61 77 76 17

e-mail: mansat.p@chu-toulouse.fr

mised, patients with rheumatoid arthritis often exert a great deal of direct pressure on this subcutaneous joint. In Gille's series [7], 2 cases of infected total elbow arthroplasty had an ulcer over the olecranon. Those with posttraumatic arthritis have frequently undergone multiple operations that compromise the vascularity of the soft tissues and thus increase the risk of wound healing complications [1, 3].

3. PATIENT PROFILE

Patient health status is very important to evaluate before treating an infected total elbow arthroplasty. Many patients with rheumatoid arthritis are medically debilitated and often immunocompromised. For those patients, the only goal for surgery may be a non-infected, pain-free elbow. The most appropriate treatment for those people may be resection arthroplasty. For those who are in relatively good health, preservation of the arthroplasty requires multiple surgical procedures and aggressive treatment associated with a high risk of complications. Thus, any treatment plan should be placed in the context of the patient's needs and their ability to undergo this kind of treatment.

4. DIAGNOSIS

The clinical presentation of an infected total elbow arthroplasty may be subtle and only recognized by maintaining a high index of suspicion [3, 4, 7]. There is not a single reliable standard test, and therefore, the diagnosis is based on clinical evaluation, serological investigation, diagnostic imaging and microbiological analysis [11-13].

4.1. Clinical factors

A detailed clinical history and physical examination constitute the most important ways to recognize a potential periprosthetic infection. The type and duration of symptoms, details of the postoperative course, the presence of comorbidities, and the types of treatments rendered should be discussed in detail. Periprosthetic infection may be diagnosed with reasonable certainty on the basis of the history and clinical presentation when there are classic signs of infection such as severe joint pain, fever, chills, or a draining periarticular sinus [1-3, 7]. However, periprosthetic infection, has an innocuous presentation in most patients and it may be difficult to diagnose on the basis of the history and physical findings alone. Systemic signs of sepsis may be absent [2, 7], while the patient may be complaining of increased pain or pain at rest. Those with an obviously infected bursa should be assumed to have a deep infection unless proven otherwise.

4.2. Serologic tests

Serologic tests (measurements of white blood-cell count, erythrocyte sedimentation rate, and C-reactive protein level) represent the first-line investigation and generally have good sensitivity, but lower specificity. However, most patients have a normal leukocyte count, but an elevated neutrophil count on differential analysis [2, 7, 13]. The erythrocyte sedimentation rate (ESR) is often elevated, but not specific, as many have systemic inflammatory disease. Elevations of the erythrocyte sedimentation rate and especially of the C-reactive protein level (CRP) after 3 months suggest the possibility of infection [11]. The C-reactive protein level was found to be a better indicator of infection than the erythrocyte sedimentation rate. An ESR > 30mn per hour has been shown to have sensitivity of 82%, specificity of 85%, positive predictive value of 58% and negative predictive value of 95%. A CRP value >10mg/l has been associated with 96% sensitivity, 92% specificity, 74% positive predictive value and 99% negative predictive value. If both the ESR and CRP are elevated, the probability of infection has been noted to be 83%, and when both are negative, infection may be reliably excluded [14].

4.3. Diagnostic imaging

Many methods of imaging have been used for the assessment of peri-prosthetic infection:

1) Plain radiographs: They are of limited value in acute infection because of the absence of reliable diagnostic features. Chronic infection can cause radiographic changes, including periostitis, osteopenia, endosteal reaction, and rapid progressive loosening or osteolysis (Fig. 1). Osteolysis and loosening may have other causes, but the possibility of infection must always be considered when these processes are rapid, particularly when there are no indicators of a mechanical cause. The determination of component fixation is critical to the treatment protocol observed. Loose or poorly fixed component obviate treatment with component retention.

2) Radionuclide bone scan: Radionuclide studies currently have a role in the evaluation of many patients who have pain at the site of an arthroplasty. In a study of 72 total joint replacements, Levitsky and co-authors [15] reported that bone scintigraphy had a percentage of 33% sensitivity, 86% specificity, 30% positive predictive value, and 88% negative predictive value. Although false-positive results lead to low sensitivity, the relatively high predictive value of a negative result makes conventional bone scintigraphy as useful as an initial screening test. A scan employing indium-111, i.e. an isotope that labels leukocytes or immunoglobulin, is more sensitive than a routine technetium-99m scan. Sher and co-authors [16] reported that indium-111 leukocyte scans had only 77% sensitivity, 86% specificity, 54% positive predictive value, and 95% negative predictive value. Combining the results of these two scans helps to distinguish

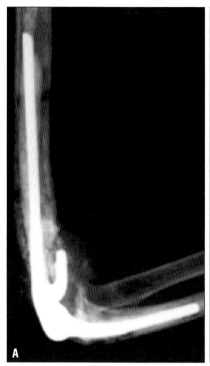
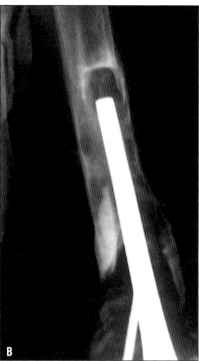

true infection from uninflamed areas of high metabolic activity such as fracture or remodeling [17] (Fig. 2).

4.4. Cultures of aspirated joint fluid

A definitive step is to aspirate the joint. To minimize the influence of ATB, joint aspiration is best performed at least two weeks after the last dose of antibiotics was given. Synovial fluid should be submitted to cell count and differential analysis, as well as culture. Recent data indicate that, in the absence of underlying inflammatory joint disease, a synovial fluid leukocyte count of greater than 1.7×10^9/L and a differential of greater than 65% neutrophils are useful cutoffs for diagnosing infected total knee arthroplasty. However, it is not known whether these cutoffs apply to other types of prosthetic joints or to patients with underlying inflammatory joint disease. The sensitivity of synovial fluid culture is 77%; occasional false-positive results may be observed [18]. The method used to culture synovial fluid must be considered. Although Gram staining may be performed on joint fluid aspirated preoperatively or intraoperatively, this test in general has relatively poor sensitivity and specificity [19-21]. There are occasions when periprosthetic infection is suspected but cannot be confirmed by joint aspiration, or others when the organism cannot be isolated. Tissue obtained from the joint capsule or periprosthetic membrane containing a high concentration of neutophils is highly suggestive of ongoing infection.

Patients are considered infected when there are positive cultures or strong clinical suspicion (based on high white blood cell count, ESR, operative observations, and so on) in the context of supportive microscopic pathology.

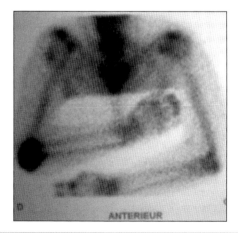

FIGURE 2. Radionuclide bone scan of an infected total elbow arthroplasty.

5. DURATION OF SYMPTOMS

Traditionally, infections have been classified according to how much time has passed since surgery because the presentation, differential diagnosis and treatment differ according to the timing of presentation. For Morrey [22], an infection is considered: (1) acute, if it developed within 3 months of the operation, (2) subacute, if it developed between 3 months and 1 year, and (3) late, if the initial recognition was made after 1 year after surgery [2, 3]. However, the time period from the index procedure to the development of infection has not been shown to correlate with infection results [10]. The duration of symptoms, as in the experience with total knee arthroplasty, were correlated with successful treatment by irrigation and debridement [23]. Therefore, delineating the onset of symptoms correlates better with the onset of infection, which has direct implications for the treatment strategy to be followed.

6. BACTERIOLOGY

Even if a microorganism is isolated from periprosthetic tissues or fluid aspiration, one may not be entirely certain that infection is present, because among the typical pathogens that cause prosthetic joint infection are also normal skin flora and intraoperative or laboratory contaminants. Furthermore, it is clear that in biofilm-associated infections, such as prosthetic joint infection, the microorganisms that live within the biofilm may be difficult to identify by use of routinely available culturing techniques, and therefore, microbiologic results alone may be insufficient to identify infection as a source of prosthesis failure [24-26]. This situation makes patient treatment very difficult. An accurate diagnosis of the reason for prosthesis failure is key to appropriate treatment strategies application. Organisms vary in virulence, adherence ability, and elaboration of extracellular components. Studies of infected orthopedic implants have shown that up to 76% of the infectious microorganisms produce a significant biofilm extracellular matrix to improve adherence to the implant [27]. Of these, coagulase-negative staphylococci have been the most common and the most dangerous biofilm producers [4, 23]. Coagulase-positive staphylococci (i.e., *Staphylococcus aureus*) are less able to form a significant biofilm than coagulase-negative staphylococcal organisms. The latter, and particularly *Staphylococcus epidermidis,* have been recognized as the primary pathogen of orthopedic-device infections owing to its unsual capacity to attach to and to colonize orthopedic implants [4, 27]. Although it is a relatively non-virulent pathogen that normally exists on the skin, it can form a tenacious bacterial biofilm that envelopes the bacteria and protects them from antibiotic penetration. This accounts for the persistence of *Staphylococcus epidermidis* and its resistance to treatment. Not surprisingly, the presence of *Staphylococcus epidermidis* has thus been associated with a high incidence of failure when prosthetic retention with irrigation and debridement is attempted [4].

The antibiotic sensitivities of infecting organisms have also been shown to vary. The sensitivity of *Staphylococcus aureus* to methicillin and cephalosporins has been reported to range between 53% and 95% [28,

29], whereas the reported sensitivity of *Staphylococcus Epidemidis* to methicillin is 70% [29, 30]. Vancomycin resistance, in particular with enterococci has been reported to be up to 23% [28]. This emphasizes the importance of identifying the pathogen before initiating antibiotic treatment.

7. TREATMENT OPTIONS

Once the diagnosis of an infected total elbow arthroplasty is either suspected or confirmed, the treatment is focused on surgical intervention. In choosing a particular treatment plan, special consideration must be given to (1) the duration of symptoms, (2) the component fixation, (3) bacteriology, and (4) the patient's health status.

Debilitated patients are best treated with excisional arthroplasty. The primary objective of treatment remains long-term infection cure, which is dependent on the complete removal of the bacteria. A secondary concern is restoration of function. All treatment plans require a minimum-6-week course of intravenous antibiotics.

7.1. Irrigation and dèbridement with retention of the components

Poor outcomes have been initially reported with this strategy. Wolfe and co-workers [3] reported 8 failures in 11 patients with this technique. Reports of the Mayo Clinic experience showed similar results, i.e. only one of nine patients had been treated successfully [2]. However, with increased awareness and earlier detection of infection, patients are often now seen acutely with well-fixed components with no apparent bone involvement. In the series by Wolfe and associates [3], 3 of 8 patients sustained fractures of the humerus or the ulna after component removal. In aseptic revisions, Morrey and Bryan [31] noted fractures in 11 of 33 subjects. The results have exemplified the difficulty in removal of the components without compromising the bone structure and have renewed interest in component retention.

Experience with infected total knee arthroplasty has demonstrated a high correlation between the duration of symptoms of infection (21 days or less) and the outcomes when component retention is applied [23]. Using this principle of symptom duration for less than 30 days, a recent study reports a 50% long-term success rate (at a mean follow-up of 71 months) [23].

Furthermore, bacteriology played a significant role, with all four patients infected by *Staphylococcus epidermidis* failing this treatment protocol, while six of the eight were successfully eradicated of the *Staphylococcus aureus* infection [2]. Therefore, treatment with debridement and component retention is dependent upon both the duration of symptoms and the bacteriologic findings.

The indications for this treatment include (1) the presence of well-fixed surgical components detected by both radiographic and intraoperative examination, (2) *Staphylococcus aureus* or other pathogen amenable to this form of treatment as suggested by bacteriology, (3) a suitable soft tissue envelope with or without use of flaps, (4) the patient medically fit to withstand the required multiple surgical procedures, and (5) duration of symptoms less than 30 days. A contra-indication to component retention is an infection caused by *Staphylococcus epidermidis*.

The technique for irrigation and debridement with component retention is performed within the context of a posterior approach utilizing the previous incision [4]. Once stability of the components is confirmed, complete disarticulation of the components including removal of the bushings follows. This is an essential stage of the procedure. The joint is debrided of all necrotic debris and copiously irrigated by pulsatile saline lavage. Antibiotic-impregnated cement beads are placed in the wound prior to wound closure. According to Morrey [4], patients return to the operating room every fourth day for repeat irrigation and dèbridement with antibiotic cement beads exchange. The number of repeated irrigation and debridement procedures is variable, but usually three or four are required. The patient concurrently receives bacteria- sensitive intravenous antibiotics for a minimum period of 6 weeks (based on serum minimal inhibitory and bactericidal concentrations).

The overall success rate of the Mayo series reported by Yamaguchi and co-workers [4] was 50%, but increased to 70% when the number of those patients infected with *Staphylococcus epidermidis* decreased. The outcome was good functional results, however, there was 43% incidence of complications, including 21% incidence of wound breakdown or triceps avulsion and 21% with peripheral nerve injury.

Recently, Mastrokalos and co-authors [32] published one case of acute infection of a total elbow arthroplasty (TEA) treated by arthroscopic lavage and synovectomy and 3-months-administration of intravenous antibiotics. A Methicillin-sensitive *Staphylococcus aureus* pathogen was isolated. After a 10-month follow-up, the patient remains free of symptoms and with blood rates within normal limits.

7.2. Staged exchange arthroplasty

Following reported success of staged exchange arthroplasty for lower extremity indications [33], this technique was successfully used for infected total elbow arthroplasties. Yamaguchi and co-authors [4] report an 80% success rate for staged revision performed at the Mayo Clinic, with the only failure occurring in patients infected with *Staphylococcus epidermidis*.

The most common indications for staged exchange arthroplasty are: (1) radiographic or intraoperative evidence of loose components with sufficient bone stock for reconstruction, (2) duration of symptoms longer than

30 days, and (3) a medically fit patient. A relative contra-indication, dependent on the surgeon and the patient, may be suggested when there is an infection caused by *Staphylococcus epidermidis*.

The surgical technique utilizes the previous posterior incision to expose the joint, with considerations to flaps for soft tissue coverage [2, 4, 34]. Arthroplasty components along with all bone cement are meticulously debrided, while preserving bone stock. Antibiotic-impregnated cement is then used as a spacer between the humerus and the ulna in order that soft tissue tension is maintained. The wound is closed and the limb is placed in a cast or hinged orthosis for 4 weeks. A concurrent 6-week treatment with sensitivity-specific intravenous antibiotics is initiated. Repeat irrigation, debridement, and biopsies of the tissues are performed as necessary. Consideration of longer staging intervals and repeat irrigation and debridement may be taken into, in the case of more resistant infections such as *Staphylococcus epidermidis*. Arthroplasty reconstruction is performed at somepoint after 6 weeks using a long-stem semiconstrained arthroplasty with antibiotic-impregnated PMMA [4].

7.3. Immediate exchange arthroplasty

There has been very little information regarding immediate exchange for infected total elbows. In Mayo series, only one case had been reported [4]. This case resulted in a failure to eradicate the infection. However, Gille and co-authors [7] recently published 6 infected TEA treated with a single-stage revision. All six cases had rheumatoid arthritis and were infected with a *Staphylococcus aureus* microorganism. The infection was acute in 2 elbows, subacute in one, and late in three. Radiologically, four of the six elbows had radiolucencies around either component when first seen for infection. Infected implants were removed, as well as all cement. A humeral fracture was observed in one case. A new implant was fixed with antibiotic-loaded cement. Appropriate antibiotics were administered for a mean of 37 days (7 to 180). The results were good in three, fair in two and poor in one. In one case, the revision prosthesis had to be removed following recurrence of infection.

Success rates of immediate exchange arthroplasty for infected total shoulder arthroplasty vary from 30 to 100% for eradication of sepsis [35-37], whereas for infected total knee arthroplasty they vary from 35 to 75%, with suggested improved results with gram-positive non-glycocalyx-producing organisms [38].

The indications for immediate exchange arthroplasty are probably very limited and at this time undetermined. The principles of the surgical treatment are similar to those of the staged revision with aggressive debridement with removal of all foreign material, antibiotic-impregnated cement fixation, and concomitant 6 to 12 weeks of intravenous antibiotic administration.

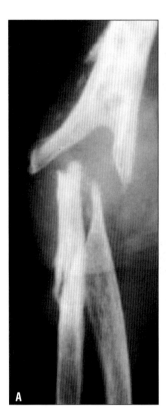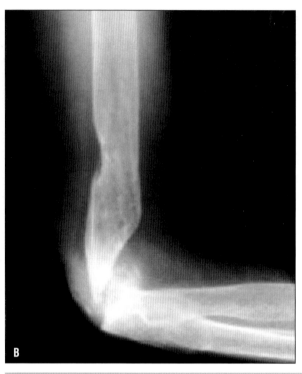

FIGURE 3. (A, B). Resection of unsalvageable total elbow arthroplasty.

7.4. Resection arthroplasty

Resection arthroplasty has been the standard of treatment for infected elbow arthroplasty and constitutes the largest treatment experience. Functional results are usually limited but can be associated with a high satisfaction rate. Moreover, with many of these patients debilitated, it is considered the treatment of choice for those medically frail and unfit to undergo extensive or multiple surgical procedures. If successful, it often provides a relatively pain-free satisfactory range of active motion with reasonable stability. This will more likely occur when the medial and lateral columns of the distal humerus are intact. If the elbow is flail or grossly unstable, it is usually non-functional and often painful [22].

The technique of elbow resection arthroplasty involves removal of the implant components through the previous incision followed by complete removal of the cement. All necrotic and contaminated tissue is excised. If remaining intact, the condyles of the distal humerus are then contoured and deepened to encircle the ulna. Sutures are passed through the humerus and through the olecranon to get some stability. Concurrent treatment with 4 to 6 weeks of appropriate antibiotic therapy is used. The limb is placed in a cast or external fixator for 3 to 4 weeks to obtain soft tissue stability (Fig. 3).

7.5. Complications

Complications following treatment of the infected elbow are usually not uncommon: fracture, triceps insufficiency, nerve injury, and skin or wound breakdown. Thus,

special attention should be given to protect surrounding neurovascular structures as well as the triceps insertion and operative wound. Hence, special consideration should be taken using triceps-on approaches and proactive planning for possible soft tissue coverage procedures. Of course, the high risk of complications and the associated morbidity are significant considerations that have to be discussed with the patient before any prosthetic salvage strategy is attempted in the context of infected elbow arthroplasty.

CONCLUSION

Infection remains a significant and severe complication of total elbow arthroplasty with an incidence above that of lower extremity joint replacements. Previously, the only treatment option was excisional arthroplasty. Recent reports of this problem suggest that both irrigation and debridement and staged exchange arthroplasty can constitute successful treatment modalities given the appropriate indications. As such, selected treatment methods may improve both the functional and satisfaction outcome of this most devastating complication.

REFERENCES

[1] Gutow AP, Wolfe SW. Infection following total elbow arthroplasty. Hand Clinic 1994;10:521-9.

[2] Morrey BF, Bryan RS. Infection after total elbow arthroplasty. J Bone Joint Surg (Am) 1983;65:330-8.

[3] Wolfe SW, Figgie MP, Inglis AE, Bohn WM, Ranawat CS. Management of infection about total elbow prostheses. J Bone Joint Surg (Am) 1990;72:198-212.

[4] Yamaguchi K, Adams RA, Morrey BF. Infection after total elbow arthroplasty. J Bone Joint Surg (Am) 1998;80:481-91.

[5] Little CP, Graham AJ, Carr AJ. Total elbow arthroplasty. A systematic review of the literature in the English language until the end of 2003. J Bone Joint Surg (Br) 2005; 87:437-44.

[6] Augereau B, Mansat P. Les protheses totales de coude. Rev Chir Orthop 2005; suppl. au n° 5; 91: 2S31-2S96.

[7] Gille J, Ince A, Gonzalez O, katzer A, Loehr JF. Single-stage revision of peri-prosthetic infection following total elbow replacement. J Bone Joint Surg (Br) 2006;88:1341-6.

[8] Figgie MP, Gerwin M, Weiland AJ. Revision total elbow replacement. Hand Clinic 1994;10:507-520.

[9] Morrey BF, Adams RA. Semiconstrained arthroplasty for the treatment of rheumatoid arthritis of the elbow. J Bone Joint Surg Am 1992;74:479-490.

[10] Poss R, Thornhill TS, Ewald FC, Thomas WH, Batte NJ, Sledge CB. Factors influencing the incidence and outcome of infection following total joint arthroplasty. Clin Orthop 1984;182:117-26.

[11] Bauer TW, Parvizi J, Kobayashi N, Krebs V. Current Concepts Review. Diagnosis of periprosthetic infection. J Bone Joint Surg (Am) 2006;88:869-82.

[12] Patel R, Osmon DR, Hanssen AD. The diagnosis of prosthetic joint infection. Current techniques and emerging technologies. Clin Orthop 2005;437:55-8.

[13] Toms AD, Davidson D, Masri BA, Duncan CP. The management of peri-prosthetic infection in total joint arthroplasty. J Bone Joint Surg Br 2006;88:149-55.

[14] Spangehl MJ, Masterson E, Masri BA, O'Connell J, Duncan C. Prospective analysis of preoperative and intraoperative investigations for the diagnosis of infection at the sites of 202 revision total hip arthroplasties. J Bone Joint Surg (Am) 1999; 81:672-83.

[15] Levitsky KA, Hozack WJ, Balderston RA, et al. Evaluation of the painful prosthetic joint. Relative value of bone scan, sedimentation rate, and joint aspiration. J Arthroplasty 1991;6:237-44.

[16] Sher DM, Pak K, Lonner JH, fenkel JE, Zuckerman JD, Di Cesare PE. The predictive value of indium-111 leukocytes scans in the diagnosis of infected total hip, knee, or resection arthroplasties. J Arthroplasty 2000;15:295-300.

[17] Palestro CJ, Swyer AJ, Kim CK, Goldsmith SJ. Infected knee prosthesis: diagnosis with In-111 leukocyte, Tc-99 sulfur colloid, and Tc-99m MDP imaging. Radiology 1991;179:645-8.

[18] Trampuz A, Hanssen AD, Osmon DR, et al. Synovial fluid leukocyte count and differential for diagnosis of prosthetic knee infection. Am J Med 2004;117:556-562.

[19] Atkins BL, Athanasou N, Deeks JJ et al. Prospective evaluation of criteria for microbiological diagnosis of prosthetic-joint infection at revision arthroplasty. J Clin Microbiol 1998;36:2932-9.

[20] Della Valle CJ, Scher DM, Kim YH, et al. The role of intraoperative Gram strain in revision total joint arthroplasty. J Arthroplasty 1999;14:500-4.

[21] Feldman DS, Lonner JH, Desai P, Zuckerman JD. The role of intraoperative frozen sections in revision total joint arthroplasty. J Bone Joint Surg (Am) 1995;77:1807-13.

[22] Yamaguchi K, Morrey BF. Treatment of the infected total elbow arthroplasty. In: The Elbow and its Disorders, 3d Edition, pp 678-684. Edited by BF Morrey. Philadelphia, W.B. Saunders, 2000.

[23] Schoifet SD, Morrey BF. Treatment of infection after total knee arthroplasty by debridement with retention of the components. J Bone Joint Surg (Am) 1990;72:1383.

[24] Tunney MM, Patrick S, Curran MD et al. Detection of prosthetic hip infection at revision arthroplasty by immunofluorescence microscopy and PCR amplification of the bacterial 16S rRNA gene. J Clin Microbiol 1999;37:3281-90.

[25] Tunney MM, Patrick S, Gorman SP et al. Improved detection of infection hip replacements: A currently underestimated problem. J Bone Joint Surg Br 1998;80:568-572.

[26] Van Pett K, Schurman DJ, Smith RL. Quantitation and relative distribution of extracellular matrix in staphylococcus epidermidis biofilm. J Orthop Res 1990;8:321.

[27] Gristina AG. Biomaterial-centred infection: Microbial adhesion versus tissue integration. Science 1987;237:1588.

[28] Garvin KL, Hinrichs SH, Urban JA. Emerging antibiotic-resistant bacteria: their treatment in total joint arthroplasty. Clin Orthop 1999;369:110-23.

[29] Masterson EL, Masri Ba, Duncan CP. Treatment of infection at the site of total hip replacement. Instr Course Lect 1998; 47:297-306.

[30] James PJ, Butcher IA, Gardner ER, Hamblen DL. Methicillin-resistant Staphylococcus epidermidis in infection of hip arthroplasties. J Bone Joint Surg (Br) 1994;76:725-7.

[31] Morrey BF, Bryan RS. Revision total elbow arthroplasty. J Bone Joint Surg (Am) 1987;69:523-32.

[32] Mastrokalos DS, Zaos KA, Korres D, Soucacos PN. Arthroscopic debridement and irrigation of periprosthetic total elbow infection. Arthroscopy 2006;22:1140e1-1140e3.

[33] Rand JA, Morrey BF, Bryan RS. Management of the infected total joint arthroplasty : Symposium on musculoskeletal sepsis. Orthop Clin North Am 1984;15:491-504.

[34] Yamaguchi K, Adams RA, Morrey BF. Semiconstrained total elbow arthroplasty in the context of treated previous infection. J Shoulder Elbow Surg 1999;8:461-5.

[35] Coste JS, Reig S, Trojani C, Berg M, Walch G, Boileau P. The management of infection in arthroplasty of the shoulder. J Bone Joint Surg (Br) 2004;86:65-9.

[36] Ince A, Seemsnn K, Frommelt L, Katzer A, Loehr JF. One-stage exchange shoulder arthroplasty for peri-prosthetic infection. J Bone Joint Surg (Br) 2005;87:814-18.

[37] Sperling JW, Kozak TKW, Hanssen AD, Cofield RH. Infection after shoulder arthroplasty. Clin Orthop 2001;382:206-16.

[38] Fitzgerald RH Jr. Total hip arthroplasty sepsis. Prevention and diagnosis. Orthop Clin North Am 1992;23:259-64.

Arthroscopic Debridement in Total Elbow Infections

Dimitrios S. MASTROKALOS*, Panayotis N. SOUCACOS

Department of Orthopaedic Surgery, University of Athens, School of Medicine, Athens, Greece

Hematogenous inoculation of bacteria is the most common cause of elbow joint infection. Exogenous inoculation of bacteria is of posttraumatic or iatrogenic origin, as for example, after elbow joint injections or postoperatively. The rate of infection after joint injections/aspirations rises usually up to 0.03%. The rate of infection after arthroscopy depends on the duration of the operation, or the number of previous operations. A number of factors may contribute to the higher rate of infection in elbow joints as compared to other joints, including that the elbow has little soft tissue coverage, the olecranon is vulnerable to trauma and that disruption of the overlying skin or an inflammatory bursitis may lead to joint sepsis. Although several methods of treatment of joint infection have been described and suggested by several authors, today it is well accepted that as soon as an elbow infection is diagnosed or even suspected, open or arthroscopic irrigation with debridement and synovectomy combined with the systemic use of the most appropriate antibiotics is the therapy of choice.

Keywords: elbow; arthroscopy; synovectomy; joint sepsis; infection; synovitis; periprosthetic joint infection.

1. INTRODUCTION

Because of its diagnostic and therapeutic importance, elbow arthroscopy has become a common surgical procedure in the last 18 years. Its popularity is increasing, and since 1988, the rate of elbow arthroscopic procedures among all arthroscopic procedures has increased in some institutions from 0.77% [1] up to 11% [2].

Indications of elbow arthroscopy include removal of loose bodies, synovectomy, tennis elbow release, debridement of osteochondritis dissecans of the capitellum, radial head excision, management of septic and non-septic arthritis of the elbow with osteophyte excision and contracture release, assessment of undiagnosed or chronic pain in the elbow, capsulectomy for arthrofibrosis, instability management and percutaneous pinning of fractures [3, 4]. Contraindications include distortion of normal bony or soft tissue anatomy and extensive heterotopic ossification. A relative contraindication is the previous surgical transposition of the ulnar nerve [3]. During the last years the indications of elbow arthroscopy have increased and the visualization of the joint is improved, but nevertheless, elbow arthroscopy is a difficult operative procedure due to the small size of the joint and mainly due to the close proximity of neurovascular structures.

2. ELBOW INFECTION

Hematogenous inoculation of bacteria is the commonest cause of elbow joint infection. Rates up to 54% have been reported [5]. As bacteria are very often spread in the blood circulation, for example, in the case of simple teeth excisions, one has to consider that predisposing factors such as diabetes mellitus, alcohol, several diseases of the liver and kidneys, tumors and chronic infections already exist. It is also experimentally shown that systemic application of cortisone raises extremely the risk of

*Corresponding Author
Department of Orthopaedic Surgery
General University Hospital Attikon
Rimini 1, 12462 Haidari, Athens, Greece
Tel: +30 210 8152818
e-mail: dsmastrokalos@gmx.net

an infectious disease [6, 7]. Rates of postoperative joint infection up to 28% are reported [8]. Exogenous inoculation of bacteria is of posttraumatic or iatrogenic origin, as for example, after elbow joint injections or postoperatively. The rate of infection after joint injections / aspirations raises usually up to 0.03% [6], although Dittrich et al. [9] report a rate of 48% and Attmanspacher et al. [7], more than 50%.

Infection rates in diagnostic or therapeutic arthroscopy vary between 0.05% and 0.4% [6, 7, 10] and in arthrotomies up to 1% [10]. Considering arthroscopic operations, it seems that the rate of infection depends on: (i) the duration of the operation, (ii) the number of previous operations, (iii) the degree of difficulty and the number of procedures during the operation, and (iv) the number of previous intraarticular injections [6].

A number of factors may also contribute to the higher risk of developing infection in elbow joints as compared with hips or knees, including that a) the elbow joint is a subcutaneous joint with little soft tissue coverage, b) the tip of the olecranon is directly under the skin and thus, it is vulnerable to trauma, and c) disruption of the overlying skin or an inflammatory bursitis may lead to joint sepsis [11].

The most common bacterium causing elbow joint infection is *Staphylococcus aureus* with rates between 40% and 80% [6, 8, 9, 12, 13], although in some cases no bacteria are found in the cultures. Bacteria are found to range between 63% and 100% [6, 8]. In cases where no bacteria are shown in the cultures, it is advisable to treat them immediately as joint infections, based mainly on clinical signs.

2.1. Clinical appearance of infection

The diagnosis of joint infection depends on the history of the patient, where special attention has to be given to potential iatrogenic or non-iatrogenic deficiency of the immune system of the patient and to any previous operations or intraarticular injections. The clinical and laboratory signs of infection are the same in the elbow joint as in all other joints. Rest and night pain are typical. The infected elbow joint appears swollen, warm with red skin and reduced function and the patient complains of fever. The diagnosis is established mainly by the rates of the C - Reactive Protein (CRP) in the blood tests, by the high ESR and the high leucocytes count, especially in the aspirated fluid. Joint aspiration, before chemotherapy is initiated, can help in identifying the bacteria involved in joint sepsis. As already reported, it is not always possible to do so. Nevertheless, more reliable than identifying bacteria in the aspirated fluid, seems to be finding the number of leucocytes, their type, CRP, LDH and the glucose-concentration [13].

Sonographic examination is sometimes helpful in determining, if there is pus only in the joint or if there is fluid around the joint and on previous surgical exposures, or whether one has to deal with a postoperative infec-

tion. Standard X-rays are always useful in diagnosing bone involvement. Indium-111-leucocytes scan and magnetic resonance imaging (MRI) with a sensivity approaching 100% are helpful only if there is suspicion that bone is involved in the infection [6].

2.2. Treatment of elbow infection

Several methods of treatment of joint infection have been described and suggested by several authors. A single full aspiration of the joint does not seem appropriate [5, 14].

Another possibility is the distension - irrigation technique as proposed by Jackson and Parsons in 1973: after irrigation and debridement follows insertion of two drains into the joint. Subsequently, the joint is distended with saline solution and antibiotics for 3 hours and then the joint is drained. This therapy lasts for about 6 to 8 days [15]. A complication of the distension and irrigation technique is the "highway" effect, i.e. the solution seeks the shortest way towards drainage. As a result, not all parts of the joint are washed out, and bacteria remain in small cavities of the joint and become resistant to antibiotics. The technique is also complicated by secondary infections due to inadequate nursing care [6].

It is today well accepted that, as soon as an elbow infection is diagnosed or even suspected, open or arthroscopic irrigation with debridement and synovectomy combined with systemic use of the most appropriate antibiotics, is the therapy of choice. It seems that systemic use of appropriate antibiotics alone [16] or with joint aspiration is not a sufficient way of treatment of a joint infection.

3. ARTHROSCOPIC TREATMENT OF ELBOW INFECTION

3.1. Indications

An acute [or early] elbow infection is an emergency and it should be treated like an emergency by operative means, arthroscopic or open, as soon as possible and so long as the general condition of the patient allows it [6, 7, 9]. It should not be postponed up to the next day. "It is always better to treat a possible joint infection twice as soon as possible than once and late" [9]. Although it is widely accepted that acute or early septic arthritis of the elbow is a clear indication for arthroscopic irrigation and synovectomy (in that way the joint-destroying process can be stopped and eliminated [17]) no specific series with arthroscopic treatment of elbow septic arthritis have been published. Concerning especially arthroscopic treatment of elbow infection, it is reported that it is effective only in the early stage of the disease, as long as no signs of cartilage and bone lesions exist [6, 7, 9].

3.2. Technique

Most surgeons prefer to use general anaesthesia because it provides total muscle relaxation, is comfortable for the patient and it allows immediate assessment of nerve function postoperatively, when the patient is awake. The standard arthroscope (4.0mm, 30°) with conical and blunt-tipped trocars and with the standard instrumentarium used for knee surgery are used. It must be noted that there is a variety of handheld and motorized instruments, which could be alternatively used. A small 2.7 mm arthroscope is not necessary, but it could be useful in narrow spaces [3]. The patient can be positioned in four ways: supine, supine-suspended, prone and lateral decubitus. A tourniquet is placed but not used. We prefer to use it at the beginning of the operation, so that we can diagnose the pathology of the joint and then we release it during irrigation and debridement. The extremity is sterilely prepared and free draped to allow manipulation. Then all bony landmarks and portals are marked. Filling of the joint with 20 mL of fluid by use of an 18-gauge needle through the lateral "soft spot" follows. There are a variety of portals which can be used in order to inspect and operate in the two main compartments of the elbow, the anterior and the posterior. The most commonly used portals for the posterior compartment of the elbow are: a) the proximal posteroradial, which is the main portal, b) the distal posteroradial, and c) the transtendinous portal. For the anterior compartment 3 portals are mainly used: a) the anteroradial, b) the antero-ulnar, and c) the proximal antero-ulnar portal. The surgeon has to decide upon whether he will use all portals or some of them. The way of how to create the portals and how to inspect and operate arthroscopically in the elbow joint is well described [3, 18]. The most important point in treating elbow infection arthroscopically is irrigation with at least 5 to 10 liters of fluid. Synovectomy takes place as in cases of rheumatoid arthritis; the only difference is that in cases of elbow joint infection, partial synovectomy is preferred, although some authors suggest that the synovial membrane should remain intact, as it is a barrier which prevents extension of the infection outside the joint [8]. For removal of adhesions, clots and synovectomy, graspers and the 3.5 or 4.5 mm shaver with the side cutting opening are usually used [9]. It is important not only to flex and extend the elbow in order to see and remove the debris and the most inflamed parts of the synovium but also to rotate the forearm in order to see and work, if necessary, around the radial head [19]. It is extremely important to see and treat all elbow joint compartments.

It is not advisable by many authors to put inflow-drainage systems after an arthroscopical procedure because of several difficulties in mobilizing the patient and because of the risk of the "highway" effect.

There is a controversy in using antibiotics in this irrigation solution. Chemical synovitis after intra-articular instillation of antibiotics [20] and toxicity to the articular cartilage with irreversible damage are reported in the literature [13, 21].

At the end of the arthroscopic procedure, collagen sponges infiltrated with antibiotics could be inserted with

an arthroscopic clamp into the joint. A drainage tube of wide diameter or two tubes with a small diameter (No 10) should be inserted into the joint and left for a short time (24 - 48 hours) but in any case no longer than 4-5 days [9].

Some authors prefer to give antibiotics (Gentamycin) injected into the joint [22], especially if there is only synovitis with no formation of clots and debris. In all the other cases, they use collagen sponges with antibiotics [9] or they totally reject their use because of a change in the pH of the joint fluid and possible chemical synovitis [13]. The appropriate systemic antibiotics should be given according to the antibiogram up to the time when CRP, leucocytes and ESR return to the normal values [6, 7, 9].

3.3. Treatment Algorithm

Arthroscopic treatment of elbow joint sepsis, including irrigation, debridement and synovectomy is a minimally invasive operative procedure which can be repeated as many times as needed. It keeps the problem of the infection in the joint without any particular risk of spreading bacteria outside the joint as might be the case with jet lavage in an open procedure.

A classification system according to the arthroscopic appearance and the radiological severity of the joint infection has been described by Gächter [7, 8, 23] (Table 1).

According to these stages of joint infection an algorithm of surgical / arthroscopical treatment has been proposed [6-9, 23] (Table 2).

Systemic use of antibiotics is obligatory according to the antibiogram, as already mentioned. Some authors give them for 4 to 10 weeks, some others prefer to give them until normalization of clinical signs and laboratory parameters [9]. In chronic cases of joint infection, arthroscopical treatment is not advisable because of the thick and sclerosed synovium, which cannot be removed with an arthroscopical resector. Open synovectomy is the best option in such cases [9, 23].

TABLE 1

Stages of joint infection according to Gächter [7,8,23].

Stage I:	opacity of fluid, redness of the synovial membrane, possible petechial bleeding, no radiological alterations
Stage II:	severe inflammation, fibrinous deposition, pus, no radiological alterations
Stage III:	thickening of the synovial membrane, compartment formation, no radiological alterations
Stage IV:	aggressive pannus with infiltration of the cartilage, possibly undermining the cartilage, radiological signs of subchondral osteolysis, possible osseous erosions and cysts.

TABLE 2	
Treatment algorithm according to Gächter [6-9, 31].	
Stage I:	arthroscopical lavage of all joint compartments + appropriate antibiotics. A single arthroscopic irrigation could be enough. In case of persistent clinical signs and high biochemical rates of infection, re-arthroscopy should take place, as soon as possible
Stage II:	arthroscopical lavage of all joint compartments with removal of all fibrin clots and partial synovectomy + appropriate antibiotics. In case of persistent clinical signs and biochemical rates, re-arthroscopy should take place, as soon as possible
Stage III:	the same as in stage II with perhaps more aggressive synovectomy. More than one arthroscopic irrigations are necessary
Stage IV:	poor or no indication for arthroscopic lavage, debridement and synovectomy. In this stage, it seems that open removal of non-vital cartilage pieces and debridement of the inflammed and cystic bone areas is the appropriate mean of treatment

3.4. Postoperative treatment

Postoperatively, the patient is allowed to move the joint and should be given analgesics. It is mandatory to start working with CPM and with systematic physiotherapy after removal of the drainage tubes. He should also be often checked clinically and his postoperative counts of Leukocytes, CRP and ESR should be checked every day or every second day. Some authors plan routinely a second arthroscopical irrigation 5 to 7 days after the 1st one, especially in the Stages II and III according to Gächter [7-9].

3.5. Complications

In a series of 473 aseptic elbow arthroscopies the most serious postoperative complication was deep infection in 4 cases (0.8%), especially in patients receiving intra-articular steroids at the end of the arthroscopy. Another one was transient nerve palsy in 10 patients (2%), considering the close proximity of nerves to the portals. In two of them, direct nerve injury was the cause. Neurological complications, including mostly transection of the ulnar nerve and compression neuropathy of the radial nerve [24] after elbow arthroscopy appear to range between 0% and 14%. Reported are also injuries to the posterior interosseous nerve [3]. Other complications are loss of range of motion, compartment syndrome and persistent drainage from portal sites [2]. Secondary cartilage lesions up to severe restriction of range of joint motion are rarely described. Change of an acute infection into a chronic one is usually the result of a delay of treatment in the acute stage of the disease [6]. Recently, complete but usually transient ulnar and radial nerve palsy following elbow arthroscopy have been reported [3, 19].

3.6. Results

Dittrich et al. in 1999 [9] reported that one arthroscopic irrigation is very often not enough to treat joint infections. Out of 97 patients treated with arthroscopic irrigation because of joint infection, only 5 patients had one arthroscopic treatment. In 36 patients, 2 arthroscopic procedures were necessary, and in 27.3, arthroscopies. In the rest of the cases more than 3 were necessary, or the patient had to be treated by an open surgery. The mean of arthroscopic irrigations was 2.9. The most difficult cases to treat are joint infections of haematogenous origin, with a mean of 4.2 revisions necessary, and then post-injection joint infections with a mean of 3.1 revisions. The authors did not report the number of revisions needed according to the stage of the infection.

Morihara et al. [25] reported excellent results 12 months postoperatively in treating shoulder infection in an infant with arthroscopic irrigation, debridement and synovectomy, using standard portals, 5 days after the onset of symptoms.

A special cause of joint infection is mycobacterium tuberculosis. Joint tuberculosis is characterized by a combination of inflammation, bone destruction - repair, including sclerosis of the bone and fibrosis of the joint capsule. The disease appears as infectious-allergic synovitis and develops into a capsule fibrosis with adhesions, causing pain and limitation of motion, which are the main indications for arthroscopic treatment (Stages I, II and III, according to Gächter) [6, 9, 23]. If necrosis of bone and soft tissue is diagnosed, it seems that the arthroscopic procedures are not indicated, or they have to be combined with open procedures (Stage IV - Gächter), in order to remove the dead bone and the dead soft tissue. Titov et al. reported excellent results by treating 13 cases of joint tuberculosis according to the above algorithm. In 11 cases, one arthroscopic irrigation with partial synovectomy and removal of adhesions was sufficient to eliminate joint infection and improving the joint range of motion, in two cases open surgery was necessary because of massive bone destruction. As in all other bacterial infections, these operative procedures were combined with the appropriate antibiotics for about 6 to 9 months [26].

Stutz et al. [23] reported excellent results in 21 out of 22 patients with joint sepsis in Stage I (Gächter) treated successfully with a single arthroscopical irrigation. The same group of authors reported that in 23% of the cases in Stage II, two arthroscopic irrigations were needed, in 23%, three, while in 6%, four. A single arthroscopy was sufficient for the rest 48%. In Stage III, the rate of successful treatment of joint infection with a single arthroscopic irrigation falls to 25%. All stage IV cases needed open debridement and irrigation. Removal of osteosynthesis hardware took place only in 1 out of 10 cases; patients with total joint replacements were not included in this study.

Jerosch et al. [27] reported on 2 cases of arthroscopic irrigation and debridement in combination with resorbable gentamycin fleeces in acute elbow infection with excellent results regarding radical elimination of infection, and functional results. The patients were treated with one arthroscopic procedure only and with systemic antibiotic therapy applied for 4 to 6 months.

4. PERIPROSTHETIC JOINT INFECTIONS

The primary goal of total elbow arthroplasty is to relieve pain, but it is also important to restore the function of the joint. Periprosthetic elbow joint infection is also an emergency which has to be diagnosed and treated aggressively, as soon as possible [28]. The bacteria mainly involved in periprosthetic elbow joint infections are staph. aureus and staph. epidermitis [11, 29]. Main predisposing factors for periprosthetic elbow joint sepsis are rheumatoid arthritis, post-traumatic arthritis and previous usage of local steroids. In a study by Morrey et al., 10.7% out of 112 cases of total elbow arthroplasties with rheumatoid arthritis were found infected [11]. 50% of 12 patients receiving steroids because of rheumatoid arthritis, developed deep infection.

Morrey et al. reported an infection rate of 9% in 156 cases of total elbow arthroplasties [11] but the rate of periprosthetic elbow infection can raise up to 12% [8], varying usually from 3% to 9% [28].

Most authors use three modes of treatment in periprosthetic elbow infection: (i) open debridement and salvage of the implant in the early stage of the disease, (ii) resection arthroplasty and (iii) arthrodesis [30]. It is advisable to try to do partial synovectomy and remove all fibrinous depositions in cases of infected joint arthroplasties. The results are good if the joint infection is at a very early stage. For some authors, arthroscopic irrigation with usually major synovectomy seems to be the preferred method for treatment of periprosthetic joint infections, especially for knee and shoulder ones that are at an early stage. Most of the literature refers to arthroscopic debridement of septic total knee arthroplasties. The rates of success vary from 20% to 90% [28].

Arthroscopic debridement is associated with decreased surgical morbidity. Inclusion criteria for arthroscopic debridement in periprosthetic joint infections are (i) a stable and well functioning prosthesis, (ii) symptoms persisting for less than a week (or less than 4 weeks [31], (iii) no immune system compromising factors, and (iv) no soft tissue involvement; a wound secretion seems to be no contra-indication for arthroscopic treatment. Absolute contraindications are previous infection in/around the elbow, concurrent remote infection and high loading requirements in young patients with traumatic arthritis [30]. Arthroscopy of infected arthroplasties might be difficult because of the "mirror" effect and the limited space in the joint compartment, and also time-consuming.

According to the joint involved, standard portals are used and the joint is irrigated with about 12 L or more of salin or bacitracin solution [50,000 U per 3L]. A suction drainage is placed and CPM is initiated immediately after the operation. Intravenous antibiotics are given for 4 to 6 weeks [31], followed sometimes by 2 to 4 more weeks of oral antibiotic administration as determined by an infectious disease consultant. Arthroscopic treatment of periprosthetic joint infection is popular in knee and shoulder sepsis.

Morrey et al. [11] reported on 14 cases with deep infection out of 156 total elbow arthroplasties. Ten of the patients were treated with resection arthroplasty with good results, 1 with debridement with a fair result, 1 with amputation with a fair result and 2 with joint replacement with fair to poor results. Yamaguchi et al. [29] report 50% of successful results in treating 14 patients with periprosthetic elbow joint infection with open irrigation and debridement. The treatment was applied in the acute stage of infection that is 0 to 80 days after the total elbow arthroplasty and between 0 and 31 days after the onset of symptoms. The joint was treated at least 3 times with irrigation and debridement. Main complications with the open irrigation and debridement were irreversible nerve injury, late fungal infection, and breakdown of the wound [29].

The difficulties of arthroscopic treatment of periprosthetic joint infections consist of inadequate access of all joint compartments, as for example that of the elbow joint, because of limited volumen of the joint, especially anteriorly.

Jerosch et al. [31] reported good results in a periprosthetic shoulder infection case treated successfully with arthroscopic irrigation, debridement and synovectomy. A local resorbable antibiotic carrier (gentamycin sponge 10x10) was inserted intra-articularly. This was a case of an early infection developed within 4 weeks without soft tissue involvement.

Wolfe et al. reported a rate of 7.3% of periprosthetic elbow infection in 164 elbows available for follow-up [30]. Out of these 12 septic arthroplasties, they treated 4 with open debridement, 6 with resection arthroplasty and 2 with arthrodesis. The authors defined as acute infection the incidence of clinical and laboratory signs within 3 months after the elbow replacement. Only in 3 cases could the implants be restored; in all the other cases, the patients had either removal of the implants and revision arthroplasties or arthrodeses with poor functional results [30].

4.1. Sample cases

We have previously reported on arthroscopic treatment of a periprosthetic elbow infection [32]. Removal of ectopic bone and joint replacement in one stage was the treatment of choice in a 65-year-old male patient with post traumatic osteoarthrosis and extensive ectopic bone formation around the right elbow. The patient received peri-operative chemo-prophylaxis and post-operative indomethacine. He was discharged two weeks after the operation with arch of elbow motion of more than 110° and with no signs of infection.

Seventy days after the elbow replacement and six days after initiation of symptoms the patient presented with signs of acute infection (erythema, swelling, warmness) around the elbow and mild fever. The CBC showed normal WBC, but elevated PLT (579.000/μL) count and the ESR (78 mm), as well as the CRP (82.5 mg/L) was elevated. The radiographic examination showed evidence of a well fixed component. Cultures of joint fluid after ultrasound guided aspiration of the elbow revealed a Methicillin-sensitive *Staphylococcus Aureus* (MSSA) strain.

An arthroscopic irrigation and debridement was performed, followed by the proper long term appropriate antimicrobial chemotherapy according to the sensitivity test of the cultures. With the patient in lateral decubitus position, under general anaesthesia and with the tourniquet placed but not inflated, arthroscopy of the anterior and posterior compartment of the elbow was performed, as described above. Aspirates and biopsy specimens were taken for Gram stain, culture and antibiotic susceptibility tests. Arthroscopic exploration showed purulent effusion and inflammatory hypertrophic synovium (Fig. 1). Arthroscopic debridement with partial synovectomy in both compartments was performed with a 4.5 mm curved shaver, taking care not to scratch the surfaces of the prosthesis (Fig. 2). The joint was then irrigated with at least 7 liters of saline solution. No antibiotics were added to the irrigating solution. Then, No 12 drainage was placed in the posterior compartment for 36 hours and all portals were sutured.

The intraoperative cultures revealed the same strain

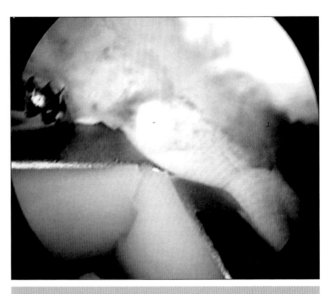

FIGURE 2. Partial synovectomy with a 4.5mm curved shaver.

(MSSA) as did the preoperative culture. The patient was treated for six weeks with iv rifampicine (600mg morning plus 300 mg in the evening) and iv fucidic acid (500 mg three times a day) and for six more weeks he received per os tbl rifampicine (600mg morning plus 300 mg in the evening) and tbl fucidic acid (500 mg three times a day).

Three months after surgery, laboratory findings returned to normal. At the 20th-month follow-up evaluation, the patient presented with neither clinical nor laboratory signs of infection. The elbow joint was pain free, and the range of motion was E/F 10°-120°. Radiologically, the implant was stable with no sign of loosening.

CONCLUSIONS

An early total elbow infection, confirmed by clinical signs and laboratory findings, should be treated as soon as possible. Arthroscopic debridement and irrigation with at least 5 liters of fluid, with or without synovectomy, is an established choice of treatment, since it is minimally invasive, can be repeated as many times as needed and keeps the infection in the affected joint, without spreading bacteria outside it. Arthroscopic debridement in total elbow infections should be followed by systemic antibiotic therapy for at least 4 weeks, according to the antibiogram. In cases of chronic elbow infections, arthroscopic treatment might have worse results than open debridement and irrigation.

REFERENCES

[1] Small NC. Complications in arthroscopic surgery performed by experienced arthroscopists. Arthroscopy 1988;4:215-221.

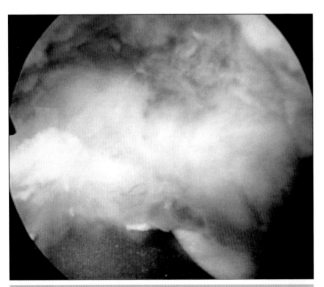

FIGURE 1. Posterolateral approach: inflammatory hypertrophic synovium.

[2] Kelly EW, Morrey BF, O'Driscoll SW. Complications of Elbow Arthroscopy. J Bone Joint Surg 2001;83-A (1):25-34.

[3] Abboud JA, Ricchetti ET, Tjoumakaris F, Ramsey ML. Elbow Arthroscopy: Basic Setup and Portal Placement. J Am Acad Orthop Surg 2006;14:312-318.

[4] Micheli LJ, Luke AC, Mintzer CM, Waters PM. Elbow arthroscopy in the Pediatric and Adolescent Popoulation. Arthroscopy 2001;17 (7):694-699.

[5] Parisien JS, Shaffer B. Arthroscopic management of pyarthrosis. Clin Orthop 1992;275:243-247.

[6] Jerosch J. Akuter Gelenkinfekt; Diagnostik und Therapie. Orthopaede 2004;11:1309-1319.

[7] Attmanspacher W, Dittrich V, Stedtfeld HW. Management bei fruhem Gelenkinfekt: Moglichkeiten und Grenzen der Arthroskopie. Trauma Berufskrankh 2003;5 (Suppl 2):213-220.

[8] Yamaguchi K, Morrey BF. Infection after total elbow arthroplasty. J Bone Joint Surg 1998;80-A(4):481-491.

[9] Dittrich V, Attmanspacher W, Stedtfeld HW. Mehrzeitiges arthroskopisches Vorgehen bei Kniegelenkempyemen. Arthroskopie 1999;12:137-143.

[10] Simank HG, Wadl B, Bernd L. Gelenkempyeme. Orthopaede 2004; 3:327-331.

[11] Morrey BF, Bryan RS. Infection after total elbow arthroplasty. J Bone Joint Surg 1983;65-A (3):330-338.

[12] Williams RJ, Laurencin CT, Warren RF, Speciale AC, Brause BD, O'Brien A. Septic arthritis after arthroscopic anterior cruciate ligament reconstruction. Diagnosis and management. Am J Sports Med 1997;25:261-267.

[13] Simank HG, Wadi B, Bernd L. Gelenkempyeme. Orthopaede 2004; 33:327-331.

[14] Wick M, Muller EJ, Ambacher T, Hebler U, Muhr G, Kutscha-Lissberg F. Arthrodesis of the shoulder after septic arthritis. Long-term results. J Bone Joint Surg [Br] 2003;85:666-670.

[15] Jackson RW, Parsons CJ. Distension - Irrigation treatment of major joint sepsis. Clin Orthop 1973;96:160-164.

[16] Riegels-Nielsen P, Frimodt-Moller N, Sorensen M, Jensen JS. Antibiotic treatment insufficient for established septic arthritis. Staphylococcus aureus experiments in rabbits. Acta Orth Scand 1989;60(1):113-115.

[17] Jerosch J, Schroder M, Schneider T. Good and relative indications for elbow arthroscopy. A retrospective study on 103 patients. Arch Orthop Trauma Surg 1998;117:246-249.

[18] Strobel M. 7. Ellenbogengelenk - Allgemeiner Teil. In: "Arthroskopische Chirurgie" Strobel, Springer Verlag Heidelberg, 1998.

[19] Nobuyuki Tanaka, Hisashi Sakahashi, Kazuya Hirose, Takumi Ishima, Seiichi Ishii. Arthroscopic and open Synovectomy of the Elbow In Rheumatoid Arthritis. J Bone Joint Surg 2006; 88-A (3): 521-525.

[20] Argen RJ, Wilson CH, Wood P. Suppurative arthritis. Arch Intern Med 117:661-666.

[21] Gachter A. Gelenkinfekt. Arthroskopische Spulbehandlung - Hints und Tricks. Arthroskopie 7:98-101.

[22] Jerosch J, Schroeder M, Steinbeck J, Halm H. Arthroskopische Therapie der bakteriellen Arthritis. Arthroskopie 8:79-83.

[23] Stutz G, Kuster MS, Kleinstueck F, Gaechter A. Arthroscopic management of septic arthritis: stages of infection and results. Knee Surg, Sports Traumatol, Arthrosc 2000;8(5):270-274.

[24] Reddy AS, Kvitne RS, Yocum LA, ElAttrache NS, Glousman RE, Jobe FW. Arthroscopy of the elbow: A long term clinical review. Arthroscopy 2000;16(6):588-594.

[25] Toru Morihara, Yuji Arai, Motoyuki Horii, Kenichi Chatani, Shinya Fujita, Daisaku Tokunaga, Toshikazu Kubo. Case Report: Arthroscopic treatment for septic arthritis of the shoulder in an infant. J Orthop Sci 2005;10:95-98.

[26] Titov AG, Nakonechniy GD, Santavirta S, Serdobintzev MS, Mazurenko SI, Konttinen YT. Arthroscopic operations in joint tuberculosis. The Knee 2004;11:57-62.

[27] Jerosch J, Hoffstetter I, Schroeder M, Castro WHM. Septic Arthritis: Arthroscopic Management with Local Antibiotic Treatment. Acta Orthopaedica Belgica 1995;Vol. 61-2:126-134.

[28] Waldman BJ, Hostin E, Mont MA, Hungerford DS. Infected Total Knee Arthroplasty treated by Arthroscopic Irrigation and Debridement. J Arthroplasty 2000;15 (4):430-436.

[29] Yamaguchi Ken, Adams RA, Morrey BF Infection after Total Elbow Arthroplasty. J Bone Joint Surg 1998;80-A,No 4:481-491.

[30] Wolfe SW, Figgie MP, Inglis AE, Bohn WW, Ranawat CS. Management of Infection about Total Elbow Prostheses. J Bone Joint Surg 1990;72-A No 2:198-212.

[31] Jerosch J, Schneppenheim M. Management of infected shoulder replacement. Arch Orthop Trauma Surg 2003;123:209-214.

[32] Mastrokalos DS, Zahos KA, Korres D, Soucacos PN. Arthroscopic Debridement and Irrigation of Periprosthetic Total Elbow Infection: A Case Report. Arthroscopy 2006 Oct;22(10):1140. el-3.

Infected Shoulder Replacement

chapter
28

George S. THEMISTOCLEOUS, Charalampos G. ZALAVRAS,
Vasileios C. ZACHOS, John M. ITAMURA*
*Department of Orthopaedic Surgery, Keck School of Medicine,
University of Southern California, LAC+USC Medical Center, Los Angeles, CA, USA.*

Management of infection after shoulder arthroplasty depends on the medical status of the patient, chronicity of the infection, and sensitivity of the infecting bacteria. Treatment options include antibiotic suppression, debridement with retention of the prosthesis, exchange arthroplasty in one or two stages, resection arthroplasty, and in rare cases arthrodesis or amputation. Culture-specific antimicrobial therapy should be administered for 6 weeks. It should be noted that eradication of infection cannot be achieved without debridement of necrotic and infected tissue and removal of foreign material. Two-stage exchange arthroplasty consisting of removal of implants and cement, placement of an antibiotic spacer, and appropriate intravenous antibiotic therapy followed by reimplantation appears to be the predominant approach to managing this challenging complication.

Keywords: shoulder; arthroplasty; replacement; infection; antibiotics.

1. INTRODUCTION

Infection is a devastating complication of shoulder replacement surgery, occurring in approximately 4% of patients having undergone shoulder arthroplasty [1]. The prevalence varies between 0% and 0.9% for primary arthroplasty and rises up to 15.4% for revision arthroplasty [2-6].

Management of a patient with an infected shoulder arthroplasty is challenging and aims to achieve control of infection and preservation of function. The currently accepted treatment options have been adapted from experience gained from treatment of infected hip and knee arthroplasty, and include antibiotic suppression, debridement with prosthesis retention, direct exchange arthroplasty, delayed reimplantation, resection arthroplasty, arthrodesis, and amputation [1, 7-9].

Limited information is available to guide management and decision making. This chapter will address the diagnosis and management of the infected shoulder arthroplasty and will present the clinical outcome of various management options.

2. RISK FACTORS

The patient's overall medical condition plays an important role in the development of infection. Host comorbidities, such as diabetes, malnutrition, chronic diseases, administration of systemic steroids, immunosuppressive agents, chemotherapy, radiation, advanced age, and presence of remote sites of infection predispose to glenohumeral sepsis and shoulder arthroplasty infection [8, 10]. The risk of infection also increases with the number of revisions performed [2-7].

*Corresponding Author
Department of Orthopaedic Surgery
LAC+USC Medical Center
1200 N State St. GNH 3900
Los Angeles, CA 90033, USA
Tel: +1 323 226 7346
Fax: +1 323 226 7346
e-mail: jitamura@msn.com

3. Mechanism

Infection in shoulder arthroplasty may result from intra-operative contamination of the surgical wound or from hematogenous dissemination of bacteria from distant sites, such as urinary or respiratory system infections.

The presence of foreign bodies in the area of the shoulder joint, such as metal alloys, polyethylene, and methylmethacrylate, provides a nidus for adhesion and colonization by bacteria, which in turn produce a glyco-calyx biofilm. Biofilm formation protects the bacteria from antibiotics and host immune responses and leads to chronicity of arthroplasty infections [11].

4. Classification

Infections after joint replacement are classified based on the time frame of their development in order to guide selection of therapy. Infections of shoulder and elbow arthroplasty have been classified into acute, subacute, and late infections, similarly to infections following hip and knee arthroplasty [12-14].

4.1. Acute infections

Acute infections appear up to 3 months after the surgical procedure in approximately 0.5% of cases [1, 4, 15], and are usually associated with wound healing problems or a wound hematoma that becomes infected [12]. Acute infections are further classified into acute superficial (not extending into the joint) and acute deep (extending into the joint) infections.

Superficial infections can be successfully treated with extra-articular soft tissue debridement, local wound care and antibiotics [16]. A more aggressive approach is required in acute deep infections with exposure, debridement, and irrigation of the shoulder joint [16].

4.2. Subacute infections

Subacute infections present between 3 months and 1 year postoperatively [17]. Removal of all foreign material, including the implant and cement, is necessary to be combined with intravenous administration of antibiotics.

4.3. Late infections

Late infections develop clinically later than 12 months postoperatively and are usually related to haematogenous or lymphatic spread of bacteria to the shoulder joint. The usual portals of entry are the oropharyngeal, genitourinary, and the gastrointestinal tract, as well as skin breaks [17]. Identification of the primary source is crucial for treatment of the shoulder infection. They often appear in patients with rheumatoid arthritis [12, 18, 19]. Late infections may also represent a chronic low-grade infection due to intraoperative contamination [20].

5. Microbiology

Approximately 50% of all late prosthetic joint infections are due to *Staphylococcus aureus,* coagulase-negative *Staphylococcus* and *Staphylococcus epidermidis. Pseudomonas aeruginosa, Candida, Propionibacterium* and *Acinebactor* have also been reported in the literature [1, 6, 17, 21, 22].

In the patients reported by Ince et al [23] Propionibacterium was unexpectedly high, being the most frequently identified pathogen after coagulase-negative staphylococci. Sperling et al [6] reported that in a series of 32 infected shoulder arthroplasties, the most common pathogens were Staphylococcus aureus (13 cases), coagulase-negative Staphylococcus (9 cases), and Propionibacterium acnes (5 cases). Jerosch and Schneppenheim [12] identified the pathogen in four out of twelve patients in their series. In three patients the infecting organism was Staphylococcus aureus and in the fourth it was Staphylococcus epidermidis.

6. Clinical Presentation

In general, the clinical picture of a periprosthetic infection is non-specific. Pain is the presenting symptom in most patients, whereas other symptoms and signs of infection, such as fever, chills, malaise, effusion, fistulae, or erythema, are rare [24].

Early infections are usually associated with persistent, moderate pain or stiffness presenting within 3 to 12 days postoperatively. Persistent wound drainage for longer than 48 hours following the procedure raises concerns for an infectious process and should not be overlooked [17, 24].

In subacute and late (chronic) infections the most predominant symptom is increasing pain that gradually evolves into pain at rest and night pain. The shoulder displays more characteristic features of infection with increasing erythema, swelling, and warmth. Patients may also have a low-grade fever [17, 24].

7. Diagnostic Modalities

7.1. Imaging studies

7.1.1. Plain radiographs
A review of plain radiographs is an essential part of the evaluation of a patient with a painful shoulder arthroplasty. Rapid failure of a cemented or cementless implant, in an otherwise skillfully performed arthroplasty, should be considered suspicious for infection [24].

Plain radiographs are usually of limited value in acute infection and, unless they show gas (infections with gas-producing organisms), they offer little in establishing a diagnosis [24]. However, they should be still used to exclude other diagnoses.

Plain radiographs become more important in late infections and usually demonstrate osteopenia of the humerus and the glenoid, widening of bone cement interfaces (component loosening is defined as a complete lucent line >1 mm around one or both components), periostitis, bone destruction, and increase of the suhacromial-humeral distance and glenohumeral distance due to fluid or soft-tissue edema. Long-standing chronic infections may also present with erosions of the periarticular bone of the humerus and glenoid [24].

7.1.2. Ultrasound, CT and MRI
Ultrasound, computed tomography (CT), and magnetic resonance imaging (MRI) have traditionally played a very limited role in the evaluation of patients with suspected periprosthetic infections.

Diagnostic ultrasound allows the documentation of fluid collections, but it is inadequate for the diagnosis of periprosthetic infection [25]. CT and MRI are of little help because of artifacts caused by the metal prosthesis [26]. Computed tomography (CT) provides better bony resolution than either plain radiographs or MRI, clearly depicting subtle bone destruction. Recently developed MRI scanning with pulse sequences reduces prosthetic artifact and may lead to an increased use of MRI in the assessment of infection [26].

7.1.3. Bone scan
Nuclear medicine studies may occasionally be helpful in evaluating the patient with a painful shoulder arthroplasty in whom the history, physical examination, and plain radiographic studies are unclear or equivocal. However, the role of bone scintigraphy for the shoulder has not been widely investigated.

Technetium-99 methylene diphosphonate (99Tc MDP) bone scans may be helpful in determining the stability of a component. Although bone scan has a high sensitivity, the low specificity for infection limits its use [27]. Indium-111-labelled white cell scan was found to have a sensitivity of 77% for infection, a specificity of 86%, a positive predictive value of 54%, and a negative predictive value of 95% [28].

7.2. Laboratory analysis
Laboratory tests that are helpful in establishing the diagnosis of an infected implant include a complete blood cell count with differential, determination of the erythrocyte sedimentation rate (ESR), and C-reactive protein (CRP). Assessment of the white blood cell count is of limited benefit as it is frequently normal. Of these tests, the CRP may be the most useful for evaluating and monitoring the patient's response to therapy [8, 12, 25, 29].

Laboratory analysis is of limited value in the early postoperative period because ESR and CRP rise as a response to surgery, with a peak usually on the second or third day [24]. However, in subacute or late infections ESR

>30 mm per hour and CRP >10 mg/l are considered critical values [30]. The sensitivity and specificity of elevated ESR for infection in total hip arthroplasty was 82% and 85%, respectively, whereas elevated CRP had a sensitivity of 96% and a specificity of 92% [31, 32]. If both the ESR and CRP are elevated, the probability of hip arthroplasty infection has been noted to be 83%, and when both are negative, infection can be reliably excluded [31, 32].

7.3. Intraoperative frozen sections
Specimens are collected from the joint capsule and the interfaces between the implant or cement and surrounding bone or both. According to Lonner et al. [33] a frozen section is considered positive if more than 10 polymorphonuclear leukocytes are identified in one high power field.

Intraoperative frozen sections are a useful tool for identifying deep periprosthetic infection, although they are subject to false-negative and false-positive results. The sensitivity and specificity of frozen sections for infection in total hip arthroplasty was 80% and 94%, respectively [31, 32]. A frozen section can also be used to assess eradication of infection during reimplantation in a two-stage revision [33].

7.4. Joint aspiration
When there is a high index of suspicion for periprosthetic infection, the shoulder should be aspirated and the fluid obtained should be evaluated for cell count and differential, and Gram stain, cultures and sensitivities should be determined [25].

Spangehl et al [31] used a cell count greater than 50,000 or a specimen with greater than 80% neutrophils as their criteria for hip arthroplasty infection. Although joint aspiration is a useful adjunct to the preoperative evaluation, a substantial number of false-positive culture results have been reported [31, 34-36]. Microbiological examination of aspirated fluid is essential both for the identification of pathogens and the determination of antibiotic sensitivities [23].

7.5. Gram stain and intraoperative cultures
Intraoperative Gram stain examination is ineffective as an intraoperative screening tool for periprosthetic sepsis, but may be helpful in selecting appropriate antibiotics for inclusion in a temporary antibiotic spacer and guiding initial empiric antibiotic therapy before obtaining the results of intraoperative cultures [31, 37].

Intraoperative cultures are presumed to be the gold standard for identifying periprosthetic infection. Intraoperatively, at least three samples must be taken before prophylactic antibiotic treatment is initiated in order that the culture of bacteria is not jeopardized. Samples must be obtained from both the capsule and the cement-bone interface in order that the rate of identification of the pathogen is increased [38].

Specimens should be sent for aerobic and anaerobic cultures. In chronic infections fungal and mycobacterial cultures may also be useful. The application of polymerase chain reaction (PCR) [39], if available, may be helpful when infection is suspected but cultures persistently remain negative [40].

8. Treatment

Treatment objectives are control of infection, alleviation of pain, and restoration of function. Selection of treatment method requires careful assessment of patient, infection, and implant factors.

Patient-related factors include the health status and expected treatment goals. The patient is classified into either an A, B, or C physiologic group, according to the system of Cierny and Mader [41]. An A host represents a patient with normal metabolic and immune status. The B host is compromised either locally (B_L) or systemically (B_S). Local compromise results from local irradiation, scarring from multiple procedures, and lymphedema. Systemic compromise results from extreme age, chronic disease, or any condition causing suppression of the immune system. The C host status is reserved for those patients in whom the risks associated with aggressive treatment would outweigh the negative aspects of the infection. Patient comorbidities must be addressed preoperatively to optimize outcome. Infection variables include the time interval between implantation and development of infection and the pathogen virulence and sensitivity to antibiotics. Finally, stability of the implant is another important factor.

Many of the techniques used in the treatment of infected shoulder prostheses have been adapted from algorithms established for the treatment of infected hip and knee arthroplasty. The six basic treatment options include antibiotic suppression, debridement with retention of the implant, exchange arthroplasty in one or two stages, resection arthroplasty, arthrodesis, and amputation [1, 7-9].

8.1. Antibiotic suppression

In elderly or frail individuals suppressive antibiotic therapy may be selected, even though the infection will not be eliminated. This method of treatment should be used when the following four criteria are met: (i) an operative procedure for prosthesis removal is not advisable because of the patient's medical condition, (ii) the microorganism has low virulence and is susceptible to an oral antibiotic, (iii) the antibiotic can be tolerated without serious toxicity, and (iv) the prosthesis is not loose [32, 42, 43].

8.2. Debridement with implant retention

Operative debridement with retention of the infected prosthesis should be reserved for acute infections in the immediate postoperative period or as an alternative for a small proportion of patients with late infection, brief duration of symptoms, gram-positive organisms sensitive to antibiotics, and no loosening of the prosthesis or excessive scarring.

Early-onset deep infection extending into the shoulder joint requires operative treatment with debridement, irrigation, and administration of antibiotics. Retention of prosthesis is possible in early postoperative deep infections if the implant appears to be well fixed [2]. This method is generally effective if treatment is initiated within 24 to 36 hours after the onset of signs of infection [8, 15, 16]. Superficial surgical wound infections that develop during or immediately after the index hospitalization are treated with extra-articular soft-tissue debridement, irrigation and a course of antibiotics [16].

A relative contraindication for debridement and attempted salvage of the prosthesis is suggested for the patient with multiple joint replacements or a prosthetic heart valve in order that the risk of metachronous infection due to those prosthetic devices is avoided [32].

8.3. One- stage exchange arthroplasty

In one-stage exchange arthroplasty thorough debridement is carried out with removal of the prosthesis, and a new prosthesis is implanted using antibiotic-impregnated cement. A course of parenteral antibiotics is administered post-operatively for a minimum of six weeks.

For one-stage exchange arthroplasty to be performed, the organism should be sensitive to antibiotics, the host should have few if any risk factors for infection, and there should be adequate bone and soft tissue support for the reconstruction of the shoulder after debridement. If these criteria are not met, a two-stage procedure is recommended.

A one-stage procedure for the management of periprosthetic infection of the shoulder has been reported by Ince et al [23] (sixteen cases), Sperling et al [6] (two cases) and Coste et al [29] (three cases). Ince et al reported the results of one-stage exchange operation as treatment for the infected shoulder arthroplasty in 16 patients. After a mean follow-up of 5.8 years, 9 patients were available for clinical examination and assessment. The one-stage exchange procedure using antibiotic-loaded bone cement eradicated infection in all 9 patients and none of them had a recurrence of infection [23].

Coste et al. [29] reported a multicenter study of 49 infected shoulder arthroplasties. One-stage exchange surgery was undertaken in three cases, with eradication of infection in all. A resection arthroplasty was performed in ten cases but the infection persisted in three of these. Two-stage exchange arthroplasty was performed in ten more cases with failure in four. The authors recommended debridement and one-stage exchange arthroplasty with concurrent administration of antibiotics.

8.4. Two-stage exchange arthroplasty with or without a cement spacer

The evolution of the treatment of infected hip and knee arthroplasty has resulted in the generally accepted approach that two-stage exchange is usually preferable for the infected shoulder arthroplasty, except for specific well-defined cases (please see section 8.3) when one-stage exchange can be performed. The two-stage technique involves removal of all foreign material (implant and cement) in combination with thorough debridement of all necrotic and infected tissues, which is followed by a 6-week course of systemic antibiotics and delayed arthroplasty. The second stage reimplantation is performed when the infection is considered to be resolved based on the clinical exam and blood tests; the ESR and CRP should approach normal levels or at least show a dramatic change toward that direction [44].

With the two-stage procedure, antibiotic therapy can be completed and a repeat debridement can be performed prior to reimplantation of a prosthesis, thereby facilitating eradication of infection [6]. Infection control has been reported at approximately 90% for hip and knee arthroplasty [10, 45]. Codd et al [7] reported on the outcome of four delayed reimplantations. Three of these patients were free of infection and had better function compared with patients who underwent resection arthroplasty.

The major disadvantage of this method is the time delay between stages, which is often associated with pain, difficult mobility and shoulder instability. Furthermore, reimplantation is often difficult because of scar formation and retraction of joint capsule, ligaments, and adjacent soft tissues.

To overcome these difficulties a temporary spacer of antibiotic-loaded cement can be inserted at the first stage and removed at the second operation [1, 2, 4, 46]. The main advantage of this treatment is that it allows for increased delivery of antibiotics to the shoulder joint, resulting in local concentrations five- to tenfold higher compared to systemic administration, while minimizing the risk of systemic toxicity [47]. Furthermore, the insertion of an antibiotic-loaded cement spacer preserves soft tissue tension and length, minimizes soft-tissue contractures, and facilitates reimplantation. The temporary spacer allows mobility and patients can tolerate physiotherapy, thus maintaining a useful range of motion as they await reimplantation [44].

Permanent retention of the cement spacer in low physical demand patients, who are unwilling to undergo major surgery or have inadequate bone stock, was recently reported to have satisfactory results [48].

8.5. Resection arthroplasty

Resection arthroplasty has been a frequently used treatment for the infected shoulder arthroplasty [6]. Because of poor functional results compared to revision shoulder arthroplasty, resection arthroplasty is considered a salvage procedure for patients with medical comorbidities and/or infections with resistant organisms. In the literature, resection arthroplasty has been reported to give good pain relief in the majority of patients [49]. Active abduction is less than 90°, external rotation is limited with moderate weakness, but patients enjoy reasonable joint stability [1, 6]. The patient should be informed that only simple everyday activities will be possible thereafter.

Reimplantation of a shoulder arthroplasty after a previous resection arthroplasty for infection can be performed with a low risk of reinfection. However, arthroplasty in this setting may be especially challenging because of the potential for bone deficits and soft tissue contractures, which can compromise the clinical outcome [50].

Sperling et al. [6] reported 32 infected shoulder arthroplasties of which 21 were treated by resection arthroplasty (group 1), six by debridement with the prosthesis *in situ* (group 2), two by a one-stage exchange (group 3) and three by a two-stage exchange (group 4). Infection persisted in 29% of the patients in group 1, in 50% of those in groups 2 and 3, and in no patient in group 4. The authors also reported that patients with a resection arthroplasty had more pain and less motion than those with an implant in situ.

Codd et al. [7] compared the results of resection arthroplasty (5 patients) versus one- or two-stage prosthesis (4 patients) in infected shoulder arthroplasties. Pain reduction was similar with both methods, however, function of the resected joint was restricted and was inferior to reimplantation.

8.6. Arthrodesis and amputation

Shoulder arthrodesis may be an option following resection arthroplasty if reimplantation cannot be performed due to insufficient bone stock. However, arthrodesis of the shoulder rarely is indicated or accepted by the patient [1].

Amputation for infected shoulder arthroplasty is exceedingly rare, but may be required to control life-threatening infection with severe loss of soft tissue and bone stock or may result from vascular injury [1].

9. CONCLUSION

The predominant approach for managing the infected shoulder arthroplasty is two-stage exchange arthroplasty, which consists of debridement, removal of implants and cement, placement of an antibiotic spacer, and antibiotic therapy followed by reimplantation. Alternative strategies include one-stage exchange arthroplasty, debridement with retention of the prosthesis, resection arthroplasty, or antibiotic suppression.

REFERENCES

[1] Cofield RH, Edgerton BC. Total shoulder arthroplasty: complications and revision surgery. Instr Course Lect 1990;39:449-62.

[2] Goss TP. Shoulder infections. In: Bigliani LU, editor. Complications of shoulder surgery.Baltimore: Williams & Wilkins; 1993. p. 202-13.

[3] Kozak TKW, Hanssen AD, Cofield RH. Infected shoulder arthroplasty. J Shoulder Elbow Surg 1997;6:177.

[4] Ramsey ML, Fenlin JM, Jr. Use of an antibiotic-impregnated bone cement block in the revision of an infected shoulder arthroplasty. J Shoulder Elbow Surg 1996;5(6):479-82.

[5] Sawyer JR, Esterhai JL. Shoulder infections. In: Warner JJP, Lannotti JP, editors. Complex and revision problems in shoulder surgery.Philadelphia: Lippincott-Raven; 1997. p. 385-98.

[6] Sperling JW, Kozak TK, Hanssen AD, Cofield RH. Infection after shoulder arthroplasty. Clin Orthop Relat Res 2001;(382):206-16.

[7] Codd TP, Yamaguchi K, Flatow EL. Infected shoulder arthroplasties: treatment with staged reimplantation versus resection arthroplasty. Orthop Trans 1996;20:59.

[8] Wirth MA, Rockwood CA, Jr. Complications of shoulder arthroplasty. Clin Orthop Relat Res 1994;307:47-69.

[9] Neer CS, Kirby RM. Revision of humeral head and total shoulder arthroplasties. Clin Orthop Relat Res 1982;170:189-95.

[10] Garvin KL, Hanssen AD. Infection after total hip arthroplasty. Past, present, and future. J Bone Joint Surg [Am] 1995;77(10):1576-88.

[11] Gristina AG, Costerton JW. Bacterial adherence to biomaterials and tissue. The significance of its role in clinical sepsis. J Bone Joint Surg [Am] 1985;67(2):264-73.

[12] Jerosch J, Schneppenheim M. Management of infected shoulder replacement. Arch Orthop Trauma Surg 2003;123(5):209-14.

[13] Wolfe SW, Figgie MP, Inglis AE, Bohn WW, Ranawat CS. Management of infection about total elbow prostheses. J Bone Joint Surg [Am] 1990;72(2):198-212.

[14] Yamaguchi K, Adams RA, Morrey BF. Infection after total elbow arthroplasty. J Bone Joint Surg [Am] 1998;80(4):481-91.

[15] Miller SR, Bigliani LU. Complications of total shoulder replacement. In: Bigliani LU, editor. Complications of total shoulder replacement. Williams & Wilkins; 1993. p. 59.

[16] Mont MA, Waldman B, Banerjee C, Pacheco IH, Hungerford DS. Multiple irrigation, debridement, and retention of components in infected total knee arthroplasty. J Arthroplasty 1997;12(4):426-33.

[17] Iannotti Joseph P, Williams GR. Disorders of the shoulder diagnosis and management. Philadelphia: Lippincott Williams & Wilkins; 1999.

[18] Poss R, Thornhill TS, Ewald FC, Thomas WH, Batte NJ, Sledge CB. Factors influencing the incidence and outcome of infection following total joint arthroplasty. Clin Orthop Relat Res 1984;(182):117-26.

[19] Wilson MG, Kelley K, Thornhill TS. Infection as a complication of total knee-replacement arthroplasty. Risk factors and treatment in sixty-seven cases. J Bone Joint Surg [Am] 1990;72(6):878-83.

[20] Maderazo EG, Judson S, Pasternak H. Late infections of total joint prostheses. A review and recommendations for prevention. Clin Orthop Relat Res 1988;(229):131-42.

[21] Lichtman EA. Candida infection of a prosthetic shoulder joint. Skeletal Radiol 1983;10(3):176-7.

[22] Settecerri JJ, Pitner MA, Rock MG, Hanssen AD, Cofield RH. Infection after rotator cuff repair. J Shoulder Elbow Surg 1999; 8(1):1-5.

[23] Ince A, Seemann K, Frommelt L, Katzer A, Loehr JF. One-stage exchange shoulder arthroplasty for peri-prosthetic infection. J Bone Joint Surg [Br] 2005;87(6):814-8.

[24] Brems JJ. Complications of Shoulder athroplasty: Infections, Instability and Loosening. AAOS Instructional Course Lectures. 51 ed. 2002. p. 29-31.

[25] Ince A, Seemann K, Frommelt L, Katzer A, Lohr JF. One-stage revision of shoulder arthroplasty in the case of periprosthetic infection. Z Orthop Ihre Grenzgeb 2004;142(5):611-7.

[26] White LM, Kim JK, Mehta M, Merchant N, Schweitzer ME, Morrison WB, et al. Complications of total hip arthroplasty: MR imaging-initial experience. Radiology 2000;215(1):254-62.

[27] Reing CM, Richin PF, Kenmore PI. Differential bone-scanning in the evaluation of a painful total joint replacement. J Bone Joint Surg [Am] 1979;61(6A):933-6.

[28] Scher DM, Pak K, Lonner JH, Finkel JE, Zuckerman JD, Di Cesare PE. The predictive value of indium-111 leukocyte scans in the diagnosis of infected total hip, knee, or resection arthroplasties. J Arthroplasty 2000;15(3):295-300.

[29] Coste JS, Reig S, Trojani C, Berg M, Walch G, Boileau P. The management of infection in arthroplasty of the shoulder. J Bone Joint Surg [Br] 2004;86(1):65-9.

[30] Spangehl MJ, Masterson E, Masri BA, O'Connell JX, Duncan CP. The role of intraoperative gram stain in the diagnosis of infection during revision total hip arthroplasty. J Arthroplasty 1999;14(8):952-6.

[31] Spangehl MJ, Masri BA, O'Connell JX, Duncan CP. Prospective analysis of preoperative and intraoperative investigations for the diagnosis of infection at the sites of two hundred and two revision total hip arthroplasties. J Bone Joint Surg [Am] 1999;81(5):672-83.

[32] Toms AD, Davidson D, Masri BA, Duncan CP. The management of peri-prosthetic infection in total joint arthroplasty. J Bone Joint Surg [Br] 2006;88(2):149-55.

[33] Lonner JH, Desai P, Dicesare PE, Steiner G, Zuckerman JD. The reliability of analysis of intraoperative frozen sections for identifying active infection during revision hip or knee arthroplasty. J Bone Joint Surg [Am] 1996;78(10):1553-8.

[34] Barrack RL, Harris WH. The value of aspiration of the hip joint before revision total hip arthroplasty. J Bone Joint Surg [Am] 1993;75(1):66-76.

[35] Barrack RL, Jennings RW, Wolfe MW, Bertot AJ. The Coventry Award. The value of preoperative aspiration before total knee revision. Clin Orthop Relat Res 1997;345:8-16.

[36] Lachiewicz PF, Rogers GD, Thomason HC. Aspiration of the hip joint before revision total hip arthroplasty. Clinical and laboratory factors influencing attainment of a positive culture. J Bone Joint Surg [Am] 1996;78(5):749-54.

[37] Chimento GF, Finger S, Barrack RL. Gram stain detection of infection during revision arthroplasty. J Bone Joint Surg [Br] 1996;78(5):838-9.

[38] Ince A, Tiemer B, Gille J, Boos C, Russlies M. Total knee arthroplasty infection due to Abiotrophia defectiva. J Med Microbiol 2002;51(10):899-902.

[39] Levine MJ, Mariani BA, Tuan RS, Booth RE, Jr. Molecular genetic diagnosis of infected total joint arthroplasty. J Arthroplasty 1995;10(1):93-4.

[40] Goldenberg DL, Reed JI. Bacterial arthritis. N Engl J Med 1985;21;312(12):764-71.

[41] Cierny G, III, Mader JT, Penninck JJ. A clinical staging system for adult osteomyelitis. Clin Orthop Relat Res 2003;(414):7-24.

[42] Goulet JA, Pellicci PM, Brause BD, Salvati EM. Prolonged suppression of infection in total hip arthroplasty. J Arthroplasty 1988;3(2):109-16.

[43] Grauer JD, Amstutz HC, O'Carroll PF, Dorey FJ. Resection arthroplasty of the hip. J Bone Joint Surg [Am] 1989;71(5):669-78.

[44] Loebenberg MI, Zuckerman JD. An articulating interval spacer in the treatment of an infected total shoulder arthroplasty. J Shoulder Elbow Surg 2004;13(4):476-8.

[45] Hanssen AD, Rand JA, Osmon DR. Treatment of the infected total knee arthroplasty with insertion of another prosthesis. The effect of antibiotic-impregnated bone cement. Clin Orthop Relat Res 1994;(309):44-55.

[46] Amstutz HC, Thomas BJ, Kabo JM, Jinnah RH, Dorey FJ. The Dana total shoulder arthroplasty. J Bone Joint Surg [Am] 1988;70(8):1174-82.

[47] Henry SL, Galloway KP. Local antibacterial therapy for the management of orthopaedic infections. Pharmacokinetic considerations. Clin Pharmacokinet 1995;29(1):36-45.

[48] Proubasta IR, Itarte JP, Lamas CG, Escriba IU. Permanent articulated antibiotic-impregnated cement spacer in septic shoulder arthroplasty: a case report. J Orthop Trauma 2005;19(9):666-8.

[49] Cofield RH. Shoulder arthrodesis and resection arthroplasty. Instr Course Lect 1985;34:268-77.

[50] Mileti J, Sperling JW, Cofield RH. Reimplantation of a shoulder arthroplasty after a previous infected arthroplasty. J Shoulder Elbow Surg 2004;13(5):528-31.

Resection Arthroplasty in the Upper Extremity

Volkmar HEPPERT*, Arrash MOGHADDAM, Peter HERRMANN, Christof WAGNER

Department of Septic Surgery, BG Unfallklinik, Ludwigshafen, Germany

Infection of the shoulder, elbow or wrist is a devastating clinical trauma for the patient that can lead to early degenerative changes, pain and limited function. Despite recent advances in joint replacement surgery, resection arthroplasty may be indicated for large joints, particularly those of the upper extremity after severe trauma complicated with infection. Preservation of motion and function are the main goals, and as a result, we no longer perform arthrodesis on these anatomical areas in our septic unit, with the exception of the small joints of the wrist. We have found that resection arthroplasty produced reasonably good results with the use of a straightforward technique. Resection arthroplasty also appears to be a valuable alternative with older patients or patients with previously failed arthroplasty or severe joint sepsis.

Keywords: infectious arthritis; endoprosthesis; resection arthroplasty; management of joint infection.

1. INTRODUCTION

Infection of the shoulder, elbow or wrist is a devastating clinical trauma for the patient that can lead to early degenerative changes, pain and limited function. Total joint arthroplasty for the treatment of sequelae of infected joints has been addressed with respect to the elbow [1]. There are several publications dealing with the role of arthroplasty in the management of previously infected joints [2, 3].

The principles of resection arthroplasty have been well established in orthopaedic surgery [1]. Before the era of endoprosthesis, resection arthroplasty was widely accepted as an option for treating complex cases. Today, it is still used in managing rheumatoid arthritis, but mostly for small joints of the wrist, hand, or foot. There are various reports on the application of resection arthroplasty after failed hip replacement, the so-called Girdlestone hip [4]. Despite recent advances in joint replacement surgery, resection arthroplasty may be indicated for large joints, particularly those of the upper extremity after severe trauma complicated by infection. To the best of our knowledge, the use of resection arthroplasty after post-traumatic infections of the upper extremity has not been previously reported.

2. THE AUTHORS' PREFERRED APPROACH

Between 2000 and 2005, 36 heterogenous patients underwent a resection arthroplasty procedure (N=36) in the upper extremity. Surgeries were performed by the first author and senior surgeon [V.H.]. There were 24 women and 12 men with an average of 77.5 years (range: 38 - 87). All patients had a history of severe infection which had been managed with surgical debridement and antibiotics administered over various time periods. At the time resection arthroplasty was performed, all the patients were still suffering from chronic infection of the joint (shoulder, elbow, or wrist).

*Corresponding Author
Chief of Septic Department
BG Unfallklinik Ludwigshafen
Ludwig Guttmann Str. 13
67071 Ludwigshafen, Germany
Tel: +49 621 68102695
Fax : +49 621 68102685
e-mail: heppert@bgu-ludwigshafen.de

Shoulder: 14 patients. In 11 cases, the infection originated from a fracture of the proximal humerus that was treated with open reduction - internal fixation (ORIF): 9 with plates and 2 with K-wires. Three infections developed following corticoid therapy. An average of 3.2 (range: 1-5) patients had undergone previous procedures on the shoulder.

Elbow: 16 patients. In 6 cases, the infection originated from a complex distal humerus fracture, with complete instability. This subgroup was surgically treated with ORIF after the injury. Four infections developed after corticoid therapy. An average of 2.9 (range: 1-4) patients had undergone previous procedures on the elbow.

Wrist: 6 patients. In all cases the infection originated from a distal radius fracture which was initially plated after trauma. An average of 3.8 (range: 1-7) patients had previous procedures performed on the wrist.

Patients were registered at the Operation Registry at our institution, which was also used for follow-up examinations. Patients were requested to return to the institution for clinical and radiographic evaluation conducted by the senior author at regular follow-up intervals. Those who were unable to return completed a standard questionnaire to evaluate function and satisfaction. The average duration of follow-up was 2.7 years (range: 1.2 - 5 years).

2.1. Evaluation of Infection

Prior to resection arthroplasty, laboratory tests were performed in order to isolate the pathogen. Blood cell counts, erythrocyte sedimentation rate and CRP were measured in all patients. Nine patients did not have a draining fistula at the time of admission, as they had undergone aspiration prior to surgery. Tissue specimens for culture and pathologic examination were obtained intra-operatively from all patients.

2.1.1. Clinical Evaluation
The results from the clinical assessment were recorded on a standard analysis form, and documented the range of motion (ROM) of all joints of the upper extremity, as well as muscle differences.

Pain was assessed using a 10-point visual analog scale (VAS; 1 point = no pain, 10 points = maximum pain). Patient satisfaction at final follow-up compared to the preoperative was also assessed using a 10-point scale (10 points = maximum of satisfaction with the result).

2.1.2. Radiographic Evaluation
Routine radiographic evaluation consisted of standard AP and lateral radiographs of the operated joint.

2.2. Operative Technique

Twenty-seven patients had all infected synovial tissue, cartilage and infected bone excised down to normal tissue in a single-stage procedure. The goal was to eradicate infection. After debridement, the resulting cavity was filled with disinfectant fluid (Lavasept®) for 10 minutes. Finally, the wound was cleansed with pulsate irrigation lavage, and a collagen sponge impregnated with gentamycin-sulfate was implanted in the resulting cavity. Nine patients with severe active infection required two surgical procedures. After debridement, the infected cavity was filled with PMMA chains; these were removed 2 weeks later [5].

A shoulder immobilizer was used postoperatively in all patients with shoulder infections for 3 weeks. Afterwards, a sling was used during the day for 10-14 days. Patients with elbow infections were stabilized with an AO fixator for 3 weeks, while patients with wrist infections were provided with a plaster cast for a total of 8 weeks. Perioperative antibiotics were administered to all patients according to the isolated pathogen. Most patients received Cefuroxim for a period of ten days, although 3 patients with MRSA infections received Vancomycin.

3. RESULTS

3.1. Complications and Reoperations

Six complications occurred in six patients, which resulted in re-operation. One patient with a shoulder infection sustained a postoperative hematoma that required revision surgery. All cultures were negative at the time of revision. Two early re-infections occurred in the elbow group. Swab cultures confirmed the presence of the initial pathogen. The infection completely resolved after the revision surgery. Three patients with shoulder infections developed a recurrent seroma, leading to draining sinus. All swabs were negative. After filling the cavity with a pedicled latissimus dorsi flap, the course was uneventful (Fig. 1).

Six patients with shoulder infections complained of severe pain during shoulder movement even after several months. These patients were treated with a pedicled latissimus dorsi flap which was fixed in the glenoid region with small titanium anchors. There were no signs of infection at the time of revision surgery.

3.2. Clinical Results

At the last follow-up examination, clinical and laboratory findings showed that all patients had good clinical results with no signs of recurrent infection.

The pain score at the time of final follow-up is shown in Diagram 1. The blue arrow represents the subgroup of patients who received a pedicled latissimus dorsi flap. The mean score for pain decreased significantly after the placement of the muscle flap. Twelve of the 36 patients had no or only mild pain during vigorous activity.

ROM scores are shown in Diagram 2. The mean abduction of the shoulder was only 35° (range: 20° -

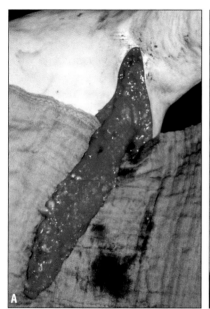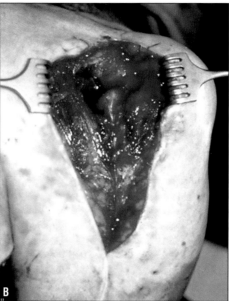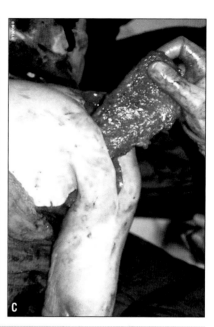

FIGURE 1. (A) Intra-operative view showing resection of the humeral head with a persistent draining sinus. The latissimus dorsi has been raised and split. **(B)** Infected cavity after debridement. **(C)** The muscle is subcutaneously tunnelled and fixed in the cavity with mitek anchors.

65°), and anterior elevation was limited (mean: 65°; range: 35°-95°). Patients with elbow infections had better functional results. Elevation was 0-25°-115°, extension averaged 25° (range: 15°-35°) and flexion averaged 115° (range: 95°-130°) (Fig. 2 and Fig. 3). Patients with wrist infections achieved an average extension of 25° (range: 5°- 35°) and flexion of 20° (range: 10°-30°) (Fig. 4). Forearm rotation was reduced by 30%. Although there were no problems of instability, patients were not able to lift heavy weights. Overhead working was no longer possible, particularly for patients with shoulder infections. Patient satisfaction scores are shown in Diagram 3. (Note that the blue arrow represents patients who had an additional muscle flap.)

4. DISCUSSION

Intra-articular infection can lead to substantial morbidity, inducing early degenerative changes, poor function and pain. The situation can get worse for the patient, if infection following trauma is combined with osteosynthesis. In these cases, surgical options include prosthetic arthroplasty, arthrodesis and resection arthroplasty.

Numerous studies have demonstrated the safety and efficacy of hip and knee arthroplasty for the treatment of degenerative joints with a history of infection [2, 4-9]. Re-infection rates have been found to range between 0% and 9.5%, with clinical results similar, but not identical to those obtained after arthroplasty of joints without a history of infection [1, 2, 5]. While prosthetic arthroplasty

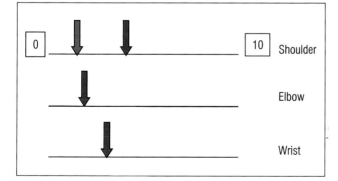

DIAGRAM 1. VAS score of pain at final follow-up (10 points = maximum pain).

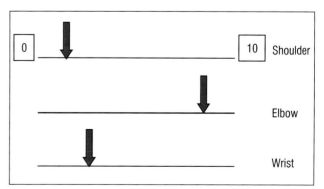

DIAGRAM 2. Range of motion (ROM) at final follow-up (10 points = unlimited function).

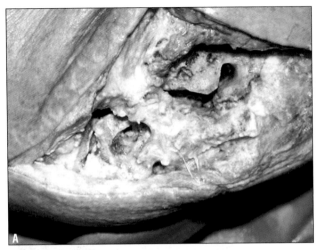

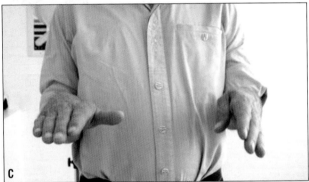

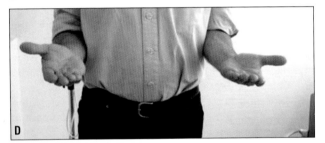

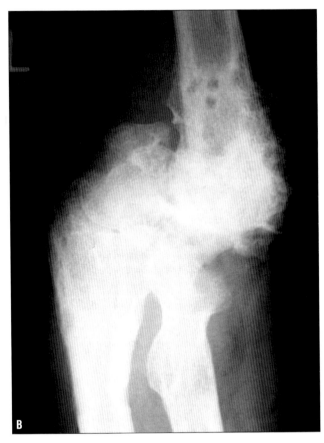

FIGURE 2. (A) Following debridement in a MRSA patient, the elbow joint is clean, but destroyed, and the bone is poorly vascularized. **(B)** Radiograph taken 18 month postoperatively. The patient was treated with external fixation and bone graft mixed with Vancomycin collagen (Biomet Company). **(C)** Post-operative view showing limited pronation, and **(D)** free supination (ROM 0-30-105).

of the hip, knee and elbow in the context of previous infection has been studied, little has been published with regard to shoulder arthroplasty in patients with a history of joint infection [3, 10-14].

Nevertheless, endoprosthesis is in, our opinion the standard procedure to follow after infection in the shoulder region. It maintains the patients' mobility, and in most cases it leaves the patient pain-free or with only moderate pain. In order to implant a prosthesis for post-infectious arthritis several precautions should be taken:

- pre-operative and intra-operative assessment to rule out active infection and determine anatomic parameters that may influence surgery
- careful decision-making with regard to prosthesis placement
- appropriate laboratory screening tests for infection
- careful aspiration of the joint
- utilizing radiographs and a computed tomography s-

can for information with regarding osseous abnormalities and determining whether glenoid resurfacing should be performed.
- Acquisition of tissue specimen intraoperatively for bacteriology and pathology (these are better than swabs).

Endoprosthesis surgery is a challenging procedure, particularly regarding the bone, which is often in the state of osteomyelitis, and the rotator cuff. In order to obtain good results and prevent subluxation after arthroplasty, the rotator cuff and the glenoid bone stock must be critically assessed intraoperatively [3, 6-9]. Notwithstanding all precautions listed above, considerable risk of re-infection still remains [6, 7, 9, 15]. Despite the fact that there are other large joints in the upper extremity, there are only few reports of the use of endoprosthesis after deep elbow infections [1, 16]. As far as we know, there are no data concern-

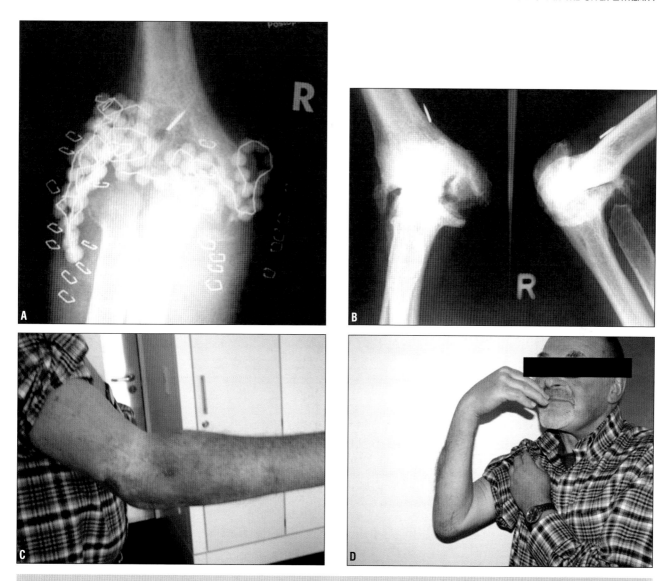

FIGURE 3. (A) 65-year-old diabetic with a 2-stage procedure. PMMA chains were placed in situ, and the wound was left open. Revision and would closure took place 2 weeks later. **(B)** Radiographs taken 3 years post-operatively. **(C)** Patient achieved good extension. **(D)** The patient is able to reach his mouth, demonstrating good flexion.

ing the wrist. Arthroplasty after infection of the joints can be performed with a moderate risk of re-infection in properly selected patients, and with regard to the challenges mentioned above, the clinical results can be variable. Despite the modern orthopaedic techniques available today, the problem cannot be solved by prosthetic arthroplasty alone.

On the other hand, arthrodesis of one of the 3 major joints of the upper extremity is also a very demanding procedure. In particular, there is still the problem of finding the correct position, especially in the area of the shoulder and the elbow, which must take into consideration each patient's individual demands. According to the literature and from our own experience, it is difficult to achieve bone consolidation in all 3 joints [10, 17]. Af-

ter a course of infection patients usually demonstrate very weak bone, while osteoporosis in older patients makes the situation even worse. Therefore, the rate of complications should not be underestimated [11].

After a deep infection in patients who have undergone multiple previous operations with extensive scarring and several fixation devices, the risk of re-infection is high. Even if the process of healing is uneventful, a large number of patients may complain of pain, inability to work [12, 14] or even sleep at night, especially in cases with shoulder or elbow arthodesis. If questions arise during either the preoperative or intraoperative assessment regarding possible ongoing infection or the ability to place a stable implant, the surgeon should consider

V. Heppert, A. Moghaddam, P. Herrmann, Ch. Wagner

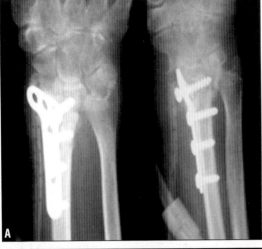

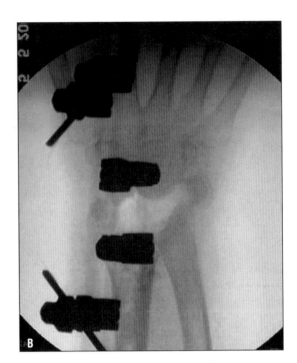

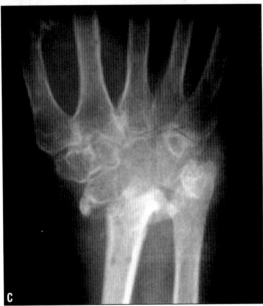

FIGURE 4. (A) 85-year-old diabetic with severe joint infection after plate osteosynthesis. (B) Radiograph taken 8 weeks post-operatively after debridement and external fixation. (C) Radiograph taken 2 years post-operatively. ROM 20-0-15.

other options, such as non-operative management or resection arthroplasty.

The main goal of lower limb reconstruction is to provide full weight bearing. In contrast, the upper extremity reconstruction is totally different: we require a functional upper limb to communicate with our environment. Thus, preservation of function and tolerable pain is what we aim to achieve for our patients after post-infectious arthritis. Most are aware of the fact that "metal and infection are poor partners" [13, 18-20]. The advantages of resection arthroplasty are:

- no implant *in situ*
- the patient requires fewer procedures in the future
- a well-defined range of motion, depending on the joint (elbow > wrist > shoulder)
- less pain

Based on the results from our study, we may critically review the goals for upper extremity reconstruction:

Satisfaction: Patients are usually not too satisfied with the result, and they are unsatisfied with the infectious arthritis itself. They complain about the compli-

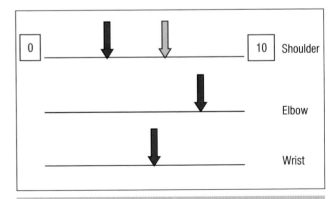

DIAGRAM 3. VAS scores of patient satisfaction with the final result.

cation (infection) and compare their current state of function to the pre-infection one. Moreover, endoprosthesis or arthrodesis will not improve patient satisfaction, as they will have limited functional outcome. Physicians are usually pleased with the results, whereas patients usually have different criteria.

Range of motion (ROM): ROM in our study was best for the elbow. Because of scaring ROM was limited to 0-25-125° (on average) for the elbow. In some cases, a noise was audible during movement, but the patients stated they had become accustomed to it. The wrist showed more limited function, but the patients were able to manage surprisingly well. Limited function seems to be much better than no function at all, on condition that there is no significant pain. None of these patients requested additional surgery (wrist fusion). The outcome was totally different for the shoulder. The average ROM was very poor and the patients were not happy with the results. The limited function achieved was attributed mostly to problems with the rotator muscles and bone deformities. Thus, in these more desperate cases, endoprostheses might not lead to better results.

Pain: In this study, pain was a problem only in patients with shoulder infections. Results were significantly better if resection arthroplasty was combined with the use of a pedicled muscle flap. The flap, which filled the previously infected cavity with well-vascularized muscle, worked like a tether and stabilized the proximal humerus. Moreover, no re-infection was observed after this procedure. Pain was not a real problem for the wrist and the elbow groups.

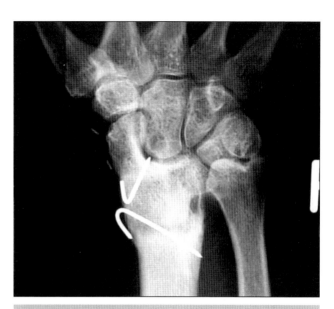

FIGURE 6. Radiograph taken 1 year post-operatively of an arthrodesis after severe joint infection of the wrist in a 42-year-old man. Good hand and wrist function were achieved by fusion of the scaphoid and the lunate to the radius. Wrist flexion at the intracarpet joint is satisfactory where the prosupination is unaffected.

5. CONCLUSION

Treatment after post-infectious arthritis of the large joints of the upper extremity remains a challenge. To our knowledge, there are no standardized procedures, and as a result, individual solutions are often provided (Fig. 5). Preservation of motion and function are the main goals, and as a result, we no longer perform arthrodesis in these anatomical areas in our septic unit with exception of the small joints of the wrist (Fig. 6).

We found that resection arthroplasty produced reasonably good results with the use of a straightforward technique. Moreover, the patients were freed from future problems regarding loosening of implant or endoprosthesis. In older patients or patients of Host B or C categories [21] where only simple operative procedures are recommended, resection arthroplasty in the upper extremity is a good alternative. Moreover, resection arthroplasty is valuable as a salvage procedure after failed arthroplasty or severe joint sepsis.

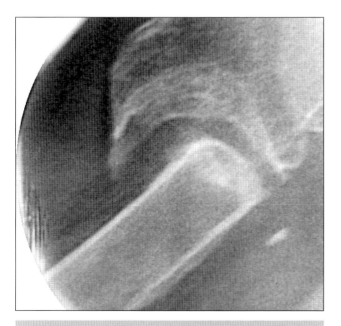

FIGURE 5. A good result is seen after resection arthroplasty of the shoulder. A "neoarthros" with limited space and acceptable stability was achieved.

REFERENCES

[1] Mileti J, Sperling JW, Cofield RH. Shoulder arthroplasty for the treatment of postinfectious glenohumeral arthritis. J Bone Joint Surg Am 2003;85-A (4):609-14.

[2] Cofield RH, Edgerton BC. Total shoulder arthroplasty: complications and revision surgery. Instr Course Lect 1990;39:449-62.

[3] Yamaguchi K, Adams RA, Morrey BF. Semiconstrained total elbow arthroplasty in the context of treated previous infection. J Shoulder Elbow Surg 1999;8 (5):461-5.

[4] Heppert V, Kessler T, Malze K, Wentzensen A. Vastus lateralis flap: an ideal procedure for definitive surgery of infected cavities of the hip. Unfallchirurg 2000;103 (11):938-44.

[5] Salvati EA, Callaghan JJ, Brause BD, Klein RF, Small RD. Reimplantation in infection. Elution of gentamicin from cement and beads. Clin Orthop Relat Res 1986;207:83-93.

[6] Brems JJ. Complications of shoulder arthroplasty: infections, instability, and loosening. Instr Course Lect 2002;51:29-39.

[7] Chin PY, Sperling JW, Cofield RH, Schleck C. Complications of total shoulder arthroplasty: are they fewer or different? J Shoulder Elbow Surg 2006;15 (1):19-22.

[8] Cofield RH, Chang W, Sperling JW. Complications of shoulder arthroplasty. In: Iannotti JP, Williams GR Jr (eds), Disorders of the shoulder: diagnosis and management. Philadelphia: Lippincott, Williams & Wilkins, 1999, pp. 571-93.

[9] Wirth MA, Rockwood CA, Jr. Complications of shoulder arthroplasty. Clin Orthop Relat Res 1994;307:47-69.

[10] Justis EJ. Arthrodesis of shoulder, elbow and wrist. 8th ed. New York: Mosby. 1992, pp. 353-361.

[11] Groh GI, Williams GR, Jarman RN, Rockwood CA, Jr. Treatment of complications of shoulder arthrodesis. J Bone Joint Surg Am 1997;79 (6):881-7.

[12] Hawkins RJ, Neer CS. A functional analysis of shoulder fusions. Clin Orthop Relat Res 1987;223:65-76.

[13] Heppert V. Wundinfektion. In Hrsg.Ewerbeck V, Wentzensen A, Holz F, Krämer KJ, Pfeil J, Sabo D (eds) Standardverfahren in der operativen Orthopedie und Unfallchirurgie. Georg Thieme Verlag, 2. 2003, pp. 807-9.

[14] Richards RR. Redefining indications and problems of shoulder arthrodesis. Philadelphia: Lippincott-Raven, 1997.

[15] Sperling JW, Kozak TK, Hanssen AD, Cofield RH. Infection after shoulder arthroplasty. Clin Orthop Relat Res 2001;382:206-16.

[16] Yamaguchi K, Adams RA, Morrey BF. Infection after total elbow arthroplasty. J Bone Joint Surg Am 1998;80 (4):481-91.

[17] Clare DJ, Wirth MA, Groh GI, Rockwood CA, Jr. Shoulder arthrodesis. J Bone Joint Surg Am 2001;83-A (4):593-600.

[18] Costerton JW, Stewart PS, Greenberg EP (1999) Bacterial biofilms: a common cause of persistent infections. Science 284 (5418):1318-22.

[19] Heppert V, Glatzel U, Wentzensen A. Postoperative and bacterial osteitis. New possibilities for therapy. Orthopade 2004;33(3):316-26.

[20] Wagner C, Kondella K, Bernschneider T, Heppert V, Wentzensen A, Hansch GM. Post-traumatic osteomyelitis: analysis of inflammatory cells recruited into the site of infection. Shock 2003;20(6):503-10.

[21] Cierny G, III, Mader JT. Approach to adult osteomyelitis. Orthop Rev 1987;16(4):259-70.

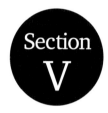

Section
V

MYCOBACTERIAL AND FUNGAL INFECTIONS

MYCOBACTERIAL AND FUNGAL INFECTIONS

chapter 30

Atypical Mycobacteria Hand Infections

André GAY[a*], **Pierre Edouard FOURNIER**[b], **Régis LEGRÉ**[c]

[a]*Service de Chirurgie, de la Main Hôpital de la Conception, Marseille, France*
[b]*Laboratoire de Bactérilogie, Hôpital de la Timone, Marseille, France*
[c]*Department of Hand Surgery, Hôpital de la Conception, Marseille, France*

The low incidence of mycobacterium tuberculosis and mycobacterium leprae in the Western world has shifted the focus on infections caused by atypical mycobacteria. Hand infections by *mycobacterium marinum* (M. Marinum) are the most frequent of the cutaneous mycobacteria infections. Hand surgeons should bear in mind this possibility when facing infected hands in high risk patients. Diagnosis of the M. Marinum infection is based on the history of water activities, the clinical examination and the epidemiological background, but has to be confirmed by the identification of mycobacteria. The role of surgical management is debated. Considering the efficiency of antibiotic treatment, surgical procedures should be limited to cases where all the infected tissues can be removed and complicated cases.

Keywords: M.Marinum; hand; infection; atypical mycobacteria; tenosynovitis.

1. INTRODUCTION

The low incidence of mycobacterium tuberculosis and mycobacterium leprae in the developed world has shifted the focus on infections caused by atypical mycobacteria. Hand infections by *mycobacterium marinum* (M.Marinum) are the most frequent of the cutaneous mycobacteria infections. M.Marinum may be present in salted or fresh water, in pools or aquariums, fish and shellfish.

Diagnosis is often delayed and incidence is probably underestimated because of a non-specific clinical presentation and, frequently, ignorance of the epidemiologic context. There is no consensus on the appropriate therapeutic treatment, notwithstanding the fact that a lot of protocols have been employed. Prognosis is most of the time benign. However, rare cases of disseminated infections have also been described.

2. ILLUSTRATIVE CASES

2.1. Case 1

A 50-year-old female office worker was admitted in an emergency unit suffering from hyperalgic tenosynovitis at the volar aspect of the left hand and wrist in the winter of 1995. In her medical history, the patient described stings in her garden and swimming pool. Clinical examination and a normal neuro-vascular test showed a hand with oedema, inflammation and pain.

A surgical synovectomy of the flexor tendons was carried out, and multiple sampling for bacteriologic and histopathological investigations were obtained. The histological examination revealed a giant cell granuloma without caseum necrosis. A direct bacteriological exam, with Ziehl Nielsen staining, revealed acid-alcoholic resistant bacillus. After three weeks of culture, Mycobacterium marinum infection was identified.

*Corresponding Author
Service du Pr Legré
Hopital la Conception
145 Bd Baille,
13385, Marseille cedex, France
Tel: +33 612 907 029
e-mail: andre_gay@hotmail.com

Antibiotic treatment with thrimetoprime-sulfametoxazole was initiated immediately, lasting for 2.5 months until apparent clinical healing. A month later, the patient presented an abscess in the thenar eminence and underwent another surgical debridement. Histology and cultures confirmed presence of *Mycobacterium marinum.* Another course of antibiotic treatment started with Rifampicin and Minocyclin and was applied for 4 months. The patient was considered then as free of disease.

2.2. Case 2

A 62-year-old female fishmonger sought medical advice in our "Hand Surgery Center" in August 1996 for a node located at the volar aspect of the right wrist. In her medical history, the patient talked about a fishbone puncture in her right wrist that had occurred five months before.

Clinical exams showed a hard node at the volar aspect of the wrist causing inflammatory reaction of the skin. No neurological or vascular disturbances were observed (Fig. 1). A surgical debridement operation (Fig. 2) with biopsies was performed (part of a histopathologic and bacteriologic exam). A direct bacteriologic examination by use of the Ziehl Nielsen stain initially showed negative results, however, after two weeks of culture, Mycobactrium marinum was isolated. The patient received antibiotic treatment with clarithromycine and ciprofloxacine for 3 months and was considered free of disease until the last follow-up after 5 years.

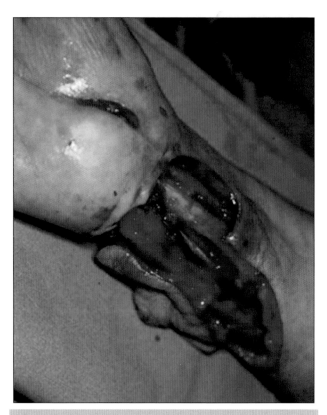

FIGURE 2. Intra-operative view.

3. EPIDEMIOLOGY

Numerous species of mycobacteria are responsible for hand infections. The most frequent ones are M. Marinum infections which are widely-spread, but nevertheless difficult to diagnose. Numerous case reports have been published, however, only three series have been reported so far. A national French investigation of 27 cases [1], an American study of 31 cases [2], and an Australian of 29 cases [3]. The incidence ranges from 0.27 [3] to 0.5 cases out of 100,000 inhabitants [4, 5]. Low frequency of this pathological entity is probably due to its mildness and non-specific symptomatology [6]. The origin of contamination is cutaneous contact. Injured skin and wounds, especially when in contact with contaminated water, for example, from an aquarium (aquarium granuloma) or a fishpond, are the most common sources of contamination. In 20% of the cases, there is positive culture. M. Marinum is often an occupational infection, found especially in divers, fishermen, fishmongers and cooks. It can affect people of all ages, but mostly those between 30 and 45 years of age [7]. Although some studies have shown higher frequency for males [1, 3], the rate is probably the same between males and females [2]. Unlike other atypical mycobacteria infections, M. Marinum infections have the same rate of occurrence in healthy and in A.I.D.S. patients [2].

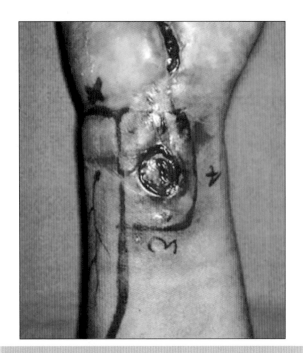

FIGURE 1. Clinical aspect.

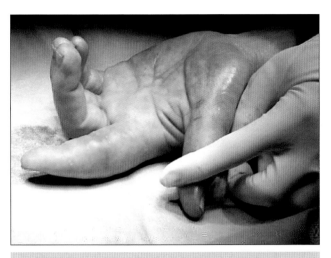

FIGURE 3. Clinical aspect of a M. Marinum finger tenosynovitis.

4. CLINICAL ASPECTS

After contamination followed by an incubation period lasting from 5 days to more than a year (mean time: 2 to 8 weeks) [1-3, 6, 7], illness manifestation is often a single painless papulo-nodular lesion (85%) that is located at the inoculation site [1-3]. Most of the time, lesions are located in the upper limb (90%): in fingers (60%) (Fig. 3) [8], in the dorsal face of the hand (15%), and rarely in the elbow. The lower limb is wounded in 10% of the cases, especially at the knee level. Rare cases of facial lesions have been described [9]. The infection begins with a nodule (66%) of progressively increasing volume, which sometimes takes a purplish-blue color. Infection can proceed toward suppuration and ulceration (nearly half of the cases), or toward the verruca aspect. In 20 to 50% of the cases, lesions can disseminate following an ascending lymphatic duct course and appear as lymphangitis

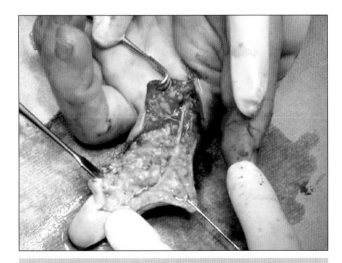

FIGURE 4. Intra-operative view of M. Marinum tenosynovitis.

and limb staged nodes [10]. Local complications in the form of tenosynovitis (Fig. 4) [11], or infectious arthritis [12-14] can occur in 10 to 40% of the cases, either as initial nodular appearance or as first signs of the disease. Tuberculin intra-dermal reaction (Mantoux) is often positive. Lesions can grow very quickly, i.e. in a couple of days or weeks, or exceptionally, their course may run undiagnosed for several years. M. Marinum can be the origin of cervical lymph nodes [5], osteomyelitis [15], sclero-keratitis [9], or generalized infection in immuno-deficients [16] or healthy subjects [17,18]. Only one fatal case of M. Marinum infection has been reported [19]. In general, the mild and non-specific clinical course and symptomatology, and the rarity of this type of infection are reasons for little suspicion and may lead to failure of diagnosis [6].

5. DIAGNOSTIC ASPECTS

Diagnosis of the M. Marinum infection is based on the history of water activities, on the clinical examination and the epidemiological background, but has to be confirmed by identification of Mycobacteria in specific cultures of mycobacteria. Several samples obtained from an abscess, nodes, joint fluid, or an open biopsy, have to be sent to a specialized bacteriological unit as quickly as possible to confirm diagnosis suspicion. A direct examination through a light microscope should be made for all samples after auramine or the Ziehl-Nielsen stain, searching for acid alcohol-resistant bacilluses. Only a few cases had positive results with immediate microscopy examination (10-20%) [1-3]. In immunodeficient people, who rarely show granulomatous reactions, the percentage of positive results is higher. If samples cannot be put in culture immediately, they could be conserved at 4°C for 24 hours maximum. M. Marinum should be cultured in particular conditions: the culture specimen should be placed in an environment rich of Loewensteinjensen, coletsos or middlebrook media, ideally at a temperature between 30 and 32°C (it is not possible to develop at 37°C). M. Marinum culture is slowly-developing (1 to 4 weeks), and its colonies are mucous and yellow after photo-induction. Cultures show M. Marinum in only 50 to 60% of cases [1-3]. Identification is based upon the culture and biochemical characteristics and can be confirmed by cell-wall fatty acids chromatography [20]. Genomic amplification by P.C.R., in case of positivity, allows confirmation of M. Marinum presence in the samples [21, 22]. There is no reliable and specific serological examination for diagnosis. As a complement to bacteriological examinations, a histological exam has to be conducted in a systematic fashion. It may show a lympho-epithelioid dermal granuloma in 60%, which in 40% of the cases is only a non-specific inflammatory dermal infiltration.

6. TREATMENT

There is no consensus on the management of Mycobacterium Marinum infections. They are naturally resistant to Isoniazide, Streptomycine and Pyrazinamide, and inconstantly sensitive to tetracyclines (Minocycline, Doxycycline) [23]. Almost all strains are sensitive to Rifampicine, Amikacine [24], Ethambutol, Trimethoprime-Sulfametoxazole [23], Clarithromycine [25] and Fluoroquinolones [26, 27]. Some infections have been successfully treated by Tetracyclines alone, or Trimethoprime-Sulfametoxazole in combination with Clarithromycine and Ciprofloxacine. However, treatment procedures applying Tetracyclines lead to failure in 10 to 20% of the cases [2]. A long-lasting antibiotic treatment is necessary, as hinted by infection recurrence after discontinuation of the treatment in case 1. Treatments with antibiotics from 3 to 18 months have been suggested [1, 3]. Edelstein suggested 6 months of antibiotic treatment or 2 months after clinical healing [2].

The place of surgical management is debatable. Considering the antibiotic treatment efficiency, surgical procedures should be limited to cases where all the infected tissues can be removed (uni-nodular early stage of the disease), and to cases complicated by arthritis or tenosynovitis.

7. CONCLUSIONS

Mycobacterium Marinum infections are not uncommon and are easily cured by adapted antibiotic therapy lasting for at least 2 months after clinical healing. The main difficulty in diagnosing lies in the need for placing the culture under specific conditions. Hand surgeons should always bear in mind this possibility when facing infected hands in high risk patients.

REFERENCES

[1] Bonafé JL, Grigorieff-Larrue N, Bauriaud R. Les Mycobacterioses cutanees atypique. Ann Dermatol Venerol 1992;119:463-470.
[2] Edelstein H. Mycobacterium Marinum skin infections. Arch Intern Med 1994;154:1359-1364.
[3] Iredell J, Whitby M, Blacklock Z. Mycobacterium Marinum infection: epidemiology and presentation in Queensland 1971-1990. Med J Aust 1992;157:596-598.
[4] Kullavanijaya P, Sirimachan S, Bhuddhavudhakrai P. Mycobacterium Marinum cutaneous infections acquired from occupations and hobbies. Int J Dermatol 1993;32:504-507.
[5] O'Brien RJ. The Epidemiology of nontuberculous mycobacterial disease. Clin Chest Med 1989;10:407-418.
[6] Hurst LC, Amadio PC, Badalamente MA, Ellstein JL, Dattwyller RJ. Mycobacterium Marinum infections of the hand. J Hand Surg 1987;12:428-435.
[7] Gluckman SJ. Mycobacterium Marinum. Clin Dermatol 1995;13:273-276.
[8] Katz D. Tenosynovite de la main a Mycobacterium Terrae. Ann Chir Main 1993;12:136-139.
[9] Schonherr U, Naumann GO, Lang GK, Bialasiewicz AA. Sclerokeratitis caused by mycobacterium marinum. Am J Ophtalmol 1989;108:607-608.
[10] Kostman JR, Dinubile MJ. Nodular lymphangitis: a distinctive but often unrecognized syndrome. Ann Intern Med 1993;118:883-888.
[11] Beckman EN, Pankey GA, McFarland GB. The Histopathology of Mycobacterium Marinum Synovitis. Am J Clin Pathol 1985;83:457-462.
[12] Alloway JA, Evangelisti SM, Sazrtin JS. Mycobacterium Marinum arthritis.Semin. Arthritis Rheum 1995;24:382-390.
[13] Harth M, Ralph ED, Farawii R. Septic arthritis due to Mycobacterium Marinum. J Rheumatol 1994;21:957-959.
[14] Jones MW, Wahid IA, Matthews JP. Septic arthritis of the hand due to Mycobacterium Marinum. J Hand Surg 1988;13: 333-334.
[15] Clark RB, Spector H, Friedman DM, Oldrati KJ, Young CL, Nelson SC. Osteomyelitis and synovitis produced by Mycobacterium Marinum in a fisherman. J Clin Microbiol 1990;28:2570-2572.
[16] Parent LJ, Salam MM, Applebaum PC, Dosset JH. Disseminated Mycobacterium Marinum infection and bacteremia in a child with severe combinated immunodeficiency. Clin Infect Dis 1995;21:1325-1327.
[17] Bodemer C, Durand C, Blanche S, Teillac D, Deprost Y. Infection disseminee a Mycobacterium Marinum. Ann Dermatol Venerol 1989;116:842-843.
[18] Vasquez JA, Sobel JD. A case of disseminated Mycobacterium Marinum infection in an immunocompetent patient. Eur J Clin Microbiol Infect Dis 1992;11:908-911.
[19] Tchornobay JA, Claudy AL, Perrot JL, Levigne V, Denis M. Fatal disseminated Mycobacterium Marinum infection. Int J Dermatol 1992;31:286-287.
[20] Parez JJ, Fauville-Dufaux M, Dossogne JL, De Hoffmann E, Pouthier F. Faster identification of mycobacteria using gas liquid and thin layer chromatography. Eur J Clin Microbiol Infect Dis 1994;13:717-725.
[21] Feddersen A, Kunkel J, Jonas D, Engel V, Bhakdi S, Husmann M. Infection of the upper-extremity by Mycobacterium Marinum in a 3-years-old boy. Diagnosis by 16S-rDNA analysis. Infection 1996;24:47-48.
[22] Takewaki SI, Okuzumi K, Ishiko H, Nakahara KI, Ohkubo A, Nagai R. Genus-Specific polymerase chain reaction for the mycobacterial DNAJ gene and species-specific oligonucleotide probes. J Clin Microbiol, 1993;31; 446-450.
[23] Forsgren A. Antibiotic susceptibility of Mycobacterium Marinum. Scand J Infect Dis 1993;25:779-782.
[24] Arai H, Nakajima H, Naito S, Kaminaga Y, Nagai R. Amikacin treatment for Micobacterium Marinum. J Dermatol 1986;13:385-389.
[25] Bonnet E, Debat-Zoguereh D, Petit N, Ravaux I, Gallais H. Clarythromycin: a potent agent against infections due to Mycobacterium Marinum. Clin Infect Dis 1994;18:664-666.
[26] Laing RB, Wynn RF, Leen CL. New antimicrobial against Mycobacterium Marinum infection. J Hand Surg 1994;131:914. Brady RC, Sheth A, Mayer T, Goderwis D, Schleiss MR. Facial sporotrichoid infection with Mycobacterium Marinum. J Pediatr 1997; 130:324,326.
[27] Saito H, Watanabe T, Tomioka H, Sato K. Susceptibility of various mycobacteria to quinolones. Rev Infect Dis 1988;10:S52.

The Tuberculous Infection of the Shoulder, Elbow and Wrist

Ferdinando DA RIN

Department of Bone Infection, Codivilla–Putti Institute, Cortina d' Ampezzo, Italy

Tuberculosis (TB) has increased over the last years, probably as a result of the increase in immigrants from countries with a higher rate of prevalence. There are about 60-70 new cases of tuberculosis every year, from which 9% pertain to the upper limb. Tuberculosis in the upper extremity is located in the wrist in 3.1% of the cases, while involvement of the elbow is rather uncommon. Common sites for tuberculosis osseous foci appear to be the epi/metaphyseal regions of the radius, ulna and humerus. Multifocal bone lesions are found in adults more frequently than children. In general, there appears to be no preferential age for TB that can appear with no specific diagnostic features. Diagnosis is based on patient history, clinical characteristics and laboratory findings. The diagnosis is often disguised by symptoms that can be variable and unpredictable. It is imperative that a biopsy and cultures be carried out for correct diagnosis. Treatment is based on an extended, multi-component, antibiotic therapy along with surgical debridement.

Keywords: bone tuberculosis; tuberculous arthritis of the wrist; tuberculous arthritis of the elbow; tuberculous arthritis of the shoulder.

1. INTRODUCTION

In the past, tuberculosis (TB) was considered a scourge from God. Until the discovery of antituberculosis drugs, such as Streptomycin that was first applied in 1945, many people died due to this disease [1]. Recently, increasing numbers of new cases have been reported even in western countries. We are witnessing an increase, not only in the typical antibiotic resistant forms, but also in the atypical mycobacteria infections [2]. This may be attributed, in part, to the influx of immigrants from countries where TB occurs at a higher frequency.

*Corresponding Author
Department of Bone Infection
Istituti Codivilla-Putti, Cortina d' Ampezzo
32043 Cortina d' Ampezzo, Italy
Tel: +39 043 6883111
e-mail: darin.ferdinando@iol.it
         darin.ferdinando@libero.it

Mycobacteria (MB) that are responsible for causing TB can be divided into typical and atypical forms (Fig. 1, 2 and Table 1).

MB is a positive gram bacillus, without a ciliary body or a capsule, having the form of a lengthened rod. Its main characteristic is being alcohol-acid resistant (detected by the use of a typical Ziehl-Nielsen stain). Another important characteristic is its high content of lipids, which makes it highly resistant to the bactericidal agents. Moreover, they have tuberculingenic action, and a specific toxic and negative chemotactic effect on leucocytes. Polysaccharides are, on the other hand, the agents that induce antigenic activity.

Two pathological types of TB have been described according to the reaction of the bone tissue [3, 4]:

a) ***Exudative TBC,*** which involves formation of an exudate that accumulates at the side of medullary spaces and causes secondary vascular alterations that lead to bone necrosis and caseation. The bone trabeculae are not resorbed and the affected tissue presents as devitalized and eroded bone.

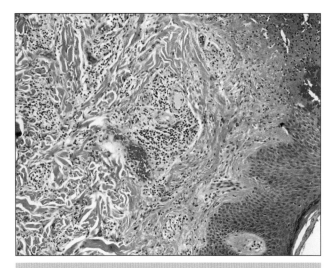

FIGURE 1. A tubercular lymphocytic and monocytic infiltrate.

TABLE 1

Types of the most frequently encountered typical and atypical mycobacteria (MB)

Typical MB
- Mycobacterium tuberculosis hominis
- Mycobacterium Bovis e Avium

Atypical MB
- Mycobacterium Kansaii
- Mycobacterium Marinum
- Mycobacterium Scrofolaceum
- Mycobacterium Flavescens
- Mycobacterium Avium complex
- Mycobacterium Xenopi
- Mycobacterium Fortuitum
- Mycobacterium Chelone

b) ***Productive TBC,*** which entails the formation of a granulomatous tissue consisting of active cells and capillaries causing lacunar resorption (decay). Histologically, this form is characterized by giant multinuclear cells with nuclei that are situated at the periphery (similar to a rosary) with compact eosinophylic cytoplasm (like cells of Langhans) which are surrounded by epithelioid elements, due to localized hyperplasia of the histiocytes. Lymphocytes-monocytes and plasma cells are also observed.

2. PATHOGENESIS

TB most commonly starts with manifestation of Ranke's primary complex (pneumonia-adenitis-lymphangitis).

Generally, this first contact resolves and the mycobacterium stays hosted in the lymph nodes which undergo calcification. In a number of cases, however, MB is dispersed into the blood, causing the so-called "secondary type tuberculosis", which can affect various organs, such as the kidney, some glands, the urinary bladder, the meninges, as well as bone. Bone infection which occurs at a rate of about 7.5%, is commonly located at the epiphysis of the long bones, the knee, the hip, or the spine, and it usually presents as arthritis. In fact, we rarely have tubercular localization on the diaphysis of the long bones [5]. In contrast, direct inoculation through an animal or human bite or by wound contamination is a common pathway for the development of mycobacterium marinum infection that is due to contact with infected water or fish sting [6].

3. CLINICAL PRESENTATION AND LABORATORY FINDINGS

Skeletal tuberculosis has an insidious onset causing light pain and fever in the evenings. Rarely will we see fistulas and, if they occur, they may appear far away from the focus, as in the case of a spondylitis, where the abscess may drain through a fistula at the inguinal space, following the anatomic channels of gravity between the sheaths and the muscles. The focus of the lesion does not appear warm or reddened, but almost normal, and thus, the tuberculous abscess is characterized as "cold abscess". The affected joint presents functional limitation and erosions apparent in the x-rays. The classical laboratory tests for pyogenic infections (ESR, CRP, and fibrinogen) are slightly elevated in tuberculosis. This can change if, in addition to the tuberculosis, there is also an over-riding infection caused by common germs. In this case, the two pathologies are combined and present signs typical of both illnesses.

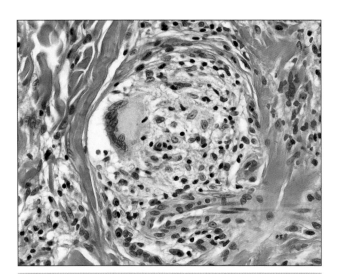

FIGURE 2. Typical tuberculae with several histiocytes. Signs of epithelioid cell formation can also be seen.

The Mantoux and Time tests are only positive for contraction of Koch's bacillus, but do not indicate disease activity. It is also important to interpret negative test results as in some cases, such as in the elderly with reduced immune defense the test could be negative. Newer laboratory tests on pus and/or expectoration, based on the method of Ligasi (Lcx), have 100% accuracy and the results are available in 7 days. Another recent examination is the TB test, the A 60, which allows for a serologic diagnosis via the titers of IgA, IgM, and IgG. The test has 80% accuracy. In addition, the identification of a 16S rRNA MB specific gene on a biopsy sample is also currently available using immunohistochemical methods.

Table 2 shows the clinical and laboratory results obtained from 30 patients with tubercular arthritis (specific) and 12 non-tubercular cases (nonspecific) of the wrist. These results show that: (i) in the case of tuberculosis the histological diagnosis is essential, (ii) it is difficult to detect the mycobacterium in a culture sample, even if it is placed in an enriched cultural medium, and (iii) the opposite is true in the case of non-tuberculus forms of infections, such as in staphylococcal arthritis.

The first findings on standard radiographic views may indicate only the presence of changes, raising suspicion for further investigation [7, 8]. The radiographic changes observed can be divided into four stages (Fig. 3).

There are various diagnostic tools, including CT, scintigraphy, MRI and fistulography. **Conventional Tomography (CT)** is useful, but rarely performed (Fig. 4). However, once it is performed it helps to discover hidden foci of infection that are not visible with standard X-rays, and to mark a possible sequestrum or the focus itself. **Scintigraphy** with labelled leucocytes is now routine when an infection is suspected, and especially when dealing with an infection that develops in two phases. **Magnetic Resonance Imaging (MRI)** is, in expert hands, a very sensitive tool that can detect an infection in progress. If there is a fistula, **fistulography** can provide some information to identify the productive focus and its characteristics.

4. DIFFERENTIAL DIAGNOSIS

The differential diagnosis of tuberculous arthritis includes the following: pyogenic arthritis and osteomyelitis; rheumatoid arthritis (adult and juvenile forms) and sieronegative arthritis; gout and pseudogout; osteoarthrosis in acute phase and osteonecrosis; bone tumor and metastasis; neuropathic joint disease; sarcoidosis and amyloidosis; and renal osteodystrophy [9].

It is also worth considering other types of infection in order to distinguish them from tuberculous arthritis. These include:
  a) Synovial types of inflammation:
    – synovitis specific
    – rheumatoid seronegative arthritis (initial phase)
    – villonodular synovitis
    – hemophilia
  b) Inflammations at the wrist level:
    – de Quervein syndrome
    – carpal tunnel syndrome
    – styloiditis
    – carpal instability
    – reflex cympatic dystrophy
  c) Inflammations at the elbow level:
    – epicondylitis
    – nervous compressions
    – overuse syndromes
  d) Inflammations at the shoulder level:
    – cuff lesions
    – subacromial impingement
    – degenerative arthritis

5. MEDICAL THERAPY

Because mycobacteria very frequently develop a resistance to drugs, the chemo-therapeutic treatment of tuberculosis is based on multi-drug therapy [10]. We use this therapy for all bacterial types and localizations, except for those cases which are resistant to classical antibiotics. Today, drug therapy remains the principal management of skeletal tuberculosis.

For a long time we have applied the following combination: Streptomycin 1gr/day; Isoniazid 400mg/day; Ethambutol 1200 mg/day; Rifampicin 600 mg/day. A maximum of 80 gr of Streptomycin is administered in addition to one daily dosage of Rifampicin that is taken in the morning on an empty stomach, for at least one year without interruption because its resumption after a break may cause hepatitis due to enzymatic induction. The

TABLE 2

Comparison of clinical and laboratory instruments in tubercular arthritis vs non-tubercular cases of the wrist.

30 cases of tuberculosis
19 cases of non-specific infection

	Specific	Non-specific
Anamnesis	10/30	12/19
Clinical presentation	10/30	14/19
Radiography	10/30	6/19
RMN scintigraphy with marked leucocytes	12/19	
Laboratory tests	6/30	19/19
Mantoux or Time Test	28/30	///////
Cultural examination	5/30	19/19
Biopsy/histology	19/30	///////

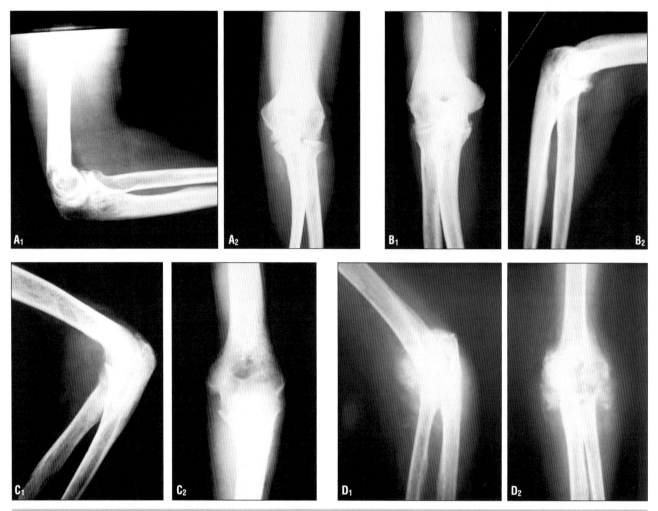

FIGURE 3. (A) Stage 1: Demineralization caused by inflammation of the synovial membrane. **(B)** Stage 2: Narrowing of the articular space due to initial destruction of the cartilage. In this stage, the synovial membrane will hypertrophy and fill the articular space, and bone erosion develops at the sites where the articular capsule is attached. **(C)** Stage 3: The entire joint is affected and presents many bone lesions, the articular space is narrowing without serious anatomical destruction of the articulation. In this stage, the joint space is filled with hypertrophic synovial membrane and pus. The articular cartilage, the capsule and the ligaments are destroyed. There could also be abscesses and fistulas. **(D)** Stage 4: Further joint destruction with disruption of the anatomical profile.

treatment must be continued for more than one year and up to 2 years, suspending only the streptomycin.

For children, the dosages are the following: Rifampicin 10-15 mg/Kg/day; Isoniazid 10-12 mg/kg/day; Miambutol 20-25 mg/kg/day; Pyrazinamide 30-40 mg/kg/day; Streptomycin 0.5 gr/day (15-20 gr max). In addition, we also apply a local infiltrate of the same drugs that are administered daily per os (Fig. 5a). The articular space is infiltrated on day 1 with Streptomycin, on day 3 with Ethambutol, and on day 5 with Isoniazid (a part of a daily dose).

The same drugs are used if there are fistulas, in combination with daily pulsating washes through the drainage tubes that are surgically applied during the debridement. This is carried out for 20 days, after which we suspend only the local therapy for 10 days.

This is considered one cycle of therapy. Normally, once 2-3 cycles are completed, X-ray imaging and clinical control is performed in order to decide whether the therapy will be continued. The local therapy lasts no more than 20 days to avoid local irritation from the introduced drugs. The discharged patient continues the therapy at home taking the following medication: Ethambutol + Isoniazid B6 4cp/day (Miazide®) for 6 days a week for a period of 1.5-2 years; Rifampicin 2cp/day of 300 mg/day (Rifadin®) for 1-1.5 years. In addition to antibiotic therapy, immobilization with special casts may be essential in very painful cases. In general, we allow joint motion, because we have noticed that if there is no local pain and inflammation, a satisfactory range of motion can be maintained, after successful chemotherapy (Fig. 5b).

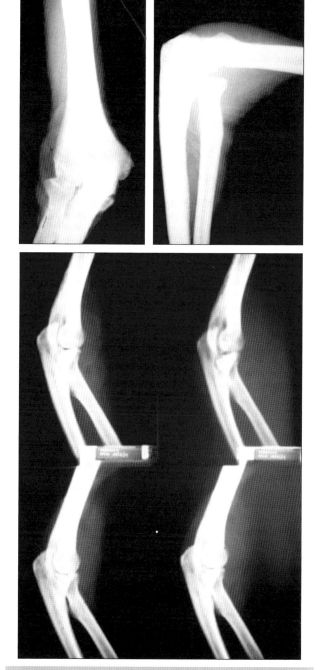

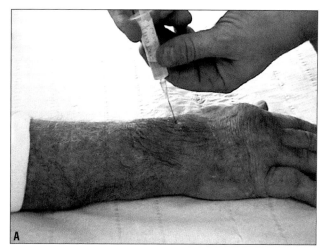

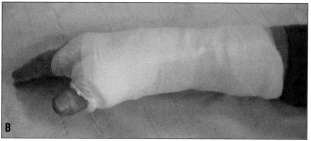

FIGURE 5. **(A)** A typical aspect of the local infiltrative therapy. **(B)** Immobiliziation aides in painful inflammatory cases.

FIGURE 4. The conventional tomography shows a lesion at the ole-cranon that is not visible on X-rays.

rheumatoid arthritis, since such an infection is more frequent to develop on the wrist site. Use of intra-artic-ular steroids is indicated, but could destroy the joint in the case of tuberculosis.

The tuberculous infection is sometimes caused by in-tra-articular rupture of an intrasynovial abscess formed among tendons, mostly flexors [14, 15]; in some cases it originates from carpal bones, from the scaphoid and/or from the lunate. From these sites, it can easily extend to all carpal bones causing diffuse carpal arthritis, which al-

6. TUBERCULOUS ARTHRITIS OF THE WRIST

According to the literature, tuberculosis of the wrist is very rare (3.1%) (Schema 1) [11]. In 1986, Martini [12] reported 2%, while Liebe et al. reported 4% in 1982 [13]. TB of the wrist should be differentiated from

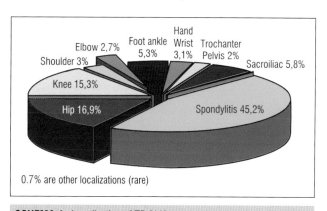

SCHEMA 1. Localization of TB [11].

so affects the radius and the ulnar epiphysis (wrist pan-arthritis) [16, 17].

In the onset of wrist tuberculosis, all patients present with diffuse pain, rigidity and dorsal swelling. If the swelling is on the volar side, the diagnosis is most often flexor tenosynovitis (Fig. 6). It has not been understood yet why mycobacterium tuberculosis affects the flexors, as it is the only place known to be affected when there is localization on tendons.

7. PHARMACEUTICAL MANAGEMENT OF WRIST TB

Pharmaceutical treatment of skeletal tuberculosis is usually preceded by joint aspiration or a biopsy that can be performed arthroscopically. When the diagnosis is confirmed, local infiltration and systemic therapy follows after two cycles of surgical debridement. Usually, this lesion leads to ankylosis, because during the painful inflammatory phase, the patient is immobilized.

Subcutaneous tendon lesions are sometimes associated with this type of infection and need to be repaired by tenorrhaphy or by surgical transfer of synergistically acting tendons, when possible. A technique often considered in cases where the first row or even the radial epiphysis is involved is proximal row carpectomy [16, 17]. This would allow some wrist motion without pain, and create some space between the residual articular surfaces. Even if the proximal epiphysis of the capitate is eroded, the presence of a fibrous pannus that reduces the contact between the capitate and radial epiphysis allows useful joint mobility (Fig. 7).

For cases with progressing infection, even those with a limited range of motion and wrist pain, arthrodesis is recommended. Certain difficulties may be encountered in that process, which are attributed to the characteristics of the affected bone and to the fact that consolidation is difficult to achieve. Osteosynthesis with plates or even autologous bone grafts is not recommended for the arthrodesis, because these materials are considered foreign bodies and may aggravate the infection itself, or could lead to sequestrum formation. Articular surface debridement and compression with an external fixator or the use of a cast after fixation of the articulation with crossed K-wires is suggested [18].

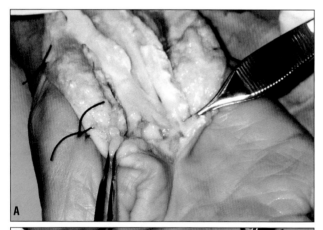
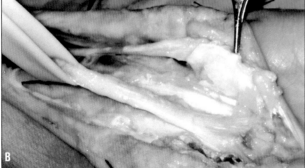
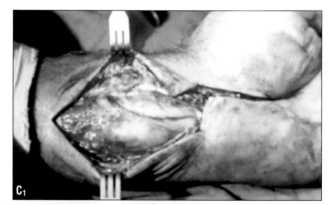
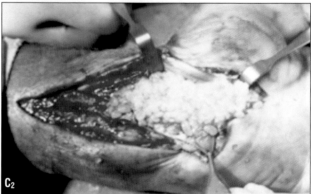

FIGURE 6. (A) A typical appearance of tuberculous flexor tenosynovitis. Surgical debridement is performed after local and systemic tuberculostatic therapy. **(B)** Median nerve isolation; the nerve is covered with granulation tissue due to the TB. **(C)** A typical "orizoid granule" presented in a case of TB of the flexors of the wrist [Courtesy of V. Mazzone (Ascoli Piceno)].

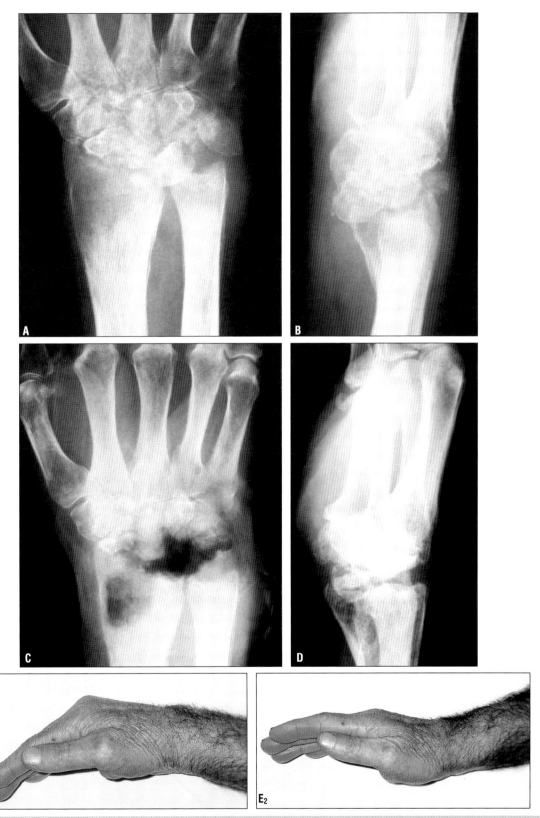

FIGURE 7. (A) Antero-posterior (AP) and **(B)** lateral radiographs showing tuberculous arthritis of the wrist with a large focus on the distal epiphysis of the radius, a prominent epiphysis of the ulna and collapse of the radius and carpal volar dislocation. **(C)** AP and **(D)** lateral radiographs taken 18 months post-operatively, showing a central gap that is bridged by the remaining distal segment of the scaphoid. On the ulnar side, the reactive fibrous pannus maintains the distance between the ulna and residual triquetral bone. **(E)** Clinical presentation 42 months post-operatively. Painless mobility was achieved in an infection-free wrist.

8. TUBERCULOUS ARTHRITIS OF THE ELBOW

The elbow is affected by tuberculosis at a percentage of only 2.7%. Martini [9], Silva [19], Eckel and Due [20]. The sites most commonly affected by osseous tuberculosis are the epi/metaphyseal region of the radius, ulna, and humerus. In many cases, the olecranon seems to be the site where the infection is first situated. Afterwards, the infection proceeds towards the joint space and rapidly destroys it. In fact, the elbow rapidly reaches a state of painful rigidity with serious functional deterioration (Fig. 8).

The therapeutic approach is initially the same as that generally adopted for the treatment of all affected articulations. An initial surgical debridement is necessary, as the patient cannot tolerate local infiltrations that will increase the articular swelling and cause pain. We have surgically treated 87 patients (Table 3). Of the 87 patients, 67% were males and 33% females. The affected elbow in 72% of patients was the right one and in 28% the left, while all the patients were right-handed. Unlike other joints, the final outcome for an infected elbow joint is fusion. The results obtained at hospital admission compared with those we had after stabilization of the illness are reported in Tables 4 and 5, respectively (radiographic stage of the lesion). Results were good for the first stage and poor for the fourth stage, especially as far as pain and motion are concerned, even with resolution of the infection. Note that even after treatment, many patients with infection in stages 2 and 3 progressed to a worse stage due to deterioration of the disease.

Additional cohorts of patients underwent only conservative treatment, reaching 67% recovery, and others spontaneous arthrodesis. Arm function after elbow arthrodesis is a severely debilitating problem for the

TABLE 3
Surgical treatment of 87 cases.

Surgical focal debridement	34
Biopsy	18
Drainage	34
Abscess drainage	8
Ulnar nerve transposition	2
Neurolysis of the ulnar nerve	1
Neurolysis of the radial nerve	1
Radial head resection	15
Prosthesis	3

patient. Even if a position of 90° is reached and maintained, the patient is not able to make full use of his hand. He uses it only "to bring up the umbrella" (see Fig. 8). Although removal of the radial head improves pronation and supination, it is recommended that a light flexion of the elbow, little beyond 90° is probably more functional for a good hand-to-face contact.

9. TUBERCULOUS ARTHRITIS OF THE SHOULDER

We found that the shoulder is affected at a rate of 3.0%, which is similar to the findings of Martini (2.5%) [9], Lafond (2.8%) [21], and Eckel and Due (3.0%) [20]. It presents with multifocal bone lesions, and adults are more frequently affected by shoulder tuberculosis than children. The joint synovium and the capsule are infiltrated by tuberculous granulomatous tissue, resulting in tuberculosis synovitis. This, in turn, invades the cortical bone through

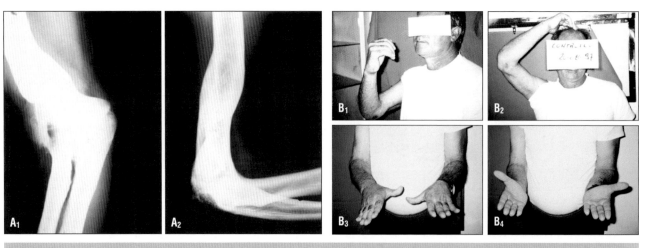

FIGURE 8. (A) An example of TB managed with ulno-humeral arthrodesis fixed at 90°. **(B)** The patient is infection free and shows good pronation and supination function.

Elbow Tuberculosis: findings at hospital admission (n= 87).

Radiographic Stage	I	II	III	IV
N° patients	9	31	33	14
Mobility	0	12	12	12
Fistula	5	16	12	5
Pain	7	28	19	14
Fever	0	2	2	0

TABLE 5

Elbow Tuberculosis: findings at follow-up and control of disease (n= 87)

Radiographic Stage	I	II	III	IV
N° patients	9	21	38	19
Mobility*	9	16	13	14
Fistula absent	9	21	16	19
Pain absent	9	21	13	14
Fever absent	9	21	16	19

*only in cases where there was improvement and valid function.

the synovial recesses near the joint capsule insertion. Initially, the infection is usually localized at the epiphysis or the metaphysis and when it extends towards the joint, tuberculous arthritis is induced.

9.1. Therapeutic management

The treatment of shoulder tuberculosis is conservative, using systemic and local multi-drug therapy [22]. In 90% of the cases the infection resolved after chemotherapy (110 cases). In 6% there were recurrences after 2 years after the completion of the therapy. This occurred in patients who received treatment with a delay of more than one year after the diagnosis or in those who were previously treated for rheumatoid joints.

Recently, we have applied endo-prosthesis [23, 24] to achieve a good degree of mobility after resolution of the infection (Fig. 9). The surgical treatment takes place after two or three cycles of antibiotics, and involves debridement of the joint, humeral head removal and sub-

stitution with temporary spacer (antibiotics plus cement). After 45-60 days, endo-prosthesis is implanted. The antibiotic cement spacer prevents the articular stumps from adhering to the bone stumps, and maintains the anatomical length of the soft tissues allowing active, though limited motion. At the same time, it carries a high load of antibiotic able to be released into the septic focus in high concentrations that could by no means be achieved through systemic administration.

In order that the antibiotics be mixed into the cement, they need a molecular structure which remains stable at temperatures ranging from 50° to 150°C. They also need to be able to stabilize when the temperature is 37°C, to be water soluble, available in powder, non-toxic, non-allergenic, able to settle in the cement molecules, to have small volume and little impact on the mechanical characteristics of the cement. They should also have a wide spectrum of antimicrobial activity that should be bactericidal, and effective even if administered in small doses (low MIC and MBC). For an antibiotic-loaded cement spacer in a tuberculous joint, we suggest succinate streptochemycin.

9.2. Results

The results from this combined management were encouraging with improvement of motion of 50% and resolution of the tubercular infection (Fig. 10). The humeral component was always implanted because of the presence of a fibrous tissue in the glenoid that functions as a pad. This choice was dictated by the following parameters: (i) the limited motion and the need to have reduced friction of the "new joint", (ii) the absence of glenoid bone able to receive the prosthesis, and (iii) the physicians' concern as to whether they should use supporting bone graft, taken for granted that they would like to be as less aggressive as possible. The ultimate goal was to avoid dissemination and/or recurrences of the infection. Seven cases were treated in this manner. Good mobilization of the shoulder was not achieved, even after resolution of infection, in only one patient. The most complex part was the release of the mobile anatomic structures, which were enclosed in a fibrous,

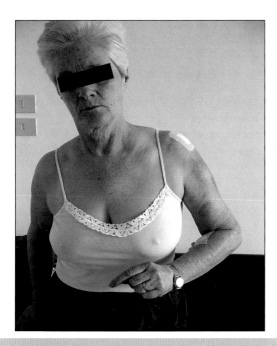

FIGURE 9. Clinical presentation of shoulder tuberculosis with painful rigidity in abduction and internal rotation.

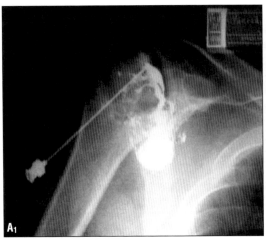
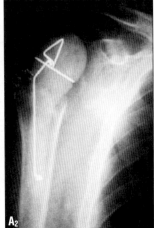
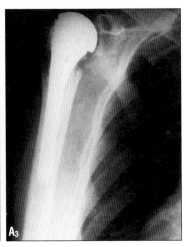

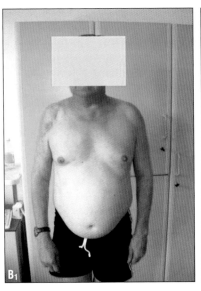
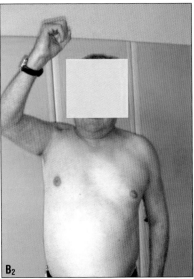

FIGURE 10. (A) A 58-year-old patient with fistulae tuberculosis [25]. After stabilization of the infection with 3 local and general systemic antibiotic cycles (antitubercular, teicoplanin and ciprofloxacin for 60 days), surgical debridement, resection of humeral epiphysis and application of a spacer were performed. The spacer was impregnated with strepto-chemycetin/vancomycin/gentamycin/clindamycin. After that, a humeral prosthesis was applied. The cement used for the stem stabilization of prosthesis was impregnated with clindamycin/gentamycin (Copal®). (B) After the prosthesis implantation the patient presented limited functional motion, infection and pain.

very thick and adhesive tissue. The patients who were selected were those treated immediately after diagnosis. It should be noted that the limitation of the shoulder motion was very well tolerated, due to mobility of the scapulo-thoracic joint.

10. CONCLUSIONS

Tuberculosis in the major joint of the upper limb may affect patients of all ages. There are no pathognomonic symptoms and signs preceding its clinical presentation. We should always bear in mind tuberculous arthritis when we manage patients with monostotic lesions or monoarticular arthritis, and more specifically with rheumatoid arthritis. Moreover, it is imperative that we should carry out a biopsy and obtain cultures that need to be tested for susceptibility to antibiotics. New laboratory tests give us the possibility to differentiate the septic types. The treatment is essentially medical in combination with polychemotherapy, applied even locally for at least one year at patient's home under medical supervision. Prognosis is better when soft tissue pathology is predominant.

For the tuberculous arthritis of the wrist, proximal row carpectomy may alleviate ankylosis. This kind of infection is always associated with flexion limitation. When the wrist function recovers, it allows sufficient motion that would serve at least for the normal hygienic needs of the patient. Arthrodesis is not easy to perform due to the destruction of the affected bone and the difficulty to apply osteosynthesis. The tuberculosis of the elbow resolves more easily than that of other articulations, but it is more incapacitating, as painful ankylosis is very frequent. Prosthesis implantation in two stages can be an alternative solution. The shoulder is a joint that even after the treatment and eradication of the infection, usually presents with severe pain. Joint stiffness both during the treatment and in later stages is generally well tolerated due to the compensatory motion of the scapulo-thoracic joint. Tuberculous arthritis remains a pathology with difficulties in management and thus, remains a challenge for both the surgeon and the patient. The surgeon should not only be familiar with different surgical techniques which are applicable to different cases, but also have broad experience both in the treatment of such infections and in upper limb surgery.

REFERENCES

[1] Waxman SA. Streptomycin: background, isolation, properties and utilization. Int Rec Med Gen Pract Clin 1953;166(7):267-80.

[2] Kozin SH, Bishop AT. Atypical Mycobacterium infections of the upper extremity. J Hand Surg [Am] 1994;19:480-7.

[3] Bergami PL, Montina S. (Ed). Tubercolosi osteoarticolare. USES Firenze. Enciclopedia Medica Italiana. Volume XV, 1989, pp. 714 - 723.

[4] Resnick D, Niwayama G. Patologia e diagnostica dell' apparato locomotore. Ed Verducci 1986;2178-2198.

[5] Jaffe HL. Metabolic, degenerative and inflammatory diseases of bones and joints (localizzazioni ossee e extrapol). Philadelphia, Lea & Febiger 1972.

[6] Aubry A, Chosidow O, Caumes E, Robert J, Cambau E. Sixty-three cases of Mycobacterium marinum infection: clinical features, treatment and antibiotic susceptibility of causative isolates. Arch Intern Med 2002;162:1746-52.

[7] Thijin CJP, Steensma JT. (Eds). Tuberculosis of the skeleton. Springer-Verlag Berlin Heidelberg, Germany, 1990.

[8] David-Chausse J. Tuberculose osteo-articulaire des membres. Encyclopedie medico-chirurgicale: appareil locomoteur. Paris, 1979.

[9] Martini M. Tuberculosis of the bones and joints. Springer, Berlin-Heidelberg- New York, 1988.

[10] Colombani S, Allaria A. Trattamento conservative della tubercolosi osteo-articolare. Relaz XLV Congresso SIOT. Firenze 26-29 Ottobre, 1960.

[11] Ghirardini GL, Da Rin F. Localizzazioni rare della tubercolosi osteo-articolare. Atti SERTOT. Vol XXIV 1982;Fasc. 1.

[12] Martini M, Ouahes M. Bone and joint tuberculosis. A review of 652 cases. Orthopaedics 1988;11:861-866.

[13] Leibe H, Kohler H, Kessler P. Osteoarticular tuberculosis. Review - current status of diagnosis and therapy. Zentralbl Chir 1982;107 (5-6):322-42 [German].

[14] Dumontier C, Maylin V, Sautet A, Lenoble E, Urban T, Apoil A. Rupture a la paume des tendons flechisseurs d'origine tuberculeuse. Rev Chir Orthop 1996;82:668-71.

[15] Esenyel CZ, Bulbul M, Kara AN. Isolated tuberculous tenosynovitis of the flexor tendon of the fourth finger of the hand. Case report. Scand J. Reconstr Surg Hand Surg 2000;34:283-5.

[16] Al Qattan MM, Bowen V, Mantkelow RT. Tuberculosis of the hand. J. Hand Surg [Br] 1994;19:234-7.

[17] Benkeddache Y, Sidhoum SE, Derrid A. Les different aspects des tuberculoses de la main: a propos d'une serie de 45 cas. Sem Hop Paris 1988;64:3031-40.

[18] Bahri H, Maalla R, Baccari F, Hamdi MF, Tarhouni IL. Tuberculose du poignet et de la main: a propos de 23 cas. La Main 1998;3: 209-11.

[19] Silva JF. A review of patients with skeletal tuberculosis treated at the University Hospital, Kuala Lumpur. Int Orthop 1980;4(2):79-81.

[20] Eckel H, Due K. Tuberculosis of the smaller joints. Rofo 1985; 142(1):19-23.

[21] Lafond EM. An analysis of adult skeletal tuberculosis. J Bone Joint Surg [Am] 1958;40-A(2):346-64.

[22] Colombani S, Montina S. IV convegno nazionale per lo studio della tubercolosi osteo-articolare. Cortina d'Ampezzo 1-3 luglio 1967.

[23] Mc Cullough CJ. Tuberculosis as a late complication of total hip replacement. Acta Orthop Scand 1977;48(5)508-10.

[24] Savoini E, Gualdrini G, Ghirardini GL, Da Rin F. La coxartrosi nelle coxiti tubercolari stabilizzate Atti SERTOT Vol XXV 1983; Fasc.1

[25] Gualdrini G, Da Rin F, Ghirardini GL. Le sovrainfezioni nella tubercolosi osteo-articolare fistolizzata. Atti SERTOT Vol XXIV 1982; Fasc.1.

Fungal Infections of the Upper Limb in Immunocompetent Patients

Ioannis A. IGNATIADIS*, Panayotis N. SOUCACOS

Department of Orthopaedic Surgery, University of Athens, School of Medicine, Athens, Greece

Fungal infections of the hand are being reported with increasing frequency. Most fungal infections are superficial and relatively benign. There are general signs and symptoms suggesting the presence of a fungal infection. The early symptoms include atypical, nonspecific signs, such as low-grade fever, night sweats, weight loss, lassitude, easy fatigability, cough and chest pain. Cutaneous mycoses are caused by fungi (dermatophytes) that infect superficial keratinized structures such as skin, hair, and nails. These are spread from infected persons by direct contact. The most common subcutaneous mycoses are sporotrichosis and phaeomycotic cysts. Sporotrichoses are the only fungal infections which involve predominantly the upper limb. They are caused by the dimorphic fungus Sporothrix Schenckii, which is a ubiquitous organism found in soil in temperate and tropical climates. Deep and systemic fungal infections are rare, but quite serious. Clinical problems from deep and system fungal infections often result in significant morbidity, and even mortality.

Keywords: mycoses; dermatophyte infection; immunocompetence; sporotrichosis; systemic fungal disease.

1. MYCOLOGY: GENERALITIES

Fungi, which include both yeasts and molds, are eukaryotic organisms [1]. Most fungi recognized today are obligate aerobes. Few are facultative anaerobes, while there are no recognized obligate anaerobic fungi. With the exception of *Candida albican,* the environment provides the natural habitat for most fungi. Candida albicans is part of the normal human flora. *Conidia,* consisting of asexual spores, are the most medically interesting fungi. Conidia, which are of the greatest significance, include the arthrospores, the chlamdospores, blastospores and the sporangiospores. The arthrospores comprise the mode of transmission of Coccidioides immitis. The chlamydospores (Candida albicans) are a quite resistant fungal category, and the blastospores and sporangiospores, such as *Rhizopus* and *Mucor,* are formed within a sac (sporangium) [1].

Despite the plethora of fungal species, fungal diseases can be readily diagnosed in laboratory. Diagnostic modes include: 1) direct microscopic examination, 2) culture of the organism, 3) DNA probe tests, and 4) serologic tests [1]. Systemic mycosis can be diagnosed with tests of presence of antibodies in patient's serum or spinal fluid. In cases where there is a suspicion of coccidioidomycosis, histoplasmosis or blastomycosis, the most frequently used diagnostic modality is the complement fixation test [1].

2. FUNGAL INFECTIONS

2.1. Patients at risk for Mycoses

Various patient populations are at risk for fungal infections. One group includes various categories of

*Corresponding Author
Department of Orthopaedic Surgery
General University Hospital Attikon
1 Rimini str, 12462, Haidari, Greece
Fax: +30 210 8152818
e-mail: soukakos@panafonet.gr

immunosuppressed patients, including: a) patients with reduced number or compromised function of polymorphonuclear leucocytes, b) organ transplant recipients, c) patients with malignant neoplasms during periods of chemotherapy, d) patients with immunologic and metabolic disorders (SLE, collagen vascular diseases), e) diabetes mellitus, f) dysgammaglobulinemia, and g) patients who have previously received treatment with corticosteroids or cytotoxic agents. In addition, it is now well recognized that various categories of immunocompetent patients are also at risk. These include: a) travelers or inhabitants of regions known to be endemic for fungal infections and b) participants in activities or occupations that bring them in direct skin contact with infected animals or contaminated materials or ingestion or inhalation of aerosols or dust contaminated with fungal spores, and c) recipients of prolonged antibiotic therapy [2].

2.2. Signs and symptoms in Mycoses

There are general signs and symptoms suggesting fungal infection. The early signs are atypical and nonspecific symptoms, such as low-grade fever, night sweats, weight loss, lassitude, easy fatigability, cough, and chest pain. Systemic fungal diseases may mimic other infections, such as tuberculosis, brucellosis, syphilis, sarcoidosis and disseminated carcinomatosis. Often they present with mucocutaneous lesions. Initial clues to the presence of a fungal infection may be provided with non-specific laboratory findings, including accelerated erythrocyte sedimentation rate, increase in C-reactive protein, elevations in γ -globulin or low-grade and persistent elevations in peripheral blood neutrophils and/or monocytes.

2.3. Categorization of fungal infections

Fungal infections may be categorized as superficial or systemic. Systemic infections may have been caused by dimorphic fungi (forms of mold in the environment), or other fungal agents formerly considered as saprobes or contaminants in immunosuppressed individuals. Opportunistic mycoses comprise the nonpathogenic fungi that can cause subcutaneous and disseminated infections in intravenous drug users or immunosuppressed individuals. Some of these nonpathogenic fungi include Aspergillus species, Candida species, and Zygomyces species [2]. Cutaneous and subcutaneous mycoses are also medical mycoses.

Cutaneous fungal diseases are caused by dermatophytes that infect only superficial keratinized structures, such as skin, hair, and nails. This is usually attributed to *Tinea versicolor* (pityriasis versicolor). A superficial skin infection of cosmetic importance is attributed to *Malassezia furfur,* while *Tinea Nigra* is an infection of the keratinized layers of the skin by the organism *Gladosporium werneckii* which is normally found in the soil.

Subcutaneous mycoses, including sporotrichosis, chromomycosis and mycetoma, are caused by fungi that grow in the soil and on vegetation. These are usually introduced in subcutaneous tissue through trauma [1].

Systemic mycosis result from inhalation of the spores of dimorphic fungi that have their saprophytic mold forms in the soil. Within the lungs, their spores differentiate into yeasts or other specialized forms. Most of these infections are asymptomatic and self-limited. Examples of these types of systemic mycosis include coccidioidomycosis, histoplasmosis and blastomycosis.

Opportunistic fungi as *Candida, Cryptococcus, Aspergillus, Mucor* and *Rhizopus* do not induce disease in most immunocompetent individuals. However, they are quite effective in inducing disease in patients with impaired defense mechanisms [1].

3. Fungal Infections of the Upper limb

3.1. Generalities in upper limb mycoses

Fungal infections of the hand are being reported with increasing frequency. Clinically, these can be usefully classified into four categories: cutaneous fungal infections, subcutaneous, deep and systemic fungal infections. Most fungal infections are superficial and relatively benign. On the other hand, deep and systemic result in serious clinical problems, which if not managed effectively, can often result in significant morbidity and even mortality [3].

3.2. Cutaneous mycoses of the hand

Cutaneous mycoses are caused by fungi that infect superficial keratinized structures, such as the skin, hair, and nails. These are referred to as dermatophytes and they are transmitted from an infected person by direct contact. Dermatophytosis, including "tinea" and "ringworm", are chronic infections favored by heat and humidity. They are characterized by pruritic papules and vesicles, broken hair and thickened broken nails. Treatment involves local antifungal creams (undecylenic acid, myconazole, etc), or oral griseofulvin. Prevention centers on keeping skin dry and cool [1].

A rare type of mycosis of the hand is referred to in the literature as *tinea manuum bullosa.* The causative organism is a zoophylic mycete, T.verrucosum. In a case report, the patient was a 36-year-old male, a crop and livestock farmer by trade, complaining of an erythematous-squamous lesion on the palm of his right hand. Mycological culture produced a profuse growth of *Trichophyton verrucosum.* Blood chemistry and immunology test results were normal. Treatment with terbinafine 250 mg per day led to clinical and mycological healing [4, 5].

Generalized dermatophyte infection is referred to as *Trichophyton rubrum* infection syndrome. Prerequisites for this diagnosis include skin lesions at the following four sites: 1) feet, often involving soles, 2) hands, often involving palms, 3) nails, and 4) at least one lesion in other location than the feet, hands or nails with the exception of the groin. In addition, diagnosis requires positive microscopic findings with potassium hydroxide preparations of skin scrapings in all four locations. Finally, identification of *T. rubrum* by culture of scrapings at three of the four locations, at least, is also necessary [5].

3.3. Subcutaneous mycoses of the hand

The most common subcutaneous mycoses are sporotrichosis and phaeomycotic cysts. Sporotrichoses are the only fungal infections which involve predominantly the upper limb. They are caused by the dimorphic fungus, *Sporothrix Schenckii*, which is a ubiquitous organism in soil in temperate and tropical climates. Sporothrix spores produce by subcutaneous implantation, a chronic granulomatous infection, with ulcers primarily and secondarily to regional adenopathy. The most common manifestation is lymphocutaneous involvement with characteristic violatious ulcerations and drain seropurulent fluid.

Patients at great risk for Sporothrix infections are home gardeners who handle soil and sharp objects. Definitive diagnosis of Sporotrichosis requires fungal cultures with the isolation of *Sporothrix Schenckii*. The standard medium for culturing is modified Sabouraud's agar. Because of the delay of clinical diagnosis that is usually related to incorrect diagnosis and treatment (usually for a presumed bacterial infection), culture of all ulcerated skin lesions for both bacteria and fungi and separate cultures grown at room temperature are mandatory. Because of the risk for atypical mycobacterial infections which have the same pattern as granulomatous infections, appropriate cultures for the isolation of these organisms should also be performed.

The drug of choice for lymphocutaneous sporotrichosis is itraconazole. Complete resolution in most patients occurs with treatment of 100 to 200mg/day for 3 to 6 months. Longer treatment periods are required for deep or disseminated infections [6]. A case of an unusual clinical course of sporotrichosis has been reported involving a 79-year-old female, employed as farmer, where sporotrichosis occurred on the patient's face at the first infection. After three recurrences of the infection near the original lesion and because medical treatment with potassium iodide and itraconazole had not been successful the facial lesion was excised. This therapeutic experience indicates the possibility that *Sporothrix Schenckii* gradually develops resistance to potassium iodide and itraconazole. After an interval of four years unexpectedly cutaneous lesions developed on the left upper limb, a previously unaffected area. She developed nodules on her left hand and forearm. The primary lesion was crusted and granulomatous, but the lesions on the hand and forearm were nodular. Lymph nodes were not palpable. Biopsy material revealed *Sporothrix*

Schenckii. The patient responded to treatment with potassium iodide (600mg/day). The cutaneous lesions completely resolved after 26 weeks of treatment [7].

A rare subcutaneous infection is the phaeomycotic cyst attributed to a darkly pigmented fungus *Exophiala, Phialophora,* or *Bantalis*. The infection occurs by traumatic implantation of wood or by intravenous catheter in an immunocompromised patient. Surgical removal is the standard treatment for this infection. Antifungal therapy alone is not clearly successful.

3.4. Deep and systemic mycoses of the hand

Deep and systemic fungal infections are rare, but very serious clinical problems that often result in significant morbidity and even mortality arise. These infections of the upper limb have three common clinical presentations: septic tenosynovitis (Fig. 1), septic arthritis, and osteomyelitis [8] (Fig. 2). Infectious disease consultation is recommended for diagnosis and treatment in both immunocompetent and immunocompromised patients to avoid recurrence of infection. Sporotrichotic septic arthritis after direct joint inoculation may be confused with inflammatory arthritis of pyogenic infection. Sporotrichosis can also produce osteomyelitis (multifocal) or tenosynovial infection (dorsal wrist tendons). Extensor tenosynovitis may cause rupture of an extensor. Flexor tenosynovitis may result in carpal tunnel syndrome or ulnar nerve entrapment.

Bursal sporotrichosis has been reported in the olecranon and also sporotrichal myositis of the biceps muscle. The basic principles of successful treatment are surgical debulking of the infecting area, combined with systemic antifungal therapy (intravenous amphotericin B or oral itraconazole) [9].

Another deep hand infection, fungal mycetoma, is particularly resistant to medical therapy and often re-

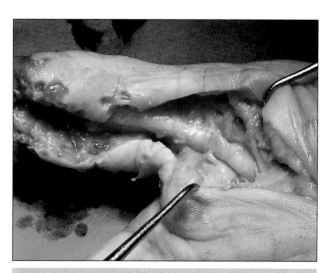

FIGURE 1. Iatrogenic Mycotic tenosynovitis in an immunocompetent patient's.

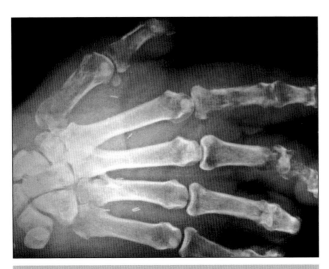

FIGURE 2. Mycotic Osteomyelitis confirmed by microscopy and culture.

quires amputation. Mycetomas are subdivided into two groups: those caused by aerobic bacteria (actinomycetomas) and those caused by fungi (eumycetomas). Actinomycetomas have usually successful antimicrobial treatment and surgery is almost never needed. Eumycetoma is caused by saprophytic soil fungi that are usually inoculated through minor injuries. The most affected countries are India, Sudan, Senegal, Somalia, Venezuela, Mexico, Yemen, and Zaire. Sporadic cases also occur in temperate regions [9]. They are usually localized on the lower extremities (70%), and the hand (12%). Eumycetomas are usually caused by maduromycete fungi, especially *Madurella mycetomatis* and *M. grisea.* The prevalence of the different fungi varies from country to country and seems to be influenced by rainfall conditions. *A. kalrae* has occasionally been reported as an opportunistic human pathogen [10].

Antifungal treatment of Eumycetoma remains unsatisfactory. Intravenous amphotericin B, oral thiabendazole, topical and intravenous myconazole, oral griseofulvin, and ketoconazole have been tried. These medications are most often used in association with surgery. They limit the size of the excision, when used before surgery, and they reduce the risk of recurrence, when used after it, for at least 6 to 12 months. Itraconazole is more potent *in vitro* against some fungi than ketoconazole, it has better tissue diffusion and a better safety profile without hepatotoxicity, even with prolonged administration.

There have been a few reports concerning itraconazole treatment of eumycetoma. Of the six cases caused by *M. mycetomatis* that have been reported, one case showed a good initial response to treatment (300 mg daily for 1 year), but recurred when treatment was stopped. Three cases of eumycetoma caused by *M. grisea* were resistant to therapy. Two cases caused by *Pseudallescheria* sp. have been described: one caused

by *P. larensae,* treated with no success and one caused by *P. boydii,* successfuly treated were also reported. Moreover, two cases caused by *Acremonium* sp, one caused by *A. kilience* and one caused by *A. falciforme,* which were treated with success. Finally, one case caused by *Fusarium* sp. was also reported, with improvement. These results suggest that the efficacy of itraconazole is variable, inconstant, and often partial.

Eumycetoma generally occurs in immunocompetent hosts, which differs from other opportunistic infections, such as the cutaneous Alternaria infection. However, despite the presence of saprophyte mycetoma agents in soil and the high frequency of trauma, cases of mycetoma are uncommon. In a study on the immunologic status of patients with mycetoma, it was found that these patients were partially deficient in cell-mediated immunity [11].

Systemic fungal diseases occur in healthy individuals and in immunocompromised patients. They include histoplasmosis, blastomycosis, coccidioidomycosis, paracoccidiomycosis and mucormycosis. All of these diseases are endemic to certain geographic areas.

Histoplasmosis is caused by Histoplasma capsulatum and is endemic in Mississippi and Ohio river valleys. Typical pulmonary calcifications on a chest radiograph, in association with positive skin or serologic testing confirm the diagnosis.

In disseminated rare cases tenosynovial infections are present or carpal tunnel syndrome, arthritis, or fatal necrotizing myofascitis in the upper extremity. A case of recurrent osteomyelitis of capitate bone was also reported. Diagnosis of *H. Capsulatum* is confirmed by measuring complement fixing (CF) antibodies and precipitin bands. A titer more than 1:32 is suggestive of active infection. A polysaccharide antigen test is available commercially and can help in diagnosis.

Critical treatment to prevent recurrence is a combination of complete tenosynovectomy, bone debridement, and prolonged systemic antifungal therapy as oral ketoconazole or itraconazole, or intravenous amphotericin B. San Joaquin Valley in California and the deserts of southwest of United States are the endemic regions of a highly infectious fungus Coccidioides immitis. This fungus has a predilection for synovium and 10% of coccidioidal infections occur in the wrist and hand. Tenosynovitis, joint infection and osteomyelitis of the hand have been reported. Osteomyelitis of a metacarpal may mimic an enchondroma. Tenosynovitis is present with chronic diffuse swelling over the dorsal or volar side of the wrist or palm. Untreated cases may lead to extensor tendon rupture and mimic rheumatoid arthritis [8]. Diagnosis may be confirmed by culture or serologic testing. Coccidioidomycosis also responds favorably to synovectomy and systemic antifungal therapy [3].

Mucormycosis is an acute and chronic fungal infection caused by fungi of the order Mucorales. The most commonly isolated agents are Rhisopus and Rhizomucor. These infections are aggressive and destructive, but fortunately, rare [8]. Rapid diagnosis and radical debridement are essential to preserve tissue devastation. The most common predisposing condition is diabetic ketoacidosis, but other such conditions include chronic renal failure, hematological malignancies, connective-tissue disorders and organ transplantation [4].

Rhisopus and Mucor infection of the hand is usually cutaneous and subcutaneous (24% of all cutaneous cases) [8]. Fifty percent of primary cutaneous mucormycosis cases occur in patients with severe trauma contaminated by soil or water. The other fifty percent involves patients with diabetes (20%), leukemia (9%), and chronic kidney failure (5%), or organ transplantation (4%). These cutaneous and subcutaneous infections are presented with progressive gangrenous cellulitis and necrosis of the wound margin. Advanced disease is indicated with black eschars and pus especially in an immunocompromised host.

In an unpublished case of a deep antebrachial and hand zygomatosis with flexor synovitis, we observed median nerve and bone involvement. An immunocompetent patient was admitted to our clinic with a recurrent flexor tenosynovitis and history of a recent superficial cutaneous infection of the ipsilateral hand related to catheter insertion involving the middle and ring fingers and the thumb. The mycosis had been misdiagnosed and previously treated by classical antibiotics for two months. With the exception of the thumb, a subungual purulent collection was present (Fig. 3). ESR and CRP were elevated. WBC count and differential was normal. Hand X-rays revealed osteolysis of the 1st ray and the phalanges of 2nd and 3rd finger. Surgical exploration revealed brownish purulent fluid in all spaces and tendon sheaths. There were fibro-purulent bands, and the median nerve was necrotic (Fig. 4). Opening of all the hand septa, synovectomy and extensive debridement, including the median nerve, were performed. The trauma was packed with surgical gauze, so as it could heal secon-

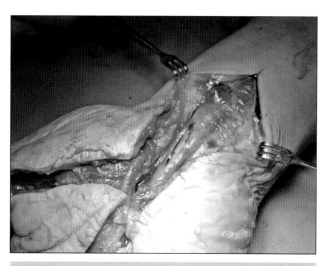

FIGURE 4. Median nerve necrosis caused by *Rhizopus oryzae* in an immunocompetent male young patient.

darily. Specimens were sent for cultures and biopsy. The cultures revealed a zycomycete, *R. orysae,* and treatment with amphotericin B was initiated. The patient underwent surgical debridement weekly and hyperbaric oxygen therapy daily for four weeks. Although two months after the initial debridement healing of the wound was satisfactory, resection of the first ray and the phalangeal bones of the index and middle finger was performed because osteomyelitis still persisted. A few weeks later, a wrist-bone subtotal carpectomy, which excluded the pissiform and trapezium, was performed. Six months after the last bone resection, the patient was found free of infection and the mycosis eradicated.

Timely and accurate diagnosis of zygomycosis can be difficult because these infections often present in an indolent and chronic manner. As a result, hand surgeons should have general awareness of the possibility, particularly since most patients are initially wrongly treated for an inflammatory condition. Definitive diagnosis can be made with a surgical biopsy and appropriate culture. Because these organisms are fastidious, good collaboration with the microbiologist is essential.

Successful treatment of deep zygomycosis of the hand requires surgical debridement and appropriate chemotherapy with amphotericin B. The surgical principles are similar to those for the treatment of common hand infections. The anatomic location of the infectious disease dictates the extent of the debridement. The underlying risk factors for developing zygomycosis should be addressed, if possible. Because long-term antimicrobial therapy is usually necessary, consultation with an infectious disease specialist is recommended. With this multimodal approach a functional, disease-free hand can be obtained. Despite al these, deep zygomycosis of the hand due to *R oryzae* is not always curable, and at least bone excision or partial amputation is needed when osteomyelitis coexists.

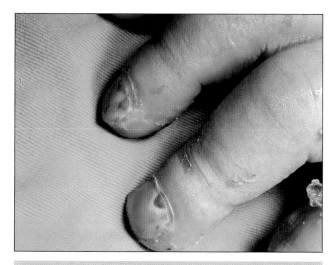

FIGURE 3. Subungual purulent collection caused by upper limb zygomatosis.

Mucormycosis can result after a forearm infection at an intravenous infusion site, an intramuscular injection in an immunocompromised patient, or a contamination of devitalized tissue after major or minor trauma [7]. Burn wounds dressed with contaminated elasticized tape have been reported with this disease [11]. *Mucor hiemalis,* a common soil inhabitant, was recovered from a diabetic gardener with a localized subcutaneous infection of a finger.

Mucormycosis has a tendency to invade deep tissues, although osteomyelitis in the hand is rare. The diagnosis is typically made histologically. It requires that tissue is examined for presence of characteristic irregular, broad, nonseptate, right-angle branching hyphae. Biopsy and smears often reveal the organisms when cultures are negative. Cultures from an excised ulcer may grow *Rhisopus, Mucor,* or *Absidia,* as well as other *Mucorales,* such as *Cunninghamella* and *Apophysomyces.*

The standard therapy for mucormycosis is prompt and aggressive surgical debridement of necrotic tissue, skin grafting and amphotericin B. Predisposing systemic factors and diabetes should be aggressively managed. Intravenous amphotericin B remains the drug of choice and should be given in full dose without the delay of increasing dose titration. The lipid formulations of amphotericin B such as Abelcet and Ambisome can be used. High doses of these agents are necessary in patients who are at risk of dying of this infection, despite their known toxicity.

CONCLUSION

The most clinically interesting fungi in hand surgery are conidia which include arthrospores, chlamydospores, blastospores and sporangiospores (Rhisopus and Mucor). Mycoses occur in immunosuppressed patients usually and in certain groups of immunocompetent patients. They can be superficial or systemic and deep.

Although deep mycoses are rare they often result in significant morbidity and long term both operative and conservative treatment. When extensor or flexor tenosynovitis and fasciitis of the hand are present care must be taken with radical surgical debridement and opening of the fascia and rapid culture or serologic testing to prevent recurrence and tissue devastation.

REFERENCES

[1] Hitchcock TF, Amadio PC. Fungal infections. Hand Clin 1989;5: 599-611.

[2] Dressler F. Infectious diseases affecting the musculoskeletal system in children and adolescents. Curr Opin Rheumatol 1993;5: 651-7.

[3] Amadio P. Fungal infections of the hand. Hand Clinics 1998; 14(4):605-12.

[4] Aste N, Pau M, Aste N. Tinea manuum bullosa. Mycoses 2003; 48:80-81.

[5] Kick G, Korting HC. The definition of Trichophyton rubrum syndrome, Mycoses 2001;44:167-171.

[6] Goodman NL. Sporotrichosis. In: AF Di Salvo, editor, Occupational Mycoses. Philadelphia: Lea & Febiger, 1989.

[7] Shinogi T, Misago N, Narisawa Y. Cutaneous Sporotrichosis with Refractory and Reinfectious Lesions in a Healthy Female. J Dermatol 2004;31:492-496.

[8] Patel MR, Malaviya GN, Sugar AM. Chronic Infections: Fungal Infections. In: DP Green (ed.), Hand Operative Hand Surgery, 5th Edition, Philadelphia, PA: Elsevier-Churchill Livingstone, 2005, pp. 106-116.

[9] Welsh O. Mycetoma: Current concepts in treatment. Int J Dermatology 1991;30:387-98.

[10] Mahgoub ES. Mycetoma. Semin Dermatology 1985;4:230-9.

[11] Degavre B, Joujoux JM, Dandurand M, Guillot B. First report of mycetoma caused by Arthrographis. Kalrae: Successful treatment with itraconazole. Am Acad Dermatology 1997;37:318-20.

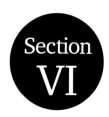

Section
VI

SPECIFIC SURGICAL TECHNIQUES

SPECIFIC SURGICAL TECNIQUES

Management of Infection in 2-stage Flexor Tendon Reconstruction

Alexandros E. BERIS[a*], Anastasios V. KOROMPILIAS[a],
Marios G. LYKISSAS[a], Gregory I. MITSIONIS[b], Marios D. VEKRIS[a],
Vasilios A. KONTOGEORGAKOS[a], Panayotis N. SOUCACOS[b]

[a]Department of Orthopaedic Surgery, University of Ioannina, Ioannina, Greece
[b]Department of Orthopaedic Surgery, National University of Athens, KAT Hospital, Athens, Greece

Two-stage flexor tendon reconstruction is a well-known and established technique for the restoration of the flexor tendons. Complications do occur, including rod buckling, rod migration, rupture of the distal end of silicone rod, synovitis, bowstringing, impingement of the proximal suture in the sheath, flexion deformity of the PIP and / or DIP joints, and infection. Infection is common in stage I due to the extensive surgical exposure that takes place in this stage, and to factors associated with the silicone rods, but uncommon in stage II. In most cases infection is treated with systemic antibiotics and/or closed irrigation of the pseudosheath. Rod removal is needed occasionally, followed by a new stage I and II procedure after 3-6 months. Infection does not appear often, but inadequate treatment may require reoperation of the two stages, which increases the possibility of failure.

Keywords: infection; silicone rod; flexor tendons; staged reconstruction.

1. INTRODUCTION

Two-stage flexor tendon reconstruction with the Hunter technique is a well known and established method of flexor tendons repair in zone II. The Paneva modification with a pedicle graft through the loop of flexor digitorum superficialis (FDS) and flexor digitorum profundus (FDP) is an advantageous modification of the Hunter technique [1].

One of the complications of both techniques is infection, which may compromise the functional outcome. The main principles of hand surgery should be followed in order to avoid infection. In the early stage of cellulitis, intravenous antibiotics and immobilization of the hand may resolve the infection. Pus formation is treated by continuous irrigation of the intrasynovial part in zone II and intravenous antibiotics administration. If the infection does not subside, removal of the rod follows and stages I and II are repeated after 6-9 months.

2. TWO-STAGE FLEXOR TENDON RECONSTRUCTION

Flexor tendon injuries in zone II is a difficult area to treat due to the fibro-osseous canal. A meticulous technique should be followed in the treatment of

*Corresponding Author
Department of Orthopaedic Surgery
University of Ioannina, School of Medicine
Ioannina, 45110, Greece
e-mail: aberis@cc.uoi.gr

zone II injuries, where adhesions may compromise the functional result. There are two ways to overcome adhesion formation: (i) two-stage flexor tendon reconstruction with a silicone rod, and (ii) placement of an autologous tendon graft.

In 1971, Hunter and Salisbury presented the preliminary results after two-stage flexor tendon reconstruction [2]. Since then, flexor tendon reconstruction has been widely accepted, but with fluctuating rates of success and complications [3-5]. In accordance with the James Hunter technique, insertion of a silicone-Dacron tendon prosthesis in a primary stage, leads to the formation of a pseudosheath with a smooth and gliding surface which allows a tendon graft to pass through it in a second stage [6-8]. In further studies, he proved that the fibro-osseous canal reconstruction in zone II allows unrestricted gliding without adhesion formation [9]. The Paneva modification of the Hunter technique refers to forming a loop between the FDP and the FDS in the first stage, and the use of the formed pedicle graft in the second stage [10]. This technique is advantageous because it permits the reconstruction of a scarred or destroyed FDP from an intrasynovial tendon (FDS) of a similar size. The above procedure leads to sufficient functional results and to reduction of donor site morbidity [1].

The indications for two-stage flexor tendon reconstruction are classified as follows: (i) Boye's categories 2-5, (ii) patients with failed primary tendon repair, and (iii) cases where the fibro-osseous canal is destroyed, as in amputations [11]. On such occasions, the application of primary or delayed primary tendon repair in zone II leads to failure, and the two-stage flexor tendon reconstruction using silicone rods is the treatment of choice.

3. INFECTION

The staged flexor tendon reconstruction is a demanding technique with risks and complications. The complications can be classified in relation to the stage in which they appear (Table 1). In stage I of the two-stage flexor tendon reconstruction, some complications are: (i) rod buckling, (ii) necrosis of the skin, (iii) rod migration, (iv) rupture of the distal end of silicone or Hunter rod, (v) synovitis, and (vi) infection. In the second stage, the following can be observed: (i) bowstringing, (ii) impingement of the proximal suture in the fibro-osseous canal, (iii) tendon grafts loose or tight, (iv) distal or proximal disruption of graft suture, (v) flexion deformity of the PIP and/or DIP joints, which is considered to be the most common complication in this stage, and (vi) infection [11, 12].

Infection is an uncommon complication that may considerably affect the outcome. The percentage of infection in the literature varies from 2.3% to 25.6% in both stage I and stage II (Table 2). Inadequate treatment may require removal of the rod and reoperation with the two-stage technique, which increases the failure rate of the flexor tendon repair. Infection is more common in stage I than in stage II, and this fact may be attributed to extensive surgical exposure of the digit, silicone rod synovitis or both.

Extensive surgical debridement should follow in order that all scar tissue of the fibro-osseous canal is removed. This could be achieved through an inverted L incision in the thenar or the opisthenar, and a Bruner incision in the digit. Reconstruction of at least the 1st, the 2nd, and the 4th pulley with different techniques is necessary. In stage II of the Hunter technique, the removal of the silicone rod and the placement of a tendon graft

---

TABLE 1

Complications during two-stage flexor tendon reconstruction.

Stage I	Management
Rod buckling	Avoid excessive obstruction of the pulleys
Skin necrosis	Zig-zag incision with angles no less than 45°
Rod migration	Xenogram prior to stage II
Rupture of the distal end	Open the volar aspect of the distal phalanx and fish out the implant with a retriever
Synovitis	Antibiotics, splinting, avoidance of passive motion
Infection	Antibiotics, closed irrigation, splinting
	Rod removal if the infection does not regress

Stage II	
Bowstringing	Meticulous reconstruction of the failed pulleys
Suture impingement in the sheath	Meticulous care when opening the sheath at the wrist level
Loose or tight grafts	With the wrist in neutral position, the finger rests in slightly more flexion than the adjacent finger
Distal graft disruption	Graft reattachment. Use the fishmouth technique
Proximal graft disruption	Antibiotics, closed irrigation, splinting
Infection	Flexion contractures prior to surgery must be corrected before performing Stage I or II
PIP and/or DIP deformity	Flexion contractures resulting from surgery should be corrected with dynamic night splints

TABLE 2

Infection in staged flexor tendon reconstruction in the literature.

Study	n (Digits)	Infection in Stage I (%)	IV antibiotics & closed irrigation (%)	rod removal (%)	Infection in Stage II (%)
Beris et al. [1]	31	6.4 (2 fingers)	3.2 (1 finger)	3.2 (1 finger)	–
Weinstein et a.l [5]	28	10.7 (3 fingers)	7.1 (2 fingers)	3.6 (1 finger)	–
Soucacos et al. [11]	109	2.8 (3 fingers)	1.8 (2 fingers)	0.9 (1 finger)	–
LaSalle et al. [12]	43		2.3% in both stage I & II		
Wehbe et al. [13]	150	4.0 (6 fingers)	unknown	unknown	0.7 (1 finger)
Amadio et al. [14]	130		15% in both stage I & II		
Frakking et al. [15]	51	–	–	–	2.0 (6 fingers)
Finsen [16]	43	13.9 (6 fingers)	11.6 (5 fingers)	2.3 (1 finger)	9.3 (4 fingers)

are completed through two small incisions, one in the volar aspect of the wrist, and one in the distal phalanx. If palmaris longus is used, a third incision for the retrieval of the tendon is centered above the wrist [6, 11].

3.1. Pathogenesis

Many authors have reported complications related to silicone rods [13-17]. According to Hunter, those materials are highly electrostatic, and as a result, they attract airborne particles and surface contaminants during their insertion [18]. This fact may lead to the adherence of several bacteria on the silicone rod surface, which may cause an increased rate of infection in the first stage of the two-stage flexor tendon reconstruction [13, 14]. Immersion of the silicone rods in saline, Ringer's lactate, or triple antibiotic solution in order that they loose their electrostatic properties is suggested [18]. Certainly, further research on the properties of the silicone rods and their ability to provoke infection is required.

Synovitis is a complication which appears only in the first stage of the two-stage flexor tendon reconstruction. Its presence may lead to infection and can influence the clinical outcome. Silicone synovitis may be attributed to the rod. On many occasions, synovitis can be treated efficiently with antibiotic administration and immobilization of the finger in the resting position. In order to minimize the effects of this complication, the surgeon should avoid contact of the silicone rods with foreign particles, such as powder on newly opened surgical gloves, and should continuously irrigate the silicone rod [18].

Two-stage flexor tendon reconstruction is considered as one of the most useful tools for an expert hand surgeon. The outcome of this technique has been compared to that of the primary one-stage grafting. The results from the comparison between the two techniques are very difficult to estimate, and sometimes, they are contradictory. This fact can be attributed to the different methods that are used to estimate the results. By using different methods of evaluation and by exclu-

ding the thumb flexor tendon reconstruction, Wehbe et al noticed that among the factors that influence the final results in the two-stage flexor tendon reconstruction, infection was not included. In their study, infection had a rate of 4% (6 fingers), which was attributed to a contaminated batch of implants [13]. In the same paper, synovitis, which was one of the most common complications in stage I, did not influence the final result [13].

The four cardinal signs of tenosynovitis are: (i) excessive tenderness just above the sheath, (ii) rigid position of the finger in flexion, (iii) symmetric swelling of the involved part, and (iv) pain when the finger is in passive extension [19]. The last sign is similar to the first and most usual symptom appearing early in the process. There is a high possibility that these four signs may be absent in immunosuppressed patients, at an early stage of infection, and in patients with inadeaquate antibiotic treatment. Infection in patients who undergo two-stage flexor tendon reconstruction is due to the common flora of the skin, and the most common isolated organism is Staphylococcus aureus [1, 14].

3.2. Treatment modalities

Acute infection of less-than 48 hours-duration may resolve with intravenous antibiotic administration. Antimicrobial drug therapy should be rationally based on culture results. While waiting for the culture results, empirical therapy consisting a combination of a second-generation cephalosporin and an aminoglycoside should be initiated. If the infection does not resolve, then closed irrigation drainage of the pseudosheath should be added to the intravenous antibiotic administration. If this procedure is to be performed, of particular importance are close observations, that should preferably take place in the hospital.

The technique described by Neviaser is used for closed irrigation drainage [20]. An exposure of the proximal end of the flexor pseudosheath is made in the region of A1 pulley by a transverse incision parallel to the distal palmar crease. A second incision is made over the region of A5 pulley. For the distal incision, an incision in the midaxial line on either side of the finger is preferred. Afterwards, a 16- or 18-gauge polyethylene catheter is passed through the proximal incision beneath the A1 pulley at a distance of 1.5 to 2 cm inside the pseudosheath. A small piece of rubber drain is placed in the distal incision so that the pseudosheath is irrigated from proximal to distal with saline and antibiotics until the fluid is clear. The postoperative irrigation program starts immediately after the wound is closed around the drain, with 30 ml of saline and antibiotics every 2 hours for the next 24-48 hours. The use of continuous irrigation with saline and antibiotics at 25 ml/h can be also equally effective. The digit is immobilized with a splint in the resting position. In case the signs of infection remain after 48 hours, irrigation is continued for 24 more hours. In our 3 patients, we used one distal volar incision over the DIP joint, and through this, the pseudosheath was approached. Two vein catheters were inserted: the first, in the proximal end of the fibro-osseous canal, and the second, 1 cm proximally to the DIP joint (Fig. 1). Through these, a continuous irrigation system was established and maintained for 48 hours.

In case the infection does not subside despite the irrigation and intravenous antibiotic administration or the infection progresses to necrosis of the pulleys and the pseudosheath, rod removal and debridement are necessary. Passive motion is initiated as soon as possible.

The patient remains under intravenous antibiotic treatment for 2 weeks and continues with per os antibiotics for the next 10 weeks. The goal is to eliminate the infection and to achieve full passive flexion of the finger so that the silicone rod can be reinserted. This takes place in a second stage I procedure, when the clinical signs and the laboratory findings are normal, usually after 3-6 months [5, 6, 8, 11].

Infection is considered as one of the most serious complications in both stages I and II as regards to the final outcome, according to several findings published in the literature (Table 2). In most cases, intravenous antibiotic administration, closed irrigation of the pseudosheath, and splinting for the painful period followed by active motion are effective. Rod removal and reoperation of stage I are applied rarely in certain cases. According to Wehbe et al, in a total of 150 fingers which were treated with the two-stage reconstruction technique, only 7 fingers presented with infection, 6 of them in stage I [13]. Soucacos et al. observed that of 109 fingers, only 3 developed infection in stage I [11]. Two fingers were treated with intravenous antibiotic administration and closed irrigation drainage of the pseudosheath, whereas in the third finger the rod had to be removed. Beris et al. found that 2 of 31 fingers demonstrated infection in the first stage, and only one of them required removal of the implant [1]. On the contrary, Amadio et al. observed that the rate of infection went up to 15% in both stages [14].

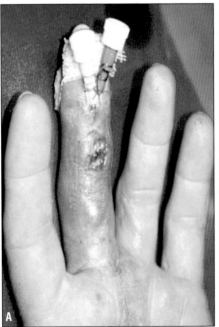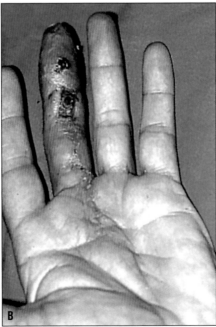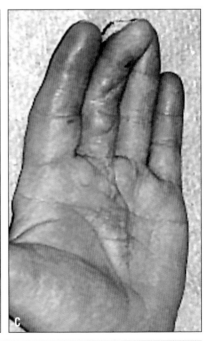

FIGURE 1. (A) An irrigation system has been introduced with two vein catheters in the distal palmar crease (distal end of synovial sheath). **(B)** 48 hours later the catheters were removed. **(C)** 15 days later the second stage of Paneva followed. The photograph shows the result one month after the second stage.

4. Conclusions

Staged flexor tendon reconstruction is an effective technique for reconstructing the flexor tendons. Moreover, it is a demanding procedure with complications in both stages. The most serious complication among others is infection in stage I. However, its treatment is usually conservative and only in a minimum of cases silicone rod removal and re-operation of the stage I procedure are required. This re-operation may be more difficult due to adhesions, and may have compromised functional results. Meticulous techniques and careful observation are essential pre-requisites in order that infection is avoided and urgent treatment is applied in case such a complication does develop.

References

[1] Beris AE, Darlis NA, Korompilias AV, Vekris MD, Mitsionis GI, Soucacos PN. Two-stage flexor tendon reconstruction in zone II using a silicone rod and a pedicled intrasynovial graft. J Hand Surg 2003;28A:652-60.

[2] Hunter JM, Salisbury RE. Flexor-tendon reconstruction in severely damaged hands. A two-stage procedure using a silicone Dacron reinforced gliding prosthesis prior to tendon grafting. J Bone Joint Surg 1971;53A:829-58.

[3] Honner R, Meares A. A review of 100 flexor tendon reconstructions with prosthesis. Hand 1977;9:226-31.

[4] Reill P. Die zweizeitige beugesehnentransplantation. Handchirurgie 1978;10:215-21.

[5] Weinstein SL, Sprague BL, Flatt AE. Evaluation of the two-stage flexor-tendon reconstruction in severely damaged digits. J Bone Joint Surg 1976;58A:786-91.

[6] Schneider LA. Flexor tendon injuries. Monographs in Hand Surgery. Boston: Little, Brown and Co., 1985.

[7] Schneider LA. Staged tendon reconstruction. Hand Clinics 1985; 1:109-20.

[8] Schneider LH. Complication in tendon injury and surgery. Hand Clinics 1986;2:361-71.

[9] Hunter JM. Staged flexor tendon reconstruction. In: Hunter JM, Schneider LH, Mackin EJ, Callahan AD, editors. Rehabilitation of the hand. St. Louis: CV Mosby Co., 1984, p. 288-313.

[10] Paneva Holevich E. Two stage tenoplasty in injury of the flexor tendons of the hand. J Bone Joint Surg 1969;51A:21-32.

[11] Soucacos PN, Beris AE, Malizos KN, Xenakis T, Touliatos A, Soucacos PK. Two-stage treatment of flexor tendon ruptures: Silicone rod complication analyzed in 109 digits. Acta Orthop Scand (Suppl) 1997;275:48-51.

[12] LaSalle WB, Strickland JW. An evaluation of the two-stage flexor tendon reconstruction technique. J Hand Surg 1983;8A: 263-7.

[13] Wehbe MA, Hunter JM, Schneider LH, Goodwyn BL. Two-stage flexor-tendon reconstruction. J Bone Joint Surg 1986;68A:752-63.

[14] Amadio PC, Wood MB, Cooney WP, Bogard SD. Staged flexor tendon reconstruction in the fingers of the hand. J Hand Surg 1988; 13A:559-62.

[15] Frakking TG, Depuydt KP, Kon M, Werker PMN. Retrospective outcome analysis of staged flexor tendon reconstruction. J Hand Surg 2000;25B:2:168-74.

[16] Finsen V. Two-stage grafting of digital flexor tendons: A review of 43 patients after 3 to 15 years. Scand J Plast Reconstr Surg Hand Surg 2003;37(3):159-62.

[17] Wilson GR, Watson JS. Migration of silicone rods. J Hand Surg 1994;19B:199-201.

[18] Hunter JM. Staged flexor tendon reconstruction. J Hand Surg 1983;8A:789-93.

[19] Kanavel AB. Infections of the hand: a guide to the surgical treatment of acute and chronic suppurative processes in the fingers, hand, and forearm. 6th ed. Philadelphia: Lea & Febiger, 1933.

[20] Carter SJ, Burman SO, Mersheimer WL. Treatment of digital tenosynovitis by irrigation with peroxide and oxytetracycline: review of nine cases. Ann Surg 1966;163:645-50.

Acute and Chronic Osteitis of the Hand

Peter BRÜSER*, Bernd von MAYDELL

Department of Hand-Plastic and Reconstructive Surgery, Malteser Hospital, Bonn, Germany

Osteitis of the hand can result in severe impairment of function due to the proximity of the infection to the peritendineal tissue, the tendons and the joints. The pathomechanisms of hematogenous, acute and chronic osteitis and a specific regimen of therapy with PMMA-beads as a spacer or Collagen sponge are illustrated. In a prospective study, 43 patients were treated, 27 because of acute and 16 because of chronic osteitis of the hand. In 11 patients, additional septic arthritis was present. The median time between the onset of infection and surgery was 4 weeks (1-4) in those cases with acute osteitis, and 9 weeks (8-96) in those with chronic osteitis. After 14 days, 39 wounds (91%) healed, and after 1 month, 42 wounds (98%). In one patient revision with implantation of new chains was necessary. Successful treatment of infections of the fingers was achieved after 1 month in 96% and after 1.5 months in 100% of the cases. The success rate at follow-up of up to 6 years was 100%, with no racurrence of infection in any of the cases.

Keywords: osteomyelitis; acute osteitis; chronic osteitis; hand infection; PMMA-beads; prospective study; treatment.

1. INTRODUCTION

In 1999, 42% of all industrial accidents in Germany caused injuries to the hand and the wrist [1]. The most frequent fractures of the hand (82%) [2] were those of the metacarpal and phalangeal bones, representing 10% of overall fractures [3].

As reported by Amine et al. [4], 6% of all infections of the hand were osteitis of the metacarpal and phalangeal bones. Reilly et al. [5] found that 57% are of post-traumatic cause, 15% of post-operative, and 15% of hematogenous. Most often the distal phalanx is infected. Chronic osteitis of the hand is reported to occur in 1-6% of the cases in general [4, 6] and in 1.7% after surgical fracture treatment [7].

Even if the prognosis of osteitis of the hand is good regarding the treatment of the infection itself, the function of the fingers, in particular, often remains impaired as a result of the proximity of the infection to the peritendineal tissue, the tendons, and the joints. Early diagnosis for prevention of this crucial complication combined with surgery and adjuvant antibiotic therapy is the basis of treatment of osteitis of the hand.

2. PATHOPHYSIOLOGY

Bacterial contamination of a wound does not always lead to an osseous infection as the conglomeration of certain prognostic factors has decisive influence on its development.

Of the local factors, macro- and microcirculation are the two most crucial important ones, since tissues with adequate physiological

*Corresponding Author
Von-Hompesch-Street 1,
53123 Bonn, Germany
Tel: +49 228 6481861
e-mail: plastischechirurgie.bonn@malteser.de

blood supply will rarely be affected. Not only compromised macrocirculation (e.g. caused by increased tissue pressure as in a compartment syndrome), but also disorders of the microcirculation are of special relevance, as they may cause thromboembolic obstruction or reduction of the capillaries and consequently, necrosis and bone infection.

General and systemic factors, referring both to age (children suffer more frequently from hematogenous, adults from post-traumatic osteitis) and to the health status of the patient (diabetes, rheumatoid arthritis, impaired blood circulation, immunosuppression etc.) may allow opportunistic microorganisms to cause infection [8].

The amount of bacterial load is of crucial importance but secondary to the kind of bacteria involved. Elek and Conen [9] proved that in damaged tissue, 10^4 organisms per gram of tissue are required to cause infection, while in the presence of an implant, only 10^2 organisms per gram. The risk of infection increases from the first moment of tissue trauma and with any delay in the operative treatment.

Any foreign material brought into the wound that is not completely inert bears the risk of inoculation and biofilm formation by bacteria, which adhere on the implants. As bacteria form an additional protective glycocalyx inside the biofilm, they become inaccessible by antibiotics administered systemically and consequently, they establish an infection that is non-treatable by antibiotics only [8].

3. Bacteriology

There is not one typical microorganism that causes osteitis. Pyogenic organisms, as well as fungi, can be the cause of the disease; *Staphylococcus* spp. and other skin organisms are the most common, however. Statistics dealing with the spectrum of causative organisms certainly are of limited value, since in the course of the infection the original organism can be displaced by competitors. The repeated exchange of organisms and the "selection pressure" caused by long-term antibiotic treatment frequently leads to polymicrobial infections.

Staphylococcus spp. is the most common aerobic organism, followed in most statistic analyses by *Pseudomonas aeruginosa, Proteus, Streptococcus* spp., *E. coli* and polymicrobial infections. A lot of cases of bone infections caused by anaerobic organisms have been reported. Due to the special demands of the processing of wound cultures, as well as the sometimes limited efficiency of the microbiological laboratories, only the frequency of such infections can be estimated. Anaerobic organisms are often found in the osteitis material and classified in advance as "sterile" [10]. Reviewing the literature, one can find numerous reports of osteitis caused by atypical organisms.

The spectrum of organisms causing hematogenous osteitis varies among the different age groups. Group B

Streptococci, *Staphylococcus aureus* and *E. coli* are found most frequently in infants younger than 12 months; in children between 1 and 16 years *S. aureus,* group A *Streptococci* and *Haemophilus influenzae* are most common. In adults *S. aureus* is most commonly found, followed by *Staphylococcus epidermidis, E. coli, P. aeruginosa* and *Candida.* Multiple other organisms should be ruled out, however, in certain regions bacteria such as *Mycobacterium tuberculosis* or *Brucella* spp. have also been found important besides pyogen organisms [11].

Infections in the bones of the hand most often occur after injury [6]. McLain et al. [12] found infections in 11% of open fractures of the hand. The spectrum of causative microorganisms did not differ substantially from that found in investigations of infections in the long bones. Special circumstances (e.g. immunocompromise, vascular impairment, systemic illness, long- term stays in intensive care units, or special mechanisms of injury such as bites or other exposure to special microorganisms) must be considered in the differential diagnosis.

4. Hematogenous Osteomyelitis

Hematogenous osteomyelitis is predominantly an illness of infants, of whom 80% are younger than 16 years [13]. Due to the vascular continuity between the epiphysis and the metaphysis in infants younger than 1 year of age, hematogenous osteitis at that age frequently proceeds through the epiphyseal cartilage into the joint, as well as through the thin cortex into the adjacent tissue. In the maturing skeleton, the epiphyseal blood supply together with the avascular cartilage become a barrier which restrains organisms from spreading into the joint. After obliteration of the epiphyseal plates in adolescence, new anastomoses between the metaphyseal and the epiphyseal vascular systems are established, possibly facilitating spread into the joint space. Hematogenous osteitis of the radius and the ulna has an incidence of 5% [14]. Reilly reports an incidence of 13% among his patients [5].

4.1. Diagnosis

Apart from observation of the local clinical signs of the infection, non-specific laboratory studies include ESR, Creactive protein, and WBC counts. Imaging studies should include ultrasound, radiograpic s and, if necessary, MRI investigations. The specificity of the sonographic findings is 93%, the positive predictive value 92%, and the sensitivity 60%. The highest specificity has the MRI, i.e. at a percentage of 100%, while its sensitivity comes up to 90% [15]. The most important differential diagnosis in children is the primary bone tumor.

For identification of the causative microorganisms, blood cultures (positive in 50% of cases), as well as aspiration or culture specimens from abscesses or joint fluid are essential. Identification of the microorganism should then be possible in approximately 90% of cases.

The basis of therapy is parenteral antibiotic administration, which should last for 3 weeks, and be continued with oral antibiotics thereafter. The German Society for Pediatric Infectiology recommends Cefuroxim, Cefotiam or Flucloxacillin for an empirical antibiotic treatment which should be applied before isolation of the microorganism [15].

Additional surgical therapy with debridement, excision of fistula or irrigation of joints is necessary whenever abscesses, fistula, or joint empyema are present.

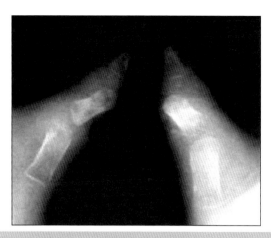

FIGURE 1. Osteitis of the thumb.

5. ACUTE OSTEITIS

The clinical term "acute osteitis" is used to signify an infection existing for up to 4 weeks, or occurring within 8 weeks after trauma. Both direct inoculations of microorganisms into the bone and/or contiguous spread from a focus of infection can be causative. *S. aureus* as the most common pathogen carries receptors (adhesins) for components of bone matrix that particularly facilitate adhesion to the bone [8]. The result is cellular inflammation and, in consequence, microthrombosis of small blood vessels, periostitis with elevation of the periosteum, osteolysis with bone marrow necrosis and finally, due to additional activation of osteoclasts, the development of a sequestrum.

The clinical findings in the early stage correspond to those of a soft-tissue infection, with the classic triad of *rubor, dolor* and *calor.* The diagnosis is particularly difficult if the infection has spread from paronychia, for instance. Therefore, it is of substantial importance to consider a bone infection if the history of the patient gives relevant indication, or if the infection persists despite antibiotic treatment. General symptoms of infection are more likely to be found in the hematogenous form.

Although leucocytosis is not always present, laboratory studies include a WBC count, as well as CRP, since they allow monitoring of the process at the same time. Identification of the causative microorganism is mandatory. However, lab results from cultures of polymicrobial infections may often deviate from clinical findings. In particular, this danger exists if the pathogen is resistant only to special substances of one group of antibiotics. False negative bacteriological findings can also result when sensitive organisms do not survive during long time intervals between sampling and culturing or when the identification is not possible because of previously applied, i.e. before sampling, systemic antibiotic treatment. When clinical suspicion arises, even sterile cultures should not exclude the diagnosis of bacterial osteitis.

Radiographic findings are not found until approximately 14 days after the onset of infection. Periosteal reactions, osteosclerosis, osteolysis or partial osteoporosis can be observed (Fig. 1).

Additional imaging studies (predominantly MRI) are most often necessary in unclear cases only (e.g., very early stages - for differential diagnosis).

6. CHRONIC OSTEITIS

The clinical term "chronic osteitis" is used if an infection lasts more than 5-7 weeks, or if the infection occurs more than 8 weeks after trauma. Typical clinical characteristics are non-healing, temporarily closing fistulae surrounded by granulation tissue and intermittent infection of the adjacent soft tissue. The fistulae are maintained by sequestrae, discharging through the fistula together with pus (Fig. 2).

6.1. Therapy

In general, conservative treatment of osteitis should only be considered in hematogenous osteomyelitis or in special situations like the very early stages of acute osteitis, as long as there is neither necrosis, melting-down tissue, nor joint affection. Treatment should include high-dose parenteral antibiotic therapy and immobilization. If this does not lead to clear improvement within a few days, surgery will be the method of choice.

Proper surgical treatment consists of debridement of the necrotic soft tissue, the necrotic parts of the bone and the inflammatory granulation tissue. The extent of the debridement will influence not only therapeutic success, but also the resulting function, since (especially in the hand) all important structures are very close to each other and also to the joints. Radical debridement means thorough resection of non-viable and/or necrotic tissue, and of granulation or scar tissue with poor blood supply. There is no indication for safety margins in the surgical

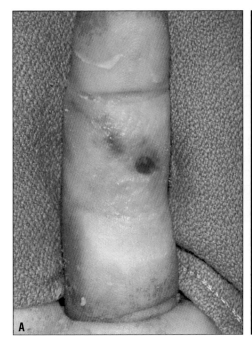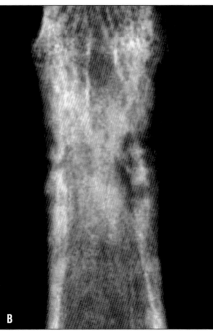

FIGURE 2. (A) Clinical aspect of a chronic osteitis with fistula. **(B)** Radiograph of the same finger with sequestrae.

treatment of osteitis of the fingers and the hand. Within the context of debridement, hydromechanical lavage is frequently necessary, in order to reduce the number of bacteria.

Every invasive treatment in a septic environment requires (ideally when the infecting organism is known) an additional local and/or systemic antibiotic therapy. Depending upon the anatomical site, Gentamicin-loaded beads or collagen sponge is used, for local antibiotic treatment.

If after debridement the bone defect is so large that

secondary bone grafting is necessary, we use the antibiotic-loaded PMMA-beads as a spacer. Otherwise, a Collagen sponge is suggested. Both carriers provide local concentration of antibiotic which is so high that even partially resistant organisms become susceptible. In a controlled study, Mendel et al. [16]. demonstrated significant reduction of organisms in an animal experiment where *Staphylococci* were apparent. Using and comparing both the carriers, the Collagen sponge proved superior to the beads. Although the additional application of Cefazolin strengthened the effect, an addi-

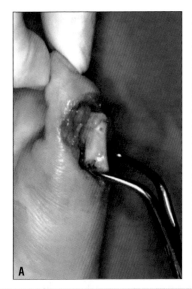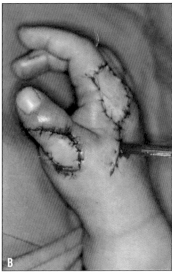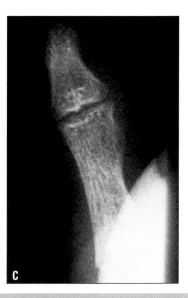

FIGURE 3. (A) Complete resection of the proximal phalanx of the thumb. **(B)** Skin cover with a Foucher's flap after filling the defect with PMMA-beads. **(C)** 5 years after reconstruction with autologous bone graft.

tional parenteral antibiotic therapy, in our opinion, is seldom if at all necessary. It may be applied only in cases of excessive infection of adjacent soft tissues.

After application of a small overflow drainage we try to close the wound without tension. Frequently, local skin flaps are used (Fig. 3). Careful and thorough debridement is important, regardless of the potential difficulty in the process of wound closure. If closure is not possible, we use an occlusive dressing (Opsite) and accomplish the definite skin closure (usually in the form of local flaps). Finally, we immobilize the hand.

Whereas many authors strongly recommend external fixation for osteitis of phalanges or metacarpals, in our experience, a simple plaster splint fixation has proven effective and thus we reckon it sufficient. If no significant improvement is obtained with this regimen within 3-4 days, revision is necessary.

In paronychia, in particular, the absence of septic arthritis of the distal interphalangeal joint should be checked. In this case, we resect the DIP joint very early and fill the defect with PMMA-beads (Fig. 4).

With any internal fixation in situ, the stabilizing effect has to be considered. Any foreign material should be removed with the exception of implants that are absolutely necessary for stabilization. Wounds in such cases should be debrided several times within a few days and controlled by examination of wound cultures in order to retain the implants until the fracture has united.

7. RESULTS

In a prospective study [17], we treated 43 patients in a period of 6 years in the way described above. The follow-up had a success rate of 100%. The ultimate goal was healing and not regaining function of the hand. Because the individual injuries were often very complex, and also function frequently improved after secondary surgery, the impairment was not evaluated.

The median age of the patients was 44 (18-72) years. In 18 cases the right hand was affected, and in 25, the left. The most frequently involved finger was the index (19 cases). In 11 patients septic arthritis appeared simultaneously. Twenty-nine patients suffered from acute, and 16 from chronic osteomyelitis. Infection occurred in 18 cases after open fractures and reimplantations, in 13 cases after paronychia, and in 12 cases after burns, osteosyntheses, or bite injuries. The time between onset of infection and surgery was a 4 weeks maximum in those cases with acute osteomyelitis, and 9 weeks (median) up to 96 weeks in the cases with chronic osteitis (Table 1).

The diagnosis of chronic osteomyelitis was made with regard to the duration of the infection (>8 weeks), if the soft tissue inflammation to a large extent had ceased and only a fistula or chronic inflammation remained; at the same time, radiological and intraoperative findings showed sequestrae, eburnation, or osteolysis. In the preoperative antibiogram *S. aureus* sensitive to Gentamycin was found in 84%, followed by polymicrobial infections of diverse organisms. In no case was Gentamycin resistance evident.

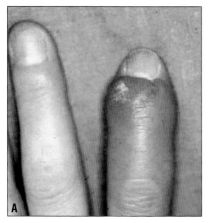
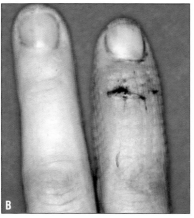

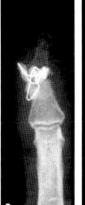
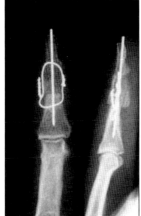
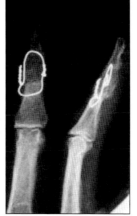

FIGURE 4. (A) Paronychia of the index finger with septic arthritis of the DIP joint. (B) 10 days after resection of the DIP joint and filling with PMMA-beads. (C) Radiographic views of the course of treatment. **Left:** Resected joint with PMMA beads. **Center:** Secondary arthrodesis with interposition of an autologous bone graft and osteosynthesis with wire suture and K-wire. **Right:** Bone union after removal of the K-wire.

In all cases, in accordance with the described standardized operation regimen, the first wound inspection after surgery took place on the second or third day. It was found that in 37 cases (86%) infection had subsided, whereas in six cases (14%) it continued.

After 14 days, 39 wounds (91%) were healed (Fig. 4a, b), while after 1 month, 42 wounds (98%). In one patient, revision with implantation of new chains was necessary due to insufficient debridement in the first place. The wound healed primarily thereafter (Table 2).

After successful treatment of the infection, in 30 cases no secondary surgery was necessary due to sufficient bone stability, and therapy was finished after 4 weeks (median).

Of 13 cases with en-bloc resections, 2 underwent surgery for a secondary stabilization and 11 for an arthrodesis (1 interphalangeal thumb joint, 5 DIP joints and 5 PIP joints). In all cases autologous bone grafts were transplanted to maintain the length of the finger. Intraosseous wire sutures were used for osteosynthesis (Fig. 4c) and all cases showed good consolidation in a time period that corresponded to the normal healing time of a primarily not infected arthrodesis. The total time of treatment with secondary operation extended to 12 weeks (median), due to the osseous consolidation or other additional injuries.

8. Conclusion

This study shows that successful treatment of osteitis of the fingers was achieved as the most substantial goal criterion after 1 month in 96% and after 1.5 months in 100% of the cases. The healing time of secondary arthrodesis was not significantly prolonged. During the follow-up period of up to 6 years there were no recurrences of infection.

TABLE 1

The sample of patients

Total number of patients	43	
Gender	Male 30	Female 13
Age (median in years)	44 (18-72)	
Location	Right 18	Left 25
Number of patients with previous operations (1-3)	17	
Acute osteomyelitis	27	
Time since onset of infection (weeks)	4 (1-4)	
Chronic osteomyelitis	16	
Time since onset of infection (weeks)	9 (8-96)	

TABLE 2

Results after treatment of acute and chronic osteomyelitis

Wound condition	Primary wound healing	Infection
2 weeks after surgery	39	4
4 weeks after surgery	42	1
6 weeks after surgery	43	–
End of treatment	**n**	**Weeks (median)**
Without secondary operation	30	4 (2-8)
With secondary operation	13	12 (12-24)

References

[1] Hauptverband der Gewerblichen Berufsgenossenschaften. BGZ Report 2/99 Arbeitsunfallstatistik, 1999.
[2] Hove LM. Fractures of the hand. Distribution and relative incidence. Scand J Plast Reconstr Surg Hand Surg 1993;27(4): 317-319.
[3] Emmett JE, Breck LW. A review and analysis of 11,000 fractures seen in a private practice of orthopaedic surgery, 1937-1956. J Bone Joint Surg [Am] 1958;40-A (5):1169-1175.
[4] Amine B et al. Chronic osteomyelitis of the metacarpals. Report of a case, Jt. Bone Spine 2005;72 (4):322-325.
[5] Reilly KE et al. Osteomyelitis of the tubular bones of the hand, J Hand Surg [Am] 1997;22(4):644-649.
[6] Stevanovic MV, Sharpe F. Acute Infections in the Hand. In: Green DP, Hotchkiss RN, Pederson WC, Wolfe SW (Eds.), Operative Hand Surgery, 5th Edition, Churchill Livingstone, New York, 2004, pp. 55-93.
[7] Duncan RW et al. Open hand fractures: an analysis of the recovery of active motion and of complications. J Hand Surg [Am] 1993; 18(3):387-394.
[8] Gristina AG, Costerton JW. Bacterial adherence to biomaterials and tissue. The significance of its role in clinical sepsis. J Bone Joint Surg [Am] 1985;67(2):264-273.
[9] Elek SD, Conen PE. The virulence of Staphylococcus pyogenes for man; a study of the problems of wound infection. Br J Exp Pathol 1957;38(6):573-586.
[10] Gunther O. Hofmann, Infektionen der Knochen und Gelenke, Elsevier, 2004.
[11] Zimmerli W, Flückiger U. Verlaufsformen und Mikrobiologie der bakteriellen Osteitis. Ortophäde 2004;33:267-272.
[12] McLain RF, Steyers C, Stoddard M. Infections in open fractures of the hand. J Hand Surg Am 1991;16(1):108-112.
[13] Dietz HG, Schmittenbecher PP, Roos R. Osteomyelitis in childhood. Monatsschr Kinderheilkd 1993;141 (8):677-688.
[14] Feigin RD, Cherry JD (Eds.), Textbook of pediatric infectious diseases. Saunders, Philadelphia, 1998.
[15] Reinehr T et al. Akute Osteomyelitis im Kindesalter. Monatsschr Kinderheilkd 1998;146:1181-1185.
[16] Mendel V et al. Therapy with Gentamicin-PMMA beads, Gentamicin-collagen sponge, and Cefazolin for experimental osteomyelitis due to Staphylococcus aureus in rats. Arch Orthop Trauma Surg 2005;125(6):363-368.
[17] Brueser P. Die Osteomyelitis im Bereich der Finger. Operative Orthopädie und Traumatologie 1993;5:60-67.

Vascularized Bone Grafts for the Treatment of Finger Osteomyelitis

Francisco DEL PIÑAL MATORRAS

Unit of Hand-Wrist and Plastic Surgery, Hospital Mutua Montañesa
and Instituto de Cirugía Plástica y de la Mano, Santander, SPAIN

Finger osteomyelitis combined with nonunion poses a challenge to hand surgeons because of the paucity of donor sites for transferring soft tissue and vascularized bone to the finger in comparison with those available for other sites of the skeleton. We present our experience in treating infected nonunion of the digits by radical debridement and immediate reconstruction by interposing vascularized bone blocks from the phalanges and metatarsals. By using this protocol we were able to clear the infection and achieve bony union in a single stage in 8 out of 9 cases. One patient required a secondary debridement. Small bone blocks taken from the toe phalanges reliably maintain their blood supply, and can be transferred and anastomosed on the digital arteries. Donor site morbidity is usually minimal, although in cases with an extended graft harvest, sacrifice of the remnant may be required.

Keywords: osteomyelitis; vascularized bone grafts; phalangeal infection; nonunion; microvascular transfers.

1. INTRODUCTION

The natural ability of the body to clear an infection depends on the interplay among local blood supply, host defenses, and the load and virulence of pathogens. Due to a "privileged" blood supply, fingers might be more resistant to infection than other parts of the body [1, 2]. As a matter of fact, osteomyelitis in the finger is a rare occurrence [3].

The foundation of treatment of osteomyelitis is based on debridement of all infected necrotic tissues, appropriate soft-tissue coverage/obliteration of dead space with flaps, and antibiotic therapy [4]. Due to their minimal soft tissue protection, which is similar to that of the ankle region, fingers are quite defenseless. Once infection is estab-

lished, there are no local flaps capable of bringing blood supply and obliterating the dead space [5]. It is not surprising hence, that posttraumatic osteomyelitis in the finger has a very poor prognosis, resulting in a more than 50% amputation rate and about 40% marked functional impairment [3].

The problem is even more complicated when there is a concomitant nonunion. Systemic antibiotics will not reach the fibrotic area, and even after control of infection, the tissue bed is so poor that conventional grafting would be very often unsuccessful. Freeland, Szabo and others [1, 2, 6] recommended a two-stage procedure: first, clearing of the infection, antibiotic impregnated beads and wound coverage, and secondly, non-vascularized bone grafting. This approach, at times successful [1, 2, 6, 7], has been found protracted or having a high failure rate [3].

Our protocol includes radical debridement and immediate bone and soft tissue reconstruction with free osteocutaneous flaps. This approach is based on Godina's and Taylor's concepts of radical debridement and vascularized bone grafting, respectively. Godina [8] proposed radical debridement and immediate coverage with free flaps in complex wounds in the extremities. Reported infection rates were low even in chronic cases. Taylor [9] introduced the vascularized bone graft as an ideal

Corresponding Author
Calderon de la Barca 16-entlo.
E- 39002-Santander. Spain
Tel: +34 942 364696.
Fax: +34 942 364702.
e-mail: drpinal@drpinal.com
        pacopinal@ono.com

method of dealing with medium-sized bone defects. Its main advantage is its rapid incorporation, similar to that of a segmental fracture. Furthermore, vascularized bone grafts resist infection, whereas similar non-vascularized bone segments would undergo resorption when infected [10]. The use of vascularized bone graft in smaller defects is reasonable in cases where failure of bone healing is likely to occur or has already occurred, such as infection or severe scarring [11-13].

2. DONOR SITES AND THE HARVESTING TECHNIQUE

The difficulty in applying this protocol is lack of available donor sites that could reliably carry small segments of vascularized bone and a compatible soft tissue paddle. Classic donor sites, such as the fibula or the scapula are impractical, and small bone graft donor sites, such as the medial condyle [14], the modified iliac crest [15], or even the radial metaphysis [16], are unable to carry a flap that suits a soft tissue defect in a finger.

Both MacFadden [17] and Isenberg [18] presented case reports in which a hemi-metatarsal was transferred successfully for reconstructing intercalated defects of the fingers. We have been able to reliably transfer small bone blocks of the toe phalanx to reconstruct complex finger defects [19]. The present study considers two donor sites for this indication: the toe phalanges and hemi- or whole metatarsal transfer.

2.1. Vascularized phalanx

The blood supply to the toes phalanges is rarely dependent on a single nutrient artery [20], but rather on tiny periosteal and capsular branches coming from the digital arteries [21, 22]. Two constant arcades encircle the neck of the proximal phalanx and the base of the middle phalanx. At the base of the proximal phalanx, branches that derive from the plantar and dorsal digital arteries and lead to the bone have been identified [21, 22].

The procedure is similar to standard toe harvesting with some particularities which are highlighted below [19]. The skin flap is designed over the bone to be harvested. Through a dorsal zigzag incision a subcutaneous vein is first dissected and isolated. The skin flap is incised on the side of the pedicle and elevated plantarwards. Taking great care is essential in order to keep intact the connections among the digital artery, the donor bone, and the vein, dorsally by including a soft tissue cuff in the vicinity of the bone. The corresponding digital nerve is separated from the digital artery, reflected plantarly, and left on the toe. The digital artery is then dissected proximally and side branches are tied off with 5/0 silk or 9/0 nylon clips, depending on their size. Traction on these tiny branches is to be avoided, as avulsion from the main digital artery may cause persistent spasm or even failure in the part to be revascularized [23]. The

digital artery is ligated distally to the bone that is to be harvested.

Once the dissection on the side of the pedicle is completed, the contralateral side is rapidly dissected out by incising the skin island and performing a subperiosteal dissection of the phalanx. The neurovascular pedicle, which would maintain the donor toe viability, does not actually need to be seen. Only nutrient branches to the bone from this pedicle need to be carefully ligated, again avoiding avulsion, as this may endanger the toe blood supply. The flexor sheath is open and the flexor tendons are reflected plantarwards. Care should be taken not to avulse the vincular tissue as this may damage the tiny rete of vessels located at this plantar aspect of the phalanx. The segment of bone to be harvested is then cut and the tourniquet released. We try to cut the exact amount of bone needed prior to disconnecting the phalanx from the toe, as afterwards it is very difficult to manipulate the small block of bone. The flap is then ready to be transferred and revascularized in the usual way (Fig. 1a).

The donor sites could be closed primarily in all cases. In our experience, the space left by the harvested bone was partially closed by axial collapse and by suturing the extensor to the flexor tendons, in a similar way to that recommended for children when non-vascularized proximal phalanx is harvested. The toe was preserved in all cases, vascularized by the contralateral pedicle (Fig. 1b inset).

2.2. Vascularized metatarsal

The metatarsals have a nutrient foramina at its distal third [21, 24], and also a rich periosteal network which is

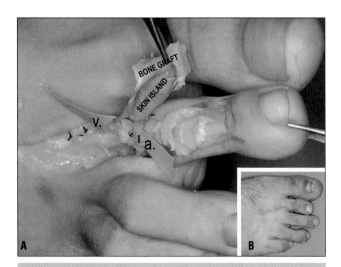

FIGURE 1. (A) A 2nd-toe middle-phalanx osteocutaneous flap elevated and pedicled on its vascular axis prior to tourniquet release (**a:** lateral plantar digital artery of the second toe; **v:** subcutaneous vein). Note that the digital nerve is not included in the flap, but preserved on the toe. **(B)** Inset: The result one year later (the hallux nail deformity is from a recent unrelated trauma).

dependent on the plantar and dorsal metatarsal arteries [24]. This vascular disposition allows harvesting a portion of the lateral aspect of the first metatarsal [17, 18], a portion of the medial aspect of the second metatarsal, or the whole of the second metatarsal [25].

The "flap elevation" technique is similar to a dorsalis pedis one, except for the fact that the first includes a piece of metatarsal. If the second metatarsal is to be fully harvested, the dorsalis pedicle is identified proximally to the web, and traced distally to the take-off of the deep plantar artery at the most proximal aspect of the web. The origin of the first dorsal metatarsal (FDMA) is identified there, and dissected out. In the vicinity of the bone to be harvested, all soft tissues lateral to this artery are left intact to protect the tiny periosteal vessels that lead to the metatarsal. Once the medial part of the dissection is completed, the lateral aspect of the metatarsal is elevated preserving only the periosteum of the bone if the whole circumference is to be included. In the case of a hemi-metatarsal, the dissection is carried over the dorsal aspect of the metatarsal, while keeping the medial attachments to the bone intact. The flap is now elevated and the tourniquet is released to let the bone be supplied with blood (Fig. 2a).

We have always used a small skin island for covering, filling the dead space and monitoring purposes. It should be borne in mind that although acceptable for a metacarpal, the thickness of the skin island would usually be too bulky for a finger.

Additionally, unless a medium size flap is to be applied (that can be designed on the axis of FDMA), a specific cutaneous perforator should be isolated and traced, or otherwise the skin island may die [26]. Technically, this is quite demanding and in order to accommodate variations, we should first incise one of the sides of the skin island, and change its location according to where a sizable skin perforator is located (Fig. 2b).

The flap is useless if the first dorsal metatarsal artery is absent (Gilbert type III) [27]. Moreover, although the bony portion will be vascularized when FDMA is located deep among the interosseous muscles (Gilbert Type II), the cutaneous paddle will not, and therefore, the use of the flap will be impracticable. Based on our experience in toe harvesting, we have noticed that Doppler is very helpful to define when FDMA is absent. It is, however, unable to differentiate a medium-sized superficially located FDMA from a normal-sized, but deep FDMA. So if there is a preoperative doubt about its presence, it is my opinion that it is wiser to try the other foot or a different donor site.

Traditionally, the dorsalis pedis is considered a second-line flap due to its significant donor site morbidity, in case a large skin flap is required. This is usually not the case for this specific application, and minimal morbidity exists only when a portion of a metatarsal is harvested (Fig. 2c). The second toe may need to be removed if a large amount of bone is needed.

3. PLANNING AND OPERATIVE PROCEDURE

3.1. Pre-operative considerations

Preoperative plain X-rays of both hands and both feet (PA in standing position) are essential. There are considerable variations in the length of the middle phalanx among patients, and sometimes, between the two feet. With the help of tracing paper, the expected bone defect is transposed to the donor site and the appropriate phalanx is elevated [23].

FIGURE 2. (A) Preoperative planning of the second hemimetarsal flap. **(B)** Flap raised. Notice that the skin island is located slightly distal to include a cutaneous perforator. Bone block is marked by arrows. **(C)** Donor site one year later. The defect in the second metatarsal has remodeled spontaneously.

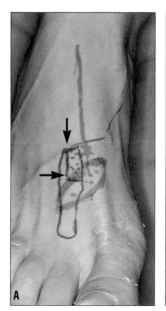
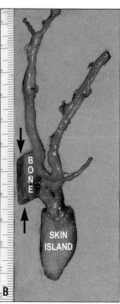
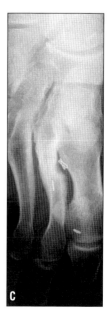

As a rule, the middle phalanx is the preferred donor site [19] as it gives the longer pedicle. Prior to its seperation from the intermetatarsal arteries, it is possible to dissect 3-4 cm of the arterial pedicle. The anastomosis of a digital artery should be carried out away from the area of the injury. Conversely, the proximal phalanx, especially if the base is to be harvested, yields a much shorter pedicle (1 to 1.5 cm of digital artery) unless the dissection proceeds proximally towards one of the metatarsal arteries. Inclusion of the parent metatarsal artery may not be beneficial as there could be major discrepancies in terms of size, compared with that of the recipient digital artery. This may be, above all, true if the dorsal metatarsal is absent (Gilbert type III), since in this case the first plantar metatarsal artery would be much more compensatory, creating a size discrepancy with the proper digital artery. For long defects we use the proximal phalanx, and only for extremely long defects, the metatarsal. Further considerations when choosing the donor site are of the need for vascularized cartilage [28] and/or skin requirements. The surgeon should be prepared to alter the plan once the definitive amount of bone is known intraoperatively.

3.2. Debridement

The bone is approached through the wound in the acute situation and through the sinus and/or previous scars in cases of chronic osteomyelitis. The sinus is excised, and any marginally viable flap, removed en block. Granulated, scarred, or denaturalized soft tissue is excised as recommended by Godina [8]. Deep cultures are taken from the bone and deep granulation tissue. The bone is excised until clear, viable, healthy tissue is met, that being the single most important step of this procedure. Ideally, in that stage no antibiotics are given. However, most of the cases examined so far involved use of antibiotics as prescribed by referring physicians. This may increase the chance of obtaining false negative cultures. The tourniquet is deflated at this stage to ensure blood supply to the bone.

3.3. Fitting and donor site closure

The flap is harvested as explained previously. It is stabilized in position by using the most convenient method, regardless of whether a previous infection had occurred in the same place. Nevertheless, K-wires (1.0 or 0.8 mm) or combinations of cerclage wire and K-wire are preferred, in order to minimally inhibit the blood supply to both the recipient and the donor bone. In the vicinity of a joint, lag-screws are preferred. The skin flap is presutured in position. The vessels are placed through subcutaneous tunnels to their recipient site. According to our experience, in the case of toe phalanges most anastomoses are carried out end-to-end, between a toe digital artery and a finger digital artery. Occasionally, a short stump of FDMA is used as a donor and anastomosed in a similar way. The veins are sutured in the web

end-to-end to a local vein. The metacarpals are pedicled on the dorsalis pedis and vena comitantes. These are sutured end-to-side to the radial artery, and end-to-end to comitants or a subcutaneous vein, respectively.

3.4. Postoperative care

Patients are administered wide-spectrum intravenous antibiotics until cultures are available, and if an identifiable organism is detected, antibiotics are changed accordingly. Within a week, in most instances, IV antibiotic therapy is discontinued and a specific oral antibiotic (Ciprofloxacin or Amoxicilin-clavulanic) is prescribed for a total of 15 days in acute infections to 4 weeks in chronic cases. Dressings are changed frequently and self-adhered compressive wrap (Coban® type) is applied afterwards, from the 5th to the 7th day, in an attempt to reduce inflammation.

The adjacent joints are mobilized after the first week. K-wires are removed no later than the 5th week, depending on the clinical presentation of union.

Patients are allowed to walk in a postoperative stiff sole shoe after 2 or 3 days when a toe phalanx is harvested, and after the third week when a metatarsal is harvested.

4. Author's Experience and Results

We have treated 4 acute and 5 chronic digital osteomyelitis cases with concomitant bony defect (11 mm to 5 cm) with the protocol indicated above (Fig. 3, 4). Defects were located at the metacarpal (1 case), the proximal phalanx (3 cases), and the vicinity of the DIP joint (5 cases). In all instances there was an associated soft tissue defect that was treated with a compound bone-soft tissue flap: 1 second metatarsal (for the longest defect), 1 hemi-second metatarsal, 3 portions of the proximal phalanx of the second toe, 3 middle-phalanxes of a second toe, and finally, 1 entire proximal phalanx and a portion of the middle phalanx of the second toe. No intraoperative or vascular complications occurred. Bony bleeding manifested itself intraoperatively in all cases. The skin island survived. Infection in an acutely infected case recurred six weeks after the operation in the distal graft-phalanx junction site, most probably as a consequence of an inadequate debridement of the distal phalanx. The infection was controlled by a new debridement, cancellous bone grafting, and a four-week course of IV antibiotic administration. The infected distal nonunion healed uneventfully, attesting to the robust blood supply of the transferred toe phalanx [10]. In another case (the second hemimetarsal), the distal bone graft-distal phalanx junction, although stable and asymptomatic, failed to show bony trabeculae crossing the junction. No finger required amputation, and in no other case the infection recurred.

Regarding the toes, only in two cases (second metatarsal, combined proximal and middle phalanx) was

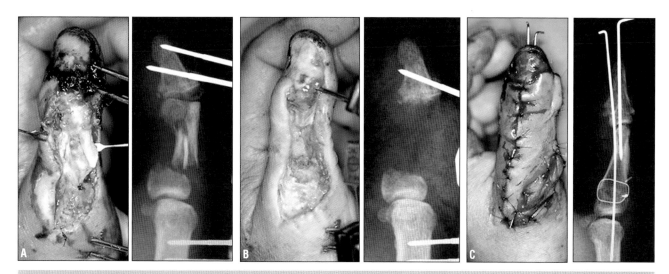

FIGURE 3. A 32 year-old male was referred 3 weeks after sustaining a crush to his thumb with severe osseous comminution. He developed purulent infection. **(A)** Infected bone and necrotic tissue were excised radically. **(B)** At a single stage, a compound osteocutaneous flap that included the entire proximal phalanx and a portion of the middle second toe was transferred. **(C)** The patient has been free of infection for 9 years.

the second toe amputated, otherwise it was shortened as explained before.

5. DISCUSSION – CONCLUSIONS

The common approach in an osteomyelitis case with nonunion is radical debridement and reconstruction with a well-vascularized osseous flap. When located in a fin-

ger, there is paucity of donor sites for transferring soft tissue and vascularized bone. The toe phalanges have constant blood supply, can give a small to moderate-size flap (our largest is 5 x 2.5 cm without sacrificing the toe), and the donor site morbidity is minimal when the toe is preserved. In our recent experience of 9 vascularized toe phalanges [19] the blood supply to the bone was reliable. The donor toe could be preserved slightly shortened, in seven out of nine cases.

The dissecting technique is demanding. When the

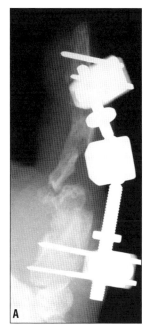
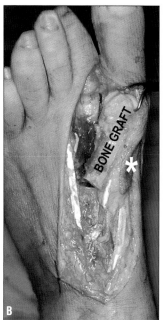
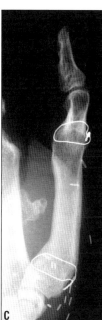

FIGURE 4. (A) A 52-year-old male was referred 3 months after sustaining a crush to his thumb. The proximal pins were discharging pus. In a single stage, the infected-scarred tissues (including the infected proximal pin tracks) were excised. **(B)** A 5-cm segment of the metatarsal was used to span the defect. **(C)** The patient has been free of infection for 10 years.

defect is longer than the length of a proximal phalanx, then a second metatarsal is our choice. The dissecting technique is easier than the phalanxone, but there is the risk of not having sufficient feeding vessels to nourish the bone when the graft is small. We were able to clear the infection in a sigle stage in 8 out of 9 cases, and move on to a second stage in the 9th. We highly recommend the technique of debridement and immediate application of vascularized bone graft for the difficult scenario of infected nonunion and osteomyelitis in the fingers.

REFERENCES

[1] Freeland AE, Senter BS. Septic arthritis and osteomyelitis. Hand Clin 1989;5:533-552.

[2] Szabo RM, Spiegel JD. Infected fractures of the hand and wrist. Hand Clin 1988;4:477-489.

[3] Reilly KE, Linz JC, Stern PJ, Giza E, Wyrick JD. Osteomyelitis of the tubular bones of the hand. J Hand Surg [Am] 1997;22:644-649.

[4] Anthony JP, Mathes SJ. Update on chronic osteomyelitis. Clin Plast Surg 1991;18:515-523.

[5] Kakinoki R, Ikeguchi R, Nakamura T. Second dorsal metacarpal artery muscle flap: an adjunct in the treatment of chronic phalangeal osteomyelitis. J Hand Surg [Am] 2004;29:49-53.

[6] Barbieri RA, Freeland AE. Osteomyelitis of the hand. Hand Clin 1998;14:589-603.

[7] Proubasta IR, Itarte JP, Lamas CG, Majo JB. The spacer block technique in osteomyelitis of the phalangeal bones of the hand. Acta Orthop Belg 2004;70:162-165.

[8] Godina M. Early microsurgical reconstruction of complex trauma of the extremities. Plast Reconstr Surg 1986;78:285-292.

[9] Taylor GI. The current status of free vascularized bone grafts. Clin Plast Surg 1983;10:185-209.

[10] Low CK, Pho RW, Kour AK, Satku K, Kumar VP. Infection of vascularized fibular grafts. Clin Orthop 1996;323:163-172.

[11] Sakai K, Doi K, Kawai S. Free vascularized thin corticoperiosteal graft. Plast Reconstr Surg 1991;87:290-298.

[12] Mattar JrR, Azze RJ, Castro Ferreira M, et al. Vascularized fibular graft for management of severe osteomyelitis of the upper extremity. Microsurgery 1994;15:22-27.

[13] Gonzalez del Pino J, Bartolome del Valle E, Graña GL, Villanova JF. Free vascularized fibular grafts have a high union rate in atrophic nonunions. Clin Orthop 2004;419:38-45.

[14] Doi K, Oda T, Soo-Heong T, Nanda V. Free vascularized bone graft for nonunion of the scaphoid. J Hand Surg [Am] 2000;25:507-519.

[15] Harpf C, Gabl M, Reinhart C, Schoeller T, Bodner G, Pechlaner S, Piza-Katzer H, Hussl H. Small free vascularized iliac crest bone grafts in reconstruction of the scaphoid bone: a retrospective study in 60 cases. Plast Reconstr Surg 2001;108:664-674.

[16] Zaidemberg C, Siebert JW, Angrigiani C. A new vascularized bone graft for scaphoid nonunion. J Hand Surg [Am] 1991;16: 474-478.

[17] McFadden JA. Vascularized partial first metatarsal transfer for the treatment of phalangeal osteomyelitis. J Reconstr Microsurg 1998; 14:309-312.

[18] Isenberg JS. Additional experience with hemi-metatarsal vascularized bone transfer for treatment of phalangeal osteomyelitis. J Reconstr Microsurg 2000;16:547-551.

[19] Piñal F del, García-Bernal JF, Delgado J, Sanmartín M, Regalado J. Vascularized bone blocks from the toe phalanx to solve complex intercalated defects in the fingers. J Hand Surg [Am] 2006;31: 1075-1082.

[20] Mysorekar VR, Nandedkar AN. Diaphysial nutrient foramina in human phalanges. J Anat 1979;128:315-322.

[21] Yoshizu T, Watanabe M, Tajima T. Étude expérimentale et applications cliniques des transferts libres d'articulation d'orteil avec anastomoses vasculaires. In: R. Tubiana (ed.), Traite de chirurgie de la main. Vol 2. Paris: Masson,1984, pp. 539-551.

[22] Chen YG, Cook PA, McClinton MA, Espinosa RA, Wilgis EF. Microarterial anatomy of the lesser toe proximal interphalangeal joints. J Hand Surg 1998;23:256-260.

[23] Piñal F del. The indications for toe transfer after "minor" finger injuries. J Hand Surg [Br] 2004;29:120-129.

[24] Shereff MJ, Yang QM, Kummer FJ. Extraosseous and intraosseous arterial supply to the first metatarsal and metatarsophalangeal joint. Foot Ankle 1987;8:81-93.

[25] MacLeod AM, Robinson DW. Reconstruction of defects involving the mandible and floor of mouth by free osteo-cutaneous flaps derived from the foot. Br J Plast Surg 1982;35:239-246.

[26] Man D, Acland RD. The microarterial anatomy of the dorsalis pedis flap and its clinical applications. Plast Reconstr Surg 1980;65: 419-423.

[27] Gilbert A. Composite tissue transfer from the foot: Anatomic basis and surgical technique. In: Daniller AJ, Strauch B, eds. Symposium on microsurgery. St Louis: Mosby, 1976, pp. 230-242.

[28] Piñal F del, García-Bernal JF, Delgado J, Regalado J, Sanmartín M. Reconstruction of the distal radius facet by a free vascularized osteochondral autograft: anatomic study and report of a case. J Hand Surg [Am] 2005;30:1200-1214.

chapter
36

Use of the Upper Tibial Corticoperiosteal Flap for Wrist Arthrodesis in Septic Conditions

Christophe MATHOULIN*, Alain GILBERT

Institut de la Main, Clinique JOUVENET, Paris, France

Progress in microsurgery has allowed the use of free or pedicled vascularized bone grafts with significant success rates. We use a free transfer of upper tibial corticoperiosteal flap for wrist arthrodesis in septic conditions. A corticocancellous flap from the anterolateral aspect of the upper third of the tibia can be used for the reconstruction of bone defect. Blood supply to the tibial diaphysis included in the flap is provided by the superior musculo-periosteal vessels. The incision on the anterolateral part of the tibia is vertical, straight, and 15-20 cm long. We used this technique in 3 cases where it was decided to perform a wrist arthrodesis with septic conditions. The patients were 3 men. The mean age was 45 (range 36 - 55). The etiologies were 2 ballistic injuries and 1 traffic injury, with sepsis in all cases. Our average follow-up was 5 years (range 3-7 years). Union was obtained in all cases on an average of 4 months (range 3-5 months). This procedure allowed the replacement of an infected poorly vascularized area by sterile bone with a good, physiologic blood supply.

Keywords: bone-loss; sepsis; vascularized bone graft; wrist arthrodesis.

1. INTRODUCTION

The close relationship between preservation of bone vascularization and bone union is well known. In the past twenty years, progress in microsurgery has allowed the use of free or pedicled vascularized bone grafts with significant success rates. Pedicled transfers were first used for lower limbs [1- 5]. For the upper limbs, Judet [3, 6] was the first to describe the use of a pedicled graft for the treatment of scaphoid nonunion.

With the development of microsurgery, free transfers were first described by Taylor [7]. Numerous clinical reports have confirmed the application of those methods [8-19]. The value of vascularized bone graft for the management of bone-loss in septic conditions is well known. This procedure allows the replacement of infected poorly vascularized bone by sterile bone with physiologic blood supply [19, 20]. We use a free transfer of the upper tibial corticoperiosteal flap for wrist arthrodesis in septic conditions. The dimensions of this flap could be 10.0 cm wide and 35 cm long.

2. TECHNIQUE

A corticocancellous flap harvested from the anterolateral aspect of the upper third of the tibia can be used for the reconstruction of bone defect.

2.1. Anatomical basis

Blood supply to the tibial metaphysis included in

*Corresponding Author

Institut de la Main, Clinique Jouvenet

6 square Jouvenet

75016 Paris, France

e-mail: mathoulin@wanadoo.fr

the flap is provided from the branches of the recurrent volar tibial artery, anterior metaphyseal and postero-lateral arteries [21]. Blood supply to the tibial diaphysis included in the flap is provided by 1 to 3 superior musculo-periosteal vessels with an average diameter of 2 mm. Dissection must be meticulous using magnifying devices (Fig. 1).

2.2. Technique

The patient is supine, with a tourniquet and an elevated buttock, making internal rotation possible. The incision on the anterolateral part of the tibia is vertical, straight, and 15-20 cm long. The incision starts 4 cm above the knee and is centered on Gerdy's tubercle. It proceeds towards the superficial fascia between the tibialis anterior and Extensor Digitorum Longus tendon. The proximal insertions of the two muscles are detached from the bone. The recurrent anterior tibial artery and the two proximal nerve branches for the tibialis anterior are separated. The anterior tibial vascular bundle is dissected over 7-10 cm, up to the last muscle-periosteal branch to the tibialis anterior. The nerve is separated from the artery.

The cortico-periosteal flap is then outlined on the cortex of the tibia. A flap up to 10 cm long can be harvested. The dimensions of this flap could be 10.0 cm in width and 35 cm in length. The borders of the cortical flap are cut with a small oscillating saw. Great care is taken in order not to damage the pedicle. The flap is then isolated on its vascular pedicle. The anterior tibial artery is ligated by its distal end to the flap. Once the pedicle is completely dissected, the bone is free (Fig. 2). Hemostasis must be very precise because the donor site can create a hematoma after this dissection. The tourniquet is released and bone circulation is checked. The pedicle must then be cut, dipped into heparinized saline, and transferred to the recipient area.

After raising the flap, the proximal muscle insertions are used to cover the donor area with a suction drain placed between the muscle and the bone. The skin is closed directly. Compressive bandages prevent a haematoma.

After preparation of the wrist, cleaning and harvesting surrounding infected tissues, the bone flap is placed into the bone loss and fixed by K-wires. The wrist arthrodesis will be fixed around the flap in accordance with the local soft tissue condition (K-wires, external fixator, plates, screws, etc.). Then an end-to-end anastomosis is performed between the anterior tibial artery and the dorsal radial artery. The vein is then sutured to the largest dorsal vein of the wrist. A cast is applied to achieve union.

3. RESULTS

We used this technique in 3 cases in which we decided to perform a wrist arthrodesis in septic condition. The

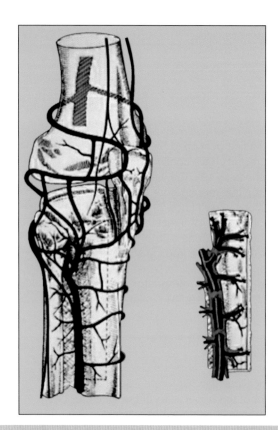

FIGURE 1. The upper tibial corticoperiosteal flap is vascularized by the branches of the anterior.

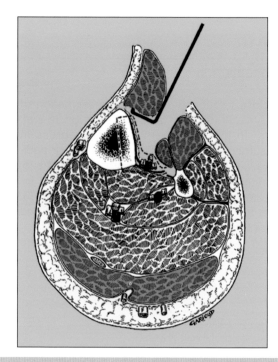

FIGURE 2. The approach is anterior, lifting the anterior tibial muscle.

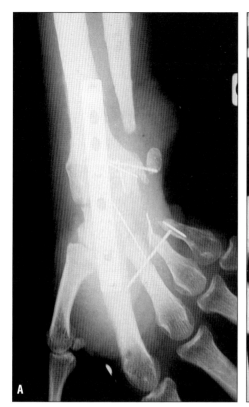 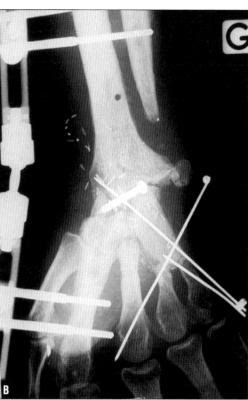

FIGURE 3. (A) Large wrist bone defect after ballistic injury. **(B)** Wrist arthrodesis with the vascularized upper tibial corticoperiosteal flap.

patients were 3 men. The mean age was 45 years (range: 36 - 55). The etiologies were 2 ballistic injuries and 1 traffic injury, with sepsis in all cases. All patients had undergone an average of 2 additional operations prior to vascularized bone grafting (range: 1-4).

The reconstructed bone segment was fixed by external fixators in 2 cases and with simple K-Wires in the third case. A cast was always placed below the elbow to achieve the union. Our average follow-up was 5 years (range: 3-7 years). The union was obtained in all cases on an average of 4 months (range: 3-5 months) (Fig. 3, 4). We did not have any problem with the donor-site, and the patients could walk the day after the surgery.

4. DISCUSSION

Bone vascularization is based on 4 interconnected arterial systems, whose specific roles have not been clearly determined yet: (i) the nutrient artery, (ii) the epiphyseal arteries, (iii) the metaphyseal arteries and (iv) the periosteal arterial network. This arterial system was first identified by Lexer [22] and was described in more detail by Brookes [23]. Although the metaphyseal and the epiphyseal networks are marked in children, Brookes feels that periosteal vascularization is not significant and that only the nutrient artery is necessary in long bone transfers. Johnson [24] showed that periosteal vascula-

rization could provide vascularization in at least 1/3 of the cortex. Also, there is microcirculation across the cortex for the bone marrow, the endosteal network and the periosteal network [25, 26]. Ostrup [27] provided experimental evidence of persistent living osteocytes during vascular transfers.

The first pedicled vascularized grafts were applied in 200 BC in India to repair facial mutilations and were reported in a Sanskrit text "the sushrista shamita" [28]. Phelps [29] and Curtis [30] developed the modern technique. Huntington [31] performed the first pedicled transfer of the homolateral fibula to reconstruct a tibial defect.

The value of vascularized bone graft for bone replacement in septic conditions is well-known. This procedure allows the replacement of the bone loss by sterile bone with intact blood supply [19]. The soft tissue around the infected bone site is often a challenge for the surgeon contemplating reconstruction in septic conditions. Dead space obliteration and skin closure may be difficult to achieve successfully. Thus, performing successful vascular anastomoses may also be a challenge because there is fibrosis around the arteries and the veins. Moreover, rigid internal fixation with screws and plates, and supplementary cancellous bone grafting are usually avoided in this setting because there is risk of exacerbation or promoting persistence of infection.

In 1992, Han et al. from Mayo clinic [32] reported a series with chronic osteomyelitis. A total of 60 patients

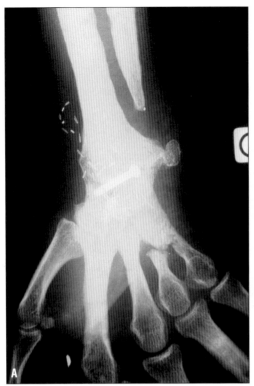

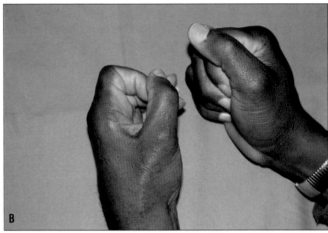

FIGURE 4. (A) Union was obtained after 4 months. **(B)** Clinical result after 3 years. Flexion allows normal use of the hand.

suffering form chronic osteomyelitis, underwent aggressive resection of obviously infected bone and soft tissue, followed by vascularized bone or osteocutaneous flap transfer for its management. All patients in this series had undergone multiple prior unsuccessful debridement and reconstruction procedures, and for practical purposes, they were considered candidates for amputations. Despite this fact, the overall success rate using vascularized bone grafting for osteomyelitis treatment is not strikingly different from rates with other indications. Following secondary bone grafting, a final union rate of 77% (46 out of 60 patients) was reported. Modest results were also reported by Weiland [18]. Of the rest, 60% experienced union with no evidence of further infection.

In our series, the infection was not so severe, and therefore, our results were better than those of using treatment of long bone osteomyelitis. We had union in all of the cases, but our series was very small. This procedure allows the replacement of infected poorly vascularized area by sterile bone with good, physiologic blood supply.

5. CONCLUSION

The use of a free transfer of upper tibial corticoperiosteal flap for wrist arthrodesis in septic conditions is a good and reliable procedure. This corticocancellous flap from the anterolateral aspect of the upper third of the tibia is vascularized by the superior musculo-pe-

riosteal vessels. This procedure, which must remain exceptional, allowed the replacement of infected poorly vascularized area by sterile bone with good, physiologic blood supply.

REFERENCES

[1] Blair VP. Surgery and diseases of the mouth and jaws. A pratical treatise on the surgery and disease of the mouth and allied structures. 3rd ed, Mosmy, Saint Louis, 1917.

[2] Harmon PH. A simplified surgical approach to the posterior tibia for bone grafting and fibular transference. Bone Joint Surg 1945;27:496-8.

[3] Judet R. Roy-Camille R. Fractures et pseudarthroses du scaphoide carpien. Utilisation d'un greffon vascularise. Actualite de Chirurgie Orthopedique 1964;4:196-214.

[4] Medgyesi S. Healing of muscle pedicle bone grafts. Acta Orthop Scand 1965;35:294-9.

[5] Medgyesi S. Observations on pedicle bone grafts in goats. Sandinavian Plast Reconstr Surg 1973;7:110-5.

[6] Judet R, Patel A. Muscle pedicle bone grafting of longbones by ostoperiosteal decortication. Clinic Orthop 1972; 87: 74-9.

[7] Taylor GI, Daniel RK. The anatomy of several free flap donor sites. Plast Reconstr Surg 1975;56:243-51.

[8] Bell DR. Congenital forarm pseudarthrosis: report 6 cases. Journal of Pediatr Orthop 1989;9:438-43

[9] Berggren A, Weiland AJ, Dorfman H. Free vascularized bone grafts: factors affecting their survival and ability to heal recipient bone defects. Plast Reconstr Surg 1982;64-A:799-811.

[10] Doi K, Tomina S, Shibata T. Bone grafts with microvascular

anastomosis of vascular pedicles. An experimental study. Bone Joint Surg 1977;59-A:809-15.

[11] Gilbert A. Surgical technique: vascularized transfer of the fibular shaft. International Journal of Microsurgery, 1979;1:100-2

[12] Goldberg VM, Shaffer JW, Field G, Davy DT. Biology of vascularized bone grafts. Orthop Clin 1987;18: 197-205.

[13] Haw CS, O'Brien BM, Kurata T. The microsurgical revascularization of resected segments of tibia in the dog. Bone Joint Surg 1978;60-B:266-9.

[14] Mathoulin C, Gilbert A, Azze RG. Congenital pseudarthrosis of the forearm. Microsurgery 1993;13:252-9.

[15] Shaffer JW, Field GA, Goldberg VM, Davy DT. Fate of vascularized and non vascularized autografts. Clinic Orthopaedic 1985;197: 32-43.

[16] Weiland AJ, Daniel RK. Microvascular anastomosis for bone grafts in the treatment of massive defects in bone. Bone and Joint Surg 1979;61A:98-104.

[17] Weiland AJ. Vascularized free bone transplants. Bone and Joint Surg 1981;63A:166-9.

[18] Weiland AJ. Clinical applications of vascularized bone grafts in Friedlaender GE, Goldberg VM (Eds), "Bone and Cartilage allografts", American Academy of Orthopaedic Surgeons, Park Ridge, IL 1991;239-45.

[19] Wood MB, Cooney WP III. Vascularized bone segment transfers for management of chronic osteomyelitis. Orthop Clin 1984;15:461-72.

[20] Wood MB, Gilbert A. (Eds) Microvascular Bone Reconstruction. Martin Dunitz, London, UK, 1997.

[21] Sanguina M, Perrotta R, Brunelli F, Gilbert A, Lassau JP. Upper tibial corticocancellous flap. Anatomy 1993;111-2.

[22] Lexer E, Kuliga P, Turek W. Unstersuchumgen uber knochenarterien. Hirchwald, Berlin, 1904.

[23] Brookes M. The blood supply of bone. Butter worth, London, 1971.

[24] Johnson RW. A physiological study of the blood supply of the diaphysis. Bone Joint Surg 1927;9:153-94.

[25] De Bruyn PPH., Breen PC, Thomas TB. The microcirculation of the bone marrow. Anatomy Reconstr 1970;168:55-68.

[26] Lopez-Curto JA, Bassingthwaighte JB, Kelly PJ. Anatomy of the microvasculature of the tibial diaphysis of the adult dog. Bone Joint Surg 1980;62A:1362-9.

[27] Ostrüp LT, Frede Rickso NJM. Distant transfer of a free living bone graft by miscrovascular anastomosis. An experimental study. Plast Reconstr Surg 1974;54:274-85.

[28] Flye MW Immunosuppressive therapy. In MX FLYE (Ed.). Principles of organ tranplantation. Saunders, Philadelphia 1989;155-75.

[29] Phelps AM Transplantation of tissue from lower animal to man. Medical Records 1891;39:221.

[30] Curtis BF, Morrey MD. Cases of bone implantation and transplantation for cyst of tibia, ostomyelitic carities and ununited fractures. Am Medi Science 1893;106:30.

[31] Huntington TW. Case of bone transference, use of segment of tibia to supply a defect in the tibia. Ann Surg 1905;4:249-51.

[32] Han CS, Wood MB, Bishop AT, Cooney WT III. Vascularized bone transfer. Journal of Bone and Joint Surgery 1992;74A: 1441-9.

Open Contaminated Wounds with Soft Tissue Loss: Management with Microvascular Flaps

Panayotis N. SOUCACOS[a*], Elizabeth O. JOHNSON[b]

[a]Department of Orthopaedic Surgery, University of Athens, School of Medicine,
Athens, Greece
[b]Department of Anatomy-Histology-Embryology, University of Ioannina,
School of Medicine, Ioannina, Greece

The vast majority of infections of the upper extremity can be successfully managed conservatively, with the use of antibiotics and immobilization. Radical surgical debridement of severe, necrotizing infections is frequently faced with compound defects which in turn, then require a series of complex reconstructive procedures. Free tissue transfer is one of the more recent techniques in the still rapidly growing armamentarium of microsurgery. Free tissue transfers allow for a one-stage reconstruction of a complex defect with concomitant functional reconstructive procedures, providing a powerful tool for the experienced microsurgeon. With the use of free flaps the goal is not only to effectively cover the wound, but also provide a solid blood supply to help vitalize the contaminated area. Moreover, the free flap serves as a clean umbrella that covers the damaged soft tissue below, allowing for secondary reconstruction procedures, when necessary.

Keywords: debridement; forearm flap; scapular flap; lateral arm flap; dorsalis pedis flap.

1. INTRODUCTION

In the 1960s, Jacobson and Suarez demonstrated that with the use of the operating microscope and refined techniques, the fine work necessary to facilitate the anastomosis of small vessels less than 1 mm in diameter was possible [1]. The use of magnification along with micro-instruments and micro-sutures opened a new era in surgery, with the establishment of a new discipline called Microsurgery. This marked the end of conventional surgery for cases of major trauma of the upper and lower extremities. After the beginning of microsurgical repair of small arteries of the digits and hands, which subsequently resulted in successful reimplantation [2-5], microsurgical composite tissue transplantation began in the 1970s and still continues to evolve. Free tissue transfers have now become routine, used alone or as part of a series of reconstructive procedures. Complex combined treatment including simultaneous management of fractures and associated soft tissue injury, "an orthoplastic approach", is now accepted for the management of complex upper extremity wounds. In this regard, the timely repair of the soft tissues with the use of free flaps, allows for optimal management of the bony and soft tissue, as well as it enables other secondary reconstructive procedures to take place [6].

Tissue coverage in the upper extremity can be

*Corresponding Author
Department of Orthopaedic Surgery
General University Hospital Attikon
Rimini 1, 12462, Haidari, Greece
Fax: +30 210 8152818
e-mail: psoukakos@ath.forthnet.gr
      soukakos@panafonet.gr

in the form of a skin graft, local tissue transfer, adjacent tissue transfer, regional tissue transfer or a free tissue transfer. The later represents the most complex of the surgical procedures and constitutes a powerful solution to complex soft tissue problems, particularly those complicated by infection. Hand infections with soft tissue loss and bony involvement are now treatable conditions.

1.1. Open contaminated wounds of the upper extremity

A large proportion of infections of the upper extremity can be successfully managed conservatively, with the use of antibiotics and immobilization. To date, cases that require minimal surgical intervention usually heal with no significant tissue deficits [7]. In contrast, however, patients with chronic posttraumatic wounds, or those with risk factors, including chronic renal insufficiency, diabetes mellitus, necrotizing infections may result in severe complex tissue loss [8-10].

Severe soft-tissue infections of the upper extremity are frequently associated with extensive necrosis of the surrounding tissues, including skin, muscles, nerves, vessels, tendons and bone. The primary goal in managing these complex acute or chronic defects has centered on infection control and limb salvage. In this regard, the first and most crucial step in the treatment of these severe soft-tissue infections is based on radical debridement of all necrotic tissue.

Traditional means of management of severe soft-tissue infections of the upper extremity required prolonged hospitalization with high cost. Despite extensive efforts, these attempts were frequently associated with significant loss of function and unstable wound coverage. Routinely, management focused on conservative topical wound treatment, once radical debridement of the infected tissues was achieved. Only after there was successful control of the infection, surgical reconstruction was attempted. Wound coverage was usually achieved with a split thickness skin graft on a granulating wound bed or a local flap for smaller areas [11-13]. The application of vacuum sealing (Vacuum-Assisted Closure) which induces granulation more rapidly has also been used as a supportive means of temporarily managing the tissue defect until a split-thickness graft or distant pedicle flap could be applied [14-16]. Overall, this type of management is characterized by multiple operative steps to reach the final result [11, 12].

More recently, energy has been focused on early definitive wound closure with one-stage reconstruction in order to reduce hospitalization and improve the functional outcome [17-20]. Recent advances in microsurgery has allowed for successful reconstruction of very complex defects after infection, with good results regarding control of infection, functional outcome, patient satisfaction and hospitalization time [21-23].

Free tissue transfer is one of the more recent techniques in the still rapidly growing armamentarium of microsurgery. Free tissue transfers allow for a one-stage reconstruction of a complex defect with concomitant functional reconstructive procedures, providing a powerful tool for the experienced microsurgeon [17, 24]. With the use of free flaps the goal is not only to effectively cover the wound, but also provide a solid blood supply to help vitalize the contaminated area. Moreover, the free flap serves as a clean umbrella that covers the damaged soft tissue below, allowing for secondary reconstruction procedures, when necessary.

2. General Considerations for the Use of Free Flaps for Contaminated Wounds

Although free flaps have been used in emergency reconstruction cases, they are more frequently used as a late procedure to cover extensive skin and soft tissue defects in upper and lower extremities, particularly to cover skin defects in open type IIIb and IIIc compound fractures. The more commonly used flaps are the latissimus dorsi muscle flap, the forearm flap, the scapular flap, the lateral arm flap and dorsalis pedis flap.

A vascularized free flap provides coverage of the wound area, as well a good blood supply to ensure viability. In addition to providing coverage and promoting healing of the wound, a good vascularized free flap also provides an adequate skin roof for secondary reconstructive procedures of either bony or soft tissue elements. The abundant blood supply provided by the flap is directed to two targets; to the flap itself and to the contaminated area.

Good candidates for vascularized flaps are those that have a pedicle that has good vessel length and diameter and is easily accessible for harvesting. Among these, are included the scapular flap, the lateral arm flap, the forearm flap, the posterior interosseous flap, the rectus abdominis flap, the dorsalis pedis flap, the homodigital or heterdigital island flap, and the venous flap. Of these, certain flaps have characteristics that make them more suitable for coverage in open contaminated wounds of the upper extremity. Characteristics of the free flap which are preferred for the upper extremity include thinness, pliability, hairlessness, non-bulkiness and proprioceptive sensibility. These requirements differ to a certain degree depending on the anatomical region of the upper extremity, in particular, for those to be applied proximal to the wrist and those for the hand and digits.

Coverage of defects in the forearm may be achieved using several different flaps. However, the most frequently used are the lateral arm and dorsalis pedis flaps for small defects and the scapular flap for medium-sized defects. The contralateral radial forearm flap, the groin flap or the latissimus dorsi flap can be used for more extensive tissue loss. It is important to note that some flaps, including the lateral arm, the radial forearm and the groin, as well as the free vascularized fibula, can also provide osteocutaneous tissue for composite tissue loss for combined bone and soft tissue defects. Forearm wounds that are too extensive to be covered by conventional type of flap or those with an inadequate recipient bed are good candidates for free vascularized soft tissue transfer. The use of a free flap provides two significant benefits in this case: the extremity does not need to be immobilized in a dependent position (as for a pedicle flap) that facilitates rehabilitation, and new vascularity is brought to the area, which significantly enhances healing.

The hand and digits require hairless, pliable and thin flaps. The dorsum of the hand can be covered using the forearm flap (free or island), the posterior interosseous flap, the lateral arm flap and the temporoparietal fascia flap. The digits, on the other hand, are best covered with the dorsalis pedis flap and the homo- or heterodigital neurovascular island flaps (uni- or bipedicled).

According to the blood supply, there are two different types of flaps: random pattern and axial pattern flaps. Random-pattern flaps receive a blood supply from several minute vessels of the subdermal or subcutaneous plexus and not from a single arteriovenous pedicle [25]. These flaps are more limited in the range of their applications, as rules regarding the width of the base of the flap must be followed in order to avoid impairment of the blood supply to the flap.

Axial-pattern flaps, on the other hand, receive their blood supply from a single constant vessel larger than those of the subdermal plexus that supplies the random pattern flap. This allows a more flexible design of the flap that is based on the vascular territory of the feeding vessel. More importantly, their axial blood supply allows for more predictable flap survival. Axial blood flow provides more resistance against bacterial inoculum [26]. Two of the more popular axial-pattern flaps that are used for the forearm include the radial artery forearm flap (also referred to as the Chinese flap) and the posterior interosseous artery flap [27, 28]. The Chinese flap is

a fasciocutaneous flap. Its blood supply is based on the radial artery, and hence requires that patient has an intact ulnar artery. In this regard, an Allen's test must be performed to demonstrate the total vascularity of the hand through the palmar arch. The posterior interosseous artery provides vascularity to the posterior interosseous flap. Its use has increased as it can be applied as a reverse flap (distal to proximal perfusion) increasing the overall potential arc of rotation. Both the Chinese and the posterior interosseous flap provide low-profile, non-bulky soft tissue coverage for either dorsal or volar forearm defects.

Venous congestion is a frequent and significant complication associated with free flap procedures [29]. Venous congestion can be the result of various factors including an inadequate anastomosis of the vein, a secondary effect to arterial insufficiency, venous spasm, venous occlusion and the absence of venous repair. Venous congestions and engorgement can potentially lead to necrosis of the flap. Leeches have been found to be effective in the treatment of venous congestion following microsurgical free flap procedures [29, 30] (Fig. 1). Since venous engorgement is a frequent cause of necrosis, the efficacy of leech therapy is of clinical significance where their application can avoid expected partial or complete loss of the flap. The usefulness of the leech appears to be related not only to immediate removal of congested venous blood, but also to the continuous flow of blood which ensues, as well as the local state of anticoagulation produced by the antithrombotic agent, hirudin [31].

3. FREE FLAPS FOR THE UPPER EXTREMITY

3.1. The lateral arm flap

The *lateral arm flap* is a thin, fasciocutaneous flap suitable for coverage of skin defects of the upper

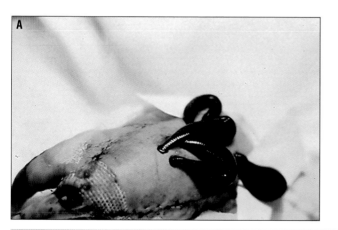
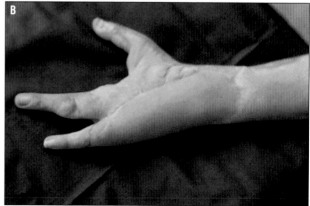

FIGURE 1. **(A)** Leeches are applied on forearm flap that developed venous congestion and threatened flap viability. **(B)** Venous congestion was successfully managed, and the flap survived.

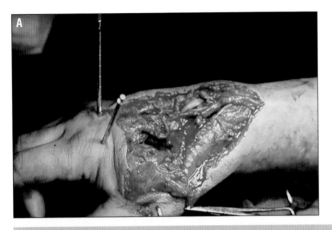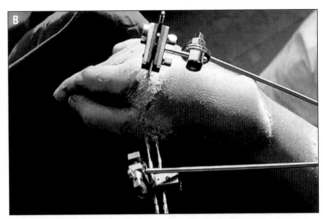

FIGURE 2. (A) Preoperative view of an extensive, contaminated wound of the dorso-lateral aspect of the wrist secondary to animal bite. The wound was thoroughly debrided to clean edges. **(B)** The soft tissue defect was successfully covered with a forearm flap. The distal end of the radial artery of the flap was anastomosed with radial artery of the donor area, so as to increase the blood supply of the hand.

extremity particularly of the dorsum of the hand. It can serve as an innervated fasciocutaneous flap or as a de-epithelized subcutaneous fascial flap. The lateral arm flap is based on the posterior lateral collateral artery and venae comitantes which have a fairly consistent vascular anatomy. The flap can be up to 8 x 15 cm² with a pedicle as long as 7 cm.

This flap is innervated by the posterior brachial cutaneous nerve, a proximal branch of the radial nerve (C5 and C6). As a result, the lateral arm flap can provide sensation, if required. In addition, sensory supply to the flap is also provided by the posterior antibrachial cutaneous nerve.

As the deep fascia is included in the lateral arm flap, it can provide good coverage for areas where tendon gliding is important and for the dorsum of the hand [32]. A vascularized bony segment up to 10 cm long and 1 cm wide can be included in the skin flap.

3.2. The forearm flap

The *forearm flap* is a fasciocutaneous flap which was developed at the Ba-Ba-Chung Hospital in the Peoples Republic of China in 1978 (Song and Gao 1982). Blood is supplied to the flap by the radial artery and the venous drainage is accomplished by either the cephalic, basilic vein or veinacometante. The flap can achieve up to a 20 cm long pedicle. This length of the pedicle facilitates the microsurgical anastomosis out of the zone of injury [33] (Fig. 2).

The forearm flap can be innervated by either the medial or lateral antibrachial nerves. As such, it can serve as a neurosensory flap. The size of the flap can reach 10x40 cm². One of the inherent disadvantages of this flap is the often unsightly donor site. This can be overcome with the use of a tissue expander (Fig. 3). In addition, preliminary tissue expansion can be used to in-

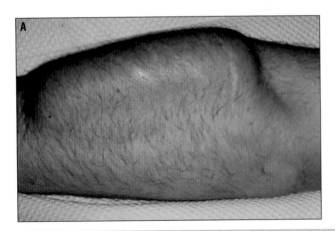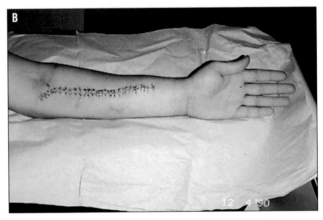

FIGURE 3. (A) A tissue expander was applied to augment the size of forearm skin. **(B)** The skin area was significantly increased with the use of the tissue expander, enabling primary suturing of the donor area without the need of a skin graft.

crease the flap dimensions, allowing direct closure of the donor defect [34].

The palmaris longus tendon and the longitudinal portions of the brachial radialis and flexor carpi radialis tendons can be included, as well. An 11-cm bony segment from the radius can also be included, however, this is related with frequent complications of fractures of the radius. No vascular impairment of the hand has been observed following sacrifice of the radial artery nor does the radial artery defect have to be bridged by a vein graft unless anatomical variations exist which indicate that the thumb and index fingers are dependent upon the radial artery for their blood supply [33].

3.3. The scapular flap

The *scapular flap* is a thin, usually hairless fasciocutaneous flap suitable for coverage of skin defects of the upper extremity particularly of the dorsum of the hand. The primary indication for the scapular flap is a defect that requires thin, relatively large cutaneous flap. The donor sites can be closed directly in scapular flaps. The blood supply of the scapular flap is based on the circumflex scapular artery and is drained by its venae comitantes. The vascular pattern of the pedicle makes it possible for several skin flaps to be raised on a single vascular pedicle. The flap can extend to 20 x 7 cm² in size and can be divided into two components based on the branches of the circumflex scapular artery: a horizontal and a vertical territory (Fig. 4).

3.4. The dorsalis pedis flap

The *dorsalis pedis flap* is also a thin, fasciocutaneous flap suitable for coverage of skin defects of the upper extremity particularly of the dorsum of the hand. This thin sensate flap is derived from the dorsum of the foot. The nerve supply comes from the branches of the deep and superficial peroneal nerves.

The dorsalis pedis receives blood supply from the dorsalis pedis artery and its terminal branch, the first dorsal metatarsal artery. The length of the pedicle can be 6 to 10 cm. The size of the flap is about 6 x 10 cm², and it can be raised in combination with the second metatarsal bone as an osteocutaneous flap (Fig. 5).

Donor site morbidity is of concern with this flap. The donor site can not be closed directly as in scapular and lateral arm flaps, rather it has to be grafted.

3.5. The neurovascular island flap

The *neurovascular island flap* can be transferred on in-

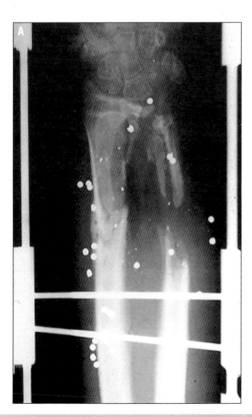
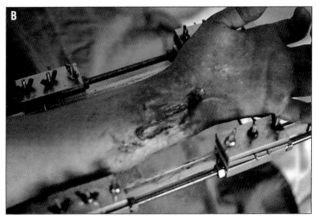
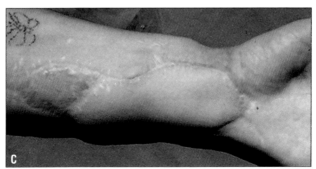

FIGURE 4. (A) Preoperative radiographs showing a severe shotgun injury at the distal third of the forearm and wrist. **(B)** View showing the infected wound with exposed tendons and severe scaring of the soft tissues. **(C)** The wound was thoroughly debrided and successful soft tissue coverage was achieved with the use of a scapular flap.

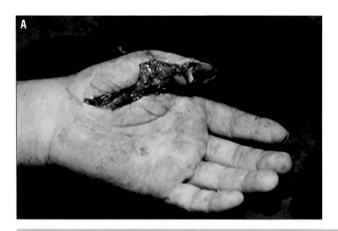

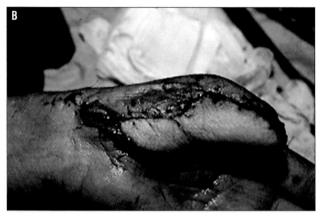

FIGURE 5. **(A)** View showing extensive skin loss and infection of the volar aspect of the tip of the thumb down to the thenar eminence in a 25-year-old laborer. **(B)** Once good debridement was achieved, the wound was covered with a dorsalis pedis flap.

tact pedicles in order to resurface critical pinch areas. The neurovascular pulp island flaps from the lateral half of the large toe provide glabrous skin similar to that of the fingertips. These are ideally suited for resurfacing the tactile pad of the thumb or fingers (Fig. 6).

These flaps can extend from the nail margin to the midline and must be mobilized on the lateral digital neurovascular pedicle. The plantar digital nerve supplying the flap provides good sensation with adequate two-point discrimination. As a result, this is one of the best free sensory island flaps available to the microsurgeon.

3.6. The temporoparietal fascia flap

The *temporoparietal fascia flap* provides a large, thin sheet of fascia derived from the temporal, parietal and occipital areas of the scalp. It provides large nutrient vessels that are anatomically consistent. This large thin sheet fascia with good vascularity is useful in reconstruction areas where large, bulky flaps are not as effective; that is, areas requiring coverage with minimal contour increase or areas requiring pliability and flexibility. The donor site of the temporoparietal fascial flap is hidden within the hairline of the scalp which gives an acceptable aesthetic result.

The excellent blood supply of this fascial flap appears to decrease the local wound contamination. In the upper extremity, it provides a thin soft tissue cover that permits early hand movement and good tendon motion underneath the cover.

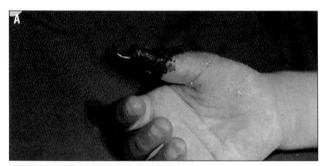

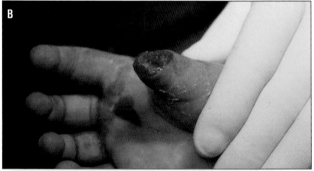

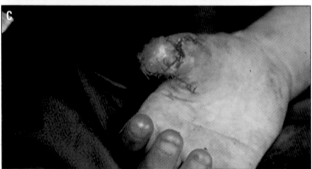

FIGURE 6. **(A)** View of thumb showing failure of replantation, with extensive necrosis and infection. **(B)** The distal necrotic part of the thumb was excised and the area was debrided. **(C)** The wound was covered and reconstructed with a homodigital neurovascular bipedicled island flap.

4. Timing of Free Flap Coverage

Free tissue transfers facilitate one-stage reconstruction of complex defects with concomitant functional reconstructive procedures [17, 24]. Although free flaps have been used successfully for managing infections in the lower extremity, there is growing support for their use in the upper extremity, as well [17, 21, 22, 24, 35-37].

Immediate flap coverage has been associated with a significant reduction of infectious complications (6%), as compared with reconstruction after 72 hours or more (17.5%), with a relatively minimal loss of flaps [Godina 1986]. Others have also demonstrated excellent results with early coverage of posttraumatic defects in the upper extremity [24, 37, 38].

Early soft tissue reconstruction, less than 72 hours after injury, is advocated for several reasons. It reduces the possibility of infection and avoids dehydration of anatomic elements. Early use of free flaps protects the neurovascular structures and creates a well-vascularized environment which in turn, promotes healing. Because this type of coverage facilitates future reconstruction that is usually required for these types of complex, extensive lesions, it also significantly improves the functional recovery of the patient.

5. MANAGEMENT OF COMPLEX CONTAMINATED WOUNDS WITH FREE FLAPS

Free tissue transfers allow for one-stage reconstruction of a complex defect with concomitant functional reconstructive procedures, providing a powerful tool for the experienced microsurgeon [17, 24]. The therapeutic strategy entails radical debridement, including a scheduled second-look intervention when necessary, and one-stage defect reconstruction with free tissue transfer.

5.1. Radical Debridement

The term debridement (from the French term *debridement*) entails the removal of soft tissues and bone that are nonviable. Debridement is performed to prevent infection, and is required for chronic wounds that have resulted from improper handling of soft tissues or infection. With the ability to transfer large, well-vascularized flaps, more radical debridement of removal of necrotic tissue is allowed.

Meticulous radical debridement to a clean margin is the first and perhaps the most important step in the management of complex contaminated wounds with free flaps [17, 35, 36, 37, 39]. In general, the same principles that are used for tumor surgery are also applied to contaminated defects. In this regard, the necrotic and infected tissues are excised to clear margins so that no potentially contaminated or devitalized tissue is remaining. Although it is important to preserve as many functional structures as possible, including nerves, tendons and vessels, these must be viable. Otherwise, persistent drainage and fistulas will form under the flap umbrella.

Damaged tissue is recognized by the presence of foreign bodies, irregular tissue consistency and its color (irregular distribution of dark red stains or hematomas). All

damaged tissue is excised with a blade. Any exposed bone is washed with antibiotic solution. Bone debridement in chromic wounds can be difficult, as it is difficult to distinguish viable bone and callus from necrotic and inflamed areas of the medullary canal. In this case, CT, bone scans and MRI may help in the preoperative planning.

Severed vessels should be dissected until normal appearing margins. Nerves are the only tissue type which requires a more conservative debridement, with only the epineurium being removed when required.

Radical debridement should be followed by careful irrigation of the wound area. Multiple irrigation with copious amounts of fluid significantly reduces the bacterial count in the wound [40, 41].

After the debridement stage is complete, normal tissue planes should be visualized. The surgeon should have no doubts concerning the viability of the wound edges. If normal tissue planes can not be visualized, then a second look procedure should be performed where the surgeon should carefully screen the wound area again, and proceed with a second debridement. This should be done by 24 hours after the initial debridement, but no latter than 48 hours [42].

In compromised wounds, hyperbaric oxygen may assist in promoting granulation tissue and stimulate angiogenesis. Wound dressings are changed under sterile conditions. Vacuum-assisted closure uses subatmospheric pressure to assist in closing the wound, and results in effective promotion of granulation tissue formation. The negative pressure that is applied to the wound helps to remove excess fluid from the interstitium at the wound periphery. This decreases the local interstitial pressure and restores blood flow to vessels that were compromised by excess pressure [15].

5.2. Single Stage Free Tissue Transfer

The management of dead space after sequestrectomy relies heavily on the use of free tissue transfer. Debridement and irrigation is followed by reconstruction of the defect with a free tissue transfer. Free muscle flaps not only provide coverage for the debrided bone and soft tissue, but they also obliterate dead space, improve vascularity and enhance leukocyte function [43, 44].

There are several flaps that play a role in hand reconstruction. Each flap type has advantages and disadvantages. The choice of the flap to be used for wound coverage is determined by the size of the wound, the type of tissue deficit, the state of the wound, the location of the wound and the length of the pedicle that is needed.

Free muscle flaps, including the latissiumus dorsi, serratus anterior and the rectus abdominis, provide good bulk for filling larger wounds, have long pedicles which allows flexibility in positioning of the flap and have large diameter vessels which allows for good microanastomoses. The most common fasciocutaneous free flaps are the lateral arm flap, the radial forearm flap, scapular flaps, dorsalis pedis and groin flaps.

References

[1] Jacobson JH, Suarez SE. Microsurgery and anastomosis of the small vessels. Surg Forum 1961;12:256-7.

[2] Kleinert HE, Kasdor ML, Romero JL. Small Blood vessels anastomosis for salvage of severely injured upper extremity. J Bone Joint Surg 1963:45:788-96.

[3] Bunke CM. Experimental digital amputation and replantation. Plast Reconstr Surg 1965:36:62.

[4] Urbaniak JR, Soucacos PN, Adelaar RS, Bright DS, Whitehurst LA. Experimental evaluation of microsurgical techniques in small artery anastomoses. Orthop Clin N Am 1977;8:249-263.

[5] Urbaniak JR. Digital replantation: a 12-year experience. In. Urbaniak JR ed. Microsurgery for major limb reconstruction. C.V. Mosby C, St. Louis 1987:12-21.

[6] Soucacos PN. Microsurgery in Orthopaedics. In: Casteleyn, Duparc J. (eds) Instructional Courses of the European Federation of Orthopaedic Surgery and Traumatology. EFORT, Journal of Bone and Joint Surgery, Vol 1: p 149-155, 1995.

[7] Tsai E, Failla JM. Hand infections in the trauma patient. Hand Clin 1999;15:373-386.

[8] Horch RE, Stark GB. The rectus abdominis free flap as an emergency procedure in exrtensive upper extremity soft-tissue defects. Plast Reconster Surg 1999;103:1421-1427.

[9] Gewin M, Wiland AJ. Vascular bone grafts to the upper extremity: indications and technique. Hand Clin 1992;8:509-523.

[10] Gonzalez MH. Necrotizing fasciitis and gangrene of the upper extremity. Hand Clin 1998;14:635-645.

[11] McCabe SJ, Breidenbach Wc. The role of emergency free flaps for hand trauma. Hand Clin 1999;15:275-288.

[12] Wood SH, Lees VC. A prospective investigation of the healing of grafted pretibial wounds with early and late mobilization. Br J Plast Surg 1994;47:127-131.

[13] Cedidi C, Hierner R, Berger A. Plastic surgical management in tissue extravasation of cytotoxic agents in the upper extremity. Eur J Med Res 2001;6:309-314.

[14] Fleishmann W, Lang E, Russ M. Treatment of infection by vacuum sealing. Unfallchirurg 1997;100:301-304.

[15] Argenta LC, Morykwas MJ. Vacuum-assisted closure: a new method for wound control and treatment: clinical experience. Ann Plast Surg 1997;38:563-576.

[16] Schneider AM, Morykwas MJ, Argenta LC. A new and reliable method of securing skin grafts to the difficult reciepient bed. Plast Reconstr Surg 1998:102:1195-1198.

[17] Godina M. Early microsurgical reconstruction of complex trauma of the extremities. Plast Reconstr Surg 1986;78:285-292.

[18] Lai CS, Tsai CC, Liao KB, et al. The reverse lateral arm adipofascial flap for elbow coverage. Ann Plast Surg 1997;39:196-200.

[19] Tung TC, Wang KC, Fang CM, et al. Reverse pedicled lateral arm flap for reconstruction of posterior soft-tissue defects of the elbow. An Plast Surg 1997:38:635-641.

[20] Germann G, Bickert B, Steinau HU, et al. Versatility and reliability of combined flaps of the subscapular system. Plst Reconstr Surg 1999; 103:1386-1399.

[21] Berthe JV, Toussaint D, Coessens BC. One-stage reconstruction of an infected skin and Achilles tendon defect with a composite distally planned lateral arm flap. Plast Reconstr Surg 1998:102:1618-1622.

[22] Germann G, Wieczorek D. Combine pedicle and free-tissue transfer to improve functional restoration of the foot: the "backpack principle" J Reconstr Microsurg 1999;15:409-413.

[23] Lutz BS, Siemers F, Shen ZL, et al. Free flap to the arteria peronea magna for tlower limb salvage. Plast Reconstr Surg 2000;105:684-687.

[24] Lister G, Scheker L. Emergency free flaps to the ypper extremity. J Hand Surg Am 1988;13:22-28.

[25] McGregor IA, Morgan G. Axial and random pattern flap. Br J Plast Surg 1973;26:202-213.

[26] Chang N, Mathes Sj. Comparison of the effect of bacterial inoculation in musculocutaneous and random-pattern flaps. Plast Reconstr Surg 1982;70:1-10.

[27] Song R, Gao Y, Song Y, et al. The forearm flap Clin Plast Surg 1982: 9:21-6.

[28] Penteato CV, Masquelat AC, Chevrel JP. The anatomic basis of the fascio-cutaneous flap of the posterior interosseous artery. Surg Radio Anat 1986;8:209-215.

[29] Soucacos PN, Beris AE, Malizos KN, Kabani CT, and Pakos S. The use of medicinal leeches, Hirudo Medicinalis, to restore venous circulation in trauma and reconstructive microsurgery. International Angiology 1994;13(3):251-258.

[30] Soucacos PN, Beris AE, Malizos KN, Xenakis TA, and Georgoulis AD. Successful treatment of venous congestion in free skin flaps using medical leeches. Microsurgery 1994;15:496-501.

[31] Soucacos PN. Management of venous congestion in trauma and reconstructive microsurgery: The significance of medicinal leeches. Schuind F, de Fontaine S, Van Geertruyden J, Soucacos PN (eds) In Recent Advances in Upper and Lower Extremity Microvascular Reconstructions. London: World Scientific Co. 34-40, 2002.

[32] Yousif NJ, Warren R, Matloub HS, et al. The lateral arm fascial free flap: its anatomy and use in reconstruction. Plast Reconstr Surg 1990;86:1138-45.

[33] Soucacos PN, Beris AE, Xenakis TA, Malizos KN, and Touliatos AS. Forearm flap in orthopaedic and hand surgery. Microsurgery 1992;13(4):170-4.

[34] Georgoulis A, Soucacos PN, Beris AE, Papageorgiou MD, Siamisis G, Vragalas V. Application of silicon tissue expanders for the direct or indirect coverage of soft tissue defects in the extremities. Acta Orthopaedica Scandinavica 1995;(Suppl 264)66:38-40.

[35] Chen S, Tsai YC, Wei FC et al. Emergency free flaps to the type IIIC tibial fracture. Ann Plast Surg 1990;25:223-229.

[36] Musharafieh R, Osmani O, Musharafieh U et al. Efficacy of microsurgical free-tissue transfer in chronic osteomyelitis of the leg and foot: review of 22 cases. J reconstr Microsurg 1999;15:239-244.

[37] Breidenbach WC III. Emergency free tissue transfer for reconstruction of acute upper extremity wounds. Clin Plast Surg 1989;16 505:514.

[38] Koschnick M, Bruener S, Germann G. Free tissue transfer: an advanced strategy for postinfection soft-tissue defects in the upper extremity. Plast Surg 2003;51:147-154.

[39] Lineaweaver WC, Hui K, Yim K et al. The role of the plastic surgeon in the management of surgical infection. Plast Reconstr Surg 1999; 103:1553-1560.

[40] Mont MA, Waldman B, Banerjee C et al. Multiple irrigation, debridement and retention of components in infected total knee arthroplasty. J Arthroplasty 1997;12:426-433.

[41] Hallock GG. The role of local fascial flaps as an adjunct to free flaps. Ann Plast Surg 1997;38:388-395.

[42] Levin LS. Debridement. Tech Orthop 1995;10:104.

[43] Mathes SJ, Alpert BS, Chang N. Use of the miuscle flap in chronic osteomyelitis: experimental and clinical correlation. Plast Reconstr Surg 1982;69:815-29.

[44] Mathes SJ, Feng LJ, Hunt TK. Coverage of the infected wound. Ann Surg 1983;198:420-9.

The Use of Pedicled Flaps for Septic Conditions of the Hand, Elbow and Forearm

Zsolt SZABO[*a], Antal RENNER[b]

[a]*BAZ University County Teaching Hospital, Miskolc, Hungary*
[b]*National Institute for Traumatology and Emergency Medicine, Budapest, Hungary*

In severe septic conditions of the upper limb one of the possible solutions is to increase the vascularity of and the blood supply to the affected tissues. This augmentation of vascularity can be achieved by use of vascularized flaps. However, there are no standard treatment strategies of proven efficiency, only some impressions and beliefs and different practices of flap usage in septic conditions of the hand. In this chapter, we review the pertinent literature and deal with such questions as: (i) Are flaps indicated for acute infection?, (ii) Does the use of a flap increase the blood supply to and thus, the healing potential of the affected tissues?, (iii) What kind of flap is the best choice?, (iv) Free or pedicled flaps? (v) Muscle or fascial flaps? Our experience with pedicled flaps in septic conditions is also presented. We conclude that pedicled fasciocutaneous flaps have very important role in the healing of septic conditions and their application should be further expanded.

Keywords: septic condition; upper limb; free flap; pedicled flap; tissue substitution.

1. INTRODUCTION

Septic conditions in the hand and upper limb have always been a serious problem for the patient and the treating physicians, and they still remain an important field of research and development. Deep knowledge of the hand and upper limb anatomy and pathophysiology of infections in those sites, as well as the understanding that such infections require specialized management are essential towards successful treatment. A simple incision and evacuation of the pus is insufficient to lead to

*Corresponding Author
Traumatology Dept. 72–76
Szentpeteri kapu
3501 Miskolc, Hungary
Tel: +0036 30 205 35 54
Fax: +0036 46 5 15 237
e-mail: zsoltszabo@axelero.hu

healing with an acceptable function. Excision instead of incision, immobilization, adequate antibiotic therapy and rehabilitation could guarantee a satisfactory outcome.

In the recent years we observed a decrease in the number of simple septic cases and an increase in the severely complicated ones. The etiology of those severe infections is diverse. Hematogenous spread and simple wounds or complex injuries with severe tissue damage vary in nature and degree of severity, and therefore require different surgical interventions. The pathogenic agents also present variability. The only common denominator is the long and expensive treatment and the questionable outcome.

There is general consensus on the necessity to perform radical excision of non-viable affected tissues. However, debridement leads to an important tissue defect and for the substitution of the defects use of different flaps is generally suggested. The concept is radical excision, wet dressing, immobilization, antibiotics, and a second surgical operation (if necessary). When the infection is eradicated, tissue substitution with an appropriate flap is performed. Following this algorithm, we can generally achieve improvement of function. In some cases, however, we had unsatisfactory outcomes despite all our efforts. The main problems encountered were:

- the surgical excision resulted in exposure of precious structures such as tendons, vessels, nerves, ligaments, bone and joints;
- the septic process had already affected precious structures, excision of which seriously influenced the functional outcome;
- despite surgical and medical treatment, the infection became chronic.

One of the possible solutions for those problems would be increasing the vascularity of and the blood supply to the affected tissues. This may result in more optimal local immune response, a greater number of white blood cells, and higher oxygen and antibiotic concentration. The vascularity can be further enhanced by using vascularized flaps.

There are some important questions to answer before flap selection and application in septic conditions. These questions are:

- Is it indicated to use flaps in acute infections?
- Does the application of a flap increase the blood supply to and the healing potential of the affected tissues?
- Which flap is the most appropriate?
- Free or pedicled flaps?
- Muscle or fascial flaps?
- What is the best time to carry out flap surgery?

Below we present the pertinent literature dealing with this subject and our experience in the field of septic trauma in the upper limb.

2. Available Literature

Employing the search engine PubMed for "infections" one could find the astonishing number of 85,500 articles. Searching for "flaps" we may obtain more than 35,000 articles. Extending our search to "flaps in infections" drastically reduces the number of articles to 2,273. Focusing on "flaps in infections of the limbs" the number will decrease to 341. "Flaps in infections of the upper limb" will give 110 articles. If we continue to look for "free flaps in infections of the upper limb" we will have 49 articles, but only 7 of them actually deal with the subject. "Pedicled flaps in infections of the upper limb" will result in 8 articles with only 3 of them dealing with the subject under investigation. Considering this paucity of literature data, we realize that there are no clear strategies of proven efficiency, only some descriptive findings and different practices of flap usage in septic conditions of the hand. Due to these findings, we were obliged to also re-

view some series reported in the literature dealing with the lower limb, as the number of such publications in relation to our topic is greater.

3. Questions to Answer

3.1. What are the indications for use of a flap in case of infection? Which type of infections? Which kind of flap is appropriate?

The use of flaps in chronic infections, especially in the lower limb is not a new concept. The first to describe the application of the muscle flap in severe forms of chronic osteomyelitis of the foot was the Russian surgeon Kernerman in 1966 [1]. The next published article was written by Hildebrandt in 1972 [2]. Both authors described the advantage of the local muscle flap application in the treatment of chronic osteomyelitis.

In the early 1980s there were numerous articles dealing with the use of flaps in chronic osteomyelitis. The authors generally accepted the idea that the success in controlling chronic osteomyelitis lies in the introduction of new vasculature, which provides nutrients, sufficient antibiotics, a fortified host defense system, and osteoprogenitor cells to the post-sequestrectomy bed. Some of them were in favor of local muscular and musculocutaneous flaps, eg. Ngoi et al. [3], Fitzgerald [4] and Mathes [5]. Others emphasized on the importance of free tissue transport to the site of the infection (e.g. Cierny [6] and Moore [7]). According to them, in case of infection a free flap should always be either a muscular or a musculocutaneous flap.

We can conclude that 20-30 years ago the use of flaps in chronic osseous infections was rather limited, and then, only muscular or musculocutaneous flaps were considered appropriate.

3.2. Local pedicled or free muscle flaps?

The advent of microsurgery in the 1980s resulted in an increasing number of reports on free muscle flap application. Some interesting comparative studies were published dealing with the advantages and disadvantages of local pedicled and free muscle flaps. In 1986, Zook [8] reported 64 flaps for wound coverage in 58 patients. In this series, there were high rates of healing for both tibial fractures and chronic osteomyelitis. The defects covered with muscle had a better outcome when muscle was covered with meshed skin grafts than with musculocutaneous flaps. The survival rate for the free flaps was 93%, and for the pedicled flaps 100%, with complication rates being higher for the pedicled flaps (45%) than for the free flaps (30%). Major complications, however, were reported for free flaps (14%), which were substantially more than those of the pedicled flaps (9%). Schuz W. [9], in 1987, reported better results with free muscular flaps than with pedicled flaps with no significant difference. At that time, first experimental studies on this subject were reported. In 1989, Richards [10] showed in a canine model the effect of muscle flap coverage on bone blood flow, following devascularization of a tibial segment. He found that blood flow to the devascularized segment of the tibia was significantly greater when the defect was covered with a muscle flap. A great number of articles reported successful outcomes with free muscle flaps. In the early 1990s the generally accepted idea was that a free muscle flap is the best way to treat chronic osteomyelitis.

3.3. Might a free muscle flap be a crucial parameter for treatment of an infection?

A perfect microsurgical technique may be performed, however, the results are not always the desired. Due to this fact, special attention has been directed to the adequacy of the debridement. Swiontkowski et al. [11] reported on the use of lazer Doppler flowmetry as an adjunct to debridement in the case of osteomyelitis. Special attention was also focused on the pathogenic flora of the infected structures. Patzakis et al. [12] in prospective studies on the results of bacterial cultures from multiple sites in chronic osteomyelitis of long bones demonstrated the different microenvironments inside the same septic site. In 1995, Guelincky [13] summarized the variety of bacterial cultures and the importance of sufficient debridement.

Radical debridement of all affected soft and hard tissues, obliteration of the dead space, and neovascularization of the involved area are of critical importance for successful management of the disease. Microvascular free tissue transfer provides the necessary tissue bulk to reconstruct the defect. The transplanted muscle can be optimally mobilized and adjusted to the defect to obliterate the dead space unlike locally transposed flaps. Smoothening the osseous cavity by a rotating drill facilitates contouring. With an optimal interface between the muscle and the wall of the cavity, small foci of infection can be eliminated. Moreover, underneath the muscle there is a more favourable environment for secondary reconstruction and bone grafting. Radical debridement combined with muscle transfer for dead space obliteration is generally accepted, my reported in the literature. Nevertheless, to achieve this goal several different treatment schedules of repetitive debridements, prolonged antibiotic administration, and finally various flap transfers have been advocated.

3.4. Bone infections are relatively well analyzed, but what about soft tissue infections?

Not with standing the relatively large number of articles dealing with chronic osseous infections, only one or two articles can be found dealing with soft tissue infections cured by flap coverage. Mathes [5] was one of the first to suggest flap application in soft tissue infections.

3.5. Is the free muscle flap still the "gold standard" in chronic bone infections? Have there been any improvements?

In the late 1990s pedicled flaps in reconstructive surgery were becoming a new trend. Well known classic flaps, such as the groin flap, the radial forearm, and the "chinese" flap were used more frequently, and new pedicled fasciocutaneous flaps were described in reports of large series. The posterior interosseous, the anterior interosseous and the kite flap were relatively new and great enthusiasm was encountered regarding their use in hand and upper limb reconstruction. In the current decade, the widely accepted method of treating chronic infections still remains the free muscle transfer. However, three main issues receive more and more attention: first, the increasing use of perforator flaps in the upper and lower limb; secondly, the significant decrease in free tissue transfers and the increasing number of pedicled flaps in tissue substitution in both the upper and the lower limb; and finally, the increasing number of studies dealing with problems related to free flap surgery. Emphasis is laid on the fact that a free flap operation lasts longer, needs special equipment and well-trained staff, and is more technically and physically demanding than the pedicled flap operation.

3.6. What is the problem with free flaps?

Rucker et al. [14] in 1999 published an *in vivo* analysis on the microcirculation of an osteomyocutaneous flap by using fluorescence microscopy. They demonstrated that even after a short 1-h ischemic time period, capillary perfusion failure and leukocyte-endothelial cell interaction are the main events indicating microvascular dysfunction after free transfer of osteomyocutaneous flaps. In their second article published in 2002 [15], they report a shutdown of perfusion of individual capillaries, resulting in significant reduction (P<0.05) in functional capillary density, not only in the subcutis, skin and periosteum, but also in the muscle itself. Their data suggest that the microcirculatory control of pedicled osteomyocutaneous flaps is maintained during critical perfusion by skeleton capillary flow but this protective regulatory mechanism is lost during the initid reperfusion period after the flap transfer. Machens [16] from Germany has published measurements of tissue blood flow by the hydrogen clearance technique, laser Doppler flowmetry and Erlangen microlightguide spectrophotometry in free tissue transfer. Khalil [17] states in his study that the restoration of blood flow to ischemic tissues causes additional damage, which is termed "reperfusion injury".

3.7. Do pedicled flaps eliminate these problems?

All tissues are susceptible to reperfusion injury, although the degree of susceptibility varies among them. Reperfusion has a broad clinical relevance especially in free tissue transfer. Thus, attention has been directed towards the use of pedicled flaps. Pinsolle [18], having 15 years of experience in reconstructive surgery at a university hospital, stated that microsurgical tissue transfers were predominant in the 1980s and decreased in the 1990s, whereas the pedicled flap had the opposite evolution. Moreover, pedicled flaps are related to a significantly lower rate of complication (18%) than free flaps (27%). Thus, he recommended use of pedicled flaps as the first choice in covering soft tissue defects in the lower limb. Several authors have demonstrated that pedicled flaps are as useful as free flaps but without the inconvenience caused by free flaps. Lee and Baskin [19] report that there has been renewed interest of surgeons in locoregional flaps for reconstruction of defects previously thought to be optimally managed by microvascular tissue transfer. Successful reconstruction by using local flaps is largely based on in-depth understanding of regional vascular anatomy. Complication rates of locoregional flaps were found similar to those of free flaps.

3.8. Do we need a muscle flap, or does a fasciocutaneous flap suffice?

Another important question to answer is whether use of a muscle flap is mandatory to obtain a good result in an infected wound. In a retrospective study, Zweifel-Schlatter M et al. [20] studied the efficacy of free fasciocutaneous flaps for the treatment of chronic osteomyelitis. They found that such flaps can be used effectively for tissue reconstruction after radical debridement in the case of chronic osteomyelitis. Yazar et al. [21] reported the outcome of a comparative study on free muscle and free fasciocutaneous flaps: both soft tissue transfers were of equal value. Free fasciocutaneous flaps were found reliable and as effective in covering defects as free muscle flaps. Moreover, they can better tolerate subsequent secondary surgical procedures. Flugel A et al. [22] reported successful use of free fascial flaps in the treatment of the hand and upper limb. They recommended their use as a valuable alternative to fasciocutaneous or muscle flaps. Since the functional results were excellent, no additional procedures were necessary. The aesthetic results seemed to be appealing.

3.9. Muscle or fascia? The importance of vascular network in neovascularization

When a muscle flap is used, its contact surface with the receiving area is the fascia of the muscle. The rich vascular network of the fascia is a guarantee for a good neovascularization, which is probably the key prerequisite for successful tissue integration in a septic environment. Several studies deal with the time required for neovascularization, which is important for flap survival in case of dissection of the pedicle. Gatti et al. [23] reported 100% survival of tube pedicles when divided after four days in experimental conditions. It should be noted that in all experimental situations the wound bed is ideal,

and obviously, the neovascularization takes place without any hindrance. However, in clinical situations the wound bed is usually far from ideal due to a variety of factors. The time required for adequate neovascularization may thus be longer in such circumstances. To prevent complications, it is recommended that division take place after the 10th day.

4. Summary of Published Data

Based on literature review, we summarize the findings as follows:
- radical excision of the infected tissue is essential for a good outcome;
- bacterial cultures obtained in a proper way from the affected tissue and an antibiogram are mandatory for selection of the appropriate antibiotic regimen;
- it is essential to achieve good blood flow towards the flap especially in the first 3-4 days. Thus, it is important to choose a pedicled flap to eliminate complications from vascular anastomoses;
- for a well-vascularized surface of the substituted tissue, a fasciocutaneous flap seems to be the best choice to avoid bulky flaps and long operations;
- flaps with antegrade blood flow should be preferred to avoid problems of venous drainage;
- in severely affected limbs it is preferable to use flaps with vascular support taken from a distant region. This may increase the blood supply of the limb, enhancing healing.

5. Authors' Preferences

We have started to use pedicled fasciocutaneous flaps in severe septic conditions of the upper limb during the last five years. Our preferences for the different levels of the upper limb are the following:
- the Foucher's kite flap for the thumb, the first web, and MP level infections and defects;
- the groin flap for extended, deep and severely contaminated wounds of the hand, wrist and forearm;
- the radial forearm flap when we need to perform composite tissue substitution or when we want to achieve increased blood supply to the hand, forearm and elbow; and
- other flaps currently used in our practice for acute trauma management and late reconstruction, since the interosseous posterior, the interosseous anterior, the ulnar forearm, and the lateral arm flaps are not used for the treatment of septic conditions.

5.1. Foucher's kite flap

The kite flap, first described by Foucher and Braun [24] in 1978, is an island flap taken from the dorsum of the index finger, and based on the first dorsal metacarpal artery with one or two veins and the terminal branches of the radial nerve. This vascular pattern is constant. The quality of its venous outflow and the good arterial inflow, together with a large arc of rotation makes this flap ideal for covering defects of the thumb, the first web space, and the MP joints. The distal point of the flap, in our practice, is extended up to the PIP joint of the index finger. During dissection special attention is directed to p-reserve a peritendinous tissue on the extensor apparatus. In this way, the defect is covered with a full thickness skin graft so that retraction and hyper pigmentation is prevented. The pedicle of the flap should be dissected with no need of visualizing the artery. A relatively thick pedicle will improve venous outflow. We have applied this flap four times for septic conditions, twice for the thumb, once for the first web space and once for the third MP joint after radical debridement. The drainage was suspended on the second day after the surgery. Intravenous antibiotic treatment was applied for five days followed by oral administration of antibiotics for a week. The infection was eradicated in all cases without complications.

5.2. Groin flap

The groin flap was first described by McGregor [25] in 1979. Anatomic studies have revealed the reliability of blood supply through the superficial circumflex iliac vessels to the skin area and subcutaneous tissue that is parallel to the inguinal ligament and lateral to the femoral artery. The axial vascular pattern allows harvest of a longer flap without compromising the vascular supply. The big advantage of the groin flap is that its size can reach 25 x 10 cm. Tubularization of the pedicle facilitates postoperative care and limits mobilization of the elbow and the shoulder. This flap is ideal for covering defects in the wrist, which is the anastomotic zone for arteries of different pedicled flaps. In case of injury around the wrist, the majority of the pedicled flaps of the forearm are compromised. The division of the pedicle requires a second operation within two weeks. Cheng et al. [26] studied the possibility of earlier division of the flap and recommended conditioning and early division after eight days. In the first cases that we treated, we performed conditioning of the flap with a rubber band placed at the base of the pedicle, but in the last 20 cases we abandoned this step and no circulatory complications occurred. The drainage was kept in place for 72 hours. We used this flap in 11 septic cases, two of which presented osteomyelitis in the ulna. One presented severe articular and osseous infection of the carpus. Eight cases presented severe soft tissue infections involving extensor and flexor tendons at the level of the forearm. All cases received antibiotics according to the antibiogram. No circulatory complications occurred. In one case where local hyperaemia and increased secretion was observed on the third day, a local antibiotic (Rifampicine) lavage system was introduced and applied for three days, followed by two days of aspiration drainage. In all cases, we observed complete disappearance of the infection. Contrary to our initial expectations, all patients tolerated well the immobilization of their upper limb and in none of the cases reduction of the range of motion of the shoulder or the elbow was observed after the division of the pedicle.

5.3. Radial forearm flap

The radial forearm flap ("chinese" flap) has been described by Yan Guofan in 1982. It is based on the radial artery and is extremely versatile. It can be alternatively elevated as an island skin flap, a free flap or as a compound forearm flap including vascularized nerve, bone and/or tendons. The big disadvantage is the sacrifice of the radial artery. Due to this and the current availability of flaps like the posterior interosseous, the anterior interosseous and the perforator flaps, we have abandoned its application, reserving it only for cases where a composite (skin, bone, tendon) flap is needed or in septic situations when the arterial inflow offered by the radial artery contributes to the healing of the infected tissues.

We used this flap in two patients with open fractures of the thumb and septic complications and in one case with severe pandactylitis of the index finger (no complications) where the wound healed completely in two weeks and healing of the affected bones was observed radiographically after three monts.

6. CONCLUSIONS

Reviewing the limited literature dealing with the application of tissue flap in the management of infections, we found the pedicled fasciocutaneous flaps to be the treatment of choice for severely infected wounds. Fasciocutaneous flaps seem to be as effective in acute and chronic infection as muscular or myocutaneous flaps. In concordance with the literature, loco regional pedicled flaps are useful and far easier to be applied compared to free flaps, and they do not have the vascular problems encountered in the latter. Even the groin flap, despite the inconvenience caused from the immobilization of the affected upper limb for two weeks, is easier to apply and has great healing potential. Finally, tissue transfer may contribute effectively to the management of upper limb infections.

REFERENCES

[1] Kernerman RP. Skin-muscle flap graft in severe forms of chronic osteomyelitis of the foot. Ortop Travmatol Protez 1966;27 (11):17-22.

[2] Hildebrandt G, Sander E. Muscle flap graft in severe forms of chronic osteomyelitis of the foot. Zentralbl Chir 1972;97 (28): 956-63.

[3] Ngoi SS, Satku K, Pho RW, Kumar VP. Local muscle flaps in the treatment of chronic osteomyelitis - the introduction of new vasculature. Injury 1987;18 (5):350-3.

[4] Fitzgerald RH Jr, Ruttle PE, Arnold PG, Kelly PJ, Irons GB. Local muscle flaps in the treatment of chronic osteomyelitis. J Bone Joint Surg [Am] 1985;67 (2):175-85.

[5] Mathes SJ, Feng LJ, Hunt TK. Coverage of the infected wound. Ann Surg 1983;198 (4):420-9.

[6] Cierny G 3rd, Byrd HS, Jones RE. Primary versus delayed soft tissue coverage for severe open tibial fractures. A comparison of results. Clin Orthop Relat Res 1983;(178):54-63.

[7] Moore JR, Weiland AJ. Vascularized tissue transfer in the treatment of osteomyelitis. Clin Plast Surg 1986;13(4):657-62.

[8] Zook EG, Russell RC, Asaadi M. A comparative study of free and pedicle flaps for lower extremity wounds. Ann Plast Surg 1986;17 (1):21-33.

[9] Schuz W, Haas HG, Klemm K. Closure of soft tissue defects in bone infections using free and pedicled muscle flaps. Unfallchirurgie 1987;13 (3): 163-73.

[10] Richards RR, Schemitsch EH. Effect of muscle flap coverage on bone blood flow following devascularization of a segment of tibia: an experimental investigation in the dog. J Orthop Res 1989;7(4): 550-8.

[11] Swiontkowski MF, Hagan K, Shack RB. Adjunctive use of laser Doppler flowmetry for debridement of osteomyelitis. J Orthop Trauma 1989;3(1):1-5.

[12] Patzakis MJ, Wilkins J, Kumar J, et al. Comparison of the results of bacterial cultures from multiple sites in chronic osteomyelitis of long bones. A prospective study. J Bone Joint Surg [Am] 1994; 76(5):664-6.

[13] Guelincky PJ, Sinsel NK. Refinements in the one-stage procedure for management of chronic osteomyelitis. Microsurgery 1995;16 (9):606-11.

[14] Rucker M, Roesken F, Schafer T, et al. *In vivo* analysis of the microcirculation of osteomyocutaneous flaps using fluorescence microscopy. Br J Plast Surg 1999;52(8):644-52.

[15] Rucker M, Vollmar B, Roesken F, et al. Microvascular transfer - related abrogation of capillary flow motion in critically reperfused composite flaps. Br J Plast Surg 2002;55(2):129-35.

[16] Machens HG, Pallua N, Mailaender P, et al. Measurements of tissue blood flow by the hydrogen clearance technique (HCT): a comparative study including laser Doppler flowmetry (LDF) and the Erlangen micro-lightguide spectrophotometer (EMPHO). Microsurgery 1995;16(12):808-17.

[17] Khalil AA, Aziz FA, Hall JC. Reperfusion injury. Plast Reconstr Surg 2006;117(3):1024-33.

[18] Pinsolle V, Reau AF, Pelissier P, et al. Soft-tissue reconstruction of the distal lower leg and foot: are free flaps the only choice? Review of 215 cases. J Plast Reconstr Aesthet Surg 2006;59 (9): 912-7.

[19] Lee RG, Baskin JZ. Improving outcomes of locoregional flaps: an emphasis on anatomy and basic science. Curr Opin Otolaryngol Head Neck Surg 2006;14(4):260-4.

[20] Zweifel-Schlatter M, Haug M, Schaefer DJ, et al. Free fasciocutaneous flaps in the treatment of chronic osteomyelitis of the tibia: a retrospective study. J Reconstr Microsurg 2006;22(1): 41-7.

[21] Yazar S, Lin CH, Lin YT, et al. Outcome comparison between free muscle and free fasciocutaneous flaps for reconstruction of distal third and ankle traumatic open tibial fractures. Plast Reconstr Surg 2006;117(7):2468-75; discussion 2476-7.

[22] Flugel A, Kehrer A, Heitmann C, et al. Coverage of soft-tissue defects of the hand with free fascial flaps. Microsurgery 2005;25(1): 47-53.

[23] Gatti JE, LaRossa D, Brousseau DA, et al. Assessment of neovascularization and timing of flap division. Plast Reconstr Surg 1984;73(3):396-402.

[24] Foucher G, Braun JB. A new island flap transfer from the dorsum of the index to the thumb. Plast Reconstr Surg 1979;63(3):344-9.

[25] McGregor IA, Jackson IT The groin flap. Br J Plast Surg 1972;25 (1):3-16.

[26] Cheng MH, Chen HC, Wei FC, et al. Combined ischemic preconditioning and laser Doppler measurement for early division of pedicled groin flap. J Trauma 1999;47(1):89-95.

Severe Osteomyelitis of the Forearm: Management with Microvascular Fibular Flaps

Bruno BATTISTON[a*], Roberto ADANI[b], Marco INNOCENTI[c], Pierluigi TOS[a]

[a]Microsurgery Department, C.T.O. Hospital, Torino, Italy

[b]Department of Orthopaedic Surgery, University of Modena and Reggio Emilia, Policlinico, Modena, Italy

[c]Microsurgery Department C.T.O. Hospital, Firenze, Italy

Severe infections at the forearm level are difficult to treat not only in terms of sterilization, but also in terms of functional restoration. Traditional radical debridement is very important, and sometimes the reconstruction of the excised tissues is difficult with conventional techniques. At the forearm level, local flaps generally are not sufficient for covering big defects. Conventional bone grafts may be resorbed or they cannot help healing when placed in an infected and hypovascular tissue bed. Therefore, bone reconstruction is a real challenge. Development of microsurgical techniques has increased the possibilities of treatment when those severe infections occur. Reconstruction of large soft tissue defects can be achieved by choosing the appropriate free flap. Vascularized fibular grafts allow the use of a segment of diaphyseal bone which is structurally similar to the radius and the ulna, and of length that would suffice to reconstruct most skeletal defects. In the upper limbs the vascularized fibular graft is indicated for patients in whom conventional bone grafting has failed or large bone defects are present (extending beyond 5 cm). When contemporary soft tissue reconstruction is needed, the fibula may give osteocutaneous and osteomyocutaneous grafts to be transferred. We report the results of a series of 22 cases of severe chronic osteomyelitis of the radius and/or the ulna treated with free vascularized fibula bone grafts. All patients were reviewed at a mean follow-up of 3 years (10-93 months); in all cases the infection never recurred. We report only one bone resorption, in the case of a double-barrel fibular transfer, which probably occurred due to vascularization failure. Even in this case, the patient was able to resume his previous occupation.

Keywords: forearm osteomyelitis; fibular free flap; microsurgery.

1. INTRODUCTION

Infections in the forearm, as in any other upper limb segment, may be acute, subacute or chronic, and may involve bone, soft tissues or both. Gene-

*Corresponding Author

Department of Orthopaedic Surgery

UOD Microsurgery

CTO Hospital, Torino, Italy

Tel: +39 011 6933301

e-mail: bruno.battiston@virgilio.it

rally, severe infections are exogenous and are caused by trauma or surgery. We will not refer extensively to etiology or diagnosis because, at the forearm level, the diagnostic approach and treatment are similar to those adopted for other anatomical sites.

The severity and extent of the infection and the type of host response are the main points of consideration in the choice of surgical strategy. The Cierny-Mader classification, based on the anatomy of bone infection and the physiology of the host, can well describe the clinical and local pathological picture [1]. Reconstruction should be carried out only after careful planning and identification of bone sequestra and dead contaminated tissues by roentgenography, sinusography, computed tomography (CT) and magnetic resonance imaging (MRI). Labeled leukocyte scans may be also useful [2].

The goal of surgery is to rule out the infection by providing a viable well-vascularized soft tissue bed. The more chronic and severe the infection, the more radical must be the debridement. Inadequate debridement may be the main reason for a high recurrence rate in chronic infections even by use of sophisticated reconstructive surgical techniques and broad spectrum antibiotics. An easy, but important step towards achieving the goal of complete and reliable cleaning is the use of methylene blue (injected in sinus tracts and on all the exposed tissues 12 hrs and immediately before surgery) making it easier to locate and remove infected tissue.

The treatment plan may follow either an *all-in-one* procedure with reconstruction of the excised tissue immediately after debridement or a *two-step* procedure with a few months delay between infected tissue excision and reconstruction. The choice, according to our experience, is dependent on the duration of the infection, the vascularization of the surrounding tissues and the host response to infection. Severe, but recent infections of well-vascularized tissues after radical debridement may be immediately reconstructed. Long-lasting infections with sclerotic tissues and poor vascularity may be treated by means of complete excision of contaminated tissues, and coverage with local or even microvascular flaps. We should wait for tendon, nerves, bone reconstruction till the moment when clinical and biological data (VES, PCR, etc.) confirm elimination of the infection. Even compromised patients with local, systemic or combined deficiencies should be checked while waiting for complete wound healing before final reconstruction.

Another reason for delaying bone reconstruction may be the need to re-establish correct bone alignment and normal relationships between the radius and the ulna. A severely shortened radius or other DRUJ malalignment in long-lasting infected nonunion with bone resorption should be treated by debridement and progressive distraction/correction using external fixation devices before proceeding to bone grafting (Fig. 1).

In the past, the remaining defect of the debrided area was either left open, while the exposed tissues were cleaned by continuous washing and medications, or it was closed with skin grafts when the infection ceased; then the defect was filled with muscle flaps and/or bone grafts of various types. Both soft tissues and osseous reconstruction was a relatively time-consuming process because it required severaltreatment stages. Treatment is particularly difficult in a region such as the forearm, which has a small muscle mass, and delicate and vital structures, such as tendons, nerves and vessels, which are superficial and poorly protected. A good success rate can be achieved in short-bone non-infected defects with cancellous or cortico-cancellous bone graft and

plate fixation only if surrounding tissues are in good condition [3].

Although traditional surgical approaches are still successful, microsurgery is the treatment of choice, since it has increased the possibilities of coverage and reconstruction. The possibility of transferring a large amount of vascularized tissue allows not only infection eradication, but also functional restoration of a segment such as the forearm, which is fundamental for normal use of the patient's hand. The surgeon can plan adequate excisions without maintaining non-viable tissues and then harvest the appropriate flap according to the needs of the debrided area. Finally, revascularized tissues are not parasites of the surrounding receiving tissues. On the contrary, they actively fight against infection and accelerate wound healing [4].

Skeletal reconstruction is a challenge to the orthopaedic surgeon. Conventional bone grafts were used with some success to cover bone defects even in infected areas [5,6] and traditional techniques as the one described by Papineau were often effective [7]. However, many of these techniques were unable to control the infection even after the bone integrity was reconstituted. Furthermore, defects extending beyond 5-6 cm were difficult to bridge by use of non-vascularized cortical or cancellous grafts [3]. The technique of bone transportation as described by Ilizarov [8] is generally effective in bone reconstruction, but there are several problems at the forearm level: tolerating the burden of external fixators for months, maintaining quality of regenerated bone and reconstituting bone continuity. Frequently, bone reconstitution does not allow good function in terms of pronation and supination [9].

In lower limbs, bone debridement may be also performed by means of partial resections thanks to the dimensions of femur and tibia. The defects may be covered with muscle flaps or cancellous grafts. On the other hand, in the infected radius and ulna the contaminated area must always be completely resected to get a healthy bed. In our experience, the vascularized fibula is the best option in reconstruction of large bone defects in the forearm, especially if they are due to severe infection. It may sufficiently reconstruct the long bones of the forearm that would result in appropriate restoration of the relative length and motion of the ulna and the radius (prono-supination) [10-16]. Preservation of the fibula vascularity avoids osteocyte necrosis, often leading to bone resorption, and is indispensable for safer and quicker integration and healing of the bone graft. Finally, its viability is important in resisting residual infection in the surrounding tissues [17-21].

2. CASE SERIES

We retrospectively studied 24 patients with infections of the forearm with bone involvement, 22 of whom had

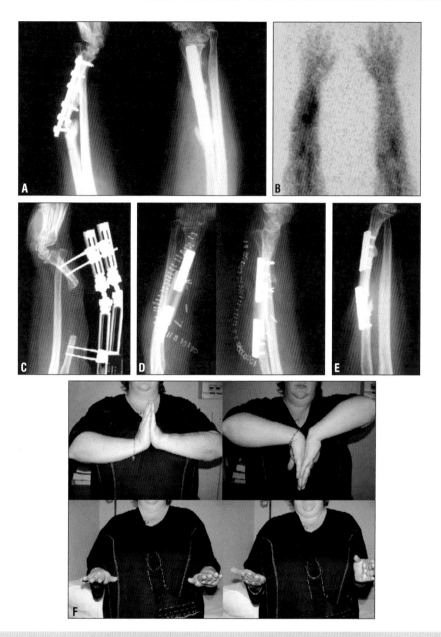

FIGURE 1. Case 18. **(A)** Infected radius nonunion with bone shortening after 4 previous surgical treatments. **(B)** Labeled leukocytes bone scan showing severe, extensive radius osteomyelitis. **(C)** First stage with bone resection and progressive distraction by external fixation to get correct DRUJ alignment. **(D)** Second stage with vascularized fibula graft (7 cm long) synthetized by double plating. **(E)** X-ray view 6 months afterwards with good bone healing. **(F)** Final functional recovery.

severe chronic osteomyelitis (Table 1) of the fourth degree, according to the Cierny-Mader classification. The patients were treated between 1992 and 2003. We did not consider minor bone infections with significant soft tissue loss in this series. In such cases, where the major problem is soft tissue loss, local and eventually free flaps are excellent options that would serve as a functional treatment.

The mean age of our patients was 35 years (16-65 years of age). All the patients had previously undergone repeated procedures with conventional treatments (debridement and bone grafting). The number of interventions ranged from 1 to 6 (mean: 3.6). The elapsed time between initial trauma and final reconstructive surgery ranged from 4 to 96 months (average: 25 months).

Two patients with bone infection and soft tissue loss

TABLE 1

Preoperative evaluation (VFG)

Case	Age (yrs)	Sex	Type of injury	Initial treatment	Previous operations
1	49	F	Closed fracture radius	ORIF	5
2	65	M	Closed fractures radius and ulna	ORIF	6
3	16	M	Open fractures radius and ulna	ORIF	3
4	24	M	Madelung's deformity	Osteotomy and bone graft	3
5	37	F	Closed fractures radius and ulna	ORIF	4
6	59	F	Open fractures radius and ulna	ORIF	4
7	30	F	Closed fractures radius and ulna	ORIF	3
8	31	F	Open fractures radius and ulna	ORIF	6
9	24	M	Open fracture radius	K wires and plaster	3
10	55	M	Open fractures radius and ulna	External fixation	5
11	37	M	Open fracture radius (gunshot)	External fixation	3
12	38	M	Open fracture ulna and radius	External fixator	4
13	31	M	Open fracture ulna and radius	External fixator	3
14	40	M	Open fracture ulna and radius	External fixator and ORIF	3
15	28	M	Closed fracture radius	ORIF	3
16	29	M	Open fracture ulna and radius	External fixator and ORIF	4
17	49	M	Subamputation - open fracture ulna and radius	Intramedullary wiring	1
18	38	F	Closed fracture radius	ORIF	4
19	25	F	Subamputation - open fracture ulna and radius	External fixator and ORIF	4
20	40	M	Subamputation - open fracture ulna and radius	External fixator and ORIF	2
21	35	M	Closed fracture radius	ORIF	4
22	46	M	Open fracture ulna and radius	ORIF	3

were debrided and subsequently had their defects covered by means of free flaps. In one case, we used a free muscle flap to cover combined extensor muscle loss (free functional gracilis) and in another, we used a fascio-cutaneous flap (dorsalis pedis) for loss of extensor tendon substance, which was associated with radius osteitis. The remaining 22 cases were treated by means of free vascularized fibula bone grafts.

In 20 cases, a two-stage treatment was performed, i.e. resection of the infected tissues in the first and free bone transfer in the second stage. In the other two cases, where the infection was more recent, one-stage treatment was performed, i.e. debridement and immediate bone transfer.

In 16 cases the bone defect was in the radius, in 5 patients in the ulna, and only in one patient in both the forearm bones, where double barrel fibular flap was used for the reconstruction. Six cases required an osteocutaneous tissue transfer with a skin pad for coverage of the bone. The length of the defect after extensive resection of necrotic bone from the septic nonunion ranged from 5 to 12 cm (mean 7.3).

The ulnar reconstruction was achieved by means of vascularized fibula twice, treating the concomitant radius

nonunion with resection and plate fixation. This procedure resulted in slight shortening of the forearm. Fibular fixation was obtained by using plates in most of the patients, i.e. in 3 cases a long plate was used, while in 14 cases two separate plates; pins, staples and screws associated with external fixation systems were used in the remaining 5 patients (Table 2).

Vascular end-to-end and end-to-side anastomosis were performed on the radial and/or ulnar artery; in 2 cases the peroneal artery was used to reconstruct the radial artery by performing vascular anastomosis both proximally and distally ("bridge graft"). In 8 cases external fixators were used in the first stage of the treatment in order that correct bone length and balance between the two bones of the forearm were achieved.

3. Results

The two patients treated for bone infection and major soft tissue problems healed without any further operation. Osteomyelitis did not recur.

All 22 patients treated with free fibula vascularized

TABLE 2

Operative treatment (VFG)

Case	Injury/VFG (months)	Site of bone defect	Graft length (cm)	Osteocuta-neous flap	Graft fixation		Complications	Additional procedures
					Proximal	**Distal**		
1	96	R	8	no	bridging plate		–	–
2	50	U	7	no	bridging compression plate		–	–
3	19	U	12	no	compression plate	compression plate	–	–
4	10	R	6	no	bridging compression plate		distal nonunion	additional cancellous graft and new distal plate
5	90	U	10	no	compression plate	compression plate	–	–
6	36	R	7,5	no	compression plate	compression plate	–	–
7	60	R	9	yes	screw and external fixator	screw and external fixator	proximal nonunion	additional proximal cancellous graft
8	48	R	8	yes	compression plate	compression plate	venous trombosis	loss of skin pad
9	24	R	8	yes	plate	plate	–	–
10	12	R	7	no	insertion of fibula into distal radius and pins fixation	compression plate	–	–
11	8	R	6	no	compression plate	compression plate	–	–
12	12	U	7	no	compression plate	compression plate	–	–
13	7	U	5	no	compression plate	compression plate	distal nonunion	additional cancellous graft and new distal plate
14	8	R	7	no	compression plate	compression plate	–	–
15	12	R	9	no	compression plate	compression plate	–	–
16	9	R	7	no	compression plate	compression plate	–	–
17	2	R/U	6 - 6	yes	U compression plate	compression plate	ulna resorption	one-bone forearm
					R compression plate	screw		
18	12	R	7	no	compression plate	compression plate	mobilization of proximal plate	–
19	14	R	7	yes	compression plate	compression plate	–	–
20	3	R	5	yes	compression plate	screw	–	–
21	7	R	7	no	compression plate	compression plate	–	–
22	9	R	7	no	compression plate	compression plate	–	–

R = radius, U = ulna

bone grafts were reviewed at a mean follow-up of 3 years (from 10 to 93 months); in all cases the infection never recurred (Fig. 2 A-D).

All patients were reviewed and classified according to the Tang system (Table 3), which is based on two assessment criteria, i.e. clinical and radiological findings.

According to Tang's classification, the following results were obtained: excellent clinical evaluation in 12 patients, good in 8, fair in 2 and poor in none; excellent radiographic evaluation in 12 patients, good in 6, fair in 3 and poor in 1.

The mean time to radiographic bone union was 4 months (range: 2.5-8 months). In 3 cases a secondary procedure was employed for an aseptic nonunion in one junction site of the graft.

At final evaluation, the elbow and wrist movements

B. BATTISTON, R. ADANI, M. INNOCENTI, P. TOS

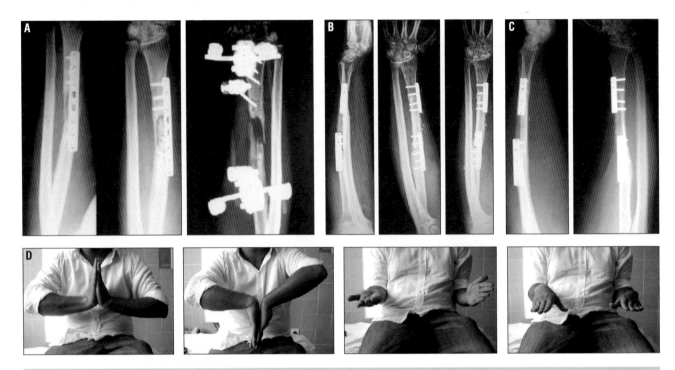

FIGURE 2. Case 21. **(A)** Severe radius infection operated on several times by means of plating, debridement and external fixation without resolution of the osteomyelitis. **(B)** Treatment with large bone resection and grafting by free vascularized fibula (7 cm). **(C)** Final bone healing 4 months later. **(D)** Clinical picture with good functional recovery.

as well as the forearm rotation were measured (Table 4). The elbow motion was satisfactory in all cases. The average pronation of the reconstructed forearm was 58° (range: 20°-80°). The average supination was 43° (range: 0°-80°). The average extension of the wrist was 38° (range: 10°-80°) and the average flexion was 38° (range: 10°-80°). The mean prono-supination loss was 35°, but the residual function was sufficient for all of the patients to return to previous activities.

No complication was registered at the harvesting site. There were no cases with fractures of the grafted bone. Distal screw loosening was seen in two patients. A second operation was necessary in three cases to remove the previous plate and replace it with a new plate associated with bone graft to achieve bone healing. In two cases the nonunions were stable, and the patients refused further operation. These patients experienced no pain and their arms could be used almost normally in common activities of everyday life. No changes occurred over time.

One patient had skin pad loss due to venous thrombosis; however, the bone healed in 8 months.

TABLE 3

Tang clinical and radiographic classification of results

Clinical results

Excellent	Ability to carry out normal work or study;
Good	Ability to carry out everyday activities with no difficulties related to the reconstructed part;
Fair	Limited ability to perform everyday activities, sometimes with difficulty;
Poor	Inability to perform everyday activities with either significant limb shortening or pain at the surgical site

Radiographic results

Excellent	Healing within 6 months with no reintervention;
Good	Healing within 1 year with no reintervention;
Fair	Healing after 1 year or reinterventions;
Poor	Nonunion after repeated surgery

TABLE 4

Clinical results - active ROM

	Forearm		Wrist	
Case	Pronation	Supination	Extension	Flexion
1	80	80	30	30
2	50	40	25	30
3	70	80	45	40
4	20	30	10	10
5	80	20	30	40
6	30	20	25	30
7	60	45	40	35
8	50	30	40	30
9	80	80	35	30
10	30	10	20	10
11	90	90	80	80
12	70	70	50	60
13	60	50	50	40
14	30	30	30	40
15	90	40	45	50
16	80	30	50	40
17	20	0	20	10
18	80	20	50	80
19	40	45	40	30
20	45	30	45	40
21	80	70	50	45
22	60	45	40	40

The patient whose results were considered poor after the X-ray evaluation had resorption of one part of the double barrel fibular graft.

4. DISCUSSION AND CONCLUSION

Severe infections of the forearm are difficult to treat not only in terms of sterilization, but also in terms of functional restoration. Traditional radical debridement is very important, but reconstruction of the excised tissues is sometimes problematic when performed with conventional techniques [22,23]. At the forearm level, local flaps generally are not sufficient to cover large defects. Skeletal integrity is another big problem. Conventional bone grafts may be resorbed and the healing process may not be easy when the graft is placed in an infected and hypovascular bed. The creation of "one-bone forearm", which can be achieved by transferring the distal radius onto the proximal ulna, may lead to complete loss of pro-supination. Its use is therefore indicated only for severe forearm trauma involving both the radius and the ulna, in the case of severe damage or functional loss of the distal radio-ulnar joint [24,25].

The development of microsurgical techniques has increased the therapeutic possibilities for these severe problems. Reconstruction of large soft tissue defects can be performed after choosing the appropriate free flap. Vascularized fibular grafts allow use of a segment

of diaphyseal bone, which is structurally similar to the radius and the ulna and of sufficient length that would allow reconstruction of most skeletal defects.

Concerning the upper limb, the vascularized fibular graft is indicated for cases of patients where conventional bone grafting has failed, or large bone defects are present (those extending beyond 5 cm). When contemporary soft tissue reconstruction is needed, the fibula combined with skin or muscle could be transferred [26].

The validity of the technique is confirmed by the results obtained in our series (Table 3): all patients returned to everyday routine activities. The possibility of preserving pro-supination, even partially, together with restored skeletal stability, undoubtedly enhanced the possibility of resuming former daily activities. Restoration of functional anatomy is one of the main advantages of this technique compared to reconstruction by Ilizarov or other techniques. No secondary fractures or recurrence of infection were found in any of the patients of the current series [27,28].

Even in other case series, the free vascularized fibular graft was successfully applied to reconstruct upper limb bone defects [29]. In Eisenshenk's experience, the transplants without a history of infection were better, compared with transplants with such a history [30]. On the contrary, in our osteomyelitis cases the healing rates were similar to series including non-infected lesions. Zimmermann suggests that there is significant early and late donor site morbidity, which should be considered when a fibula graft is opted for [31]. In our cases, the complications at donor site level were absent, while they were few at the reconstruction site (one skin pad loss, one partial bone resorption, three secondary operations for delayed healing).

In conclusion, our experience suggests that the microvascular bone transplantation for bridging infected bone defects is a distinct technique to preserve the extremities. This transplantation can survive within a weakened and infected transplant bed and helps the patients' recovery.

REFERENCES

[1] Cierny G III, Mader JT, Penninck JJ. A clinical staging system for adult osteomyelitis, Clin Orthop Relat Res 2003;414:7-24.

[2] Kaim AH, Gross T, von Schulthess GK. Imaging of chronic posttraumatic osteomyelitis, Eur Radiol 2002;12 (5):1193-1202.

[3] Ring D et a., Ununited diaphyseal forearm fractures with segmental defects: plate fixation and autogenous cancellous bone-grafting, J Bone Jt Surg Am 2004;86-A (11):2440-2445.

[4] Battiston B, Guizzi PA, Brunelli G. L'osteogenesi Riparativa Nei Trapianti Ossei Liberi Microvascolari, GIOT, Vol. XII, 2, 1986, p. 139, suppl.

[5] Brunelli G. Soft cancellous bone grafts for non-union and joint fusion. Internat. Congr. Series no. 291 (15 BN, 90, 219, 0213, 3) Orthop Surg and Traumat Tel Aviv 1972. Excepta Medica, Amsterdam.

[6] Brunelli G. Greeffes osseuses malleables a consolidation rapide, Acta Orthop Belg 1972;38:184.

[7] Papineau LJ. L'excision greffe avec fermeture retardee deliberee dans l'osteomyelite chronique, Nouv Presse Med 1973;2:2753.

[8] Ilizarov GA, Clinical application of the tension-stress effect for limb lengthening, Clin Orthop Relat Res 1990;229 (250):8-26.

[9] El-Mowafi H, Elalfi B, Wasfi K. Functional outcome following treatment of segmental skeletal defects of the forearm bones by Ilizarov application, Acta Orthop Belg 2005;71 (2):157-162.

[10] Adan R et al. Reconstruction of large posttraumatic skeletal defects of the forearm by vascularized free fibular graft, Microsurgery 2004;24 (6):423-429.

[11] Battiston B, Pontini I, Cartesegna M, Ferrero S, Sard A. La nostra esperienza nell'uso dell'osso microvascolare. Giornale Italiano di Ortopedia e Traumatologia - 2° Suppl. Vol. XXII - Fasc. 2 - Giugno 1996.

[12] Dell PC, Sheppard JE. Vascularized bone grafts in the treatment of infected forearm nonunions, J Hand Surg 1984;9A:653-658.

[13] Mattar JJ et al. Vascularized fibular graft for management of severe osteomyelitis of the upper extremity, Microsurgury 1994; 15:22-27.

[14] Lew DP, Waldvogel FA. Osteomielite, Lancet Jul 24-30 2004;364 (9431):369-379.

[15] Tang CH, Reconstruction of the bones and joints of the upper extremity by vascularized free fibular graft: report of 46 cases, J Reconstr Microsurg 1992;8:285-292.

[16] Weiland AJ, Free vascularized bone grafts in surgery of the upper extremity, J Hand Surg 1979;129-144.

[17] Dee P, Lambruschi PG, Hiebert JM. The use of Tc-99m MDP bone scanning in the study of vascularized bone implants: concise communication, J Nucl Med 1981;22:522-525.

[18] Dell PC, Burchardt H, Glowczeskie FP. A Roentgengraphic biomedical and historical evaluation of vascularized and non-vascularized segmental fibular canine autograits, J Bone Jt Surg 1984;67-A (1):105-112.

[19] Stevenson JS et al. Technetium-99 m phosphate bone imaging: a method for assessing bone graft healing, Radiology 110 1974; 391-394.

[20] Velasco JG et al. The early detection of free bone graft viability with Tc-99m: a preliminary report, Br J Plast Surg 1976;29:344-346.

[21] Portigliatti Barbos M. La marcatura fluorescente del tessuto osseo nell'uomo: messa a punto del metodo e validita sperimentale, Il Policlinico Sez Chir 1984, pp.91-95.

[22] Burchardt H. Biology of cortical bone graft incorporation, in: Friedlaender GE, Mankin HJ, Sell KW (Eds.), Osteochondral Allografts. Biology, Banking and Clinical Applications, Little, Brown, Boston, 1983, pp. 51-57.

[23] Enneking WF, Eady JL, Burchardt H. Autogenous cortical bone grafts in the reconstruction of segmental skeletal defects, J Bone Jt Surg 1980;C2-A (10).

[24] Bessy H et al. La reconstruction des pertes de substance osseuse de l'avant-bras par cubitalitasion du radius (one bone forearm), Ann Chir Main 1996;15:199-211.

[25] Peterson CA, Maki S, Wood MB. Clinical results of the one-bone forearm, J Hand Surg 1995;20A:609-618.

[26] Wood MB, Cooney WP, Irons GB. Skeletal reconstruction by vascularized bone transfer: indications and results, Mayo Clin Proc 1985;60:729.

[27] De Boer H, Wood MB. Bone changes in the vascularized fibular graft, J Bone Jt Surg 1989;71B:374-378.

[28] Allieu Y, Teissier J, Bonnel F. Etude experimentale du comportement biologique d'une greffe osscuse corticale vascularisee et problemes mecaniques. S.O.F.C.O.T. Reunion annuelle, nov. 1982, Suppl II, Rev Chir Orthop 1983;69.

[29] Malizos KN et al. Free vascularized fibular grafts for reconstruction of skeletal defects, J Am Acad Orthop Surg Sep-Oct 2004;12(5): 360-369.

[30] Eisenschenk A, Lautenbach M, Rohlmann A. Free vascularized bone transplantation in the extremities, Orthopade 1998;27(7): 491-500.

[31] Zimmermann CE et al. Donor site morbidity after microvascular fibula transfer, Clin Oral Investig 2001;5 (4):214-219.

Septic Non–Unions and Osteomyelitis in the Upper Limb Managed with Distraction Osteogenesis

Konstantinos N. MALIZOS*, Konstantinos BARGIOTAS, Theophilos KARACHALIOS, Nikolaos ROIDIS

Department of Orthopaedic Surgery and Musculoskeletal Trauma, University of Thessalia, Larissa, Greece

Osteomyelitis of the upper limp, although not as common as osteomyelitis of the tibia and femur, might be a debilitating problem and very difficult to treat. In the upper limp the most common causes of contiguous focus osteomyelitis are trauma, infected foreign bodies, perioperative infections and non-surgically induced contiguous soft tissue infections. Although the same general principles of radical debridement, adequate stabilization and soft tissue coverage used for the treatment of osteomyelitis in the long bones of the lower limp apply to humerus and forearm bones, a number of anatomical and biomechanical variations do exist and should be taken into account when planning treatment of the upper limp. Whereas shortening of the humerus might be accepted within some limits, anatomical restoration of the forearm is mandatory to achieve an acceptable functional result in cases of septic non-unions. A staged approach considering variables regarding the patient's health status, as well as local characteristics like bone and soft tissue loss and bacterial virulence, should be followed in order to treat osteomyelitis and manage successfully the consequences of the infected bone defect. Distraction osteogenesis is a valuable tool in those cases where large bone defects exist and may be combined with microsurgical soft tissue coverage techniques in order to treat infected bone and/or soft tissue loss.

Keywords: osteomyelitis; infection of the humerus; forearm infection; upper limp septic non-unions; distraction osteogenesis.

1. INTRODUCTION

Osteomyelitis and infected non-union, although less common in the upper limb, are quite debilitating for the patient and constitute a major challenge for the treating physicians. Osteomyelitis may be due to hematogenous spread or a contiguous infection focus. Hematogenous osteomyelitis usually involves the metaphysis of the long bones in children and the vertebral bodies in adults. In the upper limp the most common causes of contiguous focus osteomyelitis are trauma, infected foreign bodies, perioperative infections and non-surgically induced contiguous soft tissue infections. The incidence of this type of osteomyelitis is increasing due to the great number of motor vehicle accidents, the extensive use of fixation hardware and joint arthroplasty implants, and the increasing number of immunocompromized patients undergoing surgical procedures.

Osteomyelitis in the adult population may also result from reactivation of a quiescent focus of hematogenous osteomyelitis initially developed during infancy or childhood. Inadequate debridement, malnutrition, drug abuse, alcoholism, smoking and severe systemic or metabolic disorders may predispose to the progress and recurrence of osteomyelitis.

Bacterial factors such as genotypic variants de-

*Corresponding Author
Department of Orthopaedic Surgery and
Musculoskeletal Trauma
University of Thessalia
41110 Larissa, Greece
Tel: +30 2410 682722
Fax: +30 2410 670107
e-mail: malizos@med.uth.gr

termining the production of glycocalyx and adhesive proteins, as well as the ability of bacteria to form biofilm on hardware, have been recognized to be important in the pathogenesis of osteomyelitis. Staphylococci and pseudomonas are the most common pathogens of contiguous focus osteomyelitis and infected pseudarthrosis.

The hallmark of chronic osteomyelitis is infected dead bone surrounded by a compromised soft tissue envelope. New bone formed by the surviving segments of the periosteum and the endosteum may encase the dead bone (involucrum encasing the sequestrum).

The containment of the infection into the bone depends on the competence of the host's local and systemic defense mechanisms. Several systemic and local factors influence the ability of the host to respond to infection and treatment protocols. Patients with diabetes mellitus, chronic granulomatous diseases and sickle-cell disease are particularly susceptible to skeletal infections due to their deficient systemic and local defuse mechanisms which facilitate containment of the initial infection. Appropriate management and specific treatment selection requires a balanced judgment of a number of parameters including (i) the functional impairment, (ii) the condition of the host, (iii) the potential consequences of an aggressive surgical therapy, and (iv) the physical, psychological and financial burden of the reconstructive steps.

As in any bone infection, surgical management of upper limp infections, includes adequate drainage, extensive debridement to the point where punctuate bleeding is achieved (the "paprika sign"), and dead space obliteration with adequate healthy tissue coverage. In the presence of an infected nonunion the same principles are equally applicable, and depending on the degree of involvement of each bone segment, a variable size defect and instability are sustained after thorough debridement. In those cases where osteomyelitis is diffuse and an intercalary resection of the bone is necessary for eradication of the disease process, the skeletal stability is lost. This form of osteomyelitis may be classified as type IV according to the Cierny-Mader classification. The presence of an infected bone segment, pathological soft tissues adjoining the osseous defect, lack of skeletal integrity and, after the debridement, a variable size bone defect with a considerable degree of microbial contamination are common characteristics encountered in both conditions previously described and they are addressed with similar approaches which are described in this chapter.

In planning surgery for osteomyelitis the challenge involves bone debridement, the extent of which has been recently reinvestigated by Simpson et al. [1]. In their study, wide resection with a clearance margin of 5 mm or more was found to lead to no infection recurrence as opposed to marginal resection with a clearance margin of less than 5 mm, which developed 28% recurrence with a higher rate in type-B hosts. The debulking procedure alone led to recurrence within one year after surgery. A critical parameter, however, remains the biological competence of the host to respond to surgery and allow normal healing. Compromised local tissue conditions and osteopenia from previous trauma, surgery, irradiation or systemic conditions affecting healing such as diabetes, immunosuppression, smoking, and/or other metabolic disorders, impose additional burden and should be always taken into account in planning the reconstruction of bone loss due to infection.

In very severely infected non-unions in the upper extremity with extensive tissue loss, involvement of neuromuscular functioning units and an insensate nonfunctioning hand might pose a dilemma as to whether the patient and the surgeon should be engaged in a more lengthy attempt to salvage the limb, or amputation should be chosen, which may be further debilitating for the patient. This challenge, however, unlike that of lower extremity wounds, rarely appears in the case of upper limb infection. The poor performance of the hand prosthesis compared to that of the lower limb, is also an important parameter to consider prior to any decision.

2. ANATOMIC, BIOLOGIC AND BIOMECHANICAL CONSIDERATIONS OF UPPER LIMB NON-UNIONS

There are several anatomical and biomechanical issues that need to be considered when dealing with non-unions of the humerus and the long bones of the forearm. Although the general principle described above applies to the humerus and the forearm bones alike, special anatomic and functional considerations exist and influence treatment stategies. Whereas shortening and a degree of mal-rotation of the humerus might be acceptable, precise anatomic restoration of the forearm bones is mandatory to achieve an acceptable functional result. Unlike axial loading in the lower limb, more complex loading patterns combining bending, rotation and shear forces apply to the upper limb during daily activities.

In the majority of elderly patients the use of a single-hand-held walking aid is a necessity for their daily activities. Therefore, one should consider the parameter of time towards healing as important as the immediate rigid stabilization of the skeleton so that the patient might use his arm during the treatment course. One of the difficulties in this particular patient population is to secure skeletal stability. The bone quality may be impaired due to osteoporosis related not only to age but also to disuse of the arm. Stiffness of the adjacent shoulder and elbow joints are common secondary problems that further complicate the management.

Shortening of the humerus up to 3-4 cm does not significantly affect muscle function, and since length discrepancy is not an issue of equal severity as in the lower limb, it is finally acceptable within certain limits. A small degree of mal-alignment at the humerus level is also functionally acceptable. Although ORIF is considered the "gold standard" technique for treating non-unions of the humeral shaft, it carries the risk of injuring the radial nerve at the spiral groove and destroying the blood supply of the bone as the nutrient artery enters the shaft at the junction of the middle and distal thirds. Furthermore, in presence of infection, biofilm formation on the implants precludes the use of internal fixation devices. This also applies for the IM nailing techniques even in its newer designs like the cross locked IM nails and for techniques that improve compression and stability. However, when the resection of the infected tissues is wide enough, internal fixation devices may still be an option for skeleton stabilization.

3. MANAGEMENT STRATEGIES FOR HUMERAL SEPTIC NON-UNIONS

Although open fractures with segmental bone loss and infected non-unions of the humerus are not as common as the ones of the femur or the tibia, they are sometimes more difficult to treat [2]. Defects up to 3-4 cm can be easily managed simply by shortening and application of rigid fixation. Shortening might facilitate at the same time closure of soft tissue defects. As a result, for a small defect left after radical debridement, direct fragment apposition and mechanical stability can be immediately achieved avoiding further procedures. Similarly, soft tissue management becomes less demanding after shortening of the humerus and closure of the wound with well vascularized healthy tissue.

When chronic osteomyelitis of the humerus affects a great part of the diaphysis, or the debridement of the non-union leaves a skeletal defect of more than 4cm, it has to be dealt with according to the principles applying to any other skeletal infection lacking stability. After extensive resection of the affected tissues the wounds may be too large and complicated for primary closure or skin grafting. The fundamental principles of i) bone fixation capable of withstanding loading for a prolonged period of time until healing is complete, and ii) wound closure and dead space obliteration with healthy tissue, should be followed.

4. ALTERNATIVE TECHNIQUES

In the case of infected non-unions with a defect up to 2-2.5 times the width of the humeral diaphysis, monofocal compression with circular frames (Ilizarov) has been reported by Lammens et al. [3] who treated 6 patients with infected nonunion. Four out of 6 patients had a re-fracture which required reapplication of the frame and 4 had transient nerve palsy. Kocaoglu et al. [4] reported

on 35 patients treated with circular frames at an average of 39 months after injury. All but one non-union were healed at an average of 5.5 months. Pullen et al. [5] reported on 4 patients with severe bone loss and infection. The frame was removed at an average of 8.8 months and although re-fracture occurred in 2 out of 4 patients, eventually, union was achieved in all patients. Considering the relatively high re-fracture rate of this treatment approach, it appears that the biomechanical characteristics of callus in the humeral diaphysis after the removal of the frame are inadequate to withstand the mechanical load while the patient is engaged in routine daily activities. A staged removal of the external fixator might better prepare the callus and allow consolidation and remodeling for a short period prior to complete removal of the fixator. We have an unreported experience of 5 cases with infected non-unions and a bone defect less than 4 cm, which underwent direct monofocal compression and bone grafting from the iliac crest with a unilateral frame external fixation device. Upon the appearance of immature callus on the x-rays we started to increase the distance of the fixator from the bone by 1.5 cm to create a more elastic construct for the stimulation of the healing process. The only way to make a circular frame less rigid is to gradually remove wires or threaded pins. There was a re-fracture in one out of 5 patients. In those where a circular frame is utilized, it is suggested that it be fixed on the bone also with threaded half pins instead of tensioned wires only.

For bone defects larger than 2-2.5 times the diameter of the humerus, the bone transfer technique using a circular frame fulfills the prerequisites, restores the limb length and achieves bone integrity with minimal trauma and potential complications [6]. Although it is difficult to tolerate, especially in obese patients, circular frames can withstand more effectively rotational and shear forces than monolateral fixators and are more suitable in complex cases. Physicians should be very cautious in pin placement to avoid injury to neurovascular structures. Non-union or re-fracture at the docking site as in all long bones, radial nerve palsy due to traction or direct injury, elbow flexion contracture, and pin track infection are the commonest complications [3].

The compression-distraction technique or early autografts can be used to manage docking site non-union [7], while close monitoring of the patient can help prevent neurovascular- and joint-related problems in the course of the lengthening procedure.

In contrast to the difficulties in reconstructing large skeletal defects in the humerus when vascularized soft tissue coverage is required, a pedicled latissimus dorsi muscle or myocutaneous flap can be harvested from the ipsilateral side. This flap, if elevated completely, may be large enough to allow coverage of the entire volar or dorsal surface of the humerus with extension of the muscle into the proximal forearm. The muscular or the myocutaneous flap of the pectoralis major has a smaller arc of rotation and leaves a more noticeable scar.

5. Management Strategies for Forearm Septic Non-Unions

While a certain degree of mal-union in the humerus can be accepted, shortening and mal-union of forearm fractures has a deleterious effect on the function and cosmesis of the entire upper limb. The presence of forearm mal-alignment besides wrist deformity may cause radial head subluxation and restriction of pronation / supination. In planning of the reconstruction of segmental bone loss at the forearm it is mandatory to achieve restoration of length, alignment and the bow shape of the radius so that the forearm rotation is maintained.

Segmental defects of the forearm bones are difficult to treat with conventional methods. The combination of local infection with bone defect exacerbates the problem and poses even greater challenges [8]. Many authors believe that diaphyseal bone defects of the forearm that are smaller than 5 cm in length can be managed with corticocancellous bone grafting or non-vascularized fibular graft [9, 10, 11, 12], provided the patient has an adequate soft tissue envelope and no infection. In case of severe soft tissue loss, primary bone grafting is still the treatment of choice, combined with simultaneous soft tissue coverage [12]. Barbieri et al. [9] reported their experience of the use of autogenous bone graft and internal fixation; the most frequent complication was infection (40%). Moroni et al. [13] reported that out of 24 patients with segmental bone loss of the forearm treated with autogenous bone graft and internal fixation, 10 cases had excellent results, and Green et al. [14] claimed that the large volume of bone needed to fill a defect greater than 6 cm required multiple donor sites, a source of discomfort and morbidity for the patients.

Arai et al. [8] claimed that massive long bone defects greater than 6 cm are difficult to treat with autogenous bone graft, and therefore, other methods should be used. Long bone defects greater than 6 cm can be managed with either vascularized bone graft or bone transport using the circular frame external fixator [12, 15, 16, 17].

Vascularized bone graft was introduced in the treatment of large soft tissue and bone defects through microvascular techniques. Both fibular and iliac crest transfer have been reported with rates of success in achieving union ramging from 80% to 90%. This procedure is technically difficult, time consuming and has a consiterable complication rate both for the donor and the treated sides [18, 19]. The results of treatment by using this technique seem to be less favourable in infected cases [19] and in those with larger bone defects, where a significantly higher incidence of re-fracture is reported [20].

The technique of bone transport revolutionized treatment of high energy trauma and its consequences. It has been considered since as an ideal solution for large skeletal defects because of the fact that virtually any defect size could be bridged in a sound mechanical environment, using a versatile frame with minimal or no need for harvesting grafts from other sites of the patient's skeleton.

The system of circular frames provides rigid fixation even in osteoporotic bone and allows early active and passive motion from the first postoperative day. The Ilizarov system presents certain advantages compared with other methods of treatment, especially where there is infection and bone loss: the mechanical stimulations increase local tissue nourishment, and circular frame osteosynthesis restores the function of the injured limb, increases local blood flow and stimulates osteogenesis [4]. In 1994, Green [21] evaluated two different methods of managing segmental skeletal defects. A total of 15 patients treated with the open bone graft (Papineau) technique were compared with 17 patients treated with the Ilizarov procedure. There were many complications in the bone-grafted group such as limited graft availability, donor site morbidity and graft fractures. In the bone-transport group, the main problem was failure of the docking site to unite without supplementary grafting.

Harrington et al. [16] reported that five open fractures of the ulna with bone loss of more than 8 cm were treated by bone transport and external fixation. A satisfactory functional result was achieved, demonstrating the efficacy of this technique for difficult forearm reconstruction. Esser [22] reported a case treated with bone transport. Treatment was completed at 10 months and the only complication was transient superficial pin site infection.

Many authors have reported the use of the Ilizarov method to treat difficult reconstruction problems of the forearm. The majority of these cases are published either as case reports or they represent a small part of a various data pool that may contain - among others - oncological or congenital cases [23-25]. El-Mowafi's [24] study is the most focused, which reported results with bone transport to overcome forearm bone defects due to infection. In this series, 16 patients with defects of the forearm bones, following either debridement of osteomyelitis or of an infected non-union, were involved. The mean time from injury to the Ilizarov procedure was 11.7 months. The mean number of operative procedures before application of the Ilizarov device was 3.4. The mean length of the defects after debridement was 6.4 cm. Monofocal osteotomy was performed. The mean external fixation index, distraction index and maturation index were 41.5 days/cm, 19.8 days/cm, and 21.7 days/cm, respectively. The mean time in the frame was 8.9 months. The mean total duration of the treatment was 11.4 months. There were 14 complications in 11 patients including pin-track infection, premature consolidation, delayed union at the docking site and re-fracture. The authors concluded that the technique of bone transport is an ideal solution for treatment of a large skeletal defect in spite of the high incidence of associated problems, obstacles and true complications. In El-Mowafi's study, the complication rate was relatively high, and this may relate to the fact that patients had undergone on average 3.4 operations (range: 2 to 6) before the index procedure. These may have caused atrophy of the articular cartilage, intra-articular adhesions, contracture of the surrounding tissue and osteoporosis of the forearm bones. However, the main complication was delayed union at the docking site. Many authors [4, 15] suggest the staged use of autogenous cancellous bone graft at the docking site.

Although bone transport is an effective treatment for segmental bone loss and non-unions of the forearm [6, 26], it is at the same time a demanding procedure due to the anatomic complexity of the forearm and the potential of iatrogenic complications. Placement of k-wires and half-pins require careful planning and the surgeon must follow strictly the established guidelines based on anatomic cross-section studies. Furthermore, circular frames have to be used only in cases where no other method of treatment is indicated, while unlike the case of the lower limb, they significantly interfere with the patient's basic daily hygiene and body image.

6. SUMMARY

Osteomyelitis and infected bone loss in long bones of the upper limb are not very common but very difficult to treat. Applying the same basic principles of adequate resection of the pathological tissue, antibiotic administration (systemic and local) and skeletal reconstruction with Distraction Osteogenesis, a high rate of successful outcome is obtained. In the forearm, the reconstruction of normal anatomy is a prerequisite for full function, whereas in the humerus slight shortening or anatomical mal-alignment within narrow limits may be acceptable.

REFERENCES

[1] Simpson AH, Deakin M, Latham JM. Chronic osteomyelitis. The effect of the extent of surgical resection on infection-free survival. Bone Joint Surg [Br.] 2001;83(3):403-7.

[2] Gualda G. Gualdrini Pascarell R, Colozza A, Stagni C. Infected non-union of the humerus, Chir Organi di Movi 2000;(85):251-25.

[3] Lammens J, Baudin G, Driesen R, Moens P, Stuyck J, Smet D, Fabry G. Treatment of non-union of the humerus using the Ilizarov External Fixation, Clinical Orthop 1998;(353):223-230.

[4] Kocaoglu M, Eralp L, Tomak Y. Treatment of humeral shaft non-unions by the Ilizarov method. Int Orthop 2001;25:396-400.

[5] Pullen C, Manzotti A, Catagni MA. Guerreschi F. of Treatment post-traumatic humeral diaphyseal nonunion with bone loss. J Shoulder Elbow Surg. 2003;(12):436-41.

[6] Dendrinos GK, Kontos S, Lyritsis E. Use of the Ilizarov technique for treatment of nonunion of the tibia associated with infection. J Bone Joint Surg 1995;77A:835-846.

[7] Steinberg EL. OPINION: Illizarov externla fixation and bone transport. J. Orthop Trauma. 2004;18:470-471.

[8] Arai K, Toh S, Yasumura M et al. One-bone forearm formation using vascularized fibula graft for massive bone defect of the forearm with infection: case report. J Reconstr Microsurg 2001;17:151-155.

[9] Barbieri CH, Mazzer N, Aranda CA, Pinto MM. Use of a bone block graft from the iliac crest with rigid fixation to correct diaphyseal defects of the radius and ulna. J Hand Surg 1997;22B:395-401.

[10] Moroni A, Caja VL, Sabato C et al. Composite bone grafting and plate fixation for the treatment of nonunions of the forearm with segmental bone loss: a report of eight cases. J Orthop Trauma 1995;9:419-426.

[11] Omololu B, Ogunlade SO, Alonge TO. Limb conservation using non vascularised fibular grafts. West Afr J Med. 2002;2:347-349

[12] Stevanovic M, Gutow AP, Sharpe F. The management of bone defects of the forearm after trauma. Hand Clin 1999;15:299-318.

[13] Moroni A, Rollo G, Guzzardella M, Zinghi G. Surgical treatment of isolated forearm non-union with segmental bone loss. Injury 1997; 28:497-504.

[14] Green SA, Diabal T. The open bone graft for septic nonunion. Clin Orthop 1983;180:109-115.

[15] Dell PC, Sheppard JE. Vascularized bone grafts in the treatment of infected forearm nonunions. J Hand Surg 1984;9A:653-658.

[16] Harrington DK, Saleh M. An open fracture of the ulna with bone loss, treated by bone transport. Injury 1999;30:349-356.

[17] Harrington DK, Saleh M. An open fracture of the ulna with bone loss, treated by bone transport. Injury 1999;30:349-356.

[18] Liu X, Ge B, Wen Y. Repairing bone and soft tissue defects of the forearm with a composite segmented-fibula osteoseptocutaneous flap. Zhonghua Zheng Xing Shao Shang Wai Ke Za Zhi 1997;13: 352-353.

[19] Moran CG, Wood MB. Vascularized bone autografts. Orthop Rev 1993;22:187-197.

[20] Vail TP, Urbaniak JR. Donor-site morbidity with use of vascularized autogenous fibular grafts. J Bone Joint Surg 1996;78A:204-211

[21] Kasashima T, Minami A, Kutsumi K. Late fracture of vascularized fibular grafts. Microsurgery 1998;18:337- 343.

[22] Green SA. Skeletal defects. A comparison of bone grafting and bone transport for segmental skeletal defects. Clin Orthop 1994; 301:111-117

[23] Esser RD. Treatment of a bone defect of the forearm by bone transport. A case report. Clin Orthop 1996;326:221-224.

[24] El-Mowafi H, Elalfi B, Wasfi K. Functional outcome following treatment of segmental skeletal defects of the forearm bones by Ilizarov application. Acta Orthop Belg. 2005 Apr;71:157-62.

[25] Haidukewych J, Sperling JW. Results of treatment of infected humeral nonunions: The Mayo Clinic experience, Clinical Orthop, 2003; (414): 25-30.

[26] Ghoneem HF, Wright JG, Cole WG, Rang M. The Illizarov method for correction of complex deformities. J Bone Joint Surg 1996;78A:1480-1485.

Reconstruction of Skeletal Defects of the Upper Limb with Vascularized Bone Grafts

Konstantinos N. MALIZOS*, Michalis HANTES,
Dionysios PARIDIS, Theophanis MORAITIS

Department of Orthopaedic Surgery, University of Thessalia, Larissa, Greece

Vascularized bone grafting is an important tool for all surgeons dealing with challenging bone reconstruction problems. It should be considered when other approaches have failed or are expected to fail. Indications for the use of vascularized bone grafts in the upper extremity include bone defects after trauma or tumor resection with or without soft tissue loss, avascular necrosis, and nonunions. Bone defects or nonunion of the upper limb associated with sepsis is also indicated for vascularized bone grafts. Alternative vascularized bone grafts for upper limb reconstruction include the fibula, the iliac crest, the lateral border of the scapula, a corticoperiosteal flap from the medial femoral condyle and vascularized periosteum. The free vascularized fibula is the graft of choice for the majority of surgeons. This is because its blood supply is constant, dissection and harvesting are straight-forward, and donor site morbidity is minimal. It may be also combined with skin, fascia, and muscle to address soft tissue problems at the recipient site. Vascularized bone grafts provide structural stability, vascularity, and viable bone cells to the recipient area, which are important elements in the eradication of infection in cases of septic conditions. Treatment with vascularized bone grafts has been shown to be effective in the management of challenging reconstruction problems of the upper extremity. However, this technique requires microvascular expertise, correct fixation and immobilization of the graft and proper patient selection for a good outcome.

Keywords: reconstruction; non-union; septic skeletal defect; vascularized bone graft, fibula. ∎

1. INTRODUCTION

Septic skeletal defects pose one of the most difficult problems for reconstructive surgery of the upper limb. These become even more challenging when they are complicated by adjacent soft tissue loss. Before undertaking any reconstructive proce-dure for isolated skeletal defects, as well as for more complex bone and soft tissue loss, the general health of the patient, co-morbidities, condition of the local tissues, and function of the entire upper limb need to be carefully assessed. Previous unsuccessful attempts to treat the patient, motivation, expectations, as well as the time needed until the completion of the treatment plan, should be seriously considered by the treating physicians. A well-informed patient, who is willing to cooperate throughout the entire treatment course, is a crucial parameter for a desirable outcome.

2. BONE LOSS: ETIOLOGY & MANAGEMENT ALTERNATIVES

The etiology of bone loss may either be of a traumatic nature, as in the case of open fractures with

*Corresponding Author
Professor and Chairman
Department of Orthopedic Surgery
University of Thessalia
411 10 Larissa, Greece
Tel: +30 2410 682 722
Fax: +30 2410 670 107
e-mail: malizos@med.uth.gr

severe contamination, or lie in the course of the surgical management of a tumor or a reconstructive surgical procedure that was complicated by an infection. Infection may appear acutely in the first 2-3 postoperative weeks, with both a local acute inflammatory reaction and systemic symptoms including fever, malaise and weakness. In the majority of cases, however, in the presence of fixation implants or endoprosthesis, infection is established as a late subacute or chronic form with an insidious onset. It may appear as an infected nonunion or as osteomyelitis (Cierny-Mader I-IV) on a consolidated fracture or an "intact" bone.

The key step preceding every reconstructive procedure of either an infected humerus or forearm is the removal of not only the hardware from previous unsuccessful treatment attempts, but also all the affected soft tissues and bone up to clean margins of healthy tissue. It is equally important to obtain multiple tissue samples from various locations within the infected area for cultures and frozen sections. Patzakis et al. [1] have demonstrated that there are various microenvironments with different microorganisms inside an infected nonunion.

After one or more previously unsuccessful treatment attempts, patients presenting with septic skeletal defects of variable size, require individualized management that takes into account the size and location of the defect, the presence of an active purulent infection and function of the adjacent joints. Osteopenia and joint stiffness from disuse of the arm for several months is common, and results in difficulties with bone fixation throughout the healing period. Bone loss can be reconstructed with a wide variety of surgical methods that are aimed at both eradication of the infection and bone healing with correct length and alignment.

Distraction osteogenesis is applied mainly to tubular bone defects. It may involve a small initial shortening which can be followed by gradual callus distraction or segmental bone transport. This method has certain limitations mainly due to the anatomical location of important structures (vessels and nerves) in the upper limb. It is technically very demanding, with the additional burden of requiring a rather bulky external fixator for a long time. Modern devices with computer-assisted guidance of the distraction and the alignment of the limb have revolutionized the reconstructive procedures in cases with bone and soft tissue defects.

Grafting with autologous bone and/or bone substitutes and allograft offers an alternative for skeletal reconstruction. Autologous cancellous bone grafting is a routine procedure applied mainly to cases with non-critical sized defects. Via osteoprogenitor cells and mesenchymal stem cells of the bone marrow, it serves not only to fill the void, but also as a means of local biological augmentation of the healing process.

For skeletal defects exceeding 5-6 cm at the diaphysis or metaphysis of the humerus or forearm, treatment alternatives include non-vascularized autografts, allografts and vascularized bone grafts (VBG). In the later, the intrinsic blood supply of the graft is maintained either through an intact vascular pedicle or with microsurgical anastomosis for distant graft transfers. VBGs via their viable organic elements have the biological potential to contribute to callus formation at the host-graft junction sites. This is particularly useful when the defect is surrounded by scar tissue from previous surgeries, infection, or irradiation. Taylor et al. first reported the application of a free vascularized fibular graft in 1975 [2]. Since then, it has been applied to treat persistent nonunions, including infected nonunions, congenital pseudarthrosis, and extensive bone defects following trauma or tumor resection. This procedure converts the defect, irrespective of its length, to the equivalent of a bipolar fracture. In addition, the vessel-rich graft enhances the blood supply to the recipient site, thus, augmenting the cellular and humoral immune response and the resistance to infection.

There are several sites of the skeleton from which sizeable vascularized bone grafts can be harvested and transferred to the upper limb. These include the fibula, iliac crest, clavicle, lateral border of the scapula, ribs, part of the radius, and osteo-periosteal cortico-cancellous segment from the medial femoral condyle. The selection of the most appropriate graft is based on a number of parameters, including the size and location (diaphysis or metaphysis) of the defect, structural requirements of the recipient site (i.e. cortical or cortico-cancellous bone), availability of a longer vascular pedicle, donor site morbidity and the balance between the surgical burden and the overall benefit to the patient. This chapter reviews the indications, specific requirements for applying alternative vascularized bone grafts and their outcomes in the management of infected nonunions and/or osteomyelitis of the long bones of the upper limb.

3. Free Vascularized Fibula Graft

The fibula presents relatively low donor site morbidity and anatomical characteristics (long, straight, cortical bone) similar to the diaphyseal segments of the long bones in the upper limb. Therefore, the vascularized fibula has become the most widely used graft for the reconstruction of large defects in the clavicle, the humerus, the radius, and/or the ulna [3]. In addition, the fibula has double vascularity originating from the diaphyseal feeding vessel and the segmental periosteal branches, making it a very versatile graft. It may be osteotomized and bent or even folded to serve as a "double barrel" graft, fed by its single pedicle. Based on the peroneal artery, the fibula could also be harvested as a composite flap with nerves, muscle and skin. It is particularly useful in those cases where the radical debridement of the septic focus has left a bone defect with inadequate coverage from the adjacent soft tissues.

The surgical technique can be modified to allow harvesting of the skin as part of the flap that may also serve as a buoy for monitoring purposes. For a composite osteo-fascio-cutaneous flap, an elliptical shaped skin flap of 20 x 9 cm is dissected from the postero-lateral aspect of the leg in line with the fibula. Particular attention should be paid to incorporate the underlying fascia and to preserve the septocutaneous perforating branches of the peroneal artery. Survival of a skin flap as large as 24 x 9 cm has been reported [4].

For the osteo-muscular flap (fibula + soleus), the lateral part of the soleus muscle is dissected together with the fibula, and the perforating branches of the peroneal artery to the soleus muscle are preserved. For the fibula with the flexor hallucis longus (FHL) composite flap, the muscle may also be transferred as a functioning unit when its nerve branch is connected to a motor nerve at the recipient site (Fig. 1).

We have found that harvesting the fibular graft with an abundant periosteal sleeve extending beyond the length of the graft is very helpful. This modification requires dissection and meticulous elevation of the muscle from the periosteum for at least 2 cm at each end of the graft. The 2 cm of extra periosteum attached to each end of the graft is then longitudinally incised and sharply elevated at both ends of the fibula so that it can be reversed like a "reversed cuff of the long sleeve". This technique allows vascularized periosteum to be har-

vested at both ends of the graft. Once the graft is transfered to the recipient site, the periosteal cuff can be unfolded and placed on the junction sites to enhance periosteal callus formation. Cancellous bone grafts should also be placed at both junction sites to further augment healing. The fibular graft length utilized at the reported series varies, ranging between 6 and 26 cm [5].

4. FREE VASCULARIZED BONE GRAFT FROM THE ILIAC CREST OR RIB(S)

Vascularized grafts from the iliac crest present different structural characteristics from the fibula. These may be harvested as longitudinally curved cortico-cancellous or tricortical grafts with a length of up to 10 cm. The defect at the donor iliac crest may leave considerable morbidity, including pain or even muscle hernias. There are very few case reports or small series that describe the application of a vascularized iliac crest bone graft for the reconstruction of bone defects in the upper limb [6, 7].

The rib due to its structural properties (weak, membranous bones) and curved shape, has very limited application as a free vascularized graft for the reconstruction of long bone defects in the upper limb. In 1998, Thomas et al. [8] proposed the use of a segment of the serratus anterior muscle combined with a vascularized rib graft (SARIB) for upper limb reconstructions with multifaceted requirements. This flap was applied to five cases in their study with good results.

Lin et al. [9] reported lower (but not statistically significant) recipient-site morbidity with the fibula (22% [14/64 grafts]) compared with the rib (36% [8/22]) and the iliac crest (46% [5/11]).

5. VASCULARIZED BONE GRAFT FROM THE SCAPULA

The lateral border of the scapula although rarely used in orthopaedic surgery for vascularized bone transfer, it has been widely used in the field of mandibular reconstruction. The crest of the scapula consists of cortico-cancellous bone that can be harvested as a straight bone (up to 10 cm long) based on its 8 to 10 cm long vascular pedicle. The subscapular artery is a large vessel with an external diameter measuring 2.5 to 3.5 mm. A large adjoining flap of skin and fascia up to 25 x 15 cm can also be harvested, connected to the same vessel. However, because of the thickness of the flap and the necessity of changing the patient's position during surgery, it has not been extensively used.

In cases with proximal lesions in the arm, a vascularized scapular segment can be transferred without a microvascular anastomosis. There have been only few cases reported in the literature, i.e. a single pedicled (subscapular vessels) vascularized scapular graft to the proximal humerus simultaneously with a latissimus dorsi myo-

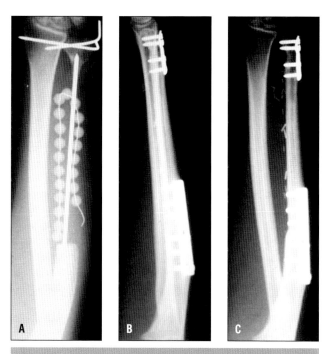

FIGURE 1. (A) An ulnar defect at "clear margins" with temporary fixation and a chain of antibiotic beads for local antibiotic delivery. **(B, C)** Four and a half years after reconstruction with a FVFG and plate and screws fixation. No recurrence of sepsis. Full arm and hand function.

cutaneous flap to replace the deltoid muscle and the overlying skin [10, 11]. Within 4 months the bone united and good flexion of the shoulder was obtained. In another case, a pedicled transfer of the lateral border of the scapula was used to reconstruct a 9-cm bone defect of the upper third of the humerus following a gunshot wound. None of the patients had shoulder dysfunction after harvesting of the scapular segment. For young women, the scapula is recommended because the postoperative scar is less conspicuous. The best use for scapular grafts is probably for infected nonunions or bone defects of the proximal humerus and humeral head necrosis [12].

6. Free Vascularized Osteo-periosteal Graft from the Medial Femoral Condyle

The free vascularized cortico-periosteal graft from the medial condyle of the femur was first reported by Sakai et al. [13]. This is a thin straightforward graft which is mainly applicable to patients with infected nonunions of the humerus and the radius without significant osseous defects after debridement. It is also suitable for those cases where other vascularized bone grafts cannot be applied due to their large size or straight configuration [13, 14]. This graft is nourished through the articular branch of the descending genicular artery and vein. Dissection is carried out after elevation of the vastus medialis without needing to open the knee joint. The size of the graft may be as large as 9 x 4 cm. It is elastic and readily conforms to the configuration of the recipient bed. It may be "wrapped" around the recipient bone, allowing a plate to be used for internal fixation.

In the small number of cases reported to date, it has been applied for infected nonunions of the clavicle and humerus. The time needed for graft union and incorporation ranged from 3 to 4 months. After graft harvesting, knee function was undisturbed [15]. One patient, however, complained of a sensory disturbance in the saphenous nerve area [3].

7. Vascularized Periosteum

Vascularized periosteum is a membrane with osteogenic potential, originating from the mesenchymal cells of its campium layer. It is elastic, flexible and adaptable to the shape of the recipient area [16, 17]. In recent reports from experimental studies, vascularized periosteum was found to be a promising alternative for the reconstruction of small skeletal defects [18-20]. Multiple donor sites for vascularized periosteum have been described, including the iliac crest, the medial distal femur, the tibial shaft, the fibula, the 10th rib, the scapula, the distal humerus and the radius or ulna, each with negligible donor site morbidity [21-25].

Vascularized periosteum can be applied as a pedicled graft in upper limb reconstruction for augmentation of bone healing at the distal half of the forearm. In a cadaveric study, the donor and the potential recipient sites of pedicled vascularized periosteal flaps from the dorsal and palmar aspect of the distal radius were systematically approached [21]. The dimensions of the vascularized periosteal flaps ranged between 1 x 2.5 cm (minimum) and 3 x 4 cm (maximum), and the length of the pedicle flaps ranged between 0.5 and 3 cm. Flaps from the dorsal distal radius can cover the distal half of the dorsal forearm when they are elevated on their proximal pedicle, while flaps from the volar surface of the radius are able to cover the distal third of the volar side of the forearm bones when based at the palmar metaphyseal arch vessels.

8. Reconstruction and Grafting of the Defect

In the presence of severe sepsis and upon intra-operative assessment during debridement, the surgeon may decide to postpone transfer of a vascularized graft to a 2nd surgical stage. In this case, the limb is stabilized with an external fixator and an antibiotic-loaded bone cement spacer or beads is/are inserted for a period of days or a few weeks (Fig. 1a). If the soft tissues adjacent to the bone defect do not provide adequate coverage of the wound primarily, it is safer to leave the wound open and apply an antibiotic bead pouch dressing for 3-4 days, and repeat this for one or two more courses until definite coverage of the soft tissue defect [26]. Wound coverage may be addressed at either a separate surgical stage with a local, regional or distal flap, or at the time of bone reconstruction by transferring a composite flap with muscle and/or skin adjoined to the vascularized bone graft.

In order that the graft pedicle is best approximated towards the recipient vessels without tension, the transferred graft may be oriented with its proximal end at either the proximal or the distal end of the recipient bone. The ideal method of stabilization should respect the vascularity of the graft and provide sufficient stability to promote healing at the host-graft construct. To avoid a stress-shielding effect on the graft, fixation should not be too rigid. Osteosynthesis with plates long enough to span the length of the defect or with one plate at each junction site supplemented by an external fixator can provide the host bone-graft construct with adequate stability. Dealing with bone defects after a chronic infection, the application of an external fixator is suggested as a safer approach. Intramedullary fixation damages the endosteal vascularity of the graft and should be avoided.

9. Complications

Systemic complications at the donor site include blood loss, hemodynamic instability, and thrombo-embolism.

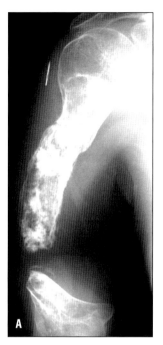
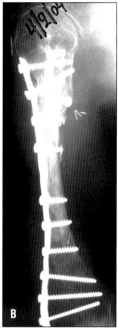
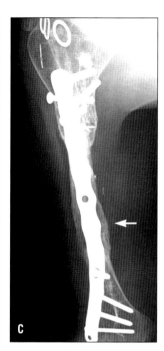

FIGURE 2. (A) Post irradiation necrosis of the humerus after Ewing Sarcoma with infected non-union. Free vascularized fibular graft bridging the defect is fixed with a thin plate spanning the entire graft length. **(B)** Postoperative X-ray of the distal graft-host junction site at 2.5-year follow-up. **(C)** Five years postoperatively, the adaptive hypertrophy of the graft is indicated (arrow).

Recipient site complications include compromised vascularity, infection, nonunion of the graft-host junction sites, and fatigue (stress) fracture of the graft. After healing and graft incorporation, stress fractures have been reported at rates ranging from 0 to 17% [27]. Donor site complications are usually minor [28-30]. However, when anatomic variations, particularly the absence of posterior and anterior tibial arteries, are not detected pre-operatively, donor site vascularity can be compromised. In the series by Vail and Urbaniak [30], the peroneal artery was the dominant artery of the foot in 1 out of 247 cases (0.4%), and a vein graft was needed to maintain the flow. The most common complication is transient muscle weakness of the flexor hallucis longus (FHL), extensor hallucis longus (EHL), or peroneal muscles, whereas contracture of the FHL after its detachment from the fibula leads to clawing of the great toe. Distal tibio-fibular fusion at the donor site in children is recommended to avoid valgus deformity of the ankle joint.

10. LOCATION-BASED APPLICATIONS OF LARGE VASCULARIZED BONE GRAFTS

10.1. Clavicle

The application of free vascularized fibular graft to treat recalcitrant nonunions of the clavicle was first reported by Wood in 1987 [29] for infected nonunions in three patients with segmental bone loss of the clavicle after an average of 3.7 failed procedures. In each case, the patient presented with pain and shoulder dysfunction. Subsequent debridement left bone loss exceeding 5 cm that was managed with autologous free vascularized

fibular grafts for salvage reconstruction. Union was achieved in all 3 cases.

In the same year, Meals and Lesavoy [31] described the use of a vascularized radius obtained from a below elbow amputated segment, to successfully reconstruct the clavicle. In a more recent report, Fuchs et al. [15] applied a free vascularized corticoperiosteal flap from the medial aspect of the femoral condyle to reconstruct infected nonunions of the clavicle with a successful outcome.

10.2. Scapulohumeral arthrodesis or glenohumeral fusion

There are a few reports with small number of cases describing the application of a free vascularized fibular graft for scapulohumeral arthrodesis either after tumor resection or for post-traumatic loss of the proximal humerus [32]. In two cases, the free vascularized fibula was augmented with allograft bone. Radiographically, bone healing was achieved at the last follow-up (2.5 years) in all patients. The author describes favorable restoration of the upper extremity function in all patients, as they were able to bring their hand to their mouth and circumduct their arm within a limited, but useful amplitude. All patients, except for those undergoing additional soft-tissue reconstruction with a pedicled latissimus dorsi muscle transfer, considered the aesthetic outcome as poor. Mean fibular graft hypertrophy was 33% at 2.5 years follow-up [32].

10.3. Proximal humerus (joint preservation)

Segmental defects of the upper part of the humerus and of the humeral diaphysis may occur from surgical resection of pathological tissue (tumor or sepsis), prosthesis failure, or as a complication of failed prior internal fixation. There are limited reconstructive options for the treatment of segmental bone defects larger than 5 cm in the proximal humerus, especially those associated with soft tissue loss. There are certain difficulties in every attempt for reconstruction at this particular site. Bone healing in this area is disturbed mainly by the absence of good vascularization and stable contact between the fragments. Free vascularized grafts, primarily from the fibula, but also from the iliac crest, provide abundant bone stock and vascularity to overcome these problems commonly encountered in the management of long bone defects with failed previous surgery. A minimum prerequisite for the glenohumeral joint salvage is the preservation of the vascularity of the humeral head.

Leung and Hung [33] in 1989 proposed the transfer of free vascularized bone from the iliac crest to repair the defect that is due to wide excision of a giant cell tumor from the proximal humerus, with satisfactory outcome. A composite osteoseptocutaneous fibular transplant for reconstruction of complex bone and soft tissue humeral defect has been applied in patients with segmental bone loss, a defect from a tumor resection, and one from failure of an allograft-prosthesis reconstruction. The fibular graft was fixed by means of intramedullary impaction, serving as an on-lay graft and a strut between the intact diaphysis and the humeral head. The average length of the segmental humeral defect was 9.3 cm. The average length of the fibular graft was 16.1 cm, and the average length and size of the skin paddle was 8.1 x 4.5 cm. The application of osteoseptocutaneous fibular transplant for combined segmental osseous and soft tissue defects of the arm is more complex than for the forearm and is associated with a higher rate of complications. The skin may serve as a buoy and allow early revision of the anastomosis after venous thrombosis.

10.4. Humeral diaphysis

Reconstruction of long defects of the humerus is challenging from several aspects, including the need to meet specific biomechanical requirements to bear not only compressive and bending forces, but also considerable rotational loading. Due to chronic disuse of their arm, patients with septic complications frequently present for reconstruction with a relatively stiff shoulder and elbow, as well as with osteopenia of the intact bone segments. Heitmann et al. [34] advocated intramedullary insertion of the fibular graft in the humeral canal and fixation with a spanning plate to optimize stability. Contemporary implants with locking screws provide biomechanical advantages, even in osteoporotic bone. Although the use of a long neutralization plate spanning the entire defect appears more appropriate, it carries the risk of recurrence of the infection. The application of an external fixator supplemented by two small plates or free screws at the fibula-host bone junction sites offer an-

other safe alternative. The retrograde orientation of the proximal part of the fibula towards the elbow, in most cases, facilitates access to the profunda brachii artery and vein. Microvascular anastomosis requires a second incision at the medial aspect of the arm, which is usually performed with 8-0 nylon sutures. First, the veins are repaired end-to-end to minimize bleeding, followed by the end-to-side anastomosis of the peroneal artery of the graft to the brachial artery. Healing at the junction sites usually takes 3.5 to 5 months. Hypertrophy of the vascularized fibula when transferred to the humerus is observed both at the endosteum and the periosteum, although it is less pronounced compared to the weight bearing bones of the lower extremity [5, 28, 35-37] (Fig. 2).

10.5. Distal Humerus

Non-unions at the distal humerus are commonly associated with an impaired mobility of the elbow joint. This is even more pronounced when the elbow has been involved in the initial zone of injury. Hattori et al. [7] and Baredjiklian et al. [38] suggested the transfer of a free vascularized bone graft from the iliac crest in combination with elbow joint release to manage these defects.

10.6. Forearm

Because the fibula matches the radius and the ulna in size and shape, FVFGs are particularly suitable for the reconstruction of large defects of the forearm. From the technical perspective, the reconstruction of the forearm presents the fewest challenges. Retrograde graft positioning may facilitate the approximation of the graft vessels to the radial or the ulnar artery for end-to-end anastomosis to either artery and to the dorsal veins. Particular attention should be paid preoperatively to the vascularity of the forearm and the hand with Doppler ultrasound and clinical examination with an Allen test. Stable fixation using plates and screws or an external fixator is decided intra-operatively after assessment by surgeons [3]. The authors prefer to increase the contact area of the graft to host forearm bone(s) by step cutting the conjoining bone ends to facilitate healing. Postoperative support with a brace may help prevent stress fractures. There is no need to wait for hypertrophy, and the patient can resume full use of the upper extremity when the graft heals in 3-4 months [39] (Fig. 3 and Fig. 4).

At a mean follow-up of 2 years, healing ranged from 89% to 96% and no recurrence of the infection was reported for septic defects in the humerus and the forearm. The number of additional cancellous bone grafting procedures required was limited. Vascularized osteoseptocutaneous fibula transfered as composite tissue offers rapid osseous incorporation, greater resistance to infection, and prompt functional recovery [27].

When there are defects in both bones of the forearm, the fibula may be applied for reconstruction of both the ulna and the radius. In this case, the graft should be har-

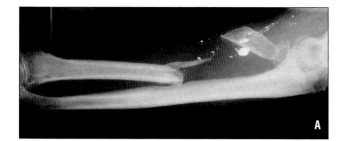

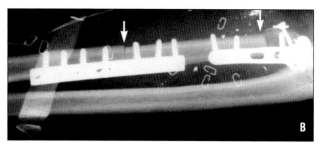

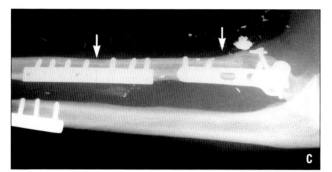

FIGURE 3. (A) Preoperative radiograph of a patient with composite skeletal (loss of proximal radius and malunion of the radial neck) and soft tissue defect (loss of mobile wad and radial nerve) after a gunshot injury and residual infection, necessitating multiple debridements. (B) Postoperative radiograph depicting the osteotomy of the radial neck and the interposition of the vascularized fibular graft and flexor hallucis longus muscle flap in the defect. (C) Three years postoperatively, the interposed vascularized fibular graft is consolidated with the proximal and distal radius.

vested to be 4 cm longer than the sum of the two defects. Duing preparation, a 4 cm segment in-between the two struts is removed after careful sub-periosteal dissection. This allows mobilization and interposition of the "folded twin-barrelled" graft into the defects, based on the same vascular pedicle. With the addition of iliac crest bone grafts at the junction sites, bone union is usually completed within 3 months at all junctions. The range of forearm rotation may be slightly limited due to the elimination of the normal bow shape of the radius [3, 27, 40, 41].

10.7. Distal Radius

Tang [5] and Muramatsu et al. [42] suggested the transfer of an autologous free vascularized fibular graft including the head in cases with loss of the distal radius.

Salibial et al. [6] applied free vascularized osteocutaneous flap from the iliac crest to repair composite defects at the distal radius, with double microvascular anastomosis.

11. "GROWING BONE" TRANSFER IN THE UPPER EXTREMITY

A vascularized transfer of the growing epiphysis, along with a variable part of the adjoining diaphysis, is probably the most effective solution in dealing with upper limb bone defects in the growing skeleton involving either the distal radius or the proximal humerus. The key feature of

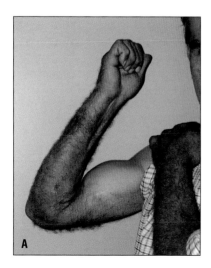

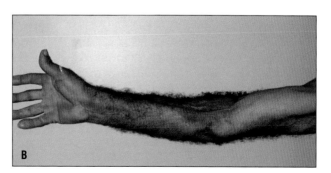

FIGURE 4. (A, B) Range of motion 3 years after the reconstruction of the skeletal-soft tissue defects and 2 years after the tendon transfers for the radial nerve palsy.

such a procedure is the ability to reconstruct the bone loss while simultaneously restoring the growth potential, provided that the blood supply of both the growth plate and the diaphysis is maintained.

The experience of Innocenti et al. [43] refers to cases with bone defects after tumor resection and a follow-up ranging between 2 and 15 years. They routinely used a graft based on the anterior tibial vessels and designed according to a reverse flow vascular model. A functional outcome with excellent results is usually achieved in distal radius reconstruction. In Innocenti's report [43] all patients regained a nearly normal range of motion on all planes and the wrist was painless and stable, whereas the articular surface underwent significant remodeling, developing a concave surface, which improved stability and range of motion.

12. FUTURE PERSPECTIVES

Current investigations are focusing on the transplantation of vascularized allograft. Although technically feasible, concerns related to the continuous use of immuno-suppression have resulted in vascularized allografts being only sporadically applied. Progress in immuno-suppression or increasing allograft tissue tolerance is a crucial step for the use of allografts in musculoskeletal reconstruction. Tissue engineering to obtain viable bone substitutes is another field of current interest in musculoskeletal research. Although both are conceptually interesting, they need further experimental investigation prior to clinical application.

REFERENCES

[1] Patzakis MJ, Zalavras CG. Chronic posttraumatic osteomyelitis and infected nonunion of the tibia: current management concepts. J Am Acad Orthop Surg 2005;13:417-427.

[2] Taylor GI, Miller GD, Ham FJ. The free vascularized bone graft. A clinical extension of microvascular techniques. Plast Reconstr Surg 1975;55:533-544.

[3] Yajima H, Tamai S, Ono H, Kizaki K, Yamauchi T. Free vascularized fibula grafts in surgery of the upper limb. J Reconstr Microsurg 1999;15:515-521.

[4] Winters HA, de Jongh GJ. Reliability of the proximal skin paddle of the osteocutaneous free fibula flap: a prospective clinical study. Plast Reconstr Surg 1999;103:846-849.

[5] Tang CH. Reconstruction of the bones and joints of the upper extremity by vascularized free fibula graft: report of 46 cases. J Reconstr Microsurg 1992;8:285-292.

[6] Salibian AH, Anzel SH, Salyer WA. Transfer of vascularized grafts of iliac bone to the extremities. J Bone Joint Surg 1987;69:1319-1327.

[7] Hattori Y, Doi K, Pagsaligan JM, Takka S, Ikeda K. Arthroplasty of the elbow joint using vascularized iliac bone graft for reconstruction of massive bone defect of the distal humerus. J Reconstr Microsurg 2005;21:287-291.

[8] Thomas WO, Harris CN, Moline S, Harper LL, Parker JA. Versatil-

[9] Lin CH, Wei FC, Chen HC, Chuang DC. Outcome comparison in traumatic lower-extremity reconstruction by using various composite vascularized bone transplantation. Plast Reconstr Surg 1999;104:984-992.

[10] Benmansour BM, Blancke D, Dib C, Gottin M, Dintimille HM. Reconstruction of a complex defect of the upper third of the humerus by pedicle transplant of the lateral edge of the scapula. A case report. Ann Chir Plast Esthet 1999;44:199-203.

[11] Seghrouchni H, Martin D, Pistre V, Baudet J. Composite scapular flap for reconstruction of complex humeral tissue loss: a case report. Rev Chir Orthop Reparatrice Appar Mot 2003;89:158-162.

[12] Yajima H, Kisanuki O, Kobata Y, Kawate K, Sugimoto K, Takakura Y. Free and island flap transfers for the treatment of motor vehicle injuries. J Reconstr Microsurg 2006;22:591-597.

[13] Sakai K, Doi K, Kawai S. Free vascularized thin corticoperiosteal graft. Plast Reconstr Surg 1991;87:290-298.

[14] Doi K, Hattori Y. The use of free vascularized corticoperiosteal grafts from the femur in the treatment of scaphoid non-union. Orthop Clin North Am 2007;38:87-94.

[15] Fucks B, Steinmann SP, Bishop AT. Free vascularized corticoperiosteal bone graft for the treatment of persistent non-union of the clavicle. J Shoulder Elbow Surg 2005;14:264-268.

[16] Canalis RF, Burstein FD. Osteogenesis in vascularized periosteum. Interactions with underlying bone. Arch Otolaryngol 1985;111: 511-516.

[17] Uddstromer L, Ritsila V, Osteogenic capacity of periosteal grafts. A qualitative and quantitative study of membranous and tubular bone periosteum in young rabbits. Scand J Plast Reconstr Surg 1978; 12:207-214.

[18] Dailiana Z, Shiamishis G, Niokou D, Ioachim E, Malizos KN. Heretopic neo-osteogenesis from vascularized periosteum and bone grafts. J Trauma 2002;53:934-938.

[19] Romana MC, Masquelet AC. Vascularized periosteum associated with cancellous bone graft: an experimental study. Plast Reconstr Surg 1990;85:587-592.

[20] Vogelin E, Jones NF, Huang JI, Brekke JH, Lieberman JR. Healing of a critical-sized defect in the rat femur with use of a vascularized periosteal flap, a biodegradable matrix, and bone morphogenetic protein. J Bone Joint Surg [Am] 2005;87:1323-1331.

[21] Dailiana Z, Malizos KN, Urbaniak JR Vascularized periosteal flaps of distal forearm and hand. J Trauma 2005;58:76-82.

[22] Penteado CV, Masquelet AC, Romana MC, Cherel JP. Periosteal flaps: anatomical bases of site of elevation. Surg Radiol Anat 1990;12:3-7.

[23] Crock JG, Morrison WA. A vascularized periosteal flap: anatomical study. Br J Plast Surg 1992;45:474-478.

[24] Bronlow HC, Reed A, Joyner C, Simpson AH. Anatomical effects of periosteal references. J Orthop Res 2000;18:500-502.

[25] Badran HA, Safe I, el Fayoumy S. Simplified technique for isolating vascularized rib periosteal grafts. Plast Reconstr Surg 1990;86: 1208-1215.

[26] Stevanovic M, Sharpe F, Itamura J. Treatment of soft tissues problems around the elbow. Clin Orthop Relat Res 2000;370:127-137.

[27] Pederson WC, Person DW. Long bone reconstruction with vascularized bone graft. Orthop Clin North Am 2007;38:23-35.

[28] Mattar Junior J, Azze RJ, Ferreira MC, Starck R, Canedo AC. Vascularized fibular graft for management of severe osteomyelitis of the upper extremity. Microsurg 1994;15:22-27.

[29] Wood MB. Upper extremity reconstruction by vascularized bone transfers: results and complications. J Hand Surg [Am] 1987;12: 422-427.

[30] Vail TP, Urbaniak JR. Donor-site morbidity with use of vascularized autogenous fibular grafts. J Bone Joint Surg [Am] 1996;78: 204-211.

[31] Meals RA, Lesavoy MA. Vascularized free radius transfer for clavicle reconstruction concurrent with elbow amputation. J Hand Surg [Am] 1987;12:673.

[32] Tomaino MN. Scapulohumeral arthrodesis for post-traumatic proximal humeral loss using vascularized fibular transplantation and allograft bone. J Reconstr Microsurg 2000;16:335-340.

[33] Leung PC, Hung LK. Bone reconstruction after giant-cell tumor resection at the proximal end of the humerus with vascularized iliac crest graft. A report of three cases. Clin Orthop Relat Res 1989; 247:101-105.

[34] Heitmann C, Erdmann D, Levin LS. Treatment of segmental defects of the humerus with an osteoseptocutaneous fibular transplant. J Bone Joint Surg [Am] 2002;84:2216-2223.

[35] Malizos K, Zalavras CG, Soucacos PN, Beris AE,Urbaniak JR. Free vascularized fibular grafts for reconstruction of skeletal defects. Am Acad Orthop Surg 2004;12:360-369.

[36] Wood MB. Free vascularized fibular grafting-25 years' experience: tips, techniques, and pearls. Orthop Clin North Am 2007;38:1-12.

[37] Gerwin M, Weiland AJ. Vascularized bone grafts in the upper extremities: indications and techniques. Hand Clin 1992;8:509.

[38] Beredjiklian P, Hotchkiss R, Athanasian E, Ramsey, Matttew L, Katz MA. Recalcitrant nonunion of the distal humerus: treatment with free vascularized bone graft. Clin Orthop Relat Res 2005; 435:134-139.

[39] Safouri Y. Free vascularized fibula for the treatment of traumatic bone defects and non-union of the forearm bones. J Hand Surg [Br] 2005;30:67-72.

[40] Chen SH, Jeng SF, Liu HC. Functional reconstructions of a massive defect in the two forearms bones. J Trauma 1990;30:49-54.

[41] Adani R, Delcroix L, Innocenti M, Tarallo L, Celli A, Ceruso M. Reconstrustion of large posttraumatic skeletal defects of the forearm by vascularized free fibular graft. Microsurg 2004;24:423-429.

[42] Muramatsu K, Ihara K, Azuma E, Orui R, Goto Y, Shigetomi M, Doi K. Free vascularized fibula grafting for reconstruction of the wrist following wide tumor excision. Microsurgery 2005;25:101-106.

[43] Innocenti M, Delcroix L, Romano GF, Capanna R. Vascularized epiphyseal transplant. Orthop Clin North Am 2007;38:95-101.

Index